Livestock Nutrition

Livestock Nutrition

Analytical Techniques

Prof. Dr. Gopal Krishna
M.V.Sc., Ph.D. (India), Ph.D. (Norway)
AvH Fellow (Germany), NORAD Fellow (Norway)
NAVS Fellow (India), ANA Fellow (India)
Retired Prof. and Head
Department of Animal Nutrition
CCS-HAU, Hisar (Haryana)

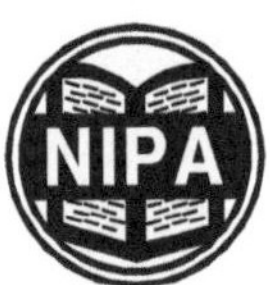

New India Publishing Agency
Pitam Pura, New Delhi-110 088

Published by
Sumit Pal Jain *for*
New India Publishing Agency
101, Vikas Surya Plaza, CU Block, L.S.C. Mkt.,
Pitam Pura, New Delhi- 110 088, (India)
Phone: 011-27341717, Fax: 011-27341616
Mobile : 09717133558
E-mail: info@nipabooks.com
Web: www.nipabooks.com

ISBN : 978-93-80235-96-7

Typeset at: Harminder *for* Laxmi Art Creation
Printed at: Jai Bharat Printing Press, Delhi

Dedicated to
the sweet and cherished memory of
respected mother **Late Smt. Gayatri Devi**
and
father **Late Shri Om Prakash Gupta**
beloved parents of
Prof. Dr. Gopal Krishna

PERIODIC CHART OF THE ELEMENTS

I A	II A	III B	IV B	V B	VI B	VII B	VIII	VIII	VIII	I B	II B	III A	IV A	V A	VI A	VII A	Inter Cases
1 H Hydrogen 1.0078																1 H Hydrogen 1.0078	2 He Hellium 4.0026
3 Li Lithium 6.841	4 Be Beryllium 9.0218											5 B Boron 9.0218	6 C Carbon 12.011	7 N Nitrogen 14.0067	8 O Oxygen 15.9994	9 F Fluorine 18.9884	10 Ne Neon 20.178
11 Na Sodium 22.9898	12 Mg Magnesium 24.305											13 Al Aluminium 26.9815	14 Si Silicon 28.088	15 P Phosphorus 30.9738	16 S Sulphur 32.06	17 Cl Chlorine 35.453	18 Ar Argon 39.848
19 K Potassium 39.098	20 Ca Calcium 40.08	21 Sc Scandium 44.959	22 Ti Titanium 47.80	23 V Vanadium 50.944	24 Cr Chromium 51.996	25 Mn Manganese 54.9380	26 Fe Iron 65.847	27 Co Cobalt 58.9332	28 Ni Nickel 58.71	29 Cu Copper 63.546	30 Zn Zinc 65.38	31 Ga Gallium 68.72	32 Ge Germanium 72.59	33 As Arsenic 74.9216	34 Se Selenium 78.96	35 Br Bromine 79.904	36 Kr Krypton 83.80
37 Rb Rubidium 85.467	38 Sr Strontium 87.62	39 Y Yttrium 88.909	40 Zr Zirconium 91.22	41 Nb Niobium 92.9064	42 Mo Molybdenum 95.94	43 Tc Technetium 98.9062	44 Ru Ruthenium 101.07	45 Rh Rhodium 102.9055	46 Pd Palladium 106.4	47 Ag Silver 107.888	48 Cd Cadmium 112.40	49 In Indium 114.82	50 Sn Tint 118.69	51 Sb Antimony 121.75	52 Te Tellurium 127.60	53 I Iodine 126.9045	54 Xe Xenon 131.30
55 Cs Cesium 132.9064	56 Ba Barium 137.34	57 *La Lanthanum 138.9155	72 Hf Hafnium 178.49	73 Ta Tantalum 180.9478	74 W Wolfram 183.85	75 Re Rhenium 186.2	76 Os Osmium 190.2	77 Ir Iridium 182.22	78 Pt Platinum 195.08	79 Au Gold 196.9685	80 Hg Mercury 200.58	81 Tl Thallium 204.37	82 Pb Lead 207.2	83 Bi Bismuth 208.9804	84 Po Polonium (209)	85 At Astatine (210)	86 Rn Radon (222)
87 Fr Francium (223)	88 Ra Radium 226.0254	89 +AC Actinium (227)															

* Lanthanum Series

58 Ce Cerium 140.12	59 Pr Praseodymium 140.9077	60 Nd Neodymium 144.24	61 Pm Promethium (145)	62 Sm Samarium 150.4	63 Eu Europium 151.98	64 Gd Gadolinium 157.25	65 Tb Terbium 158.9254	66 Dy Dysprosium 162.50	67 Ho Holmium 184.9304	68 Er Erbium 167.26	69 Tm Thulium 168.9342	70 Yb Ytterbium 173.04	71 Lu Lutetium 174.97

+ Actinium Series

90 Th Thorium 232.0388	91 Pa Protactinium 231.0359	92 U Uranium 238.028	93 Np Neptunium 237.0482	94 Pu Plutonium (244)	95 Am Americium (243)	96 Cm Curium (247)	97 Bk Berkelium (247)	98 Cf Californium (251)	99 Es Einsteinium (254)	100 Fm Fermium (257)	101 Md Mendelevium (258)	102 No Nabellium (255)	103 Lr Lawrencium (256)

Numbers in parentheses ( ) are mass numbers of most stable or most common isotope

Atomic weights (1969) based on Carbon - 12

(including IUPAC revision 1971)

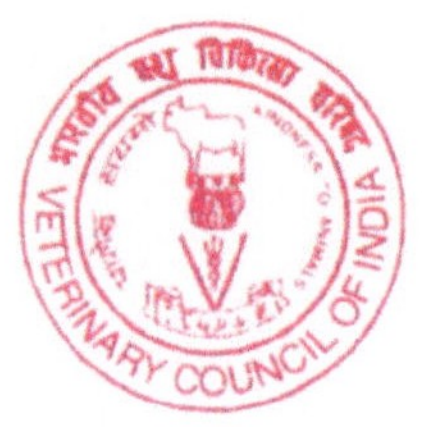

Veterinary Council of India

(Statutory body of Government of India)
'A' Wing, 2nd Floor, August Kranti Bhawan
Bhikaji Cama Place, New Delhi-110066
Ph. : 011-26162292, 26184149
Fax : 011-26182434
e-mail : vciinfo@hub.nic.in
nmohanty1@yahoo.co.in

Lt General (Dr.) Narayan Mohanty
PVSM, AVSM, VSM (Retd.)
President

D.O. No. 8-1/2011–VCI/2011 Dated : 20 July, 2011

Dear Prof. Krishna,

I am in receipt of your request dated 14th July, 2011 for a "Foreword" for your proposed Compendium on Livestock Nutrition : Analytical Techniques. I extend my sincere heart felt compliments to you for having initiated to put in place a document containing Analytical Techniques with your vast and rich experience for about four decades. I convey my best wishes to you for your success in your endeavour.

With warm regards

Yours sincerely,

(Lt. General (Dr.) Narayan Mohanty)
PVSM, AVSM, VSM (Retd.)

Prof. (Dr.) Gopal Krishna
M.V.Sc, Ph.D (India), Ph.D (Norway)
AVH Fellow, NAVS Fellow
House No. 790, Sector-55
Faridabad-121004
Haryana

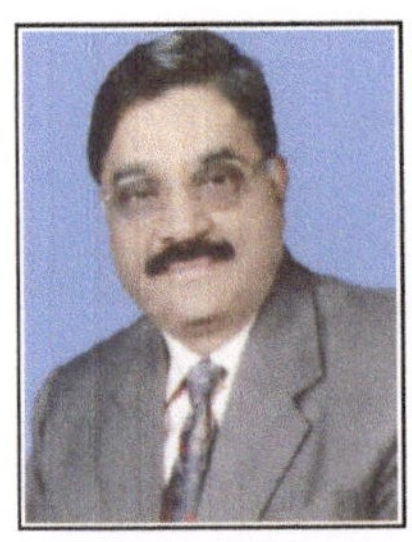

प्रो. कृष्ण मुरारी लाल पाठक
उपमहानिदेशक (पशु विज्ञान)
Prof. K.M.L. Pathak
Deputy Director General
(Animal Science)

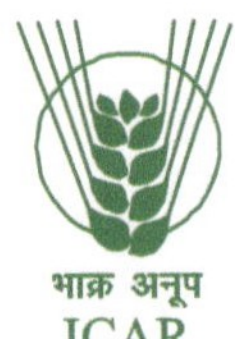

भारतीय कृषि अनुसंधान परिषद
कृषि भवन, डा. राजेन्द्र प्रसाद मार्ग
नई दिल्ली–110 114
Indian Council of Agricultural Research
Krishi Bhawan, Dr. Rajendra Prasad Road
New Delhi-110 114

Foreword

I am glad to go through the contents of publication entitled **"Livestock Nutrition: Analytical Techniques"** which fulfill the requirements of syllabus of BVSc & AH, M.V.Sc Ph.D (Animal Nutrition), M.Sc, Ph.D (F&N), M.V.Sc., Ph.D (APT), M.Sc., Ph.D (Food Technology) degrees of Indian as well as Asian subcontinent agricultural universities.

Looking towards an urgent need of an important compilation which includes lucidly the procedures of different chemical and physical methods of analysis of feeding stuffs and animal tissues, body fluids and excreta, this publication is written in a very systematic and illustrative way. A good attempt has been made to compile within one cover different methods for analyzing of biological substances of importance in nutritional research.

The author has 37 years experience in animal nutrition research along with 5 years training abroad at World Famous Weende Experiment Station, University of Gottingen, Germany, Agricultural University of Norway, AS-NLH, Hannah Research Institute, Ayr Scotland (UK). I am sure this compendium will be useful not only for students but will also be a handy reference book for research workers in the field of nutrition.

(K.M.L. Pathak)

Foreword

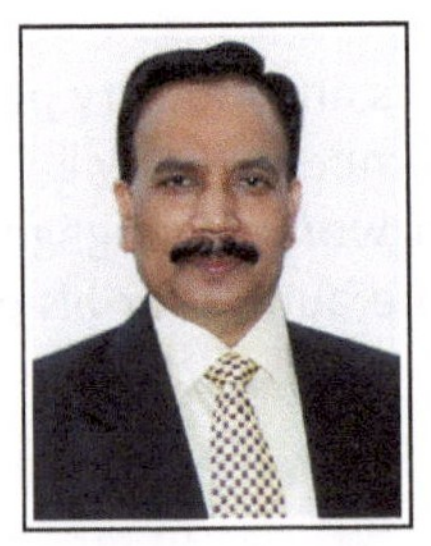

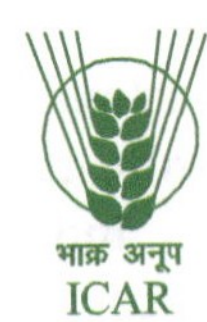

प्रोफेसर (डा.) ए.के. श्रीवास्तव
निदेशक
Prof. (Dr.) A.K. Srivastava
Director

राष्ट्रीय डेरी अनुसंधान संस्थान
National Dairy Research Institute
(मान्य विश्वविद्यालय)
(Deemed University)
(भारतीय कृषि अनुसंधान परिषद्)
(Indian Council of Agricultural Research)
करनाल–132 001 (हरियाणा) भारत
Karnal-132 001 (Haryana) India

संदर्भ सं. / Ref. No. 1-1/Dir./11/428
दिनांक / Dated 29/8/11

Foreword

I am pleased to note that the publications entitled **"Livestock Nutrition : Analytical Techniques"** have been written by Dr. G. Krishna and published by New India Publishing Agency, Delhi. The coverage of contents is very good and it will fulfil the requirements of syllabus of undergraduate, postgraduate and Ph.D students of veterinary, agriculture and allied subjects in animal nutrition.

The volume include the detailed procedures of different chemical and physical methods of analysis of feeding stuffs, animal tissues and biological materials. The language of book is very systematic, simple, understandable and lucid. It has been realised that the failure for adopting the uniform techniques for sampling, processing and analysis of biological materials is biggest concern for proper evaluation of data, compiled in different laboratories not only on chemical composition of feeds, but also on the bio-availability and utilization of feed nutrients through GIT. Routine analytical techniques namely preparation of solutions, proximate principles of feeds and processing of samples for chemical analysis, have been covered in tracer techniques dealt with in details. In measuring, fluorescence, polarization and spectrum, gas chromatography, atomic absorption spectrophotometry, flame photometry has been presented very nicely. In estimation of minerals, analysis of milk etc. have been discussed in details. The author is endowed with an excellent international exposure and four decades of research and teaching experience in India and other countries like Germany, Norway and Scotland. The book is a very handy reference book for students, research scholars, teachers and industry people engaged in animal nutrition research. I am sure that the compendium will find a promising place in the shelves of students and research workers engaged in advancement of science of animal nutrition. I congratulate the author for his great efforts.

AKSrivastava

(A.K. Srivastava)

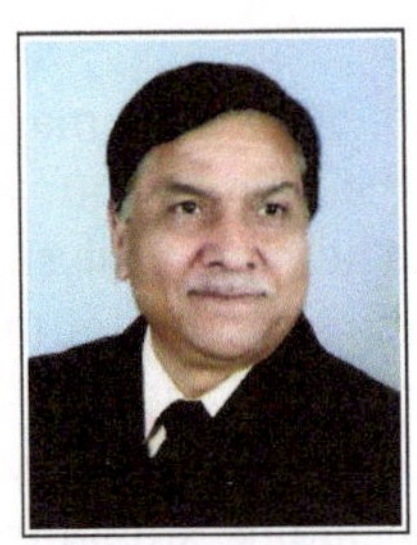

प्रो. महेश चन्द्र शर्मा
निदेशक
Prof. M.C. Sharma
Director

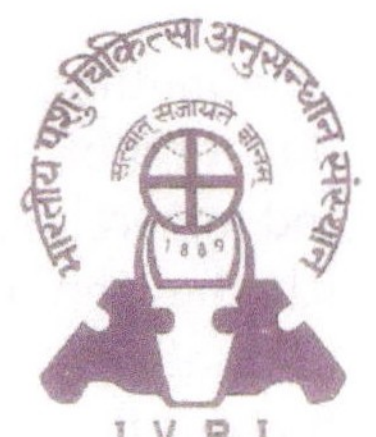

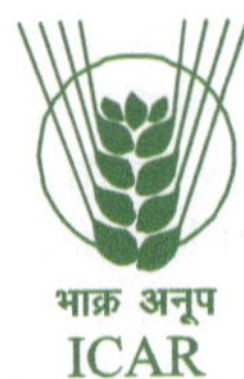

भारतीय पशु–चिकित्सा अनुसंधान संस्थान
इज्जतनगर–243 122, बरेली (उ.प्र.) भारत
Indian Veterinary Research Institute
Izatnagar-243 122, Bareilly (U.P.) India

Foreword

In strengthening the rural economy and income of livestock owners in this country, the livestock sector plays a pivotal role, as the contribution of this sector is estimated about 8% of Gross domestic product (GDP) and about 26% to the overall agricultural production in India. In the arid areas, the contribution of livestock to Agriculture GDP is as high as 70 per cent while in Semi-arid areas the contribution is over 40 per cent. In livestock rearing, the feed constitutes about 70% of the total cost of livestock production, which speaks itself the importance of animal nutrition in sustainable and economic livestock production.

The animal nutrition remains an integrated science encompassing the biochemistry, microbiology, physiology and other allied subjects. The analytical techniques involved in animal nutrition needs to be well documented in order to meet the requirements of research workers, teachers and students engaged in the livestock production, in general and the animal nutrition, in particular. I am extremely happy to learn that the eminent animal nutritionist of our country Prof. **Gopal Krishna** has prepared a comprehensive compilation related to animal nutrition and allied sciences in the form of a Compendium **"Livestock Nutrition : Analytical Techniques"**. The compendium includes the routine analytical techniques used in animal nutrition research along with different tracer techniques. The book deals with advanced analytical techniques like chromatography, spectroscopy and calorimetry techniques.

The book also includes the methods for determination of degradability of human and animal foods, fractionation of bacteria and protozoa from the rumen liquor, quality control in feed and mineral mixture processing industries, chemical analysis of milk etc., along with the general biochemical techniques. This valuable compilation is highly informative and provides almost all the analytical methods that are required for animal nutrition research, and therefore, it would be immensely useful for the animal scientists, teachers and research workers including students engaged in animal nutrition and allied subjects, I sincerely believe.

I congratulate and sincerely thank Prof. Gopal Krishna for taking this mammoth and painstaking task of preparing this comprehensive and need-based compendium, and hope that it would serve as an indispensible source of knowledge and help to the students, researchers and teachers in the country and abroad as well.

M.C. Sharma

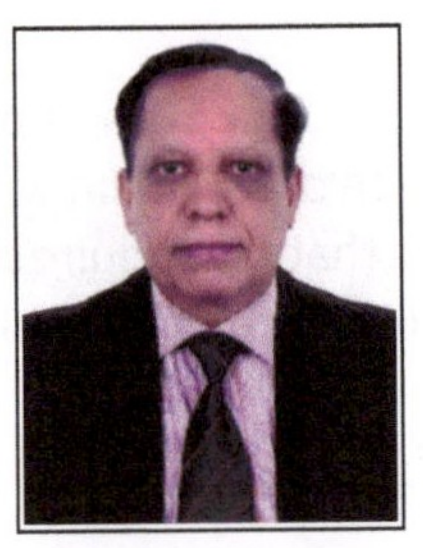

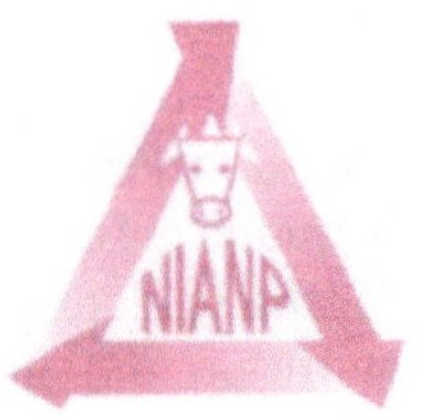

Dr. K.T. Sampath
Director

National Institute of
Animal Nutrition and Physiology
Adugodi, Bangalore-560 030, Karnataka

Foreword

Animal Nutrition, as an integrated science of chemistry, biochemistry, physiology, microbiology and other allied subjects deals with the nature of nutrients and establish their role in metabolism. For the preparation of balanced and economical rations detailed knowledge of the nutritional characteristics of various feedstuffs is a basic requirement. In this pursuit of scientific teaching and research Analytical Techniques play an important role. There are wide varieties of techniques used for the analyses of samples like from simple weighing (Gravimetric analysis) to titrations (titrimetric) to very advanced techniques using highly sophisticated instrumentation. It has long been felt that the failure of adopting uniform techniques for sampling, processing and analysis of biological materials have stood in the way of comparison of the data among different laboratories within the country as well as abroad.

The mammoth task in preparing this laboratory manual incorporating almost all important aspects of methods of analysis in Animal Nutrition, orderly presentation is highly commendable. The topics covered ranged from routine analysis in Animal Nutrition Laboratories to the latest techniques required for specialized studies. The topics have full relevance in the present day livestock scenario and would definitely contribute in updating the knowledge of students and researchers to understand the latest techniques in feed evaluation.

The rich experience of the author himself in teaching and research in India and many of the best research institutes abroad has gone into the creation of this manual, is laudable. I am sure this manual provides latest analytical methods that are required for the students, teachers and scientists engaged in teaching and research in Animal Nutrition and allied subjects.

I wish to extend my appreciation and good wishes.

K. T. Sampath

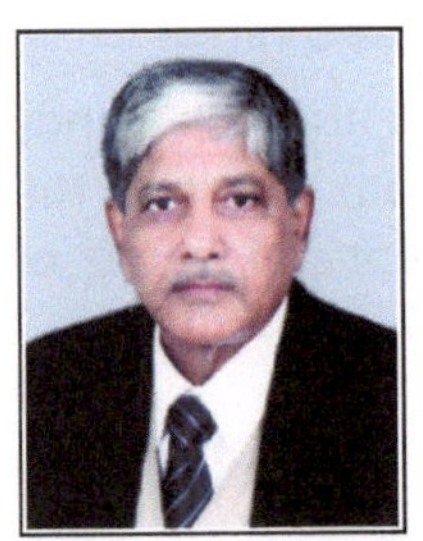

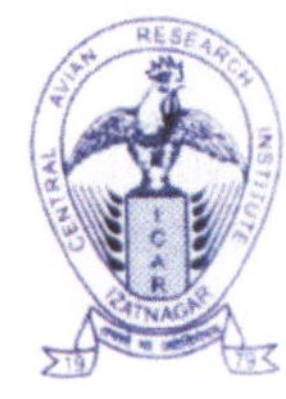

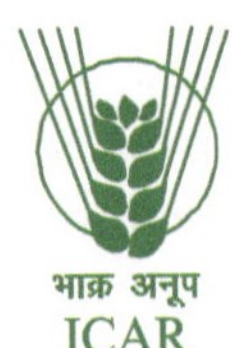

केन्द्रीय पक्षी अनुसंधान संस्थान
इज्जतनगर–243 122, बरेली (उ.प्र.)
Central Avian Research Institute
Izatnagar-243 122, Bareilly (U.P.)

EPABX : 0581-2303223, 2300204, 2301220, 2310206
Director : 0581-2301261 (O) : 2301493
(R) Fax : 91-0581-2301321
e-mail : cari_director@rediffmail.com
website : www.icar.org.in/cari/index.html

डा. आर.पी. सिंह
निदेशक
Dr. R.P. Singh
Director

दिनांक / Dated : 2 August, 2011

Foreword

I am very glad to go through the contents of publication entitled "Livestock Nutrition : Analytical Techniques" which is aimed at fulfilling the requirements of graduate and post-graduate degree courses of Indian as well as Asian Sub-continent Agricultural Universities.

Looking towards an urgent need of an important compilation which includes lucidly the procedures of different chemical and physical methods of analysis of feeding stuffs, animal tissues, body fluids and excreta, this publication is written in a very systematic and illustrative way. It has long been felt that the failure of adopting uniform techniques for sampling, processing and analysis of biological materials had stood in the way of proper evaluation of the data compiled in different laboratories regarding not only chemical composition of feeds, but also on the absorption and utilization of feed nutrients by the experimental animals. The attempt made by the author to compile different methods for analyzing biological substances of importance in nutritional research within one cover is highly commendable.

The author is of international repute having 37 years experience in Nutrition Research along with 56 months abroad training at world famous Weende Experiment Station, University of Goettingen, Germany, Agricultural University of Norway, As-NLH, Norway and Hannah Research Institute, Ayr. Scotland (U.K.). His vast experience has been included in this compendium.

This compendium will be useful not only for students but will also be a handy reference book for research workers in the field of Nutrition. I am sure that the Compendium will find a promising place in the shelf of every student and worker of Nutrition.

R. P. Singh

PREFACE

This compendium serves as a ready reference to the scientists engaged in nutritional biochemistry research and teaching. To meet this objective, an attempt has been made to portray latest developments in the analytical and tracer techniques used in nutritional biochemistry research and teaching.

The metric system of weights and measures is used throughout this compendium. At present some very good laboratory manuals, written by eminent authors on the theory and practices of chemical biochemistry and nutritional aspects, are available. I however, have not come across, so far, any suitable manual published in India or the Asian subcontinent, etc. to the teacher and students for their practical classes on this important subject, elaborated in a simple way.

During my 40 years experience as teacher, I felt that a considerable amount of time apparently turned to no account, while notes, explanations, directions, etc. are being given to the students. This compendium is written with the object of filling this long felt want. With the help of the material given in this compendium, the students and demonstrators will be able to come prepared to the laboratory with what they have practically to do, and the laboratory assistance would have all the preparation work classes ready at hand all times.

Now a days scientists have realized the importance of use of tracer techniques in exploring the changes taking place in every facet of body metabolism and nuclear techniques is the only tool which may provide accurate information about the nutrient metabolism and transportation. Therefore, this compilation aims to provide all the research techniques. Nuclear research laboratories already established in India and Asian subcontinent could use these elaborative techniques specially mentioned in this compendium.

An attempt has also been made to incorporate into this compendium a variety of important source materials that are normally scattered in many different publication. The techniques described herein represent personal preference. I am aware that there may be serveral satisfactory alternate approaches in every case, where there is a controversy, therefore, my approach to the problem has been outlined some what dogmatically in the belief that in certain circumstances a single point of view is better than serveral without selection.

This compendium will be of great assistance to the candidates appearing for the post of Senior Scientist, Principal Scientist and Head of Department at ASRB (ICAR), State Agricultural Universities, ICAR Junior/Senior Fellowship Examinations, UPSC, Dholpur House, Delhi, IAS written examination etc.

Author concluded during interview at ASRB (ICAR), Delhi that most of the candidates were not having exposure to the basic fundamentals of Analytical Techniques, Costly instruments functioning and principles of handling equipments of Nutrition research laboratories. This compendium will upgrade technical knowledge of teachers and research scientists engaged in the area of Nutrition subject.

The compendium deals with well known important techniques viz. Gas Chromatography, atomic absorption spectrophotometry, flame photometry direct and indirect calorimetry. Conway diffusion techniques and *in vitro* technique etc. Author has made an appempt to explain the principles, operation techniques, presentation and calculation of data of above named instruments. Laboratory techniques are subject to continuous modification and improvement and this collection will be no exception. Many will wish to add to or adapt them for their own purposes. But it is with the intention of providing a starting point that this compendium has been prepared. All the methods which are described, have been in regular use and therefore may be relied upon to yield positive results.

The compendium deal with General techniques related with nutritional biochemistry area. A special chapter on quality control in feed and mineral mixture processing Industries is written with an emphasis towards the importance of quality control programme so as to manufacture products of an international standard.

I trust that this compendium will challenge the mind of a student and develop in him a scientific attitude one in which he obtains his facts from the experimental evidence and draws his conclusions logically from the facts observed.

Since the compendium is primarily meant for research Scientists and teachers engaged in the area of Nutrition, exhaustive details have been avoided. But nearly all necessary practical work is included, and it is hoped that it will serve the purpose for which it is written. It is possible that inspite of my best efforts this compendium has still some shortcomings and faults.

I greatfully look to our generous and indulgent readers and fellow teachers to provide to us any fault for omission that may have crept however inadvertently. There is nothing to offer in this publication, nor is any claim made for originally in the essential and basic subject matter, but approach to the demonstration and performing various research methodologies, its manner of treatment and presentation is entirely based on my own experiences.

The author would like to thank Norwegian Agency for Agriculture Development (NORAD), Norway and Alexander von Humboldt Foundation (AvH Stiftung), Germany for providing financial assistance in the form of Post Doctoral Fellowship to the author Prof. Dr. G. Krishna enabling him to learn various Analytical and Tracer Techniques during 56 months abroad visit to World renowned laboratories of Norway, Germany and U.K.

With deep sense of gratitude and profound privilege, I would like to extend my heartfelt thanks and appreciation to my wife, Smt. Usha Rani Varshney for her patience, inspiration and constant cooperation throughout the period of preparing manuscript of this publication.

The financial assistance and valuable support of the publisher is most gratefully acknowledged.

Finally my appreciation goes to those former students in nutrition subject classes, who through their questions and suggestions have helped me in a grand way to prepare this compendium. It is to them to the students yet to come that I dedicate this compendium. I trust that this publication will challenge the mind of a student and develop in him a scientific attitude.

The author will like to thank his Guide Late Prof. Dr. S.N. Ray, Ex Director, National Dairy Research Institute, Karnal (Haryana) India, who made his foundation very strong to learn advanced Research Techniques under his able guidance.

I hope that students, teachers and fellow scientists will be informing their valuable suggestions required for the improvement of this compendium from time to time.

Gopal Krishna

General Precautions

General Precautions while Working in Nutrition Research Laboratories

1. Laboratory should have efficient ventilation and exhaust facilities and it should be neat and clean.
2. Reagents and chemicals should be kept in the properly labelled bottle on the shelf and these should be kept in a systematic way giving a very good look to the visitor.
3. Near the glassware washing sink, chromic acid prepared according to the following formula, should be kept in one litre capacity cylinder. Pipettes after using should be kept in this chromic acid solution at least for overnight and then should be washed.

   Preparation of Chromic Acid

   Weigh 60 g potassium dichromate on physical balance and transfer to a 1000 ml pyrex beaker, add 300 ml ordinary water, mix it thoroughly using glass rod, heat the solution to boil and dissolve potassium dichromate. Allow the solution to cool and then add commercial sulphuric acid slowly to one litre capacity cylinder.
4. Every day, used glassware should be washed using detergent powder and then rinsed with distilled water and these should be kept in an

oven for overnight at 100°C. Next day remove the glassware and transfer to a wooden almirah specified for it.

5. Freshly procured chemicals should be arranged in an alphabetical order in the steel almirah and these should be entered in the subsidiary register of respective laboratory.

6. Systematic breakage record register should be maintained where each worker should mention the item (glasware) broken and sign. This may help the worker to be more careful in future while using glassware.

7. Workers should put on white drill laboratory coats, while analysing any material in the laboratory. While using commercial acids, it is advisable to use acid-proof hand-gloves from the safety point of view.

8. While working in Kjeldahl digestioin room, every worker should use fume-protecting face mask which are manufactured by several companies of India.

9. Distilled water bottles should always be corked to prevent it from the contamination of atmospheric ammonia. Distilled water used in nitrogen or ammonia estimation work should be free from ammonia and it should be checked using Tashiro's indicator. Ammonia free distilled water always gives rose pink colour when tested with a drop of Tashiro's indicator, otherwise green colour will appear in the case of ammonia contaminated water.

10. Worker should remember by heart that **"water, should never be added in the acid"**. Always acid is added in the water. The beaker of 2L capacity should be surrounded by cold water and kept in the sink; then the job of adding acid in the water should be started.

11. During summer season, ammonia bottle should be opened after keeping it in the ice for two hours, Otherwise there may be chances of injury to the worker.

12. Analytical balance pan and platform should always be cleaned using camel hair brush, before starting the job of weighing. Adjustment of balance should be checked before starting the weighing.

13. Every instrument should have log book. The worker should try to record the timings of use of instrument in the log book and sign.

14. Worker should be honest and sincere while recording the final results of analysis. Every sample should be analysed in duplicate and final result should be in the range with ± 0.5 to 0.8 percent error.

15. Worker should never be allowed to smoke in the laboratory because there are chances of catching fire due to inflammable chemicals.

16. Fire extinguishing equipment should always be present in the laboratory so as to take care of the accidental firing.
17. After use, filter paper should be thrown away in the waste-paper basket. Floor of the laboratory should be neat and clean. Working table should also be cleaned daily.
18. The wastage of electricity, gas and water in the interest of country should be avoided.

Special Precautions While Analysing Sample for Trace Elements

1. The introduction of foreign substance during the preparation of the sample and in the course of analysis may have more serious consequences in trace analysis than in any other type of analysis, and hence special attention must be paid to this source of error.
2. Serious contamination of plant material can occur in mechanizing in Wiley and Hammer mills. Hand grinding with a porcelain mortar and pestle does not result in appreciable contamination by iron copper, zinc, boron, cobalt, manganese, molybdenum, calcium, sodium, magnesium, phosphorus, sulphur or potassium. A grinding mill with nylon rollers has been devised which should permit preparation of plant samples without appreciable contamination by trace elements.
3. According to the experience of Sandell (1959):

   It is not wise, in trace analysis, to use glassware which has been used previously in macro analysis.Thus, one should certainly not employ in a trace molybdenum determinaion a beaker which earlier was used for precipitation of phosphorus as ammonium phosphomolybdate. Glassware treated with dichromate sulphuric acid cleaning solution tenaciously retains tracers of chromium after thorough rinsing.
4. The ordinary distilled water of the laboratory frequently contains such relatively large amount of certain metals that its use in trace analysis is out of question. According to Sandell (1959) distilled water can be tested for the presence of copper, zinc, lead, cadmium, mercury, and other reacting metals by adding a drop of pure concentrated ammonia to 10 ml of the sample in a 25 ml glass stoppered tube and shaking vigorously with 1 or 2 ml of 0.001 per cent dithizone in carbon tetrachloride. If the dithizone is pure (free from its yellow oxidation produce, diazone) and heavy metals are absent, the carbon tetrachloride layer will be colourless. Less than 0.1 per cent of reacting metal will impart a faint colourless (red, orange, etc.), to the carbon tetrachloride.
5. It is always advisable to use all glass double distilled water equipment for trace element work. Some metals like chromium require organic

matter and other reducing impurities free water, which could be obtained only when it is passed through ion exchange resins.

6. Perchloric acid, nitirc acid, sulphuric acid, amyl alcohol and other important reagents should be distilled in all glass distillation apparatus.

7. All the digestion (wet ashing or dry ashing) should be done under fuming cupboard having sliding glass doors. It is advisable to do digestion work in the micro-kjeldahl flask covered with glass funnels having glass wool. micro digestion bench either electrically operated or having gas microburners should be used for heating purpose.

8. The blank determination should be carried through all the steps of determination proper. A zero blank is not necessarily an indication that all is well. Such a result may be the cause for suspicion reagent is combining with the desired constituent and preventing its reaction with the colour reagent. For example a trace of sulphide may lead to low results in the determination of various heavy metals with dithizone by forming sulphides that once inert toward the colour reagent. The presence of such an interfering substance will be revealed if the standards are subjected to the same treatment as the sample.

9. Sandell (1959) has reported that dilute solutions of metal ions may undergo a serious loss in strength on standing as a result of adsorption or cation exchange with, the glass container. The loss is greatest in neutral of slightly basic medium (such as may result from attack of poorly resistant glass), but may occur as well, but to a smaller extent, in slightly acidic solution. The weaker the solution the greater will be the relative decrease in concentration.

10. According to Sandell (1959), it is usually best to prepare standard solution in two stage. A moderately strong solution (for example, 0.1 percent) is prepard in 0.1 to 1 N acid. This solution should be stable for a long time, especially if kept in Pyrex, and from it the more dilute standard solution (conveniently 0.001 percent of metal) may be obtained by dilution. The latter solution should be made slightly acidic (0.1 N or so if permissible) and strored in Pyrex.

11. As per observations of Lewin (1953), fungus growth may remove metals from solution, as demonstrated for strontium.

12. Solutions in organic solvents should never be stored in polyethylene bottles.

13. Sampling of material should be done carefully. The plant sample should not be contaminated with soil or dust.

14. Sandell (1959) has reported that in dry ashing, insoluble material (for example, silica) may retain heavy metal tenaciously. Finally, there is some danger of contamination of samples in dry ashing by atmospheric dust or by substance volatilized from the interior of surface. One should be more careful while following dry ashing procedure.

References

Lewin, S.Z., P.J. Lucchesi and J.E Vance, (1953). *J. Am. Chem Soc*, 75: 6058.

Sandell. E.B. (1959). *Colorimetric Determination of traces of metals*, 3rd edn., New York, London: Interscience Publishers Inc.

Thiers, R.E. (1957). *Contamination in trace analysis and its control*, Vol. V, p, 273. New York, London: Interscience Publishers, Inc.

❐❐❐

CONTENTS

Chapter - 1

Standard Solutions - Definition and Preparation of Solutions of Various Strength of Common Acids, Alkalies and Alcohol

Normal Solution in Analytical Chemistry

A normal solution is that one that contains one equivalent weight expressed in grams (one gram equivalent weight) to be dissolved substance per litre of solution, or one gram-milliequivalent weight per millilitre.

In the case of acid a 1N solution contains 1.008 gram of replaceable hydrogen per litre of solution. A 1N solution of a base is one that contains 17.008 of hydroxyl per litre. A 1N solution of a precipitating agent contains a weight of precipitating ion equivalent to 1.008 hydrogen. The quantity of pure reagent necessary per litre of 1N solution of a precipitating solution is calculated by dividing the gram molecular weight by the valency of the precipitating ion. In case of normal solution of oxidising and reducing agents, the amount is calculated by dividing the gram molecular weight by the total valency change in the ion concerned.

Determination of Equivalent Weight

An equivalent weight of a substance is that weight equivalent in reacting power to an atom of hydrogen.

Milliequivalent weight is one-thousandth of the equivalent weight.

Gram- equivalent weight is the equivalent weight expressed in gram and is, therefore, that weight equivalent in reacting power to a gram-atom (1.008g) of hydrogen. A gram-milliequivalent weight is one-thousandth of the gram-equivalent weight.

Equivalent Weight of an Acid

$$\text{Equivalent weight of an acid} = \frac{\text{Molecular weight}}{\text{Basicity}}$$

Basicity of an acid is equal to the number of replaceable hydrogen atoms present in one mole of the acid.

$$\text{Hence, Equivalent weight of HCl} = \frac{36.46}{1} = 36.46$$

$$\text{Equivalent weight of } H_2SO_4 = \frac{98}{2} = 49$$

$$\text{Equivalent weight of } (COOH)_2.\ 2H_2O = \frac{126}{2} = 63$$

Equivalent Weight of an Alkali

$$\text{Equivalent weight of an alkali} = \frac{\text{Molecular weight}}{\text{Acidity}}$$

Acidity of an alkali is equal to the number of replaceable hydroxyl group present in one mole of the alkali.

$$\text{Hence, Equivalent weight of NaOH} = \frac{40}{1} = 40$$

$$\text{Equivalent weight of KOH} = \frac{56}{1} = 56$$

$$\text{Equivalent weight of } Ba(OH)_2 = \frac{315}{2} = 157.5$$

$$\text{Equivalent weight of } Na_2CO_3 = \frac{126}{2} = 63$$

Equivalent Weight of Oxidizing Substances

Gram-equivalent weight of an oxidizing substance is that weight of the substance in grams which is equivalent to 8g of available oxygen.

Equivalent weight of $KMnO_4$ in acidic medium can be determined as follow:

$$2KMnO_4 + 3H_2SO_4 = K_2SO_4 + 2MnSO_4 + 3H_2O + 5\ O$$

2 (39+55+64) = 316   5 (16) = 80

This shows that,

316g of $KMnO_4$ can give 80g of oxygen for oxidation or 316g of $KMnO_4$ can give 5 atoms of oxygen for oxidation.

So. $2KMNO_4 = 5\ (O) = 10H$

that is, Equivalent weight of $KMnO_4 = \frac{Mol.wt.}{5} = \frac{158}{5} = 31.6$

For example, Equivalent weight of $KMnO_4$ in alkaline medium.

$2KMnO_4 + H_2O \rightarrow 2MnO_2 + 2KOH + 3\ O$

KMnO4 = 3 (O) = 6H

For example, Equivalent weight of

$$KMnO_4 = \frac{\text{Molecular weight}}{3} = 52.7$$

Molar and Formal Solution

A gram molecular weight (or gram mole, or simply mole) of a substance is its molecular weight expressed in grams. Thus, a mole of K_2SO_4 (molecular weight = 174.3) is 174.3 gram. A mole of nitrogen gas (N_2) is 28.016 grams of the element.

A formula weight is that weight in gram corresponding to the formula of the substance as ordinarily written. In most cases it is identical to the gram molecular weight or mole, but occasionally the true molecular weight of a compound is a multiple of the weight expressed by the formulas as ordinarily written in a chemical equation. Practically in all the reactions of analytical chemistry formula weight and gram molecular weight are the same.

A millimole is one-thousandth of a mole: a milligram-atom is one thousandth of a gram-atom.

A molar solution is one containing a gram molecular weight of solute in a litre of solution (not of water). A formal solution is one containing a formula weight of solute in a litre of solution. The two concentrations are usually identical in value.

A litre of molar (abbreviated M) sulphuric acid solution contains 98.08 gram of H_2SO4; a litre of half molar (0.5000M) sulphuric acid solution contains 49.4 grams of H_2SO_4. These do not refer to 98.08 grams and 49.04 grams of ordinary concentrated sulphuric acid but to pure hydrogen sulphate. (Concentrated sulphuric acid contains about 96 per cent of hydrogen sulphate)

The advantage of expressing concentrations in term of the molar or formal solution is that volumes of reacting solutions of the same concentration bear simple relations to one another. For example, one litre of 1M H_2SO_4 will neutralize 2 litres of 1M NaOH (or 1 litre of 2M NaOH).

Volumetric Analysis

Titration

The process of adding one solution of known strength to another so that the reaction is just completed, is known as titration, since in titration we find the strength of unknown solution by measuring its volume with the help of burette, pipette and measuring flask, it is also termed as volumetric analysis.

Standard Solution

A standard solution is one whose strength or concentration is known.

Titre

A titre is define as the weight of solute contained in 1 ml of soultion or the weight of any substance which will react with or be equivalent to 1 ml of the solution. If any titre is known, any other desired titre can be calculated by means of chemical factors since titres are weight of pure substances represented by each millilitre of solution. The relationship between titre and normality is shown by the expression.

$$\text{Normality} = \frac{\text{Titre}}{\text{Gram - equivalent weight of substance in term of which the titre is expressed}}$$

It is seen that titre of normal solution is its milliequivalent weight.

End Point

The point at which the reaction is complete is termed the end point (the equivalence point or stoichiometric point). The end point that is, the point at which the titration is just completed can be found out by some change in colouration or a coloured precipitate developed during the reaction either by one of the reagents added or by the addition of an auxiliary reagent known as the indicator.

Indicator

When the reaction between two solutions is completed, then the slight excess of one solution is revealed by the colour change in the solution. This stage of reaction is known as end point.

Indicator indicates the end point generally by a change of colour of the solution. Indicator is that substance which indicates the physico-chemical condition of a chemical reaction.

There are three types of Indicators

(a) Internal Indicator

(b) External Indicator

(c) Self Indicator

Here we describe only the internal indicator.

Internal Indicator

This is a chemical substance which is added to the volumetric flask in which titration is carried out, for example, phenolphthalein, methyl orange, starch, etc.

They may be further divided according to the types of reactions in which they are used: (1) Acid-base indicators, (2) Precipitation indicators. (3) Redox indicators. (4) Adsorption indicators.

Acid-base indicators: The indicators used in acidimetry and alkalimetry are either weak organic acids (indicator acids) or weak organic bases (indicator bases), the dissociated form of which has a colour different from that of the undissociated form. *A basic indicator must posses a coloured cation while an acid indicator must posses a coloured anion.*

Precipitation indicators: They are employed in the fractional precipitation of two insoluble salts by the same reagent, for example, in the case of silver nitrate-sodium chloride titration, potassium chromate is used as a precipitation indicator.

Redox Indicators: The acid-base indicators are employed to mark the sudden change in pH during acid-base titrations. Similarly, an oxidation-reduction (Redox) indicator should mark the sudden change in the oxidation potential in the neighbourhood of the equivalence point in an oxidation-reduction titration. *One of the best oxidation-reduction indicators is the orthophenanthroline ferrous ion.*

Adsorption indicators: Surface of the molecules of certain substances (Indicators) have got a property of adsorption. They adsorb certain ions at the equivalence point and a typical orientation is developed at the surface which gives a charcteristic colour change indicating the end point. The substance employed are either acid dyes, such as those of the fluorescein series, for example, fluorescein, dichloroflorescein, and eosin which are utilized as the sodium salts, or basic dyes, such as those of rhodamine series which are extensively applied as the halogen salts. In addition to these, several other compounds have been recommended for different titrations. Table 1 gives the various internal indicators and their pH range.

Table 1 : Indicators And their pH Range

pH Range	Indicator	Acid Colour	Basic colour
1.3 to 3.0	Tropeoline O	Red	Yellow
3.1 to 4.4	Methyl orange	Pink	Yellow
4.2 to 6.2	Methyl red	Red	Yellow
6.0 to 7.6	Bromothymol blue	Yellow	Blue
8.2 to 10.2	Phenolphthalein	Colourless	Pink
10.0 to 12.0	Alizarine yellow	Yellow	Violet

Mode of Expressing Concentration

Grams Per Unit Volume

By this method, concentration is expressed in terms of the number of grams (or milligrams) of solute in each litre (or millilitre) of solution. This method is simple and direct, but is not a convenient one from a stoichiometric point of view, since solutions of the same concentration bear no simple volume relations to each other when they enter into reaction. Substance react on a molecule-to-molecule basis and not on a gram-to-gram basis.

Percentage Composition

By this method concentration is expressed in terms of grams of solute per 100g, of solution. A 10 per cent solution of a given salt is made by dissolving 10 grams of the salt in 90 grams of water.

Specific Gravity

The specific gravity of the solution of a single solute is a measure of the concentration of the solute in the solution. Thus, a solution of sulphuric acid of specific gravity 1.14 at 15°C contains 19.6 per cent H_2SO_4 by weight.

Volume Ratio

Occasionally the concentration of a mineral acid or of ammonium hydroxide is given in terms of the volume ratio of the common concentrated reagent and water. Thus H_2SO_4 (1:3) signifies a solution made by mixing one volume of the commonly used concentrated H_2SO_4 (sp. gr. 1.84) with three volume of water. This method is cumbersome, particularly in work requiring calculations from the volumes used.

Preparation of Solutions

In order to reduce solutions from a higher to a lower concentration, the following simple formulae are helpful

1. Concentration of solution desired x volume of solution desired

   ----

   Concentration of solution on hand

   = Volume of solution on hand to be diluted to the desired volume.

2. If one ml of solution of percentage composition (W/V) is diluted to the same number of ml as its percentage, it is a 0.1 percent solution. Similarly, X ml diluted to the same number of ml as its percentage is a X percent solution.

3. Volume of reagent per litre of final solution.

   100 x molecular wt normality

   = ---

   Percent x sp. gravity x the gram equivalent /mol wt.

Table 2 Gives description of normality of concentrated acids.

Table 2 : Normality of Concentrated Acids

	Specific Gravity	**Approx Nomality**	**Approx Percentage by weight**
Acetic acid glacial	1.05	17 N	99.5
Hydrochloric acid	1.16	12 N	36
Nitric acid	1.42	16 N	70
Sulphuric acid	1.84	36 N	96

General Standard Solutions Used in Analytical Work

1. *N/10 Sulphuric acid, 3 N/7 sulphuric acid.*
2. *N/7 Sodium hydroxide.*
3. *N/7 Nitric acid.*
4. *N/10 Potassium Permanganate.*
5. *2.04 N Sulphuric acid (2.04 N).*
6. *1.78 N Potassium hydroxide (1.78 N).*
7. *2.5 N Sodium hydroxide*
8. *0.225 N H_2SO_4 (1.25 gram H_2SO_4/100 ml).*
9. *0.313 N NaOH (1.25 gram NaOH/100 ml).*

Preparation of N/10 Sulphuric Acid, 3 N/7 Sulphuric Acid Solution

For the preparation of N/10 H_2SO_4, dissolve approximately 3 ml of commercial sulphuric acid in one litre distilled water, titrate it against N/10 sodium carbonate (standard solution) using methyl orange indicator. For the preparation of 3 N/7 sulphuric acid, dissolve approximately 14 ml of sulphuric acid in one litre distilled water, titrate it against 3 N/7 sodium carbonate (standard solution) using methyl orange indicator. Dry sodium carbonate at 100°C for the 12 hours in oven before using.

Preparation of N/7 Sodium Hydroxide

For the preparation of N/7 sodium hydroxide, dissolve about 6 g sodium hydroxide in one litre distilled water, titrate it against 3 N/7 sulphuric acid standardized previously using phenolphthalein indicator.

Preparation of N/7 Nitric Acid

For the preparation of N/7 nitric acid, dissolve approximately 9.5 ml nitric acid in 1 litre distilled water, titrate it against N/7 NaOH standard solution using phenolphthalein indicator.

Preparation of N/10 Potassium Permanganate Solution

Potassium permanganate solution is always prepared as a secondary standard due to the following reason:

Ordinarily even pure distilled water contains traces of organic matter, which reduce the $KMnO_4$ solution; and that is the reason that the solution should be well boiled and kept for some time before standardization.

About 3.2g of $KMnO_4$ crystals are dissolved in 1 litre of distilled water. It is then boiled for 10-15 min. and then allowed to stand for few days. It is then filtered through glass wool. The filtrate is transferred to an amber coloured bottle. Titrate N/10 $KMnO_4$ stock solution with N/10 oxalic acid standard solution in the presence of dilute sulphuric acid. When acidified $KMnO_4$ is titrated against oxalic acid. $MnSO_4$ is one of the products of reaction which acts as a catalytic agent. Hence the reaction which is slow in the beginning accelerates slowly. The brown turbidity is due to manganese oxide produced as a result of reduction of $KMnO_4$ in the absence of sufficient amount of dil. H_2SO_4 or the rapid addition of potassium permanganate in the titration flask.

$$2KMNO_4 + 3MNSO_4 + 7H_2O \rightarrow K_2SO_4 + \underset{\text{(Brown)}}{5MnO_2H_2O}$$

$$2KMnO4 + 2H_2O \rightarrow K_2O + \underset{\text{(Brown)}}{2MnO_2\,H_2O} + 3O$$

Preparation of 2.04 N Sulphuric Acid or 10 Percent Sulphuric Acid

Dissolve 58 ml Sulphuric acid (94 percent, sp. gr. 1.835 at 15ºC) in 1000 ml distilled water, titrate it with 2.04 N Na_2Co_3. Actually, titre value of 10 ml of 2.04 N H_2SO_4 should neutralize 10 ml of 2.04 N sodium carbonate. 2.04 N sodium carbonate is prepared by dissolving 27.03g sodium carbonate in 250 ml distilled water.

Preparation of 2.5 N Sodium hydroxide or 10 percent sodium hydroxide

Dissolve 105.26g sodium hydroxide (95 percent NaOH) in 1 litre distilled water and titrate it against 2.04 N sulphuric acid. Actually, 10 ml of 2.04 N H_2SO_4 should neutralize 8.1 ml of 2.5 N sodium hydroxide.

Perparation of 2.225 N H_2SO_4 (1.25g H_2SO_4/100ml)

Dissolve 7.2 ml sulphuric acid (94 percent H_2SO_4, sp. gr. 1.835) in 1 litre distilled water and titrate it against 0.313 N Na_2CO_3 standard solution.

Preparation of 0.313 N NaOH (1.25g NaOH/100ml)

Dissolve 13.16g sodium hydroxide (95 percent NaOH) in 1 litre distilled water and titrate it against 0.225N H_2SO_4.

Annexure 1 : Atomic Weights

Name	Symbol	Atomic Number	Atomic Weight *
Actinium	Ac	89	(227)
Aluminium	Al	13	26.9815
Americium	Am	95	(243)
Antimony	Sb	51	121.75
Argon	Ar	18	39.948
Arsenic	As	33	74.9216
Astatine	At	85	(210)
Barium	Ba	56	137.34
Berkelium	Bk	97	(247)
Beryllium	Be	4	9.0122
Bismuth	Bi	83	208.980
Boron	B	5	10.811
Bromine	Br	35	79.909
Cadmium	Cd	48	112.40
Calcium	Ca	20	40.80
Californium	Cf	98	(249)
Carbon	C	6	12.01115

Contd...

Cesium	Cs	55	132.905
Cerium	Ce	58	140.12
Chlorine	Cl	17	35.453
Chromium	Cr	24	51.996
Cobalt	Co	27	58.9332
Copper	Cu	29	63.54
Curium	Cm	96	(247)
Dysprosium	Dy	66	162.50
Einsteinium	Es	99	(254)
Erbium	Er	68	167.26
Europium	Eu	63	151.96
Fermium	Fm	100	(253)
Fluorine	F	9	18.9984
Francium	Fr	87	(223)
Gadolinium	Gd	64	157.25
Gallium	Ga	31	69.72
Germanium	Ge	32	72.59
Gold	Au	79	196.967
Hafnium	HF	72	178.49
Helium	He	2	4.0026
Holmium	Ho	67	164.930
Hydrogen	H	1	1.00797
Indium	In	49	114.82
Iodine	I	53	126.9044
Iridium	Ir	77	192.2
Iron	Fe	26	55.847
Krypton	Kr	36	83.80
Lanthanum	La	57	138.91
Lead	Pb	82	207.19
Lithium	Li	3	6.939
Lutetium	Lu	71	174.97
Magnesium	Mg	12	24.312
Manganese	Mn	25	54.9380
Mendelevium	Md	101	(256)
Mercury	Hg	80	200.59
Molybdenum	Mo	42	95.94
Neodymium	Nd	60	144.24
Neon	Ne	10	20.183
Neptunium	Np	93	(237)

Contd...

Nickel	Ni	28	58.71
Niobium	Nb	41	92.906
Nitrogen	N	7	14.0067
Nobelium	No	102	–
Osmium	Os	76	190.2
Oxygen	O	8	15.9994
Palladium	Pd	46	106.4
Phosphorus	P	15	30.9738
Platinum	Pt	78	195.09
Plutonium	Pu	94	(242)
Polonium	Po	84	(210)
Potassium	K	19	39.102
Praseodymium	Pr	59	140.907
Promethium	Pm	61	(147)
Protactinium	Pa	91	(231)
Radium	Ra	88	(226)
Radon	Rn	86	(222)
Rhenium	Re	75	186.2
Rhodium	Rh	45	102.905
Rubidium	Rb	37	84.47
Ruthenium	Rub	44	101.07
Samarium	Sm	62	150.35
Scandium	Sc	21	44.956
Selenium	Se	34	78.96
Silicon	Si	14	28.086
Silver	Ag	47	107.870
Sodium	Na	11	22.9898
Strontium	Sr	38	87.62
Sulphur	S	16	32.064
Tantalum	Ta	73	180.948
Technetium	Tc	43	(99)
Tellurium	Te	52	127.60
Terbium	Tb	65	158.924
Thallium	Tl	81	204.37
Thorium	Th	90	232.038
Thulium	Tm	69	168.934
Tin	Sn	50	118.69
Titanium	Ti	22	47.90
Tungsten	W	74	183.85
Uranium	U	92	238.03

Contd...

Vanadium	V	23	50.942
Xenon	Xe	54	131.30
Ytterbium	Yb	70	173.04
Yttrium	Y	39	88.905
Zirconium	Zr	40	91.22
Zinc	Zn	30	65.37

Adopted by the International Union of Pure and Applied Physics (1960) and by the International Union of Pure and Applied Chemistry (1961)

Value in parentheses or brackets denote mass numbers of selected radioactive istopes. Those in parentheses are for the isotopes of longest known half-life; those in brackets are for istopes that are better known than the corresponding isotopes of the longest half-life. All atomic weight value are based on the atomic mass $^{12}C = 12$.

Source: Pharmacopeia of the United States of America, 17th Revision (1965).

Annexure 2 : Solutions of the Various Strength of the Common Acids, Alkalies & Alcohol

Source : Official Methods of Analysis of the Association of Official Agricultural Chemists, 10th edn., (1965). Reproduced by Courtesy of the U S, Pharmacopeial Convention and the Association of Official Analytical Chemists respectively.

(a) *Hydrochloric Acid Solutions :* Specification requires not less than 35 percent HCI by wt. sp. gr. = 1.1778 at 15°C. Mix with H_2O and dilute to 1 litre.

HCl Strength Desired	**Hydrochloric Acid Required**		
g/l	**g**	**ml**	
5	14.29	12.13	
10	28.57	24.26	
20	42.85	36.39	
20	57.14	48.52	
36.46	104.17	88.45	1 N solution
50	142.86	121.29	
100	285.71	242.58	
150	428.57	363.88	
200	571.43	485.17	
222.6	636.00	539.99	Constant boiling
278.4	795.43	675.35	sp. gr. 1.125
300	857 .14	727.75	

(b) *Sulphuric Acid Solutions*: Specification requires not less than 94 per cent H_2SO_4 by wt. sp. gr. = 1.835 at 15°C. Pour acid into excess of H_2O and dilute to 1 litre.

H_2SO_4 Strength Desired g/l	Sulphuric Acid Required g	ml	
5	5.32	3.0	
12.5	13.29	7.2	For crude fiber
20	21.28	11.6	
30	31.91	17.4	
40	42.55	23.2	
49	52.13	28.4	1 N solution
100	106.38	58.0	
150	159.57	87.0	
250	265.96	144.9	
300	319.15	173.9	
400	425.53	231.9	

(c) *Nitric Acid Solutions* : Sepcification requires not less than 68 percent HNO_3 by wt., sp. gr. = 1.4146 at 15°C. 1 ml conc. HNO_3 contains about 0.96g HNO_3 Mix with H_2O and dilute to 1 litre.

HNO_3 Strength Desired g/l	Nitric Acid Required g	ml	
5	7.35	5.2	
10	14.71	10.4	
20	29.41	20.8	
30	44.12	31.2	
40	58.82	41.6	
50	73.53	52.0	
63	92.65	65.5	1 N solution
70	102.94	72.8	
100	147.06	104.0	
150	220.59	156.0	
200	294.12	207.9	
300	441.18	312.9	

(d) *Ammonia Solutions* : Specification requires not less than 27 percent NH_3 by wt., sp.gr. = 0.9 Mix with H_2O and dilute to 1 litre.

(e) *Ammonia Solutions* : Specification requires not less than 27 percent NH_3 by wt sp. gr. = 0.9 Mix with H_2O and dilute to 1 litre.

NH_3 Strength Desired g/l	Reagent Ammonia Required g	ml
5	18.52	20.6
10	37.04	41.1
15	55.55	61.7
20	74.07	82.3
25	92.59	102.9
50	185.18	205.8
75	277.77	308.6
100	370.37	411.5
150	555.55	617.3
200	740.74	823.0

(f) *Sodium Hydroxide Solutions*: Specification requires 95 percent NaOH in sticks or pellets of caustic soda. Dissolve in H_2O and dilute to 1 litre.

NaOH Strength Desired g/l	Sodium Hydroxide Required Grams	
12.5	13.16	For crude fiber
30	31.58	
40	42.11	1 N solution
50	52.63	
75	78.95	
100	105.26	
150	157.89	
200	210.53	
250	263.16	
300	315.79	

(g) *Alcoholic Solutions*** : Specification requires 95 percent C_2H_5OH by vol. sp. gr. = 0.810 at 25°C. Mix with H_2O and diliute to 1 litre.

Alcohol Strength Desired ml/l	Alcohol Required g/l	ml/l
50	42.63	52.6
100	85.56	105.3
150	127.89	157.9

200	170.52	210.5
250	213.16	263.2
300	255.78	315.9
400	341.04	421.1
500	426.32 (proof)	526.3
700	596.84	736.8

** Alcohol of any desired strength may be obtained by taking number of ml 95 percent alcohol equivalent to desired strength and diluting solution to 95 ml. For example: To obtain solution of 70 percent alcohol, take 70 ml 95 percent alcohol and dilute to 95 ml.

Annxeure 3 : Equivalent Weight of Commonly Used Chemicals

Name of the Chemical	Equivalent Weight
Sodium hydroxide	40.005
Potassium hydroxide	56.104
Sodium carbonate	53.002
Ammonia	17.032
Hydrochloric acid	36.465
Sulphuric acid	49.040
Oxalic acid	63.034
Potassium pemanganate	31.605
Sodium chloride	58.454
Potassium chloride	74.553
Potassium bromate	119.012
Potassium dichromate	49.035
Sodium thiosulphate	248.20

Chapter - 2

Conversion Factors

The Metric System

At present metric system is followed to calculate final results in analysis work. This system is quite simple in nature as well as in principle. The units of the metric system are: (1) the metre (linear measure), (2) the litre (measure of capacity), and (3) the gram (measure of mass.)

One litre is the volume of pure water at 4°C and 760 mm pressure which weigh 1 kilogram (kg). One litre equals 1000.027 cubic centimetres (Cm^3) for most work, the units "millilitre", "cubic centimetre" and used interchangeably.

At present there are three different temperature scales in common use. These are: the Fahrenheit (F), used chiefly in English-speaking countries. the centigrade (C), used universally in scientific work and the Absolute (T) or Kelvin (K) scale, differing from the centigrade only in the position of the zero point, its divisions being of the same size. its zero point is -273°C. The kelvin scale is used especially in dealing with very high or very low temperature and in computations involving the laws of gases. The following formulae can be used for converting one scale to another:

1. $\frac{(°F - 32)}{180} = \frac{°C}{100}$

2. $^{o}T = {^{o}K} = {^{o}C} + 273$
3. $^{o}F = (1.8 \times {^{o}C}) + 32$

Definition of Milliequivalent and Millimole

A milliequivalent is one-thousandth of an equivalent and is the same as millimole when the valency is 1. Millimoles may be calculated by dividing millgrams per litre by the formula weight. For example, 78 mg of ions per litre present 78/39 = 2 millimoles, 2 milligram equivalent. Here 78 mg of K ions present in one litre of the solution and the atomic weight of potassium is 39 (or formula weight) so 78/39 =2.

Expression of Figures in Terms of Logarithms

A logarithm is an exponent which must be applied to number, known as the base, in order to produce any given number. In the common system of logarithms, the base is 10. Thus, in the expression $10^2 = 100$, the exponent 2 is the logarithm of 100, when the base is 10. The above expression, in terms of logarithms, can be written.

$\text{Log}_{10'}\ 100 = 2$

which states that "The logarithm of 100 at the base 10 is 2." The relation of exponents to logarithmic forms for some whole numbers as exponents is shown below:

Note that the logarithm of 10 is 1, that of 1 is 0, and that for negative exponents there result corresponding negative logarithms. A logarithm is composed of two parts: (1) the mantisa, which is found in logarithm tables and is placed to the right of the decimal point and (2) the characteristic, which is placed to the left of the decimal point. The mantisa gives the antilogarithm or the number of which it is the logarithm.

The characteristic locates the decimal point in the antilogarithm.

Exponents	Logarithims
$1 = 10^{o}$	= 0
$10 = 10^{1}$	= 1
$100 = 10^{2}$	= 2
$1,000 = 10^{3}$	= 3
$0.1 = 10^{-1}$	= -1
$0.01 = 10^{-2}$	= -2
$0.001 = 10^{-3}$	= -3

Annexure 1 : List of Multiples And Submultiples Prefixes and Symbols

Multiple and Submultiples	Prefixes	Symbols
1,000,000,000,000 = 10^{12}	tetra	T
1,000,000,000 = 10^{9}	giga	G
10,00,000 = 10^{6}	mega	M
1000 = 10^{3}	kilo	K
100 = 10^{2}	hecto	h
10 = 10	deca	da
0.1 = 10^{-1}	deci	d
0.01 = 10^{-2}	centi	c
0.001 = 10^{-3}	milli	m
0.000 001 = 10^{-6}	micro	µ
0.000 000 001 = 10^{-9}	nano	n
0.000 000 000 001 = 10^{-12}	pico	p
0.000 000 000 000001 = 10^{-15}	femto	f
0.000 000 000 000 000 001 = 10^{-18}	atto	a

Practical Utility of Logarithm

Following figures written on left side may be expressed in log form as expressed on the right side.

2, 380, 000, 000	2.38×10^{9}
238	2.38×10^{2}
0.238	2.38×10^{-1}
0.000000238	2.38×10^{-7}

Selected Prefixes of Measure from the Metric System and Relations among Them

Prefixes	Abbreviation
deci - One-tenth, 1/10, 0.1, 10^{-1}	(d)
centi - One-hundredth, 1/100, 0.01, 10^{-2}	(c)
milli - One thousandth, 1/1,000, 0.001, 10^{-3}	(m)
micro - One-millionth, 1/1000, 000, 0.000001,10^{-6}	µ*

* µ is the Greek letter. When used alone it means 1 micron; when used a prefix it means micro.

Annexure 2 : List of conversion Factors Used in General Analysis Work

To Convert From	To	Muliply By
%	mg/kg	100000
kcal/g	kcal/kg	1000
kcal/100g	kcal/kg	10
mg/100g	mg/kg	10
g/100g	%	1
ppm	mg/kg	1
IU/100g	IU/g	0.01
μg/100g	mg/kg	0.01
g/kg or mg/g	%	0.1
IU/kg	IU/g	0.001
mg/100g	%	0.001
mg/kg	%	0.0001
ppm	%	0.0001
Therms per pound	kcal/kg	2204.6
Therms/100 pound	kcal/kg	22.046
Kcal/Ib	Kcal/kg	2.2046
μg/Ib	μg/kg	2.2046
mg/Ib	mg/kg	0.2046
g/Ib	%	0.22046
IU/Ib	IU/g	0.002205
μg/Ib	mg/kg	0.002205
mg/Ib	%	0.00022
μg crystalline Vitamin A alcohol/kg	IU/g	0.00333
μg crystaline Vitamin A alcohol per 100g	IU/kg	0.0333
μg crystalineVitamin A alcohol/g	IU/g	3.33
μg vitamin A acetate /kg	IU/g	0.002906
μg vitamin A acetate /100g	IU/g	0.02906
μg vitamin A acetate /g	IU/g	2.906
μg vitamin A palmitate/kg	IU/g	0.001818
μg vitamin A palmitate/100g	IU/g	0.1818
μg vitamin A palmitate/g	IU/g	1.1818
μg beta-carotene per kg	IU/g	0.001667
μg beta-carotene per 100g	IU/g	0.01667
μg beta-carotene per g	IU/g	1.667

Contd...

% CaO	% of Ca	0.715
% Fe_2O_3	% of Fe	0.699
% K_2O	% of K	0.830
% Na_2O	% of Na	0.742
% MgO	% of Mg	0.603
% P_2O_5	% of P	0.436
% SO_2	% of S	0.500
mg/kg Cu_2O	mg/kg Cu	0.888
mg/kg MnO	mg/kg Mn	0.774
% of Protein	% of total Protein %	0.01
% of ash	% of total ash %	0.01
ppm of ash	mg/kg of total ash %	0.01

Source : Harris. L.E., 1970, "An international record system and procedures for analysing samples," Nutrition Research Techniques for Domestic and Wild Animals, Vol. 1 Highland Drive Logan, Utah.

Annexure 3 : Weight-Unit Conversion Factors

Units Given	Units Wanted	For Conversion Multiply By
Pound	g	453.6
Pound	kg	0.4536
oz	g	28.35
kg	Ib	2.2046
kg	mg	1,000,000
kg	g	1000
g	mg	1000
g	μg	1,000,000
mg	μg	1,000
mg/g	mg/Ib	453.6
mg/kg	mg/Ib	0.4536
μg/kg	μg/Ib	0.4536
Mcal	kcal	1,000
kcal/kg	kcal/Ib	0.4536
kcal/Ib	kcal/kg	2.2046
ppm	μg/g	10,000
ppm	mg/kg	10,000

Contd...

ppm	mg/Ib	0.4536
mg/kg	%	0.0001
ppm	%	0.0001
mg/g	%	0.1
g/kg	%	0.1

Source : Nutrient requirements of domestic animals No.3 Nutrient Requirements of Dairy Cattle, 4th rev. edn., 1971, National Academy of Sciences, D.C., p. 47.

Annexure 4 : Weight and Other Measurement Equivalents

1 Ib = 453.6g = 0.4536kg = 16 Oz
1 oz = 28.35g
1kg = 1.000g = 2.2046 Ib
1 g =1000 mg
1 mg = 1,000 µg = 0.001g
1 µg = 0.01 mg =0.000001 g
1 µgper g or 1 mg per kg or mg litre is the same as ppm
1 mg/g. mg/ml means parts per thousand
1 cm = 0.3937 inch
1 inch = 2.5399 cm
1 metre = 3.2808 feet
1 feet = 0.3048 metres
1 Cu. cm = 0.0610 cu. inch
1 litre =0.2199 imp. gallons
1 oz = 28.3495 grams
1 millimicron (m µ) = 10^{-9}m = 19^{-7} cm =10 angstroms (Å)
1 angstrom (Å) = 10^{-10} m = 10^{-8} cm = 100 micromicrons (µ µ)

Temperature Equivalents
To convert Fahrenheit temperature into Centigrade; subtract 32 and multiply by 5/9.
To convert centigrade temperature into Fahrenheit: multiply by 9/5 and add 32.

Chapter - 3

Proximate Principles in Feed

General Views about Weende's System of Analysis

A team of scientists under the leardship of Henneberg and Stohmann of (University of Göttingen, Germany) developed proximate principles analysis system in the sixties of last century at Weende's Experimental Station (Germany), located at the University of Göttingen. Main components of different fractions in the proximate analysis of foods are moisture, ash, crude protein, ether extract, crude fiber, and nitrogen-free-extract. These workers emphasized that carbohydrates could be grouped into: (1) the starches and the sugars, and (2) coarse fibrous fractions. Later on an insoluble residue after boiling the fat free food sample first with dilute acid and then with dilute alkali was obtained based on the acid stomach digestion and the subsequent alkaline intestinal digestion of consumed food. At the end of digestion insoluble organic residue was denoted as crude fiber.

In Weende's system of analysis "*Soluble carbohydrate*" was called *Nitrogen-free-extract (NFE)*.

Dry Matter

Dry matter is calculated by weighing after drying to constant weight in an oven at 103-105°C. Generally, molasses, milk or feeds with a high moisture content is preferably dried in two steps, increasing from 50°C to 105°C after 24h. Hay, grasses and silages are usually predried at 60-70°C and roots in small cut samples at 70-80°C, while starchy feeds can stand120-140°C. Silage suffer losses of volatile components in oven drying. The method of toluene distillation permits a correction to be made from titrable acids in the distillate. Moisture in molasses may be estimated by "Dairy Search" method developed at NDRI, Karnal (Haryana) release bound water by treatment with hydrochloric acid and then extracted with xylol (Krishna *et al.*, 1972). Some laboratories adopt Karl Fischer (1935) method for the estimation of moisture in molasses.

For green fodders the samples should be taken from the field when there is no dew on the fodders. The plants should be harvested little above the ground level (2-3 cm) and brought to the laboratory where the plants are cut into smaller pieces (2-3 cm size). It is better to have all the parts represented. About 1-2 kg sample may be prepared and 100g sample in a clean dry pre-weighed tray may be taken and is kept in the oven overnight at 100°C.

Objectives for Determining the Moisture

1. Determination of moisture is essential in bulk purchasing the feed ingredients when the grain crops is harvested, normally the moisture content is high.
2. In storing, the feed ingredients determination of moisture is essential. The safe limit for storage is 15 percent moisture. Feeding stuffs containing more than 15 percent moisture should not be stored as it may develop the undesirable moulds and fungus or may even catch Fire due to hot fermentation.

Crude Protein

According to Weende's food analysis scheme, nitrogenous fraction of food may be divided into two portions- Protein and non-protein. Protein is made up of dispensible amino acids-glutamic acid, aspartic acid, alanine, serine, proline, hydorxy proline; semidispensible amino acids-arginine, glycine, histidine, cystine, tyrosine; indispensable amino acids-lysine, trytophan, leucine, phenylalanine, methionine, threonine, isoleucine, valine. Another part of non-protein nitrogen consist of urea nitrogen, ammonia nitrogen, uric acid nitrogen, free amino acids, amines, etc. Overall protein may be divided into two portion-true protein and non-protein nitrogen. *True protein nitrogen is estimated by Stutzer reagent method (Where protein is precipitated with cupric hydroxide in alkali conditions) while non-protein nitrogen fractions, for example, urea nitrogen, ammonia nitrogen are estimated accurately by Conway (1957) diffusion technique*. In general, pure proteins yield 5.25-5.75 cal. of gross energy per gram.

Crude protein is estimated by Kjeldahl digestion procedure, where organic matter is digested by heating with concentrated sulphuric acid. From the N-containing organic molecules ammonium sulphate is formed. The amount of ammonia is estimated by distillation, and then titrated against standard acid solution. In Kjeldahl method following steps are involved.

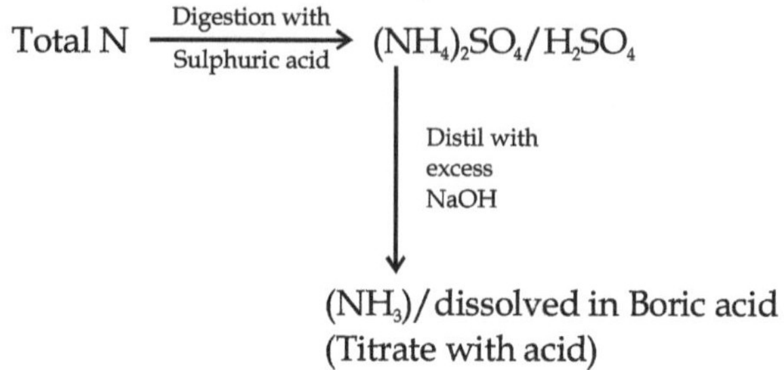

Crude protein = N× 6.25 where N is nitrogen percent, Factor 6.25 is based on the fact, that protein contains 16 percent nitrogen.

Factors in different feeding ingredients for conversion of N into CP

Meat (general factor)	N× 6.25
Milk and dairy products	N× 6.38
Flour	N× 5.70
Gelatine	N× 5.55
Egg	N× 6.68

N.B. : The above factors are recommended by Conway (1957).

Crude Fat

Crude fat is also known as ether extract. This is combination of simple fat-fatty acid esters, compound fat, neutral fat, sterols-Pseudo fat (Vitamins A.D_2, E, K) and Carotene. Fat is estimated by extraction with petroleum ether (boiling point 40°-60°C) by extraction with ether in a Soxhlet extractor. Too high values may be encountered with silages, and sometimes oil cakes due to oxidized fat or calcium soaps in faeces which are not completely extracted. The treatment with acid ahead of the extraction of faeces, and when the feedstuffs are extracted with a better solvent (Chloroform-methanol, benzene-methanol, ether-methanol, acetone or isopropyl alcohol), it gives better results. Part of the fat of feeds particularly polar lipids, which are integrated in the cell structure, is not easily extracted. The faeces of animals sometime contain fattly acids bound to calcium and may escape the assay in this way. *A series of analyses conducted in the department of Animal Nutrition (Agricultural Universtiy of Norway) Ås-NLH, NORWAY, revealed that the yield of extractable fat is increased by pretreatments with hydrochloric acid (HCI). Generally gross energy of crude fat is 9.40 kcal/g feed.*

Generally, two methods of extracting the fat from biological samples are followed. In the first method, weight of extracted material is recorded after evaporating the solvent and loss in weight of the moisture-free sample following its extraction is known as crude fat. In the second method difference in the weight of oil flask is recorded which is denoted as crude fat. The second method gives more accurate results.

Carbohydrate

Carbohydrate portion of biological material is made up of two parts- nitrogen-free-extract and crude fiber. Nitroge-free-extract is also known as soluble carbohydrate which consists of water soluble vitamins. Mono-saccharides (simple pentose hexose sugars), Oligosaccharides (compound sugars), Polysaccharides (starches).

Table 1 : Effects of the Weende's Crude Fiber Procedure On Fat-Free Food

Constituent	Boiling with 1.25 percent H_2SO_4	Subsequent boiling with 1.25 percent NaOH
Protein	Partial extraction	Complete extraction
Starches and sugars	Hydrolysis and extraction	-
Cellulose	rare effects	rare effects
Hemicellulose	Variable extraction	Extensive but highly variable extraction
Lignin	rare effects	rare but highly variable

Sources : Crampton, E.W. and L.E. Harris, 1969, Applied Animal Nutrition, 2nd edn., W.H. Freeman and Company, San Francisco.

Insoluble carbohydrate (crude fiber) is mainly polysaccharides consisting of hemicellulose and cellulose. Actually, residue of a feed that, is insoluble after, successive boiling with dilute alkali and dilute acid is known as a crude fiber and contains besides cellulose a part of nitrogen also. It has been noted that Weend crude fiber may be a misleading index of the overall digestibility of a feed, because crude fiber itself is at least as highly digested as the soluble carbohydrate (nitrogen-free-extract). Crude fiber gives an indication of bulkiness of a feed. As per Weende's method, some of lignin, pentosans and part of the cellulose are dissolved and included in calculations of NFE. Dietary fiber is considered to be plant-cell skeletal remains that are resistant to digestion. Although primarily cell walls consisting of cellulose, lignin, and the hemicelluloses, dietary fiber also includes soluble polyaccharides such as pectin, plant gums, and mucilages.

Generally, gross energy yield from carbohydrate is 4.15 kcal/g.

Ash

The residue from burning any biological material in furnace at 500°C is called ash.

Organic Matter

This is calculated by deducting the ash percent from dry matter.

Nitrogen Free Extract (NFE)

This is calculated as below:

100-(ash+crude protein+crude fat+crude fiber)

Main Features of Weende's System of Analysis

1. Lignin is indigestible and dissolved into the nitrogen-free-extract (NFE) by the use of sodium hydroxide.
2. Carbohydrate is divided into two factions. That is, highly digestible (NFF) less digestible (crude fiber).
3. The highly digestible fraction calculated by difference is supposed to represent available carbohydrate.
4. It is a vary simple scheme of analysis which is accepted worldwide.

References

Conway. E.J. (1957). *Microdiffusion analysis and volumetric error* (4th ed.), Crossby, Lockwood and Son Ltd. London.

Fisher, K. (1935). Angew. *Chem* 48: 394.

Krishna, G., M.N. Razdan and S.N. Ray, 1972 *"Dairysearch" method for moisture determination in molasses, Proceeding Second World Congress on "Animal feeding,"* held at Madrid (Spain), pp. 691-94.

Paliwal, V.K.; Yadav, K.R. and Krishna, G. (1981). Note on proximate nutrient composition of Agro-Industrial by products of Haryana State. *Indian J. Anim. Sci.* 51 : 1173-76.

Chapter - 4

Preparation of Samples for Chemical Analysis

Chemical changes occur during oven-drying because of the direct effect of high temperature, or of enzymic or bacterial changes during the early stages of drying, or of loss of volatile consitituents. Feeds containing molasses should be ground in a mortar.

Dried materials should be ground to pass 1 mm sieve. Samples expected to moisture during the treatments are usually predried. If wet samples are used directly in the assay, sufficient large quantity has to weighted out. In the first stage, roughages about 250-1000g are used, somewhat dependent upon homogeneity and moisture content of the wet material. These samples are weighted into trays and dried in draft oven at 60-70°C. The dry samples are then again weighed, determined the moisture content. The trays are then left to equilibrate in air at room temperature for two days. before a second reweighing of the trays with samples. Then the sample is milled and filled into airtight containers and labelled as dry samples.

A series of experiments have been conducted to demonstrate the effect of mode of preparing and drying the sample on the chemical constituents. The main chemical constituents of biological materials affected by the above processes are sugar, soluble carbohydrate (Jones, 1962), *in vitro* cellulose digestion (Johnson *et al.*, 1962) available protein and available lysine, crude fiber (Harberts and Immink, 1959) acid-detergent fiber (Van Soest, 1965a), ligin (Mc Dougall and Delong, 1942) and volatile constituents. It has been observed that non-enzymic browning reaction is the main cause for increasing yields in fiber and lignin because the products of the browning have solubiliy characteristics similar to that of lignin. Sugar values are lowered because of degradation of sugar residues in the browning reaction. It is recommended that drying in such cases should be done below 50°C to avoid problems, but in determination of volatile constituents, prior drying must be avoided. *It is a well-known fact that volatile substances of silages have a higher calorific value, and their loss in drying by conventional sample preparation may be the reason why the digestible energy of silages sometimes appears to be more effciently utilized than those of other forages* (Ekern and Reid, 1963). Actual energy content of silage can be determined on fresh matter with bomb calorimetry by using a suitable primer such as *dimethyl formamide* or *butyl cellosolve* (Coppock and Van Soest, 1959; Fenner and Archibald, 1959). *It is always advisable to estimate nitrogen in fresh excreta, since significant portion of nitrogen is lost in drying.*

Some of the laboratories suggest that silage dry matter should be correct on the assumption that 80 percent of the formic, acetic, butyic, propionic and valeric acid are lost during oven-drying at 103-105°C (Saue, 1968).

Herbage

Bulk sample is first mixed as well as possible and a 150g sub-sample is taken. This is thoroughly macerated with 150 ml of water and 5 ml toluene in bottom-drive macerator. Herbage samples, however, give a 2-Phase mix, with fibers floating in a dilute solution of cell contents which is very diffcult to sample. To overcome this, 5g of bentonite are added before maceration. This absorbs the aqueous phase and the fiber disperses uniformly in the resulting paste, allowing accurate sub-sampling.

Faeces

Out of faeces mix, sub- samples are weighted for chemical analysis, and at the same time other samples (approximately 10g) are taken for determination of the dry matter content of the macerate; these are dried to constant weight in an oven at 100°C. The toluene or thymol reduces bacterial losses during handling and drying.

Silage

Sample of silage should be taken randomly from silo pit and mixed homogenously in mixer. Sub-samples of silage should be treated in the same way as in the case of herbage.

References

Coppock, C.E. and P.J. Van Soest (1959). ARS 44-45. Agriculture Reserach Service, US Deptt. Washington. D.C.

Ekern, A. and J.T. Reid. (1963). *J.Dairy Sci.* 46: 522.

Fenner. H. and J.G. Archibald, (1959). *J. Dairy Sci.* 42: 1995.

Harberts C.L. and H.J. Immink, (1959). Mededeling, O 87, I.B.S. Jaarback, P. 159. Institute Voor Biologischen Scheikundig onderzoek Van Landbouwgewassen, Wageningen.

Johnson, R.R. B.A. Dehority, H.R. Conrad and R.R. David, (1962). *J. Dairy Sci.*, 45: 250.

Jones. D.I.H. (1962). *J. Sci. Food Agr.*, 13: 83.

Mc Dougall, D. and W.A Delong, (1942). *Can. J. Res.*, 20: 20.

Saue, O. (1968). Tech Bull., 135, Instt. Anim, Nutr. Agricultural University of Norway. Ås-NLH, Norway.

Van Soest. P.J. (1965a). *J. Assoc. off. Agr. Chem.*, 48: 785.

Chapter - 5

Processing and Weighing of Biological Samples

A biological sample received in the laboratory should be processed as below:

Fresh Green Sample: During metabolism trial period it is always advisable to take a sample of fresh green fodder daily so as to avoid chemical composition variation from place-to-place in a field. Take about two and half kilo sample from the bulk, cut the whole plant including the stem and stalks with a pair of scissors into small pieces and mix thoroughly. Weigh about 100g accurately in the aluminium tray $23 \times 15 \times 6$cm approximately for estimation of moisture. It is always recommended to weigh the sample immediately in the laboratory so as to avoid the losses of moisture.

Semi Dried Sample: In this case first determine the moisture content, then dry the material in the sun or in an oven, powder and store in bottle. Dry feed may be straight away powdered and stored for analysis in every case the moisture content of the final sample should always be determined for expressing the proximate principles on a dry matter basis.

Weighing of Sample for Proximate Principles Analysis

1. For moisture and ash estimation, weigh 10-12g for all concentrate, 10-12g for dry roughages, 5-6g for dried green fodder and fodder leaves.

2. For moisture, fat and crude fiber, weigh 2g for oil seeds and oil cakes, 3-5g for cereal grains and pulses, 2-3g for dry green fodder, fodder leaves and straw.
3. For crude protein and true protein estimation, weigh 0.5 to 1g oil cakes, 1.5 to 2g for seeds and grains, 2-3g for dry green forages and fodder leaves, 6-10g for dry roughages, 10-12g for fresh green leaves and forage.

☞ **Notes**

1. *After weighing, samples should always be kept in dessiccator.*
2. *For weighing the powdered samples from 2-5g weighing bottles up to 50 ml capacity could be used or aluminium scoop should be used.*
3. *It is always advisable to weigh the correct amount of sample by difference for each determination, but exact weight should known.*
4. *If contamination is a problem between samples such as when working with trace minerals or insecticides, use a separate weighing bottle and spoon for each sample.*
5. *Do not weigh exact amount of sample. This takes more time to weigh and results in errors in sampling.*
6. *In case of liquid samples, it is always advisable to stir sample well if sediment is on the bottom.*
7. *It is recommended that same pipette should be used to deliver a separate sample into the container after proper washing.*
8. *Always use glass pestle and mortar to grind the biological samples in trace element work.*

Chapter - 6

Dry Matter Content of Herbage Faeces, Silage and Molasses

Dry matter is generally defined as the constant weight a sample attains when heated at 100°C (occasionally 150°C). This definition , suitable for inert materials such as sand, has three main lacunae when applied to biological materials.

1. In these materials, water is present in various states ranging from extraneous moisture as rain or dew, through water present in cell sap, water present in various physico-chemical and chemical combinations.

2. Biological materials contain active respiratory enzymic systems which continue to function during the early stages of drying; in fact, as the material heats up, activity will be enhanced until it is stopped either by denaturation of the enzymes or by desiccation. Besides altering the chemical composition of the material, such activity will lead to loss of dry matter.

3. Most biological materials contain organic compounds which are volatile at 100°C and which are, therefore, lost on drying. This leads to an under-estimation of dry matter content, for example, in the case of faeces, silage and molasses.

General Methods of Drying

Low-temperature Drying

Some laboratories adopt low temperature drying using vacuum drying oven (temp. 30°C, 16 mm mercury pressure). This type of drying will reduce losses of volatile labile compounds, losses due to prolonged enzymic activity are likely to be large.

High temperature Drying

Most of the laboratories adopt high-temperature drying using oven at 100°C. In this case there are losses of volatile or heat-labile components.

Freeze Drying

Where it is desirable that changes in chemical composition should be kept to a minimum during drying, freeze-drying has to be employed, but this cannot be used to determine dry matter content as the sample does not come to a standard end point. It has been observed that more volatile organic compounds may also be removed during the process.

Estimation of Dry Matter in Forages, Faeces and Concentrates

Apparatus

(1) Aluminium moisture cup with lid, (2) Hot air oven, (3) Metal tongs, (4) Asbestos sheet, (5) Desiccator (6) Analytical balance and (7) Weight box.

Procedure

Weigh accurately about 5g of the material in an empty aluminium dish. having a diameter of at least 50 mm and a depth of about 20 mm, shake the dish until the contents are evenly distributed. Place the dish in an air oven maintained at 105°C ± 2°C and dry for at least two hours. Cool in a desiccator and weigh. Repeat the process of heating, cooling and weighing until the difference between two successive weighings is less than 1mg. Preserve the dried material for the determination of crude fiber and acid insoluble ash.

$$\text{Moisture, percent by weight} = \frac{100(W_1 - W_2)}{W_1 - W}$$

Where, W_1 = Weight in gram of the dish with the material before drying.

W_2 = Weight in gram of the dish with the dried material

W = Weight in gram of the empty dish.

(DM) = 100 -Moisture percent

Reference: IS: 2052-1958, Indian Standards Institution BIS Specification for Compounded Feeds for Cattle, First revision.

Example : Name of sample -Cotton ginning trash
W = 18.472 g
W1 = 23.472 g
W2 = 23.112 g

Dry Matter Content of Herbage and food material

Moisture, percent by weight grams

$$= \frac{100(23.472 - 23.112)}{23.472 - 18.472}$$

= 7.2 percent moisture

Dry matter = 100-7.2
= 92.8 percent dry matter.

Estimation of Dry Matter in Molasses and Silage

As mentioned earlier, dry matter determination of heat sensitive or heat unstable material by oven drying always gives the underestimated figure. Moisture is ordinarily considered as being held in organic materials in much the same manner as water is held in a wet sponge. Drying in an oven at times sets free water held by surface phenomena, water, of crystallization and water of constitution, it may drive off water, which is the result of chemical reactions involving extreme changes in constitution. Inherent errors in the method of oven drying are the result of oxidation during heating, loss of volatilization of substances other than water and sealing in of water by varnish-like films.

A feedstuff may contain from a trace to as high as 50 percent of reducing sugars and their presence is an immediate indication that decomposition may occur. Most feedstuffs contain proteins which react with reducing sugars. This reaction is accelerated by heat and often results in decomposition which is measured as moisture in the usual moisture method. The magnitude of decomposition is dependent upon a number of factors such as type of reducing sugars, the character of the nitrogenous material and temperature employed in a moisture test.

Some laboratories follow Karl Fischer (1935) method, which is based upon the oxidation of sulphur dioxide by iodine in the presence of water, where in a magnetic stirring device, electrodes, circuity for dead stop end point detection are needed. This is a complicated and is a costly procedure.

In the case of other methods, for examples toluene distillation method, there complete dextrinization and disintegration of carbohydrate moiety, specially in the case of heat unstable and sensitive materials like molasses.

Method I

Determination of Dry Matter in Silage and Molasses by Toluene Distillation. (Method of Dewar and McDonald, 1961)

The dry matter in silage and molasses is calculated from the volume of water removed by distillation in the presence of toluene. A titrimetric determination of the total acidity of the distillate is used to correct the measured volume of the distillate for the volume occupied by volatile acids.

Apparatus

(1) Dean and Stark assembly, (2) Electrical heating mantles, (3) Liebig condensers, (4) Reduction adapters, (5) Round bottomed flasks (with ground glass joints-one litre capacity).

Reagents

(1) Ethanol, (2) Phenolphthalein indicator, (3) Sodium hydroxide 0.1 M and (4) Toluene.

Procedure

1. Weigh 70-80g of silage and molasses into the flask and add 400 ml of toluene
2. Heat the moisture of silage and molasses with toluene and adjust the controller until the toluene boils steadily. After 90 min, and subsequently at 15 min. intervals, note the volume of aqueous phase in the receiver. When two consecutive equal reading are obtained, discontinue the heating, allow the receiver and its contents, to cool to room temperaure and record the volume of the aqueous phase.
3. Pipette 10 ml of the aqueous phase into a 100 ml conical flask. Add 40 ml ethanol, previously neutralized to phenolphthalein and titrate with 0.1 M sodium hydroxide using phenolphthalein indicator.

Cacluation

Obtain the dry matter (DM) in the silage from the expression

$$DM = 100 - \frac{99.8V}{W} \times \frac{(1-ft)}{10}$$

Where, V = total volume of aqueous phase (ml).

W = weight of silage taken

t = titre (ml 0.1 M sodium hydroxide).

f = A factor dependent on the constituent acids of the sample but which for practical purposes may be taken as 0.00555

Method II

"Dairyserch" Method for Moisture Determination in Molasses (Method of Krishna *et al.*, 1972) developed at NDRI, Karnal (Haryana), India

A simple method was developed at NDRI, Karnal (Haryana) to estimate moisture in molasses by disintegrating the carbohydrate moiety with the help of hydrochloric acid and completely extracting thereby boundwater with the help of xylol. Newly developed method helped in the recovery of 95-98 percent of added distilled water in the molasses.

Procedure

10-15g molasses is weighed in the distillation flask of Dean and Stark assembly, 25ml of xylol (AR) and 3 ml hydrochloric acid (AR) are added. It is mixed completely by shaking and kept overnight in a moisture free place. The contents are distilled on the bath at 120°C temperature for 15-20 min only. The water in the receiver is allowed to separate from the xylol by moving a spiral copper wire up and down in the condenser and receiver occasionally, thus, the layer of water is setteld at the bottom of recevier. The receiver is immersed in water at about 27°C for at least 15 min or until xylol layer is clear and then volume of water (actual water and acid water) is noted down. The value of three (hydrochloric acid) is deducted out of total volume recorded and result is calculated cited as below:

$$\text{Moisture content, percent by weight} = \frac{100\,VD}{W}$$

Where V = Actual volume of water (ml) (Volume of water) observed from the receiver-3). as 3 ml Hcl was used

D = Specific gravity of water at the temperature at which the volume of water is read.

W = Weight in gram of the material taken for the test. In this method, efficiency of recovery of added water is 95-98 percent.

Method III

Moisture in Molasses

(Method of Karl Fischer, 1935)

Apparatus

(1) Biuret with automatic zero reservior for reagent, (2) Magnetic stirring device, (3) Titration Vessel, 300 ml Berzelius with stopcock attached to side at bottom for withdrawing excess solution is recommended. (4) Electrodes and (5) Circuitry for deadstop end point detection.

Reagents

Karl Fischer Reagent: This reagent is available from laboratory supply houses or it may be prepared as follows:

Dissolve 133g I_2 in 425 ml dry pyridine in dry glass stoppered bottle. Add 425 ml dry methanol or ethylene glycol monomethyl ether. Cool to 4°C in ice bath and bubble in 102-105g SO_2. Mix well and let stand for 12h stopcock (leakage is less when ethylene glycol monomethyl ether is used). The reagent is reasonably stable, but restandardize for each series of determinations.

Anhydrous Methanol: Reagent grade CH_3OH containing < 0.1 percent water. Prepare methanol by distilling over magnesium.

Procedure

Add about 120 mg H_2O from weighing pipette or other suitable device and titrate with Karl Fischer reagent.

Calculate c = mg H_2O/ml reagent.

For titration of molasses c = about 5 mg/ml. Weigh quantity of molasses, estimate to give 20-40 ml titre in titration apparatus and titrate.

$$\text{Percent } H_2O = \frac{c \times \text{ml reagent}}{\text{g sample} \times 10}$$

Drain excess liquid and repeat with succeeding samples. It time lapse occurs between titraion of samples, adjust liquid in titration vessel to end point by titration with reagent before adding next sample.

Moisture in Dehydrated Vegetables

(Method of Karl Fischer, 1935).

Apparatus

Same as metioned above

Reagents

Formamide : Practical grade.

Karl Fischer Reagent: This reagent is available from laboratory supply houses or it may be prepared as follow:

Dissolve 84.7g resublimed I_2 in 269 ml reagent, grade pyridine (0.1 percent H_2O) in one litre Pyrex glass-stoppered bottle. Add 667 ml of dried absolute methanol (preferably < 0.05 percent H_2O). To this add 64g of sulphur dioxide gas. To avoid appreciable heating add the SO_2 slowly at the rate of about 40g/h. Stopper solution tightly and store 2-3 days before use.

Some commercial methanol is suitably dry for use in the reagent. If it is found necessary to dry the available supply, add 5 g of magnesium turnings to each litre and after the initial vigorous reaction subsides, distill off the alcohol. Take care or keep the distillation system free from contamination by atmospheric moisture.

Procedure

Determine the water equivalent of the Karl Fischer reagent and the blank titre of the formamide daily, or each time a series of determinations is made, because immediate reaction decrease the reagent's effective strength. To determine the blank, titrate 10 ml of formamide in 2.0 ml Erlenmeyer flask. To the same flask add using a weight burette, 70-100 mg of water and titrate. Calculate the water equivalent of the reagent- mg H_2O/ml reagent. (It is advisable to average at least three blanks and water equivalent value for each standardization. The net titre of the flasks should check within 0.1 ml and the range of the water equivalent value should not exceed six parts per thousand:. Carry out all titration drop by drop near the end point until an end point constant for 30 seconds is obtained. Grind the samples of dehydrated vegetables to pass a 40 mesh sieve and store in small tightly sealed containers. Weigh samples of approximately 500 mg of the ground material into a dry glass-stoppered 250ml Erlenmeyer flask which contains a stirrer. Add 10 ml of formamide with slight agitation to disperse the sample and prevent clumping. Heat for 40 seconds on hot plate held at 150 ± 10°C. Release the stopper slightly and gently rotate the flask during the heating. Cool to room temperature and titrate (Because of the viscous nature of some of the sample-formamide mixture, it is sometimes expedient to rotate or agitate the flask slightly during the titration in addition to using the magnetic stirrer). Calculate the percent water as follows:

$$\text{Water percent} = \frac{100\ (\text{Sample titre minus blank titre})\ (\text{Water equivalent})}{(\text{Sample weight in milligrams})}$$

☞ Notes

1. *Usually besides methanol and formamide listed above, pyridine, dioxane and dimethyl formamide are employed as sample solvents.*
2. *Direct titration usually gives total water, that, is , free plus hydrated water. When a suitable water-miscible liquid can be found in which the samples is insolube, free water can be determined by extraction with this liquid and titration of the extract.*
3. *Instead of weighing out portions of water for standardization of the Karl Fischer reagent, finely ground sodium tartrate dihydrate (1-1.5g) dispersed in 50 ml of pretitrated methanol may be used as a standard.*

4. *It has been observed in the case of dehydrated plant material, for examples, spices, contain active aldehyde and ketones that react with the methanol in Karl Fischer reagent to form water.*
5. *Methyl cellosolve (ethylene glycol monomethylether) may be used as a substitute for methanol in the Karl Fischer reagent and formamide as the sample solvent.*

Method IV

Now-a-days, several companies have started manufacturing instrument for monitoring moisture percent in biological materials, one example of such type of instruments is *Barbender Moisture Tester,* which is combination of drying oven, desiccator and analytical balance. The percentage of moisture is read directly on a scale. Another instrument, the speedy Moisture Tester, depends on the reaction of calcium carbide with the water of the sample. The pressure of the evolved acetylene is read on a dial directly calibrated in percent of moisture. Some instruments measure the conductivity of the sample. One such instrument is the *Tag-Heppenstahl Moisture Tester* used for determination of moisture in grains. Another instrument called Tag Dielectric instrument, measures the dielectric properties of the sample. *Recently instruments have also been devised using nuclear magnetic resonance principles, radio-frequency power absorption, microwaves as sensors, and other properties of matter, etc.*

Comparison of Methods for Determination of Silage Dry Matter

Brahmakshatrriya and Donker (1972) have published an interesting paper comparative study of various methods. *Their study confirmed that toluene distillation (corrected) is the most accurate method for determining dry matter in silage.*

References

Brahmakshatriya R.D. and J.D. Donker, (1972). *J. Dairy Sci.,* 54: 1970.

Dewar, W.A. and P. Mc. Donald, (1961). *J. Sci. Food Agr.,* 12: 790.

Fischr. K. (1935). *Angew Chem.* 48: 394.

Krishna. G., M.N. Razdan. and S.N. Ray, (1972). "Dairysearch" method for moisture determination in molasses. *Proc. Second World Congress on Animal feeding* held at Madrid (Spain), P. 691.

Chapter - 7

Dry Matter and Partial Dry Matter

The dry matter content of feed samples and other materials is expressed on three aspects as fed, partially dry, and dry.

As fed refers to the feed as it is consumed by the animal, the term as collected is used for materials which are not usually fed to the animal, that is, urine, faeces, etc. If the analysis on a sample is affected by partial drying the analyses are made on the as fed or as collected sample. Similar terms: Air dry, that is hay: as received: fresh; green and wet.

Partially dry, reports to a sample of "as fed" or "as collected" material that has been dried in an oven (usually with forced air) at a temperature usually about 60°C of freeze-dried and has been equilibrated with the air; the sample after these processes would usually contain more than 88 percent dry matter (12 percent moisture); some materials are prepared in the way so that they may be sampled, chemically analysed and stored. This analysis is referred to as "partial dry matter" percent of "as fed" or "as collected" sample. The partially dry sample must be analysed for dry matter (determined in an oven at 105°C) to correct subsequent chemical analyses of the samples to a "dry" basis. This analysis is referred to as "dry , percent of partial dry sample similar term - "Air dry" is also used.

Dry refers to a sample of material that has been dried at 105°C until all the moisture has been removed. Similar terms 100 percent dry matter or moisture free is also used. if dry matter (in an oven at 105°C) is determined on an "as fed" sample, it is referred to as "dry matter of as fed sample." If dry matter is determined on a partial dry sample it is referred to as "dry matter of partial dry sample." It is recommended that analyses be reported on the "Dry" basis (100 percent dry matter or moisture free), and in addition the "as fed dry matter" should be reported (Harris, 1970).

Flow Chart For Process sampling "Samples as fed" or "as collected"

↓

↓	↓
Sample contains more than 88 percent dry matter	Sample contains less than 88 percent dry matter
Grind, using a one mm sieve	Determine partial dry matter percent on as fed sample
Determine dry matter directly at 105°C	Dry in a force draft oven at 60°C or freeze-dry
This is known as "as fed" dry matter (or "as collected" dry matter or as collected sample)	Let it come to equilibrium with moisture in air
	↓
	This analysis is referred to as partial dry matter of "as fed" or "as collected" sample
	↓
	Grind immediately, using a one mm sieve
	↓
	Determine dry matter at 105°C. This analysis is referred to as dry matter percent of "partial dry" sample
	↓
	"as fed" dry matter (or "as collect dry matter) = Partial DM percent on as fed sample × DM (percent) of partial dry sample × 100

Source : Harris L.E., 1970, *Nutrition Research Techniques for Domestic and Wild Animals*, Vol. 1, 1408, Highland Drive Logan, Utah.

Reference

Harris , L.E., E.W. Crampton and J.M. Asplund, (1969). "Feed description and methods for reporting nutritive value, "Techniques and procedures in Animal Science Research, *Monograph, American Society for Animal Science, 49 Sheridan Ane. Abbany, New York,* pp. 157-65.

Chapter - 8

Gross Energy Value of Herbage, Faeces, Urine, Milk, Meat and Silage

Calorimetry

The process of measuring the amount of heat generated by the combustion of a substance is known as calorimetry. The first successful calorimeter using oxygen under pressure for the combustion of substance in a closed vessel was devised by Berthelot in 1881. Subsequent development by Mahler in 1992, Atwater in 1899, and Parr in 1912, served to improve and to reduce the cost of the original Berthelot apparatus by variations in mechanical details.

Type of Bomb Calorimeter

1. *Isothermal oxygen bomb calorimeter.*
2. *Adiabatic oxygen bomb calorimeter*
3. *Ballistic oxygen bomb calorimeter*

Isothermal Oxygen Bomb Calorimeter : The rise in temperature of the calorimeter bucket may be observed while the jacket temperature remains constant. The temperature of the jacket may be adjusted continually during a test to keep it equal to that of the calorimeter bucket throughtout.

Adiabatic Oxygen Bomb Calorimeter : In this type of calorimeter, there is no need of radiation correction and requires only the observation of the initial and final calorimeter temperatures and jacket temperature is kept equal to inner calorimeter temperature throughout. *This type of bomb calorimeter differs from Isothermal type in the sense that in the latter case observations of temperature before, between and after the initial and final temperatures are required.*

Ballistic Oxygen Bomb Calorimeter : A known weight of a sample is ignited electrically and burned in an excess of oxygen in the bomb and the maximum temperature rise of the bomb is measured with the thermocouple and galvanometer system. By comparing this rise with standard sample of known calorific value is burnt, the calorific value of the sample material can be determined. *In this case calibration constant is calculated by combusting benzoic acid in bomb calorimeter. Calorific value is estimated by multiplying galvanometer deflection due to sample with calibration constant.*

Standards Used in Calorimetry

Five repeat tests are recommended to give an accurate mean value. Single standardizing tests at regular intervals are recommended as a check for the satisfactory functioning of the apparatus.

Benzoic Acid: It has a calorific value of 6.32 kcal/g. In any case use sufficient material to give a heat release of 4 kcal. In this case 0.7 g (benzoic acid) having calorific value 6.32 kcal/g may be used. This material is not appreciably hygroscopic. burns easily and completely and may be readily compressed into pellets for ease in handling.

Naphthalene: It has a calorific value 9.614 kcal/g

Sucrose: It has a calorific value 3.95 kcal/g

Note : Naphthalene and sucrose were not found satisfactory for standardizing purpose.

Operation of Isothermal Bomb Calorimeter

Reagents

1. Benzoic acid (Heat of combustion 6.318 kcal/g) available from
   (a) National Bureau of Standards. Washington D.C.
   (b) Toshniwal Brothers, New Delhi.
2. Standard alkali solution. The washings from an oxygen Bomb test must be titrated with a standard alkali solution to determine the acid correction. Usually 0.0725 N sodium carbonate solution is recommended. This is prepared by dissolving 3.84 g Na_2CO_3 in water and diluting to one litre

   This solution is equivalent to 1 kcal/ml.
3. Methyl orange or methyl red indicator.

Setting up the Calorimeter

Insert the thermometer into plain jacket calorimeter and adjust the support so that the bulb extends about halfway to the bottom of the water jacket. This requires that approximately 16 cm of the thermometer be below the top of the cover.

Ignition of Sample

When ready to fire charge, press the button and hold it down while the pilot light glows. The light will go out when the fuse has burned. Release the button as soon as the light goes out, usually within one or two seconds. If the light has not gone out at the end of this period, probably the fuse was not properly arranged or there is a short circuit in the apparatus.

Oxygen Filling

Relief Valve: Clockwise rotation rises the relief pressure, and unscrewing or turning counter clockwise lowers the pressure at which the valve will open. The adjustment will remain indefinitely at any desired setting.

Procedure for Filling Bomb Calorimeter with Oxygen

1. To charge the bomb with oxygen. place it in the bench socket and make certain that the screw cap has been turned down hand-tight.
2. Remove the inlet valve thumb nut and attach the filling tube, drawing the union nut down moderately tight with a wrench.
3. Close the control valve on the filling connection and open or "Crack" the oxygen tank valve not more one-quarter turn.
4. Open the filling connection valve slowly.
5. Observe the gauge and allow the pressure to rise slowly until the desired point is reached, say 25 atmosphere, then close the control
6. Relieve the gas presssure in the connecting tube, pushing sideways on the black plastic ball knob under the relief valve.
7. The gauge should return to zero at once leaving the bomb charged with oxgyen to the maximum pressure previously indicated.
8. If, by accident, the oxygen pressure introduced into the bomb should ever exceed 40 atmosphere, as would happen if the full tank pressure of a relatively full oxygen cylinder should reach the bomb, do not under any circumstances, ignite the charge.

The Calorimeter Water: On a solution or trip balance, determine the weight of the completely dry oval bucket, then add 2000 g of distilled or demineralized water. Prior to weighing, the water should be brought to a temperature 3.0 to 3.5°C below that of the calorimeter jacket. This initial adjustment generally will ensure a final temperature slightly above that of the jacket. Some operators use a lower initial temperature so that the calorimeter temperature remains below that of the jacket.

Assembling

1. Set the filled bucket in the jacket with the long axis of the oval, in line with the operator, and with the bomb locating boss in the bottom positioned nearest the operator.
2. Grasp the bomb valve between the thumb the forefinger, and lower the bomb into the water, taking care to avoid jarring or disturbing the contents. Set the bomb with its feet spanning the locating boss and turned so that the electrode terminal is near the insulated ignition wire.
3. Attach the thrust terminal to the bomb electrode and shake back into the bucket all drops of water adhering to the fingers.
4. Place the cover on the jacket with the thermometer toward the operator. Lower the cover into position. using care to avoid striking the thermometer against anything.
5. The locating pin at the rear of the cover should fall into the hole in the top rim of the jacket, thereby properly aligning the assembly.
6. Put on the rubber driver belt and start the motor. The stirrer will turn at the proper speed if the electric supply to the motor corresponds to that stamped on the Parr motor name plate.

Instructions for the Care and Handling of Calorimetric Thermometer

Each new thermometer must be tested for entrapped gas and examined carefully with a reading lens to check for mercury separations and gas bubbles.

Mercury Separations: Cool the bulb with a mixture of salt and ice to draw the mercury into lower part of the contraction chamber. Gently tap the stem until all of the entrapped nitrogen has been removed from the mercury reservoir; then warm while holding the thermometer vertically. If there are droplets of mercury in the expansion chamber which cannot be removed by cooling, they will have to be collected by raising the main thread to the top of the capillary. This is done by heating the bulb in warm water but not above 60°C. As mercury enters the expansion chamber, snap the top of the stem with a finger and then cool slowly.

Caution

The thermometer is easily broken by forcing and appreciable amount of mercury into the expansion chamber. Always store this type of thermometer in a vertical position, bulb down.

Temperature Observations

1. Run the motor for five minutes to attain thermal equilibrium but do not record temperature during this period. Adjust the thermometer reading lens and be prepared to take temperature readings as soon as equilibrium is indicated by a slow, uniform rise.
2. Read and record the calorimeter temperature to the nearest 0.005°F (0.002°C) at one minute intervals for exactly five minutes.
3. Then press the button on the ignition unit to fire the charge at the start of the sixth minute record the exact time and temperature at the firing point. After firing, approximate 20 seconds will elapse before the mercrury starts to rise. The rate of rise will be rapid during the first few minutes and decrease as the calorimeter approaches maximum temperature.
4. If the net temperature rise can be estimated from previous tests with similar samples, take 60 percent of expected rise and add it to the observed temperature at the firing point. Locate this temperatue on the thermometer scale and record the time when the mercury column reaches this point.
5. If the approximate temperature rise cannot be estimated, record the temperature readings (taken without the magnifier) at 45, 60, 75, 90 and 105 minutes after firing. The time required to reach 60 percent of the total rise can then be computed by interpolation after the test is completed.
6. After the period of rapid (about 4 to 5 min. after firing) adjust the reading lens. and record temperatures to the nearest 0.005°F (0.002°C) at one minute intervals, has been constant for five minutes. Usually the temperature will reach a maximum then drop very slowly.
7. The difference between successive readings must be noted and reading continued, at one minute intervals, until the rise of temperature change becomes uniform and constant over a period of five minutes.

☞ Note

If the intial water temperature is low, or if the heat of combustion of the sample is less than expected, the final temperature (due to combustion), may not be above that of the jacket. In this event the temperature will not reach a maximum, but will continue to rise slowly during the final period. This is permissible, but it requires that the effect of the additional heat input be accounted for in the radiation calculation.

Opening the Calorimeter

1. After completing the reading, stop motor, remove the belt and lift the cover from the jacket. Clean the thermometer bulb with a cloth to remove any water, and set the cover on the support stand. It is not necessary to remove the thermometer from its holder. but care should be taken to guard against breakage. Disconnect the firing connection from the bomb terminal and lift bucket and take bomb out of the jacket.
2. Replace the cover and thermometer on the empty jacket to measure its temperature for the next test.
3. Lift the bomb out of he bucket and relieve all residual pressure. This should be done slowly and at a uniform rate, such that the operation will require not less than one minute.
4. After all the pressure has been relieved, remove the screw cap, lift out the bomb head and place it on the support stand. Examine the interior of the bomb for soot or other evidence of incomplete combustion and discard the test if any is found.

The Acid Titration: Wash all interior surface of the bomb with a jet of distilled water and quantitatively collect the washing in a beaker. Titrate with standard alkali solution. using methyl orange or methyl red indicator. Save the soultion, remaining after the titration for determining the sulphur content of the sample. In computing the correction for acid formation it is assumed that all of the acid titrated is nitric acid (HNO_3) and that the heat of formation of 0.1 N HNO_3 under bomb conditions is 13.8 kcal per mol. Obviously, if sulphuric acid is also present, part of correction for sulphuric acid is included by a separate computation based upon the sulphur content of the sample.

The Fuse Correction: Carefully remove all unburned pieces of fuse wire from the bomb electrodes, straighten them and measure their combined length in centimeters. Subtract this length from the initial 100 cm and enter this value on the data sheet as the net amount of wire burned. The correction is then computed for the burned position by assuming a heat of combustion of 2.3 kcal/cm for Parr 45 (No. 34 B adn S gauge chromel C).

The Sulphur Correction : The sulphur content of the sample should be determined if it exceeds 0.1 percent. This is accomplished by a gravimetric or turbidimetric analysis of the solution remaining after the acid titration. A correction of 1.4 kcal must be applied for each gram of sulphur converted to sulphuric acid. This is based upon the heat of formation of 0.17 N H_2SO_4 which is 72 kcal/ml. But a correction of 2×13.8 kcal per mol. of sulhpur is included in the nitric acid correction. Therefore, the additional correction which must be applied for sulphur will be $72 - (2 \times 13.8) = 44.4$ kcal per mol.

or 1.4 kcal/g of sulphur. For convenience, this is expressed as 14 kcal for each percentage point of sulphur per gram of sample.

Radiation Correction : This method is based upon the work of Dr H.C Dickinson of the National Bureau of Standards, who observed, that the point of transition from the period of heat gain to the period of heat loss occures at a point of time when the temperature rise has reached 60 percent of its total amount. Calculation : The following data should be available at the completion of a test in the Isothermal calorimeter.

a = Time of firing.

b = Time (to nearest 0.1 min.) when the termperature reaches 60 percent of the total rise.

c = Time at beginning of period (after the temperature rise) in which the rate of temperature change has become constant.

t_a = Temperature at time of firing, corrected from thermometer scale error.

t_c = Temperature at time c, corrected for thermometer scale error.

r_1 = Rate (temperature units/min) at which the temperature was rising during the five minutes period before firing.

r_2 = Rate (temperature units/min.) at which the temperature was falling during the five minutes period after time c.

It the temperature was rising instead of falling after time c, subtract the quantity r_2 (c-b) instead of adding it when computing the corrected temperature rise.

C_1 = Millilitres of standard alkali solution used in the acid titration.

C_2 = Percentage of sulphur in the sample.

C_3 = Centimetres of fuse wire consumed in firing.

W = Energy equivalent of the calorimeter in calories per degree Fahrenheit or Centigrade.

m = Mass of sample in grams.

Temperature Rise : Compute the net corrected temperature rise t, by subsituting in the following equation:

$t = t_c - t_a - r_1, (b - a) + r_2 (c - b)$

Thermochemical Correction : Compute the following for each test:

e_1 = Correction in calories for heat of formation of nitric acid

C_1 = If 0.0725 N alkali was used for the titration.

e_2 = Correction in calories for heat of formation of sulphuric acid (H_2SO_4) = (14) (C_2) (m)

e_3 = correction in calories for heat of combustion of fuse wire.
= (2.3) (C_3) when using Parr 45C10 nickel chromium fuse wire.
= (2.7) (C_3) when using No. 34B and S. gauge iron fuse wire.

Gross Heat of Combustion

Compute the gross heat of combustion (H_g) in cal/g by substituting in the following equation:

$$H_g = \frac{tw - e_1 - e_2 - e_3}{m}$$

Where tw is not corrected temperature rise

Example I

Objective

Estimation of gross energy of wheat straw using Isothermal bomb calorimeter (Parr Bomb, USA)

Weight of sample (m)-0.5g

Temperatue record nearest to 0.005°F

Time	Temperature Prior to Firing
1st min.	76.2
2nd min.	76.2
3rd min.	76.2
4th min.	76.075
5th min.	76.15
Start of 6 th min. exact time of firing	
□	76.5
45 s	76.55
60 s	76.70
75 s	76.80
90 s	76.95
105 s	77.05
2nd min.	77.10
3rd min.	77.175
4th min.	77.225
a	6th min.
b	90 s
c	4 min.
ta	76.5

Contd...

te	77.225
r_1	0.02°F
r_2	0.004°F
C_1	3.15
C_2	0.17
C_3	8.27
W	1356 kcal/°F

$$H_g = \frac{tw - e_1 - e_2 - e_3}{m}$$

Where tw is net corrected temperature rise

$$e_1 = C_1$$

$$e_2 = (14)\ (C_2)\ (m)$$

$$e_3 = 2.3\ (C_3)$$

$$tw = tc - ta - r_1\ (b - a) + r_2\ (c - b)$$

$$tw = 77.225 - 76.5 - 0.02 - (76.95 - 76.50) + 0.004\ (76.025 - 76.950)$$

$$= 0.725 - (0.02)\ (0.45) + (0.004)\ (-\ 0.925)$$

$$tw = 0.725 - 0.009 - 0.0037$$

$$= \frac{tw - e_1 - e_2 - e_3}{m}$$

$$= \frac{(0.7133)(1356 - 3.15) - (14 \times 0.017)(0.5)(2.3)(8.27)}{0.5}$$

$$= \frac{965.8788 - 23.361}{0.5} = \frac{942.5178}{0.5}$$

$$= 1885.0356 \text{ cal}$$

$$= 1.885 \text{ kcal}$$

(In one gram) wheat straw = 3.770 kcal (Gross energy)

Example II

Objective

Estimation of grosss energy of hominy feed using Isothermal bomb Calorimeter, Toshniwal-Brothers (P) Ltd. India:

1. Wt of pelleted hominy feed consisting 59.32 percent DM = 1.420 g
2. Wt of dry matter in the pellet = 0.842 g
3. Wt of fuse wire = 0.023 mg

4. Wt of thread = 0.007 mg
5. Wt of unburned wire = 0.022 mg
6. Bucket temperature = 33°C
7. Jacket temperature = 33°C
8. Value of alkali used = 2.9 ml

Cooling Correction

The cooling correction includes the effects of the heat interchange between the vessel and the jacket due to conduction, convection and radiation, and of the heat of stirring and evaporation. This is minimized by having:

(a) The temperature of the water in the vessel below that of the water in the jacket at the time of firing and within ± 1.0°C preferably ± 0.5°C, of it at the end of the chief period;

(b) A low heat of stirring; and

(c) A low loss by evaporation

The correction may be applied using the Regnault Pfaundler formula or the Dickinson formula. In determining the water equivalent the same formula has to be used. No cooling correction is necessary when using adiabatic type water jacket, provided that the thermal conditons of the determination are substantially the same as those in the determination of the heat capacity, that is the firing temperature and heat release are approximately constant and the length of chief period is fixed.

Dickinson Correction

In place of the Regnault-Pfaundler cooling correction which is cumbersome the Dickinson Correction may be adopted, provided that it has also been employed to find the water equivalent or the heat capacity of the apparatus.

$$\text{Cooling correction} = V' (T_a - Tb) + V'' (T_n - T_a)$$

Where

To = the time in min.% at temperature (to)

Tn = the time in min.% at temperature (to)

Ta = the time in min.% at temperature (to + 0.60) (tn - to)

n = number of minutes in the chief period (5 to 10 min.)

V′ = rate of fall of temperature per min.% in the preliminary period (if the temperature is rising during the preliminary period then V′ is negative)

V″ = rate of fall of temperature per minute in the after period

to = average temperature during preliminary period

tn = average temperature during after period

(tn-to) = the temperature rise

Table 1 : Record of temperature prior to and after firing

Time (Min.)		Temperature (°C)	
1.		1.080	
2.		1.100	
3.		1.105	Prior of firing V′ -0.0075
4.	to	1.110	
5.		1.111	
6.		1.900	
7.		2.450	
8.		2.710	
9.		2.740	
10.		2.750	
11.		2.755	
12.		2.758	
13.	tn	2.758	After firing V″ = 0.0075
14.		2.757	
15.		2.756	
16.		2.756	
17.		2.755	

V′ = 0.0075

V″= 0.00075

$(t_n - t_o)$ Temperature rise = 1.648

60 percent of it = 0.9888

= t_0 + 60 percent

= 0.9888 + 1.110 = 2.0988

= 0.9888 + 1.110 = 2.0988

If 2.70°C rise in temperature is in 3 min.

Then 1°C rise in temperature will be = $\frac{3}{2.710}$

Then 2.0988°C rise in temperature will be

$$= \frac{3 \times 2.0988}{2.710}$$

= 2.323 min.

T_o = 4 (time in minutes at temperature To)

T_n = 13 (time in minutes at temperature Tn)

T_a = 4 + 2.323 = 6.323 (time in min.)

$T_a - T_o$ = 6.323 - 4.000 = 2.323

$T_n - T_a$ = 13.000 - 6.323 = 6.677

$V' (T_a - T_o)$ = 0.0075 (2.323)

$V'' (T_n - T_a)$ = 0.075 (6.677)

Cooling Correction

= V' (Ta - To) +V'' (Tn - Ta)

= 0.0174225 + 0.00500775

= 0.0224

Un-corrected temperature = 1.648°C

Corrected temperature = 1.6704°C

Heat energy-1.6704 × 2524.22 = 4216.457 kcal

1. Nitrogen correction = 1.43 × 2.9 = 4.147 kcal
2. Wire correction = 0.335 × 0 = 0 kcal
3. Thread correction = 4.180 × 7 = 29.260 kcal

Total = 33.407 kcal

Net-heat energy production
= Heat energy - total of nitrogen, wire and thread correction
= 4216.457 - 33.407 kcal = 4183.050 kcal

If 0.842g sample have gross energy = 4183.05 kcal

Then 1 g sample will have gross energy $\frac{4183.05 \times 1}{0.842}$ = 4967.99 kcal

Result : The given sample of hominy feed contained 4.96799 Mcal/kg gross energy.

Estimation of Energy Equivalent Factor for Istothermal Bomb Calorimeter

Definition: The water equivalent is the weight of water which is equivalent in effective heat capacity to the entire system (calorimeter vessel containing a specified weight of water, calorimeter bomb charged with oxygen, fuel and water, thermometer and stirrer).

Standardization Procedure: Use a standard benzoic acid pellet weighing neither less then 0.9 nor more than 1.1g. Determine the corrected temperature rise t from the observed test data, also titrate the bomb washings to determine the nitric acid correction and measure the unburned fuse wire.

Compute the energy equivalent using the following equation

$$W = \frac{Hm - e_1 + e_3}{t} \text{kcal}/^{\circ}\text{C}$$

Where,

W = energy equivalent of calorimeter in kilo calories per degrees centigrade.

H = heat of combustion of standard benzoic acid in cal/g.

m = mass of standard benzoic acid sample in g.

t = corrected temperature rise in degree C.

e_1 = correction for heat of formation of nitiric acid in kilo calories.

e_2 = correction for heat of combustion of firing wire in kilo calories.

Example

Standardization with 0.955 g benzoic acid sample (6.319 kcal/g) produced a net corrected temperature rise of 2.609°C. The acid titration required 2.8 ml of 0.1 N standard alkali and 7.5 cm (18.4 mg) of nichrome wire and 8 cm (5 mg) of cotton thread during combustion.

Substituting the values in the Equation:

H = 6.319 kcal /g

m = 0.955 g

e_1 = (2.8m) (1.43 kcal/ml) = 4.0 kcal

e_2 = (18.4mg) (0.335 kcal/mg)+ (5mg) (4.180 kcal/mg)

= 6.2 + 20.9 = 27.1 kcal

t = 2.609°C

$$W = \frac{(6.319)(0.955) + 4 + 27.1}{2.609}$$

= 2325 kcal/°C is energy equivalent of calorimeter

Operation of Adiabatic Bomb Calorimeter

The most interesting point in this device is that there is no temperature differential between the inner vessel and the water in the outer vessel, so that the observed temperature rise of the inner vessel is also the "true" temperature rise. There is no need of cooling correction and only two temperatures viz., need prior and after burning sample be noted down.

The world famous Gallenkamp Co. have started manufacturing adiabatic automatic bomb calorimeter. The basic requirement is for an automatic device to raise the temperature of the water in the outer jacket (which in the isothermal system is assumed to remain at constant temperature) at exactly the same rate as the water in the inner vessel is heated by combustion of the sample in the bomb.

Actual Procedure

A known weight of sample is placed in the dish. This is placed inside the bomb with the ignition wire fitted, the bomb sealed and then charged with oxygen at 25 atmosphere pressure. The bomb is then immersed in the water in the inner vessel (a fixed weight of water is used), the electric firing leads are attached and the adiabatic lid is fitted. There are four holes in this lid through which pass the stirring mechanism, thermometer (in the present model two thermometers are used, graduated to 0.01°C and read to 0.002°C giving a total temperature range of 15°-24°C) and one thermistor element. The water in the outer vessel, in which the second thermistor is located, is cooled slightly by adding tap water. As soon as the temperature in the inner vessel becomes effectively constant adiabatic control is switched on which rapidly raises the temperature of the water in the outer vessel and lid to that of the inner vessel. The temperature of the latter is then recorded (it should be changing by less than 0.002°C per minute at this stage) and the sample ignited electrically. After a time-lag of 30s the temperature of the water in the inner vessel begins to rise, and almost immediately the control starts heating the water in the outer vessel, switching itself off and on as the temperature of this water tends to rise above, and then lag behind that in the inner vessel. Maximum temperature is reached in 13 min. with this equipment. The temperatures are recorded after 13 and 14 min. and should agree to within 0.02°C. The control is then switched off and the bomb removed, emptied and recharged with another sample for a further determination. The water in the inner vessel is only charged after 3-4 determinations, as the equipment can safely be used well above ambient temperature/however, the inner vessel must always be weighed and any loss of weight resulting from removal of water adhering to the bomb made good before each fresh determination.

During the "chief period" of the determination the operator is free to carry out the preparation and weighing of other sample; alternatively, if large number of determinations have to be made, one operator can readily supervise two calorimeters at the same time.

Causes of Poor Combustion

(a) *Excessive, rapid admission of gas to the bomb during changing, causing part of the sample to be blown out of the cup.*

(b) *Loose or powdery condition of the sample in the cup.*

(c) *The use of a sample containing coarse particles.*

(d) *Use of an ignition current too low to ignite the charge or too high, causing the fuse to break before combustion is well under way.*

(e) *Insertion of the fuse wire loop below the surface of a loose sample. Best results are obtained by barely touching the surface of the sample or even hanging the wire slightly above the surface.*

(f) *Use of not enough oxygen to burn the charge completely or conversely, the use of a very high initial gas pressure which may retard development of the required turbulence during combustion.*

Example

Objective

Estimation of gross energy (GE) of silage (predried) by adiabatic bomb calorimeter

Observations		Sample I	Sample II
1.	Wt of crucible+sample+cotton and primer	6.3941 g	8.8558 g
2.	Wt of crucible	5.5514 g	7.9325 g
3.	Wt of sample+cotton or primer	0.8427 g	0.9233 g
4.	Wt of cotton or primer	0.0070 g	0.0070 g
5.	Final temperature	20.742°C	21.188°C
6.	Initial temperature	19.218°C	19.522°C
7.	Uncorrected temp. rise	1.524°C	1.666°C
8.	Thermometer correction	-°C	-°C
9.	Corrected temp. rise	-°C	-°C
10.	Total heat capacity	2470 kcal	–
11.	Total heat release	3764 kcal	4115 kcal
12.	Heat from cotton	34 kcal	34 kcal
13.	Heat from chromium	3 kcal	3 kcal
14.	Constant heat gain	37 kcal	37 kcal
15.	Primer heat gain	O kcal	O kcal
16.	Corrected heat gain (sample)	3727 kcal	4078 kcal
17.	GE from 1 g sample	4460 kcal	4451 kcal

Source : Krishna G. (1973) Lic. Agric. Ph.D. Thesis, Agricultural University of Norway, Ås-NLH, Norway

Operation of Ballistic Bomb Calorimeter (Gallenkamp)

Procedure

Weigh about one g of any biological sample in bomb crucible and place it on the support pillar in the base of the bomb, take 5.08cm length of sewing cotton, insert one end of the cotton between the coils of the firing wire and dip the other end into the centre of the sample in the crucible. A standard length of cotton should be used for each test so that sealing ring is in position in its groove, lower the bomb body on to the locking ring and turn the body until its thread engages that in the ring. Turn the locking ring until it clamps the bomb body to the base. Hand tightening is quite adequate to compress the sealing ring completely into its groove and seal the bomb. Plug the thermocouple into the hold in the top of the bomb body.

For routine tests, assuming that the valve of the oxygen cylinder is open, close the pressure release valve on the bomb and open the valve on the front panel of the control box about 1/4 turn. Allow the pressure to rise to 25 atm. in about 20 seconds and then close the valve. This pressure has been found adequate to ensure the complete combustion of the recommended amount of sample material.

By means of the "Galvo Zero" knob on the control box bring the light spot index of the galvanometer to zero and leave for about 30 seconds to check that the temperature is stable, that is, that the zero does not drift. Press and release the firing button. The button starts turning clockwise showing the timer is working and after about 10 to 15 s increasing deflections on the pressure gauge and then the galvanometer showing that the firing has been successful. Note the maximum deflection of the galvanometer.

Immediately after the maximum deflection has been recorded, the gases can be released from the bomb through the pressure release valve at the right of the base of the bomb. Remove the body of the bomb and fill it with cold water, rinsing out two or three times place the next sample in position, then dry the bomb body taking special care that the thermocouple hole is dry.

Calibration of Ballistic Bomb Calorimeter Using Standard Benzoic Acid

The purpose of this calibration is to establish the relationship between the galvanometer deflection and the amount of heat released by the combustion of the sample. Thermochemical grade benzoic acid is the recommended standard material but any other pure material of known calorific value can be used. *In any case sufficient material should be taken to give a heat release of 4 kcal with benzoic acid, calorific value 6.32 kcal per gram, about 0.7 gram is required.*

Calculation

For simplicity only one standardizing test is considered, in practice the calibration constant Y would be the mean of at least 6 standardizing tests.

Galvanometer deflection with benzoic acid = Q_1

Galvanometer deflection with no sample = Q_2

Galvanometer deflection due to benzoic acid = $Q_1 - Q_2$

GE release from Wgram of benzoic acid = $6.32 \times W$ kcal (Gross energy)

Calibration constant 6.32 WZ $(Q_1 - Q_2)$ = ZY kcal/scale division.

Galvanometer deflection with test sample = Q_3

Galvanometer deflection with no sample = Q_2

Galvanometer deflection with test sample = $Q_3 - Q_2$

GE release from Z (gram) of test sample = $(Q_3 - Q_2)$ Y kcal

GE of test sample = $(Q_3 - Q_2)$ Y/Z kcal/g

☞ **Note**

This fact is based on the comparative study conducted by the author of this compendium it is found that among all the existing calorimetry systems, only Isothermal system gives more accurate result of analysis.

Some Manufacturers of Different Bomb Calorimeters

1. **Isothermal Type Bomb Calorimeter**
   (i) Toshniwal Brothers (P) Ltd, New Delhi (India)
   (ii) Parr instrument Compnay, 211 Fifty-third Street, Moline, Illinois (USA).

2. **Adiabatic Type Bomb Calorimeter**
   (i) Gallenkamp Co., USA.
   (ii) Parr Instrument Company, 211 Fifty-third Street, Moline, Illinois (USA).

3. **Ballistic Bomb Calorimeter**
   Gallenkamp Co., USA

Processing of Biological samples for Burning in Bomb Calorimeter.

1. Faecal Sample

It is necessary to burn the solid samples in an oxygen bomb. They should be air-dry and and ground until all particles will pass a 70 mesh sieve. It has been experienced that heat-drying of faeces may lead to considerable lossses of energy. However, low temperature drying of faeces, while it may reduce losses of volatile constituents, may lead to other losses resulting from bacterial activity. *Some laboratories adopt vacuum drying technique, where crucible* and *contents are placed in a vaccum desiccator over silica gel in a refrigerator at 5°C. Most samples of faeces are dry enough to ignite after 24 h drying. Freeze drying of faeces sample may also be adopted.*

It is always advisable to prepare Pellets of 1.1-1.2 g because excessive rapid admission of gas to the bomb during charging, causes part of the sample to be blown out of the cup. It has been observed that loose or powdery condition of the sampe in the cup prior to ignition causes ejection due to violence of combustion.

2. Herbage and Feed Samples

With adequate care herbage should lose a negligible proportion of its dry matter content during oven drying . About 1.2-1.4 g of sample, giving a gross-energy of approximately 6000 kcal/kg dry matter similar to that released from the benzoic acid used for calibrating the calorimeter, is then pelleted and weighed immediately. At the same time a second sample is taken and oven dried at 100°C to estimate the moisture content of the pelletd sample. This method of determining the amount of dry matter in the pellet has been adopted because (a) during pelleting of ovendried sample, appreciable amounts of moisture may be absorbed. and (b) a pellet made from milled grass equilibrated in air tends to break up it is subsequently ovendried to determine its dry matter content.

3. Silage

Volatile constituents are lost when silage is oven-dried, resulting in under estimation of the dry matter and energy contents of fresh silage. About 5g fresh silage sample is taken in capsule and approximately 1 g benzoic acid is added, sample is combusted inside the bomb following the usual procedure. Because the energy content of the silage is found by difference, precision is lower than with dried samples, but this is fully justified because of the inevitable losses of volatiles occurring when silage is oven-dried. *In the place of benzoic acid, other such primer such as dimethyl formamide or butyl cellosolve may also be used.*

4. Milk Samples

About 10 g milk sample is taken in capsule, simultaneously same amount of milk is taken in another silica crucible for dry matter estimation. Both the samples are dried in vacuum drying oven over silica gel at about 20°C and a vacuum of about 15 mm Hg pressure. Dried sample is combusted inside the bomb according to usual procedure. Nitrogen is estimated simultaneously in both samples (taking same amount as taken for bomb calorimetry). Standard factors may be used to correct for the calorific value of volatile nitrogen.

5. Minced Meat Sample

About 2g of minced meat sample is weighed in capsule and combusted directly without drying and adding primer.

6. Urine Sample

When urine is dried in the capsule as such it forms a sticky layer on the base which will not ignite in the bomb. *Another method is that a weighed quantity of acidified urine is evaporated to dryness on a dried and weighted cylindrical piece of cellulose. After this drying, which is best done at room temperature in vacuo, the piece of cellulose with urine-residue is placed in the bomb to measure the calorific value. For a complete oxidation of the urine-residue about two-third of the energy must be produced by the cellulose and about one-third by the urine residue.*

Defect in Cellulose Method

1. *Determination of the combustion value of urine is based upon a difference-determination with an unfavourable ratio of cellulose/urine.*
2. *Method with cellulose is very laborious, the cellulose pieces must be dried to constant weight, urine must be added gradually to the cellulose.*
3. *Burning with cellulose is not complete.*

Use of Polyethylene foil (pep) for Burning Urine

Netherland worker (Nijkamp, 1965) developed a new technique using polyethlylene-foil. Polyethylene-foil (Pef.) can be used as a container for the evaporation of the urine. Polyethylene, having a very high heat of combustion undoubtedly causes a higher burning temperature than cellulose. Confirmation of this assumption can be found in the fact that during a determination with cellulose, less nitric acid is formed (0.2-0.3 mg equivalent) than during a determination with polyethylene-foil (approximately 0.5 mg equivalent).

Polyethylene burns so fiercely, that it strongly promotes the complete oxidation of the urine-residue. To bring about a complete burning of the urine-residue, it is enough that one-third of the energy is produced by the Pef. and two-third by the urine.

Actual Procedure of Using Polyethylene Foil

According to standardized method (Nijkamp, 1965) so much material is burnt in the bomb that about 5000 kcal are formed. For the determination of the combustion value of the urine this means that about 1.7 kcal must be produced by Pef. *The heat value of Pef. being about 11 kcal/g, this means that about 155 mg of Pef. must be used. This should be 0.015 mm thick. 120 cm^2, as this foill generally weighs between 140 and 170 mg.*

Procedure 1

About 20 g urine sample is weighed in a Pef-tube and dried in vacuum desiccator over dilute sulphuric acid for 48 h at room temperature. Polyethylene-foil tube as described, is placed in a 25 ml beaker in such a way that the middle part of the tube lies on the bottom and both open ends are upwards. Volatile nitrogen absorbed in dilute sulphuric acid is actually estimated by Kjeldahl method mentioned in this compendium.

Following published factors are used to calculate calorific value of volatile nitrogen and added to the calorific value of urine estimated by bomb calorimeter.

1. *In non-ruminants except poultry. 5.4 kcal/g urinary nitrogen. This factor corresponds to a heat of combustion value of urea of about 2.54 kcal/g. Some of the recent handbooks erroneously list the heat of combustion value of urea as 2.14 kcal*
2. *In poultry, 8.22 kcal/g nitrogen.*
3. *In ruminant 7.45 kcal/g nitrogen.*

National Institute of Animal Physiology, Copenhagen, Denmark, follows aforesaid procedure to estimate actual calorific value of urine. It has been experienced that results are underestimated by about 30 percent if calorific value of volatile nitrogen is not included in this procedure.

Procedure 2

About 20g urine sample is weighed in a Pef-tube and dried in vacuum drying oven at a temperature of about 20°C and a vacuum of about 18 mm Hg pressure, over silica gel. The samples are taken in duplicate simultaneously and dried sample is combusted in bomb calorimeter and other sample is processed for the estimation of nitrogen by Kjeldahl method. The nitrogen should also be estimated in the same quantity of fresh urine, by deduction, loss of volatile nitrogen may be calculated. The standard factors mentioned in procedure 1 should be applied to calculate the calorific value of volatile nitrogen.

These polyethylene foil or tube/or bags may be obtained from M/s British Visqueen Ltd, Six Hills Way, Stevenage, Herts, and M/s Walter Coles and Co. Ltd. London. S.E. 17.

☞ Notes

1. *The vacuum must be introduced not too swiftly, since the acidified urine contain much dissolved carbon dioxide.*

2. *If a larger quantity of urine is used (for urine with low specific gravity a second portion of urine can be weighed in the same tube after evaporation of the first portion).*

Whether Acidification of Urine is Necessary before Drying and Combustion

Netherland worker, Nijkamp (1965) concluded that the results for combustion value and carbon-determination in the alkaline urine were considerably lower than those in the acidified urine. It is most probable that observed losses occur during the evaporation of the alkaline urine to dryness. He observed that the evaporation to dryness of alkaline urine causedconsiderable determination of the heat of combustion, it is necessary to use acidified urine. Later on a problem was felt with HCI also, since it gives too high results. Probably the excess HCI is oxidized in the bomb to chloride, according to the exothermic reaction, $4Cl+O_2 \rightarrow 2H_2O+2Cl_2$. The chloride formed in this way will then react with some heat production with the metallic wall of the bomb, this wall thus being attacked severely. *He tried sulphuric acid to acidify urine in various concentrations and concluded that addition of 0.2 ml sulphuric acid (1:1) to about 18 g urine is sufficient for the complete combustion of urine.*

However, urine sample meant for carbon estimation should be preserved with sodium fluoride it is not good to add acid in the urine sample dried, specially for the estimation of carbon. because carbon in the chemically bound CO_2 is removed by the acidification.

Carbon Estimation in Biological Sample

Carbon content of the urine can be determined reliably in connection with a calorimetric determination. In that case the content of the bomb is passed through a suitable set of absorption tubes. It proved to be sufficient to use only four tubes, Tube 1 contains drierite dried for at least 8 at 200°C tube 2 contains calcium chloride also dried for at least at 200°C; tubes 3 and 4 contain a sodium hydroxide mixture, which can be prepared in the following way; in wide necked bottle 7 ml of water are added to 80 g of soda lime. This wet soda lime then is added to 350 g of sodium hydroxide flakes, which are crushed somewhat finer for a very short while in a morter. All these are mixed carefully in a closed bottle. The filling of tubes 3 and 4 demands some experience since a U-tube with the NaOH mixture easily becomes stopped up during the analysis. Measures to prevent this blocking are: (a) filling the U-tubes loosely, (b) tapping lightly the filled U-tubes in a horizontal position so that there is some separation between the coarse and fine particles, (c) placing a thin roll (diam, about 0.3-0.4 cm) of metal gauze in the U-tube over the total length. Instead of the NaOH mixture the much more expensive soda asbestos can be used. Soda asbestos as well as the NaOH mixture becomes easily blocked. The gas stream from the bomb can be led through this absorption system at a high rate. namely about 0.3 l/min. so that emptying and washing the bomb tubes takes 40 min. only.

It has been experienced that the results for combustion value and carbon determination in the alkaline urine are considerably lower than those in the acidified urine. Thus, for the determination of the heat of combustion and carbon content it is necessary to use acidified urine.

Reference

Krishna, G. and Ranjhan, S.K. (1975). Calorific value of Indian feeds for Swine and Poultry. *Indian J. Nutr. & Dietetics.* 12: 148-150.

Krishna, G. (1975). A view to the calorific value of Indian feeds of poultry. *Indian Poultry Review* 6 : 453-454.

Krishna, G. and Ranjhan, S.K. (1977). Calorific value of Indian feeds and fodders for Cattle. *Indian J. Anim. Sci.* 47: 299-363.

Krishna, G. and Ranjhan, S.K. (1977). Calorific value of Indian feeds and fodders for sheep. *Indian J. Anim. Sci.* 47: 283-285.

Krishna, G. Razdan, M.N. and Ray, S.N. (1973). "Dairy Search" formula for the estimation of calorific value of milk in *Bos Indicus* in the tropical/subtropical region. *International Research Communication.* 73-11: 32-49-4.

Krishna, G. Razdan, M.N. and Ray, S.N. (1977). Studies on energy and protein requirements of Zebu (*Bos Indicus*) *Z. Tierphysiologie and Tierernährung und Futtermittelkde.* 38: 281-284.

Krishna, G. (1985b). Major mineral components and calorific value of Agro-Industrial by products and tropical wastes. *Agricultural Wastes,* 13: 149-154.

Nijkamp, H.J. (1965). *"Some remarks about the determination of the heat of combustion and the carbon content of urine"* fide EAAP, publication No. 11, Editor, Blaxter, K.L., Academic Press, London, New York , pp 147-57.

Chapter - 9

Ether Extract and Crude Fiber in Feeds and Fodders

Apparatus and Reagents

1. *Soxhlet extraction asembly. This consists of 3 parts (a) condenser at the top, (b) the soxhlet or extractor in the middle, and (c) the receiver flask at the bottom. The 3 parts are assembled by means of their grounds glass interchangeable joints (Fig. 1).*
2. *Extraction thimble.*
3. *Petroleum ether (B.P. 40°C to 60°C)*
4. *Constant temperatue bath or six heater hot plate with temperature controlling device.*

Procedure

Preparataion of Thimble

Take about 8×8 cm piece of Whatman filter paper No.1 and wrap it around wooden stick (2 cm) diameter, tie it with thread so the thimble may not be opened easily during extraction.

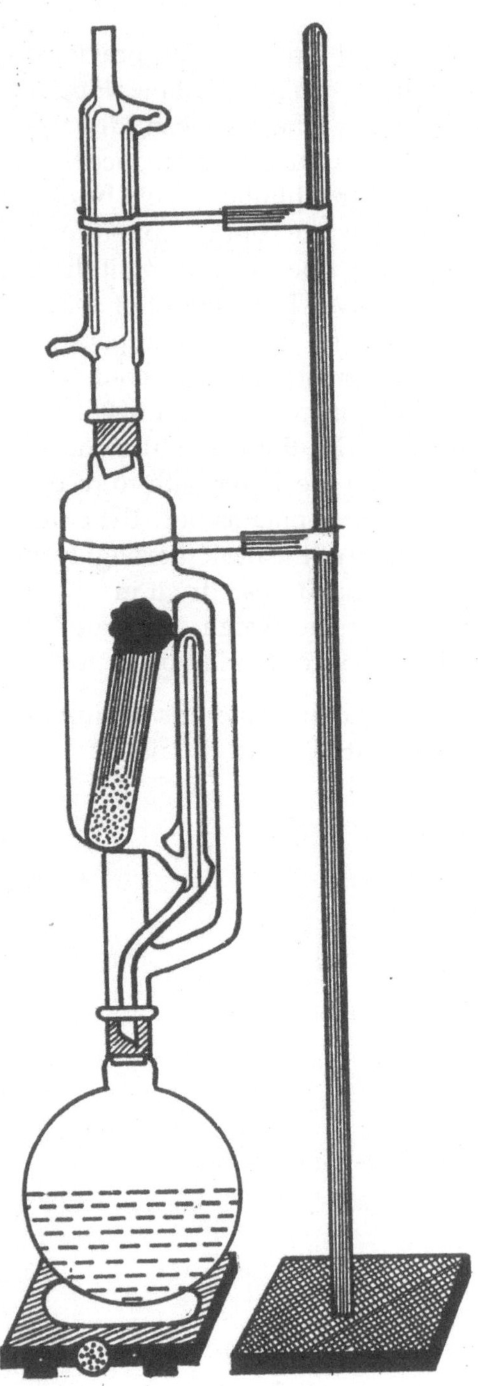

Fig. 1 : Soxhlet extraction assembly for estimation of ether extract

Actual Method

Weigh about 2-5 g material already dried previously in a moisture cup and transfer it in a previously prepared thimble. Plug the mouth of thimble with fat free absorbant cotton. Take the clean, dry receiver flask from the soxhlet assembly and weigh it accurately. Introduce the thimble with sample into the soxhlet. The height of the thimble should be of such size that highest point of it should remain below the bent of siphon. Assemble the apparatus and fill soxhlet with petroleum ether by pouring it through the condenser at the top by means of glass funnel. The amount of solvent taken is about 1½ times the capacity of the Soxhlet. Place the apparatus on a water bath at 60°C, fix by clamps to retort stand and start cold water circulation in the condenser. Extract for eight hours roughly (about 250 times). After extraction is over, remove the thimble with the material from soxhlet. Assemble the apparatus again and heat it on the water bath to recover all the ether from the receiver flask. The flask now contains only the crude fat. Disconnect the receiver flask, wipe the outside of the flask thoroughly with a clean dry cloth to remove the film of moisture and dust, dry it in a hot air oven at 100°C for one hour, cool in a desiccator and weigh. Preserve the extraction thimble with the material in a desiccator for crude fiber determination.

Reference : IS: 2052, 1979 Indian Standards Institution, (BIS) Specification for Compounded Feeds for Cattle, Third revision.

Calculation

Ether extract

1. *Weight of empty oil flask* = W
2. *Weight of empty oil flask + oil* = W_1
3. *Weight of dried material taken* = M

Ether extract percent $= \dfrac{W_1 - W}{M} \times 100$

Example : Name of sample - Gram chuni

W = 133.020g

W_1 = 133.148 g

M = 1.854 g

$$\textit{Ether extract percent} = \frac{(133.148 - 133.020) \times 100}{1.854} = 6.903 \text{ percent ether extract}$$

$$= 6.903 \text{ g}/100 \text{ g dry matter}$$

☞ **Notes**

1. *Wipe out the external surface of oil flask with toilet paper and weigh the flask atleast three times after warming it in the oven atleast for one hour.*
2. *Never calculate the result of ether extract analysis by observing the difference in the weight of thimble. We could never get the correct result by following this wrong method.*

Determination of Crude Fiber

Crude fiber is determined as that fraction remaining after digestion with standard solutions of sulphuric acid and sodium hydroxide under carefully controlled conditions.

Reagents

1. *2.04 N sulphuric acid or 10 percent sulphuric acid (see Chapter 1)*
2. *2.5 N sodium hydroxide or 10 percent sodium hydroxide (see chapter 1.)*
3. *Ethyl alcohol.*

Apparatus

1. 1 litre capacity spoutless beaker covered with bulb condenser filled with water (Fig. 2)
2. Stick filter (Fig. 3)

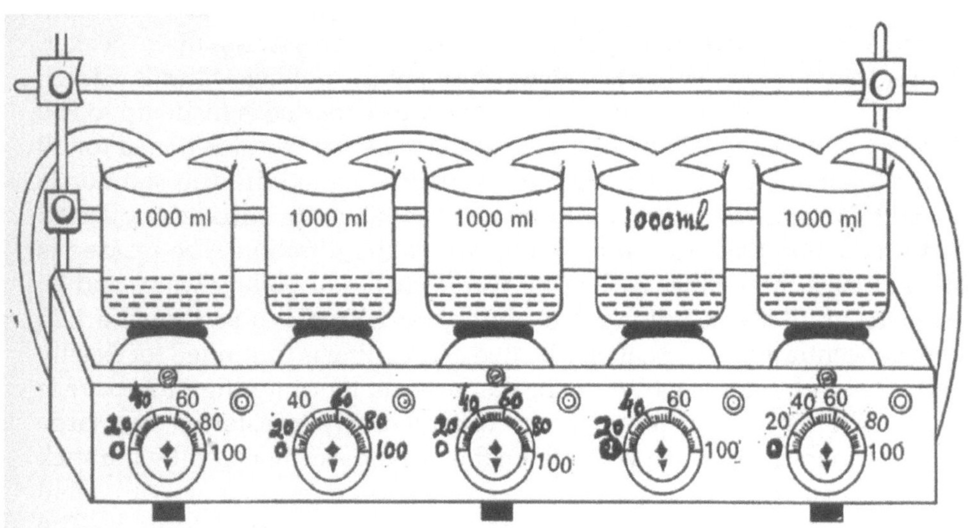

Fig. 2 : Apparatus used for the estimation of crude fiber.

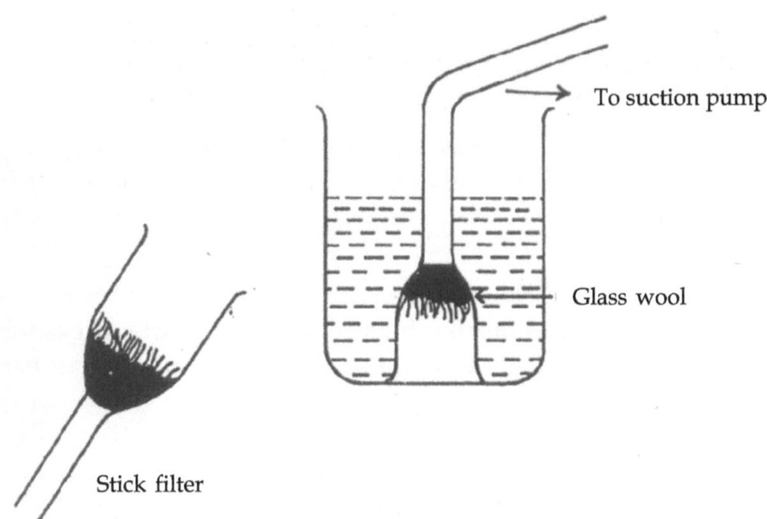

Fig. 3 : Practical demonstration of use of stick filter in filteration job.

The stick filter is a 20 cm long heavy wall glass tubing, inner diameter 0.2-0.3 cm. The 3 cm of one end are widened to give an inner diameter of 0.9 cm. The opening is fitted with glass wool to give the appearance of a small broom, with a 2 cm thick brush.

Procedure

Weigh accurately about two grams of the dried material and extract the fat for about 8 h with petroleum ether using a soxhlet or other suitable extractor. Transfer the fat free material to a one litre capacity spoutless beaker. Two hundred ml level is marked with glass pencil. Boiling water is added, then 25 ml, 10 percent sulphuric acid is mixed and volume is made up to 200 ml level so as to make 1.25 percent concentration. This liquid is boiled for 30 min. as shown in Fig. 9.2. At the end of the boiling period the acid solution is removed by means of suction, through the stick filter. The filtrate is collected in a clean suction flask to control efficiency of the filtration. The residue is washed at least three times by boiling water, then add boiling water and 25 ml 10 percent alkali and dilute it to the mark (200 ml) so as to make 1.25 percent concentration. The beaker is heated and boiling is continued for exactly 30 min. The stick filter is left in the beaker and another filtering procedure is repeated. The resulting residue is then quantitatively transferred to a large porcelain crucible. The wash water from the beaker is drained off by the stick filter. Finally the fiber cake is extracted and dried by moistening with small portions of ethanol, which are permitted to drain between additions. The glass wool is then removed from the stick by means of forcep, and is left with the residue inthe crucible. Material sticking with the glass tube are gently brushed down into the crucible.

Dry the crucible alongwith material and glasswool at 100°C to constant weight cool and weigh. Incinerate the contents of the crucible at 600°C ± 20°C for two hours in a muffle furance untill all the carbonaceous matter is burnt. Cool the crucible containing the ash in desiccator and weigh.

Reference : IS: 2052 1979, Indian Standards Institution, BIS Specification for Compounded Feeds for Cattle, Third revision.

Calculation

Crude fiber (on moisture free basis) percent by weight.

$$= \frac{100(W_1 - W_2)}{W}$$

Where,

W_1 = Weight in gram of procelain crucible and contents before ashing.

W_2 = Weight in gram of porcelain crucible containing glass-wool and ash.

W = Weight in gram of the dried material taken for the test.

Example

Name of sample - Dried faeces of sheep

W_1 = 26.524 g

W_2 = 25.760 g

W = 1.852 g

$$= \frac{100(26.524 - 25.760)}{1.852}$$

= 40.712 percent crude fiber

= 40.712 g/100 g dry matter

References

Paliwal, V.K., Yadav, K.R. and Krishna, G. (1981). Note on proximate nutrient composition of Agro - Industrial by products of Haryana State, *Indian J. Anim. Sci.*, 51 : 1173-76.

Chapter - 10

Nitrogen and Crude Protein in Feeds and Fodders

Crude Protein Estimation

Principle

The nitrogen of protein and other compounds is transformed into ammonium sulphate by acid digestion with boiling sulphuric acid. the acid digest is cooled, dilute with water, and made strongly basic with sodium hydroxide. The released ammonia is distilled into a boric acid solution or standard sulphuric acid solution. When boric acid is used to collect ammonia then is the titrated with standard sulphuric acid or standard hydrochloric acid. When standard sulphuric acid is used to collect ammonia then it is titrated with standard sodium hydroxide solution.

Equipments

1. *Macro-Kjeldahl nitrogen digestion and distillation apparatus*
2. *Kjeldahl flask (650 ml.)*
3. *Erlenmeyer flask (500 ml.)*
4. *Two burettes*

Reagents (For Acid/Alkali) Titration Method

1. *Potassium sulphate or Anhydrous sodium sulphate*
2. *Copper sulphate*

3. *Concentrated sulphuric acid sp. gr. 1.84*
4. *Sodium hydroxide solution -Dissolve about 450 g of sodium hydroxide in 1000 ml of water*
5. *Standard sulphuric acid = 0.5 N*
6. *Standard sodium hydroxide solution = 0.25 N*
7. *Methyl Red indicator solution : Dissolve 1 g of methyl Red in 200 ml of rectified spirit, 90 percent by volume.*

Procedure

Transfer carefully about 2 g of the prepared sample, accurately weighed, to the kjeldahl flask. Add about 10 g of potassium sulphate or anhydrous sodium sulphate about 0.5 g of copper sulphate and 25 ml or more, if necessary, of concentrated sulphuric acid. Place the flask in an inclined position, and heat below the boiling point of the acid until frothing ceases. Increase heat until acid boils vigorously, and digest for a time after the mixture is clear or until oxidation is complete (about two hours). Cool the contents of the flask. Transfer quantitatively to the round-bottom flask with water, the total quantity of water used being about 200 ml. Add a few pieces of pumic stone to prevent bumping . Add carefully the sodium hydroxide solution in quantity which is sufficient to make the solution alkaline by the side of the flask so that it does not mix at once with the acid solution but forms a layer below the acid layer. Assemble the apparatus taking care that the tip of the dip tube extends below the surface of the standard sulphuric acid solution in the receiver (Fig. 1). Mix the contents of the flask by shaking and distill until all the ammonia has passed over into the standard sulphuric acid solution. Titrate with the standard sodium hydroxide solution.

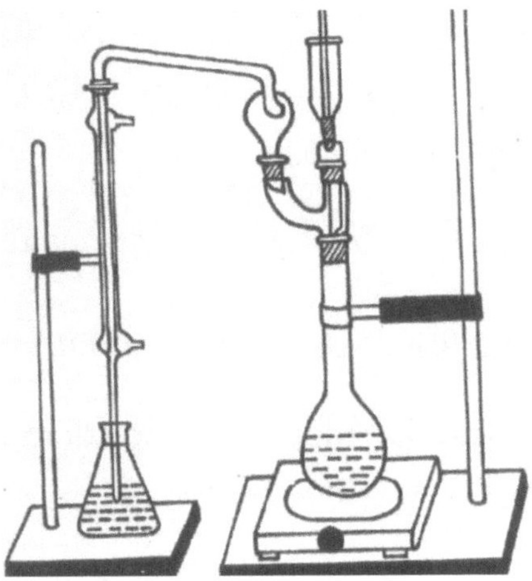

Fig. 1 : Macro-Kjeldahl distillation apparatus for distilling nitrogen

Carry out a blank detrmination using all reagents in the same quantities but without the material to be tested.

Calculation

Total nitrogen, percent by weight (on moisture-free basis)

$$= \frac{0.014(B-A)N \times 100}{W(100-M)/100} g/100g$$

Where,

B = Volume in ml of the standard sodium hydroxide solution used to neutralize the acid in blank determination.

A = Volume in ml of the standard sodium hydroxide solution used to neutralize the excess acid in the test with the material

N = Normality of the standard sodium hydroxide solution

M = Moisture percentage

W = Weight in grams of the material taken for the test.

Example: **Name of sample** - *Undecorticated cottonseed cake*

B = 9.8 ml

A = 3.8 ml

N = 0.25 N

W = 0.5 gram

M = 5 percent

Nitrogen percent $= \frac{0.014(9.8-3.8)0.25 \times 100}{0.5(100-5)/100}$

= 4.42g/100g dry matter

Crude protein percent = $N \times 6.25$

= 4.42×6.25

= 27.62 g/100g dry matter

☞ **Note**

We can use 0.5 N hydrochloric acid in the place of 0.5 N sulphuric acid.

Reagents for Boric Acid Titration Method Using Micro-Kjeldahl Distillation Assembly

Boric Acid Indicator

Put 20 g of the purest boric acid into a one litre flask and add 200 ml alcohol and about 700 ml distilled water. The boric acid is brought into solution by shaking

and 10 ml of mixed indicator is added. On mixing, the whole contentis brought to the desired end point of faint reddish colour which usually requires the addition of little N/10 HCI and then the mixture is made up to the mark. This solution should be kept in ammonia free atomsphere. Try to prepare fresh solution every week. Remove small amount of boric acid solution in a separate bottle and cork the bottle tightly after taking out the solution.

Reagents

1. *Mixed Indicator : This contains Bromocresol green 0.033 percent and Methyl Red 0.066 percent in alcohol. It keeps indefinitely.*
2. *N/100 Hydrochloric acid or N/100 sulphuric acid.*

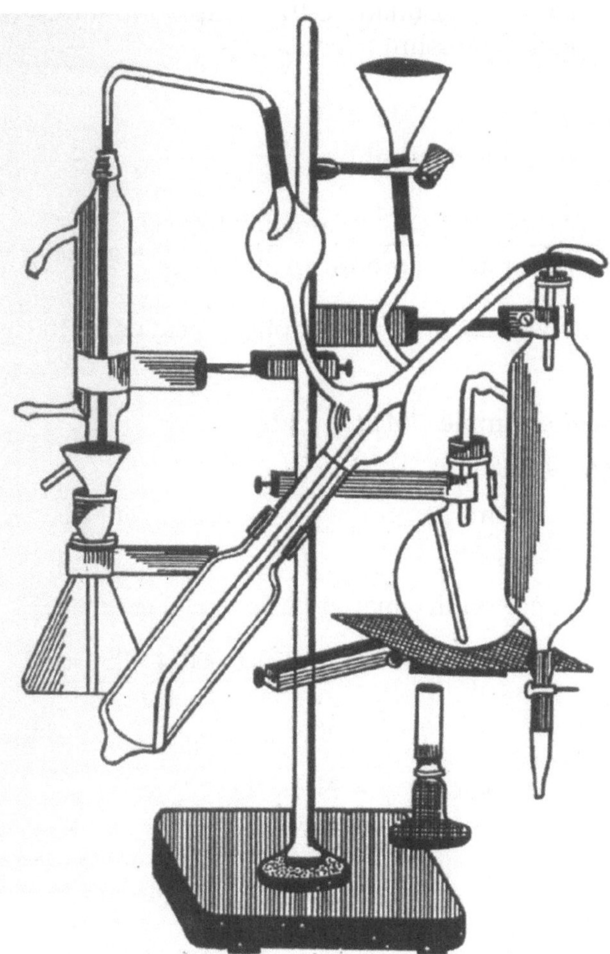

Fig. 2 : Micro-Kjeldahl distillation apparatus for distilling nitrogen.

Procedure

Any biological material is digested as mentioned in the previous method. The digested material is made up to a volume of 100 ml in a volumetric flask. Five ml aliquot is taken in the receiver of distillation apparatus. (Figure 10.2) about 10 ml of 45 percent solution of sodium hydroxide is added till the blue colour is formed. Released ammonia is collected in 10 ml 2 percent boric acid solution. Faint reddish colour of boric acid starts changing to green colour since the released ammonia is absorbed by boric acid solution. Released ammonia is allowed to distill till the original volume of 10 ml of boric acid becomes 30 ml. Green coloured boric acid solution is back titrated with N/100 sulphuric acid or N/100 hydrochloric acid using microburette, used volume of this standard solution is noted down.

After the completion of distillation, the sample in the receiver is taken out by creating a negative pressure of cooling.

Calculation

Total nitrogen, percent by weight

$$= \frac{\text{Titre value (A)} \times 0.00014 \times \text{Volume made} \times 100}{\text{Aliquot taken} \times \text{Wt of substance on dry matter basis}} = \text{g}/100\text{ g}$$

Titre value (A) = Volume of N/100 sulphuric acid or N/100 hydrochloric acid used.

Example : Name of sample - *Malt sprout*

1. Titre value (A) = 21.85 ml
2. Volume made = 250 ml
3. Aliquot taken = 5 ml
4. Weight of substance on dry matter basis = 4.50 g

Total Nitrogen percent $= \dfrac{21.85 \times 0.00014 \times 250 \times 100}{5 \times 4.50}$

$= 3.39$ g/100g

Total crude protein percent $= \text{N} \times 6.25$

$= 3.39 \times 6.25$

$= 21.187$g/100g

☞ Notes

1. *In nitrogen estimation, ammonia free distilled water should be used, if traces of ammonia are present then distill blank water and find out concentration*

of traces of ammonia by titration of distillate with N/100 Hcl and deduct this concentration of ammonia from sample reading of N/100 Hcl used in titration.

2. *Distill N/10 Ammonium thiocyanate with every set to know the recovery of Ammonia as usual done with sample tested. Five ml of N/10 Ammonium thiocyanate should be equal to five ml of N/10 Hcl if ammonia recovery is 100 percent.*

Biuret Method for Protein Content in Wheat

(Method of Johnson, R. M. and W.T. Greenway, 1971)

A rapid biuret method for protein content in grain was reported in the March, 1971 issue of Agricultural Research USA. This method rquires 35 min. to complete an anaylsis.

This test consists of combining 1 g of finely-ground grain , 1 g powdered cupric carbonate with 100 ml of alkaline-alcohol solution, heating and stirring to 60°C, stirring for an additional 2 min. at room temperature, filtering and reading percent transmittance at 550 nm.

Reagents

1. *Alkaline-alcohol solution- Place 5.61 g potassium hydroxide pellets in 1000 ml volumetric flask, add 600 ml isopropyl alcohol, and make up to volume with distilled water.*
2. *Cupric carbonate (reagent grade)*

Apparatus

(i) Udy clone mill-with 0.024′ screen or equivalent

(ii) Balance (accurate to within 0.01 g).

(iii) Hot plate magnetic stirrer combination.

(iv) Magnetic stirrer

(v) Vacuum filter assembly (No. 2A Buchner funnel with 9 cm glass fiber filter).

(vi) Colorimeter (any photoelectric colorimeter set at 550 nm may be used).

(vii) Automatic pipette, 100 ml.

Procedure

1. Grind 30 g representative sample in udy mill
2. Weigh 1.00 ± 0.01 g of the blended finely ground grain into 250 ml Erlenmeyer flask.

3. Add 2 ml of isopropyl alcohol and swirl.
4. Pipette 100 ml of alkaline-alcohol solution into flask (0.1 N KOH, 60 pecent IPA).
5. Add 1.00 ± 0.01 g of powdered cupric carbonate. Stopper with 2-hole stopper containing a thermometer.
6. Heat to 60°C on combination hot plate magnetic stirrer.
7. Stir on magnetic stirrer at room temperature for two minutes.
8. Prepare Buchner funnel for filtering by placing a glass fiber filter in funnel.
9. Filter through glass fiber filter in Buchner funnel and collect about 30 ml of clear filtrate.
10. Read percent trasmittance of the filtrate at 550 mμ in a 5 x 10 mm sample cell and establish a standard curve (conversion chart) by selecting 35 or more samples covering the protein content range to be encountered. Obtain meter readings by the rapid method and by the Kjeldahl method. From the two sets of values calculate the regression equation for the standard curve.

Precautions

1. Since different lots of the same grade of cupric carbonate from a specific manufacturer vary, a new standard curve must be prepared for each lot.
2. The udy Analyzer can be modified by changing the filter to 550 mμ and the sample cell to 0.5 cm path length.
3. As uniformity in results between colorimeter has not been established, each lot should construct a separate standard curve and conversion chart for each instrument.

References

Agarwala, O.N. and Krishna, G. (1988). Evaluation of protein requirement of adult sheep for maintenance. *Indian J. Animal Nutrition.* 5 : 218-221.

Johnson R. M. and W. T. Greenaway, (1971). *Five minute biuret method for protein content in wheat*, Bulletin USDA, ARS, Market Quality Research Division, Beltsville, Maryland 20705.

IS: 2052-1979 *Indian Standards Institution.* (BIS) *Specification for compounded Feeds for Cattle, Third revision.*

Chapter - 11

True Protein in Feeds and Fodders

True Protein Estimation

True protein nitrogen is also termed a *Albuminoid nitrogen* in animal feeds and fodders and human foods. If material (Such as seeds, seed residue or oil cake) is rich in alkaline phosphates, 1-2 ml of 10 percent solution of potash alum is added to decompose them. If this is not done Cu_3 (PO_4) and free alkali may be formed and the protein-copper precipitate may partially dissolve in the alkaline liquid.

Reagents

1. *Saturated solution of potash alum.*
2. *Stutzer's reagent - (Preparation). In a wide mouth stoppered bottle dissolve 40 g of pure copper sulphate into two litres of water. Add 10 ml of glycerine and sufficient quantity of 30 percent sodium hydroxide solution which will give mixture just alkaline reaction to litmus (Dissolve 30g of sodium hydroxide in about 100 ml of water) and add the whole solution to the copper sulphate and shake the bottle thoroughly.*

Allow the precipitates to settle and siphon the supernatant liquid. Pass the precipitate through filter paper into 5 cm diameter funnel and allow to drain. Collect the precipitate with a horn spatula and transfer in into a glass mortar. Rub the precipitate thoroughly with a glass pestle after adding 3 ml of glycerine and a little water. Transfer the whole thing with about 600 ml of water in a wide mouth stoppered bottle, shake well and filter. The process is repeated till the filtrate is free from alkali and sulphate. Finally, collect the precipitate and add 30 ml of glycerol and enough water till the mixed emulsion comes to the level of 320 ml which has previously been marked on the container bottle.

Procedure

Weigh a quantity of sample usually taken for crude protein estimation and transfer it into 250 ml beaker, add 100 ml of boiling water, mix the content thoroughly with a glass rod. Place the beaker with the content in a water bath in such a way that the major portion of the beaker, inserted through the opening of the surface of the plate, is submerged in hot water, leave the beaker thus for half an hour during which stir vigorously, with a glass rod, the contents in the beaker a number of times; remove the beaker from the water bath and add 5 ml of saturated solution of potash alum and 10 ml Stutzer's reagent and stir thoroughly. Allow the mixture to stand for six hours and allow to cool down, filter and wash with cold water several times till it becomes free from sulphate.

Transfer the filter paper with the precipitate into a Kjeldahl's flask and estimate nitrogen content as mentioned in Chapter 10.

Total Non-protein Nitrogen (NPN)

Total NPN in any biological material may be estimated as below:

Total NPN = Total crude protein nitrogen - True protein nitrogen.

Reference

AOAC, (1965). Official methods of analysis of the Association of Official Agricultural Chemists 10th ed. AOAC. Benjamin Franklin Station. Washington, D.C. p. 329.

Krishna, G. and Günther, K.D. (1987). Nutrient Composition and amino acid Content of some Agro-Industrial byproducts and wastes used as livestock feeds. Z. *Landwirtschaftliche Forschung*. 40 : 277-280.

Krishna, G., Paliwal, V.K. and Yadav, K.R. (1980). True protein and non protein fractions in Agro-Industrial Wastes/by products in Haryana State. *Haryana Agricutural Univ. J. Res.* 11 : 458-462.

Chapter - 12

Non-Protein Nitrogen Fractions in Biological Materials

1. Ammonia Nitrogen by Distillation Method

Method I (For Animal Feeds)

Reagents

1. *Mangnesium oxide (carbonate free)*
2. *Standard sodium hydroxide 0.25 N*
3. *Standard sulphuric acid 0.5 N*
4. *Methyl red indicator*

Weigh accurately 2 to 4 g of the prepared sample. Shake it with water and filter. Wash the residue thoroughly with water. Transfer the filtrate to the distillation flask and dilute to about 200 ml with water. Add about 5 g of the magnesium oxide, Connect the flask to the condenser by means of the connecting bulb tube and distill about 100 ml of liquid into the receiver containing standard sulphuric acid and methyl red indicator solution, Titrate the contents of the receiver with the standard sodium hydroxide solution. Carry out a blank determination using all reagents in the same quantities but without the material to be tested.

Ammonical nitrogen, percent by weight (on moisture free basis)

$$= \frac{0.14(b-a)N \times 100}{W(100-M)/100} g/100g$$

where

b = Volume in ml of the standard sodium hydroxide solution used to neutralize the acid in blank determination.

a = Volume in ml of the standard sodium hydroxide solution used to neutralize the excess acid in the test with the material.

N = Normality of the standard sodium hydroxide solution.

W = Weight in gram of the material taken for the test.

M = Moisture percentage.

Method II (For Rumen Liquor)

Approximately 10 ml rumen liquor, accurately weighed, are added to 50 ml of N/6 sulphuric acid in a 100 ml flask and the mixture is transferred to a 500 ml volumetric flask with N/6 sulphuric acid; 50 ml 10 percent sodium tungstate are added and the volume is made up to the mark with N/6 sulphuric acid. After standing for at least 24 h the mixture is filtered and aliquot of the filtrate is taken for analysis.

Various trial experiments showed that the rumen liquor could remain in the 100 ml flask with sulphuric acid for at least two day before it is made up to 500 ml after that any time between 24 and 49 h could lapse before filtration takes place without any measurable change in the analytical results.

Aliquot of the filtrate from the Tungstate precipitation is neutralized with N NaOH using Phenol Red as indicator. Two ml N NaOH are then added in excess and the mixture is distilled for 10-15 min in a current of steam, the distillate being collected in N/50 acid. This procedure gives results identical with those obtained when the acid aliquot is rendered alkaline by addition of solid magnesium oxide.

2. Urea Nitrogen by Distillation Method

Method I (For Animal Feeds)

Reagents

1. *Calcium chloride solution : Dissolve 25 grams* $CaCI_2$ *in 100 ml* H_2O.
2. *Urease solution : Prepare fresh solution by dissolving standardised urease in water so that each 10 ml neutralized solution will convert N of* $\geq$ *0.1 gram pure urea.*

   Standardization : To determine alkalinity of commercial urease preparation, dissolve 0.1g in 50 ml water and titrate with 0.1 N HCI, using Methyl red.

Add same volume 0.1 N HCI to each 0.1g urease in preparing urease solution. To determine enzyme activity, prepare about 50 ml neutralized 1 percent solution. Add different amounts of solution to 0.1 g sample of pure urea and follow with enzyme digestion and distill as in determination. Calculate activity of urease preparation from amount of this urease solution that completley converted urea as determined by complete recovery of nitrogen by distillation.

3. *Defoaming solution. Dissolve 50 g diglycol stearate in 375 ml of benzene, 75 ml of alcohol, and 250 ml of dibutyl phthalate. Warm, if necessary.*
4. *Standard sulphuric acid, 0.5 N or 0.1 N when amount of nitrogen is small.*
5. *Standard sodium hydroxide solution, 0.25 N or 0.1 N*
6. *Methyl red indicator solution. Disslove one gram of methyl red in 200 ml of rectified spirit.*
7. *Magnesium oxide (carbonate free) freshly ignited, heavy type.*

Procedure

Weigh accurately about 2g of the prepared sample in Kjeldahl flask. Shake it with about 250 ml of water. Add 10 ml urease solution, put the stopper tightly and let it stand for one hour at room temperature; or 20 min at 40°C. Cool to room temperature, if necessary. Use more urease solution if feed contains greater than 5 percent urea (approximately equal to 12 percent protein equivalent). Rinse stopper and neck with few ml of water. Add 2g of magnesium oxide (heavy type), 1 ml of calcium chloride solution, and 5 ml of defoaming solution. Connect the flask to the condenser by means of the connecting bulb tube and distill about 100 ml of the liquid into the receiver containing standard sulphuric acid and methyl red indicator solution. Titrate the contents with the standard sodium hydroxide solution. Carry out a blank determination using all reagents in same quantities but without the material to be tested.

Calculation

Total ammoniacal nitrogen (urea and ammoniacal nitrogen), percent by weight (on moisture free basis.)

$$= \frac{0.14(B - A)N \times 100}{W(100 - M)/100} g/100g$$

Where

B = Volume in ml of the standard sodium hydroxide solution used to neutralize the acid in blank determination.

A = Volume in ml of the standard sodium hydroxide solution used to neutralize the excess acid in the test with the material

N = Normality of the standard sodium hydroxide solution.

W = Weight in gram of the material taken for the test.

M = moisture percentage.

Crude protein, percent by weight = 6.25 (X - Y) (on moisture free basis)

Where X = Percent by weight of total nitogen

Y = Percent by weight of ammoniacal nitrogen.

Method II (For Rumen Liquor)

Aliquots of tungstate filtrate are neutralized and in the estimation of ammonia. 10 ml 0.6 percent KH_2PO_4 is added as a buffer, followed by 5 ml of a 30 percent alcohol urease extract. The mixture is incubated at 40-45°C for 20 min. Two ml N NaOH is then added and the mixture is distilled in a current of steam for 10-15 min. The distillate is collected in N/50 acid and back titrated with alkali.

3. Colorimetric Methof for the Determination of Urea in Serum and Urine (Based on Berthelot Reaction)

Method of Berthelot 1959

Principle

The principle on which the urea determination is based, is the liberation under standard conditions of ammonia from urea with the help of the enzyme urease. Urea + $H_2O \xrightarrow{\text{Urease}}$ ammonia + carbon dioxide. According to the principle given by Berthelot (1959), with the help of sodium hypochlorite and phenol in an alkaline medium, the ammonia formed is converted into indophenol.

$$\text{Ammonia + sodium hypochlorite + phenol} \xrightarrow{\text{(Catalyst)}} = \text{indophenol}$$

By introducing the catalyst disodium pentacyanonitrosyl ferrate (disodium nitroprusside). Lubochinsky and Zalta (1954) have modified the reaction, making it more rapidly quantitative.

In alkaline medium the indophenol formed is coloured blue. The intensity of this the colouration is a measure of the quantity of ammonia formed from the urea and can be determined colorimetrically at 630 nm.

The urea concentration of the sample to be examined can be calculated easily from the relatiohship between this optical density and the optical density of urea standard solution determined at the same time.

Peters and Van Slyke (1946) have drawn up a formula giving the correlation between the urea and the rest nitrogen content.

Rest N = 1.07 × Urea N + 10

The conversion of urea N into urea is given by the equation

Urea = 2.14 × Urea N

The method is extremely suitable for routine determinations for manual as well as automated techniques.

Reagents

1. *Liquid phenol, 85 percent*
2. *EDTA buffer, pH 6.5.*

   One gram of EDTA disodium salt dihydrate is dissolved in 90 ml of demineralized water. The pH is adjusted to exactly 6.5 with sodium hydroxide and the volume is diluted with distilled water to 100 ml. This solution is stable indefinitely.
3. *Urea nitrogen standard 20 mg/100 ml.*

   428 mg urea dissolved in a cold saturated solution of benzoic acid in demineralized water to produce a final volume of one litre (Stable indefinitely).
4. *Urease solution.*

   20 mg of urease dissolved in EDTA buffer to a final volume of 50 ml. It can be kept for a few weeks at 4°C.
5. *Phenol solution*

   5 ml of liquid phenol is placed in a measuring cylinder (do not pipette with the mouth). Twenty five mg of sodium nitroprusside is added and dissolved by adding demineralized water to produce 200 ml. It can be kept for 2-4 days at 4°C in the dark. The reagent must not come into contact with the skin.
6. *Sodium hydroxide solution, 5 N.*
7. *Hypochlorite stock solution 0.14 N.*

   Sodium hypochlorite stock solution can be purchased or prepared according to the directions of Weller (1962). The concentration is estimated as follow: 1 ml of the stock solution is dissolved to 100 ml with demineralized water. To 50 ml of this solution is added 1g potassium iodide dissolved in a small amount of water, 5 ml of a 25 percent hydrochloric acid solution and 3 drops of starch solution. Then the solution is titrated with 0.1 N thiosulphate until colourless.

The concentration of hypochlorite solution is calculated according to the following formula.

$$\text{Active chlorine} = \frac{V \times 3.546 \times 200}{1000} g/100ml$$

Where V is the volume (ml) of thiosulphate used. The solution is diluted to produce a 0.014 N (0.5g active chlorine/100ml) stock solution. It is stable indefinitely.

8. *Hypochlorite-sodium hydroxide solution.*

   Naocl , 0.07 N; NaOH, 2.5 N. Equal parts of 0.14 N hypochlorite solution and 5 N NaOH are mixed.

Procedure

Mixtures	T	TB	S	SB
Urease solution. ml	0.5	—	0.5	—
Serum, plasma, ml	0.02	0.02	—	—
Standard solution, ml	—	—	0.02	0.02

T = Testing Sample, TB =Testing Blank Sample, S=Standard Sample, SB=Standard Blank Sample

Incubate 20 min at 37°C or 30 minutes at room temperature

Phenol solution , ml	10	10	10	10
Urease solution , ml	—	0.5	—	0.5
Hypochlorite solution, ml	1.0	1.0	1.0	1.0

After 10 min. at room temperature, read against demineralized water at 540, 546 and 590 nm. The colour is stable for 2 h.

Calculation

$$\text{mg, urea nitrogen/100 ml} = \frac{A(T) - A(TB)}{A(S) - A(SB)} \times c(S)$$

$$\text{mg, urea nitrogen/100 ml} = \frac{A(T) - A(TB)}{A(S) - A(SB)} \times 20$$

Where A is spectronic 20 value

☞ Notes

1. *Preparation of ammonia-free distilled water can be done with the help of a cationic exchanger.*
2. *Both the concentrated phenol solution and the concentrated hypochlorite solution are corrosive and poisonous; do not pipette by mouth and avoid contact with skin.*

3. *Haemolytic sera cannot be examined because of the formation of colours, which are not identical with those obtained with the urea standard.*

4. *The urine sample should first be diluted 1:500 with ammonia free aqua dest or ammonia free physiological saline.*

5. *It is sufficient to carry out one reagent blank and one standard determination per series of serum or urinary tests.*

6. *Use clean and in particular ammonia free glassware. Avoid atmospheric contamination with ammonia.*

7. *The Beer-Lambert law is valid upto to a concentration of about 200 mg of urea nitrogen/100 ml. Higher concentrations should be analysed with half the stated sample volume and the results are multiplied by 2. For lower concentrations, it is advisable to read at 578 nm and for very low concentrations, at 645nm.*

8. *Multiply the result of urea nitorgen by 2.14 so as to get the result in terms of urea.*

9. *The urine is collected with 5 ml of thymol isopropanol to prevent bacterial hydrolysis of urea.*

10. *Coulombe and Lavreau (1963) have developed and published a new semi-micro method for colorimetric determination of urea.*

4. Colorimetric Method for the Determination of Ammonia in Serum and Urine

(Based on Berthelot Reaction)

Method of Berthelot, 1859

Principle

In this method. we do not use urease enzyme.

Reagents

Most of the reagents are same as mentioned under urea estimation procedure.

Ammonia standard (20 mg of ammonia nitrogen / 100 ml) : 944 mg ammonium sulphate dissolved in demineralized water and made up to one litre. It is stable indefinitely if frozen.

Procedure

Mixture	T	RB	S
Demineralized water, ml	0.5	0.5	0.5
Urine, ml	0.02	–	–
Demineralized water, ml	–	0.02	–
Standard, ml	–	–	0.02
Phenol solution, ml	10.0	10.0	10.0
Hypochlorite NaOH solution, ml	1.0	1.0	1.0

After 10 minutes at room temperature, measure the absorbance between 540 and 580 nm against water. The colour is stable for 2 h

Calculation

$$\text{mg Ammonia nitrogen/100 ml} = \frac{A(T)-A(RB)}{A(S)-A(RB)} \times 20$$

$$\text{mg Ammonia /100 ml} = \frac{A(T)-A(RB)}{A(S)-A(RB)} \times 24.3$$

$$\text{mg Ammonia } (NH_4^+)/\text{ 100 ml} = \frac{A(T)-A(RB)}{A(S)-A(RB)} \times 25.7$$

$$\text{mEq (m moles) Ammonia} = (NH_4^+)/100\text{ml}$$

$$= \frac{A(T)-A(RB)}{A(S)-A(RB)} \times 1.43$$

Where A is spectronic 20 value

☞ Note

Add 5 ml of thymol isopropanol solution to urine, it prevents the splitting of urea by bacterial urease.

We should analyse urine as such as well as in 1:10 dilution.

Method of Ammonia Nitrogen Estimation in Rumen Liquor, Silage extract, Serum and Food extract etc.

(Method of Cook, 1976)

Principle

Light blue colour is developed when ammonia nitrogen is reacted with sodium nitroprusside, phenol and sodium hypochlorite and intensity of colour is measured against standard ammonia nitrogen at 650 nm using spectrophotometer.

Reagents

1. *Reagents A : 10.0 g phenol.*

   0.05 g sodium nitroprusside

   Make up the volume to 1 litre with water, store in the cold in a dark bottle (keep for 1 month)
2. *Reagents B: 5.0 g sodium hydroxide*

   8.4 ml sodium hypochlorite solution (containing 4 to 6% available chlorine). Make up volume to one litre with water. Store in the cold in a dark bottle. Keep for one month.
3. *Standard solution: (i) Weigh 707.8 mg ammonium sulphate and dissolve in 100 ml water, this will give concentration of ammonia nitrogen 03 mg N/0.2 ml. (ii) Working Solution: Dilute stock solution 100 times, this will give concentration of 3 µg N in 0.2 ml diluted solution.*

Method

Take 10 ml sample, add 2 ml 50 percent Trichloroacetic acid (TCA), mix and allow to stand, Then centrifuge at 3000 rpm for 15 min. use, supernatant, diluted ten times if necessary/and develop colour as decribed below:

1. Take triplicate (ammonia free distilled water washed) test tubes.
2. Add 0.2 ml of diluted samples to 5 ml Reagent A and mix.
3. Add 5 ml Reagent B and mix.
4. Incubate at 37°C for 15 min.
5. Measure optical density at 650 nm against ammonia free distilled water.

Example

Spectrophotometer Reading

	Set I	Set II	
Sample 1	a – 0.167	b – 0.164	Average 0.164
Sample 2	a – 0.271	b – 0.255	Average 0.236
Sample 3	a – 0.320	b – 0.320	Average 0.320
Standard	a – 0.445	b – 0.454	Average 0.446

Standard

It has been observed that 3 µg N in 0.2 ml gives optical density 0.446.

Then 1 µg N in 0.2 ml gives $\frac{0.446}{3} = 0.148.$

In the case of **sample 1**, O.D. will be $\frac{0.164}{0.148} = 1.108.$

10 ml of solution is effectively 1 ml effluent (R.L.)

Then concentration of ammonia nitrogen

$$= \frac{1.108 \times 10 \times 100}{0.2 \times 100} = 5.5 \text{ mg N/100 ml effluent.}$$

(i) Therefore sample 1 contained 5.5 mg ammonia nitrogen per 100 ml effluent.

(ii) Therefore sample 2 contained 8.885 mg ammonia nitrogen per 100 ml effluent.

(iii) Therefore sample 3 contained 10.81 mg ammonia nitrogen per 100 ml effluent.

5. Colorimetric Method for Determination of Urea in Animal Feeds

(Method of Watt and Chrisp 1954)

Principle

Urea is extracted from the sample with approximate 0.02M hydrochloric acid and determined spectrophotometrically with 4 dimethylamino-benzaldehyde. Extraction with acid inhibits the activity of any urease naturally present. Colour is removed with charcoal and nitrogenous substances are precipitated with zinc ferrocyanide.

Reagents

(i) Charcoal, decolourizing powder, activated.

(ii) Dimethlaminobenzaldehyde solution: Dissolve 4g of dimethylamino-benzaldehyde in 20 ml of hydrochloric acid, approx. 36 percent m/m HCI, and dilute to 200 ml with propanol-2-01.

(iii) Hydrochloric acid, approx. 2M-Dilute 1 vol. of hydrochloric acid, approx. 36 percent m/m. HCI, to 6 Vol.

(iv) Hydrochloric acid, approx.0.02M-Dilute 1 vol of approx. 2M hydrochloric acid to 100 vol.

(v) Potassium ferrocyanide solution, 10.6 percent m/V.

(vi) Sodium acetate trihydrate, solution, 13.6 percent m/V.

(vii) Urea working standard solution, 5 mg/ml of Urea Dissolve 1 g of urea in water and dilute to 200 ml.

(viii) Zinc acetate solution-Dissolve 21.9 g of zinc acetate dihydrate in water, add 3 ml of acetic acid, glacial and dilute to 100 ml.

Preparation of Standard Graph

(a) Measure 0, 5, 15, 20 and 25 ml of urea working standard solution into six 250 ml volumetric flasks (b) Add 150 ml of approximate 0.02 M hydrochloric acid and shake at intervals over a period of 30 min. Add 10 ml of sodium acetate solution, mix and add 1 g of charcoal and mix. Allow to stand for 15 min. Add 5 ml of zinc acetate solution and mix. Add 5 ml of potassium ferrocyanide solution, mix dilute to 250 ml. Filter through a 15 cm Whatman No. 2 filter paper. Reject the first few ml of filtrate. Pipette 10 ml of the filtrate into a 50 ml volumetric flask, add 10 ml of dimethylaminobenzaldehyde solution, dilute to 50 ml and allow to stand for 10 min. Measure the absorbance in a 40 mm optical cell at 435 nm (c) Construct a graph relating absorbance to mg of urea present. The absorbance corresponding to 0 and 5 mg of urea and calculate absorbance against 0.15 and 0.75mg urea respectively.

Examination of Feeding Stuff

Transfer 5g of sample. ground to pass a 1 mm sieve, into a 250 ml flask. Continue as in b commencing at "Acid 150 ml of approx 0.02 M hydrochloric acid...." and ending at "..... in a 40 nm optical cell at 435 nm."

Calculation of Result

Read from the standard graph the number of mg of urea equivalent to the absorbance and multiply by 5. The result gives the g/kg of urea in the sample.

☞ **Note**

The solution after filtration should be colourless.

With highly coloured samples the weight of charcoal may be increased to 5 g.

6. Creatinine and Creatine in Urine, Blood Plasma and Tissues

Introduction

The most widely used method for the determination of creatinine is based upon the formation of a red colour with alkaline picrate. This reaction which was discovered by M. Jaffe and adapted for quantitative use by Folin appears to depend on the formation of a red tautomer of converted to creatinine (Its anhydride) by heating with acid. Folin originally employed a solution of potassium dichromate as an artificial standard, but subsequently he recommended the use of creatinine solution of known concentration and the practice is now generally adopted. Procedures are given below for the determination of creatinine and creatine in urine, blood plasma and of creatine in tissues.

Method for Preformed Creatinine in Urine

A standard creatinine solution containing 1 mg of creatine/ml is prepared by dissolving 1 g of creatinine, or 1.602 g of creatinine zinc chloride in 0.1 N hydrochloric acid to one litre.

A convenient quantity of the urine, say 1 ml is transferred to a 100 ml volumetric flask and 1 ml of the stock standard (containing 1 mg creatinine) to another similar flask. To each flask, 20 ml of a saturated aqueous solution of picric acid and 1.5 ml of a percent W/V aqueous solution of NaOH are added. After 10 min., each solution is diluted to the mark with water and the relative intensities of the colours are compared in a colorimeter. If the reading of standard and unknown differ by more than 50 percent, the determination should be repeated with a more suitable amount of the sample. If photoelectric instrument is used, the zero adjustment is made with a reagent blank. Alternatively the zero setting can be made with water and blank is read separately and subtracted from the standard and unknown.

Method for Total Creatinine in Urine

To a suitable quantity of the urine, say 1 ml, contained in a 300 ml conical flask is added 20 ml of a saturated aqueous solution of picric acid and the flask and its contents are weighed to the nearest 0.1g. About 130 ml of water is added and the liquid is boiled gently for 45 min. and then more rapidly until the volume is reduced to about 20 ml. After cooling, sufficient water is added to restore the flask and content to the original weight and 1.5 ml of 10 percent sodium hydroxide are added. After 10 min. the solution is rinsed into a 100 ml volumetric flask and made to the mark,comparing the colour with that of a standard prepared above.

Calculation of Creatine

The difference between the figures for "total creatinine" and preformed creatinine represents the creatine (expressed in terms of creatinine). This may be multiplied by 1.16 to express the result in terms of creatine itself.

Method for Serum Creatinine and Creatine Estimation

Procedure 1

Five ml serum is placed in a flask, followed by 40 ml of N/12 sulphuric acid and 5 ml of 10 percent W/V aqueous solution of sodium tungstate hydrated ($Na_2WO_4.2H_2O$) and the mixture thoroughly shaken and filtered.

Into each of four tubes is placed, 8 ml of the filtrate and 8 ml of water is placed in a fifth tube to serve as a blank. The mouths of two of the four tubes containing filtrate are covered with tin foil and the tubes are autoclaved at 15 pound pressure (115° to 120°C) for 20 min. removed and allowed to cool. To each of the five tubes is then added 4 ml of an alkaline picrate solution, freshly prepared by adding 1 volume of 10 percent W/V aqueous sodium hydroxide to 5 volumes of a 1.175 percent W/V aqueous solution of picric acid. (On standing for a few minutes this alkaline picrate forms a flaky precipitate that makes measurement difficult).

After 20 min. reading are made at 520 nm. The colour remains unchanged for at least two and half hours. A calibration curve is constructed with solutions containing known amounts of creatinine.

Procedure 2

Duplicate 3 ml samples of serum are placed in centrifuge tubes. To the first (X) is added 3 ml of water and to the second (S) 3 ml of a creatinine solution containing 2 mg per 100 ml (prepared by dilution with water of a stock solution containing 0.5 g of creatinine in one litre of 0.1 N hydrochloric acid). After mixing, 3 ml 5 percent aqueous sodium tungstate is added to each. followed, after again mixing 3 ml of 0.33 N sulphuric acid. The contents of the tubes are mixed, and centrifuged after 10 min. To 6 ml samples of protein free fluid from X and S, 6 ml of water (to serve as blank) are added to 4 ml of a fresh mixture of equal parts of 0.75 N aqueous sodium hydroxide and saturated picric acid. The mixtures are allowed to stand and the optical densities are measured after 25 to 30 minutes (spectrum blue given filter No. 603). X is read against the blank B and the standard S against X.

It there is insufficient serum for the preparation of a standard in serum, a standard in water is prepared within 6 ml of creatinine solution (0.5 mg per 100ml) and 4 ml of alkaline picrate. This is read against the blank B. A correction must be made to allow for the fact that in serum filtrate creatinine give approximately 90 percent of the density given in water.

In the serum creatinine concentration is greater than 3 mg per 100 ml, the serum filtrate must be diluted. Appropriately higher concentrations of creatinine solution must be added to the serum used for preparing the standard and the filtrate from this is diluted in the same way.

Method for Plasma Creatinine Using Lloyd's Reagent

A protein free 'filtrate' is prepared by pipetting 0.5 ml of plasma or serum and 1 ml of water into a 1.3 x 100 cm tube mixing with a glass rod adding 1 ml of 20 percent trichloroacetic acid with continuous stirring and spinning down the precipitated protein. Two ml of the supernatant fluid is placed in a 13 x 100 ml tube, and quantities of a standard solution (for example, 0.5, 0.1, 1.5 and 2.0 ml) of an aqueous soultion containing 0.25 or 0.5 mg of creatinine per 100 ml placed in a similar tube and diluted to approximately 2 ml with water. In this case water (2 ml) serve as a blank. To each tube are added 0.2 ml of a saturated aqueous solution of oxalic acid and 15 to 20 mg of Lloyd's reagent. The tubes are stoppered and inverted or shaken occasionlly and are then centrifuged and the clear supernatant fluid is aspirated off through a fine tipped glass tube and discarded. Into each tube are pipetted 2 ml of an alkaline picrate solution, prepared on the same day by mixing 5 parts of approximately 0.04 M, (that is, 0.92 per) picric acid solution with 1 part of 10 percent sodium hydroxide and then diluting with 12 parts of water. The tubes are stoppered and well shaken to suspend the Lloyd's reagent, allowed to stand for at least 10 min with occasional shaking fluid in each tube is then measured at 250 nm. The colour is stable for at least two hours at room temperature.

Method for Animal Tissues

An alkaline picrate reagent and standard creatinine solutions are required.

1. The alkaline picrate solution: Mix 5 volumes of a saturated aqueous solution of pure picric acid (about 1.2 percent W/V) with 1 volume of a 10 percent W/V aqueous solution of sodium hydroxide. The solutions of acid and alkali should be stocked separately and the mixture freshly made just before use.
2. A creatinine stock standard, containing 1 mg creatinine per ml is prepared by dissolving 1.602 g of creatinine zinc chloride in 0.1 N hydrochloric acid and diluting with the same solvent to one litre.
3. A diluted standard is made by treating a suitable volume of the stock standard with 10 ml of 0.1 N hydrochloric acid and diluting with water to one litre.

Procedure

Tissues or organs should be removed as promptly as possible after the death of the animal. If abundant material is available it should be run through a meat chopper in order to produce a uniform sample, but in the case of small organs it will generally be sufficient to cut into small pieces with scissors. Portions weighing approximately 1 g (or if the creatinine content is high it may be necessary to operate on smaller quantities are transferred to tarred 50 ml glass stoppered) Erlenmeyer flasks which are at once closed to prevent evaporation of moisture and again weighed. The material in each flask is treated with 20 ml of 2 N sulphuric acid and the vessels are covered with tin foil and heated for 45 min. in an autoclave at 15 Ib pressure. After cooling, each solution is transferred to a 100 ml volumetric flask with the aid of 40 to 50 ml of water and 15 ml of 2 N sodium hydroxide is added, followed by 5 ml of a 10 percent aqueous solution of sodium tungstate. The mixture, which should now be faintly acidic to congro-red indicator, is diluted to the mark with water and well shaken. After being allowed to stand for 5 min. the solution is filtered and 10 ml of the filtrate treated with 5 ml of alkaline picrate solution. Alternatively if the colour is too deep for satisfactory matching, suitable, quantities of the filtrate should be diluted to 10 ml with water and treated with 5 ml of alkaline picrate solution. As early as possible at the same time, suitable quantities of the diluted standard solution (say from 1 ml upwards) are diluted to 10 ml with water and mixed with 5 ml of the alkaline picrate solution. After standing for 10 minutes in order to permit the colour to develop fully the sample is matched against a series of standards by direct visual observation or alternatively is compared with a standard of closely similar intensity by means of colorimeter.

Total creatinine – preformed creatinine = creatine (as creatinine). To convert creatine expressed as creatinine into the amount of creatine itself, multiply by 1.16 (Total creatinine – Preformed creatinine x 1.16 = Creatine).

7. Uric Acid in Poultry Excreta

Introduction

About 80 percent of the urinary nitrogen of the chick is present as uric acid. Bose and Ghosh (1945) determined the uric acid content of poultry excreta by utilizing the difference in iodine titre before and after treatment with uricase. One of the most critical steps in the determination of uric acid appeared to be its complete extraction from the excreta. Hutchinson (1941), extracing with 0.5 percent lithium carbonate, reported that warming was essential to put the urates into complete solution. Bose (1944) extracted at room temperature for up to one and half hours after detecting some loss of uric acid following hot extraction with lithium carbonate.

The method consists of a simple extraction and dilution, followed by absorbance measurements before and after reaction with uricase.

Reagents

1. *Lithium carbonate : (0.5 percent solution)*
2. *Glycine Buffer. 0.1 M, pH 9.2 ± 0.1 : The glycine solution was adjusted to the desired pH with 10 N NaOH.*

3. *Uricase : Usually it is advisable to procure pure uricase type II soluble powder from Sigma Chemical Company, St Louis, Missouri. It is dissolved in 0.1 M glycine buffer. This preparation was stable for about a month when stored in a refrigerator.*

4. *Uric acid purification : One gram of commercial uric acid is dissolved in 120 ml of the 0.5 percent lithium carbonate solution, 80 ml of water are added and the mixture is warmed to 60°C. It is then cooled, acidified with hydrochloric acid and allowed to stand for one hour. After filtering, the precipitate is washed with 50 ml of water, and the entire procedure is repeated. The uric acid is dissolved in 2 l of boiling distilled water, cooled to room temperature, filtered and the precipitate washed first with cold water and then with absolute ethanol. After the ethanol evaporates, the precipitate is dried at 100°C for three hours and stored in a desiccator.*

5. *Uric acid standard : The standard stock solution of Folin (1930), as modified by Buchanan et al. (1945), is made by dissolving 100 mg of the purified uric acid in 12 ml of 0.5 percent lithium carbonate, in a 100 ml volumetric flask, at 60°C. After preparing solution, the sample is cooled and made up to volume with water. Serial dilution of this stock solution is made with glycine buffer so as to give concentrations of uric acid between 1 and 10 μg per ml. A standard curve is prepared by plotting absorbance at 292 nm on concentrations of uric acid. This standard should be prepared fresh daily.*

Procedure

One gram sample of the fine ground excreta is quantitatively transferred to 250 ml volumetric flask. The neck of each flask is washed with two 25 ml portions of 0.5 percent lithium carbonate solution. After extracting for half an hour with frequent swirling of the samples. the flasks are made up to volume with distilled water and mixed by inversion. A portion was centrifuged to remove solids, and a 1 : 10 dilution of an aliquot of each samples is made with the glycine buffer. One ml aliquot of each of the diluted uric acid samples is pipetted into 15 ml tubes. A blank is prepared, using 1 ml of glycine buffer and 9 ml of uricase solution. The blank tube is covered with paraffin paper and mixed gently by inversion, taking care to see no bubbles are formed which interfere with the extinction reading. Cell corrections for possible changes in absorbance of uricase solution are obtained by reading the blank solution at 292 mμ before and after incubation. Extinction reading on test samples are made by adding 9 ml of uricase solution from a fast flow serological pipette, mixing as above, transferring a portion to a 1 cm silica cell, reading, and returning solution to original test tube. After becoming familiar with the technique, it takes approximately 40 seconds from the time of the enzyme addition to the extinction measurement. After all the samples are read, they are then incubated at 45°C for four hours. A pan of water in the incubator is kept to prevent evaporation from the tubes. After the incubation period, cell corrections are again made, using the incubated blank solution followed by the terminal extinction readings of the samples.

Calculation

$$\text{mg uric acid/gram excreta} = \frac{\text{E(initial)} - \text{E(terminal)} \times \text{dilution factor}}{\text{k} \times \text{sample wt} \times 1000}$$

where,

E = Corrected extinction reading

Dilution factor (see text) = $250 \times 10 \times 10 = 25{,}000$

K = Change in extinction/ µg of uric acid/ml was obtained from the calibration curve. On a Beckman DU Spectrophotometer, a value of 0.075 is obtained.

References

Berthelot, M.P. (1859). *Rep Chim. Appl.,* 1: 202.

Bose, S. (1944). *Poultry Sci,* 23: 130-34

Bose, S. and D.B. Ghosh, (1945). *Poultry, Sci.,* 24: 146-49.

Buchanan, O.H., W.D, Blcok and A.A Christman, (1945). The metabolism of the methylated purines. I., *J. Biol. Chem.* 157: 181-87.

Cook, A.R. (1976). *J. Gen. Microbiol,* 92: 32.

Coulombe, J.J., and L. Lavreau, (1963). *Clin, Chem.* 9: 102.

Follin, O. (1904). *Zeitsch. Physiol., Chem.,* 42: 223.

Follin, O. (1930). *J. Biol. Chem.,* 86: 1790.

Follin, O. and J.L. Morris, (1914). *J. Biol. Chem,* 17: 469.

Hutchinson, J.C.D. (1941). *Biochem. J.* 35: 81-90.

IS: 2052-1979 Indian Standards Institution, (BIS) *Specification for Compounded Feeds for cattle.* Third revision.

Krishna, G. Paliwal, V.K. and Yadav, K.R. (1980). True protein and non protein fractions in Agro-Industrial Wastes/by products in Haryana State. *Haryana Agricultural Univ. J. Research.* 11 : 458-462.

Krishna G. (1979). A note on menace of urea adulteration in Indian Poultry feeds. *Poultry Guid* 16 : 59-62.

Lieb, H. and M.K. Zacher, (1934). *Zeits, Physiol. Chem.,* 223: 169.

Lubochinsky, B and J.P. Zalta, (1954). *Bull Soc. Chim Biol.,* 36: 1363.

Pearson, R.M. and J.A.B. Smith, (1943). *Biochem. J.,* 37: 142-49.

Peters, J.P. and D.D. Vanslyke, (1946). *Quantitative Clinical Chemistry, Interpretations.* Vol. 1, Williams and Wilkins, Baltimore.

Pudelkiewicz, W.J. M.W. Stutz and L.D. Matterson, (1968). *Poultry Sci.* 47: 1274-77.

Watt, G.W. and J.D. (1954). *Crisp, Anal. Chem.,* 26: 452.

Weller, H. (1962). *Romtgen Lab. Praxis* 15: 77.

Chapter - 13

Total Ash and Acid Insoluble Ash in Feeds and Fodders

Definition

The residue of incineration at 550-600°C is the crude ash.

Reagent

Dilute hydrochloric acid -approximately 5 N prepared from concentrated hydrochloric acid. Dissolve 445 ml conc. hydrochloric acid (about 36 percent HCl) in one litre distilled water.

Procedure for Total Ash Estimation

Take a vitreosil crucible in oven at 100°C for six hours, remove and keep it in a desiccator and weigh up to constant weight. About 5-10 g of sample is taken in the weighted vitreosil crucible. The material in the crucible is charred on a low flame and the crucible is then kept in muffle furnace and temperature is allowed to raise to 600°C and kept constant for two hours. It is removed on cooling and kept in a desiccator and weight of crucible is taken.

Observations

1. Weight of empty vitreosil crucible = 39.120 g
2. Weight of crucible+material = 44.120 g

3. Weight of material = 5.0 g
4. Dry matter content in material, percent = 92.38 g
5. Weight of material on dry matter basis = 4.62 g
6. Weight of ash and crucible = 39.690 g
7. Net weight of ash = 0.570 g

Percent of total ash $= \dfrac{\text{Wt. of ash} \times 100}{\text{Wt. of material on dry matter basis}}$

$= \dfrac{0.570 \times 100}{4.62}$

= 12.337 percent on dry matter basis

Procedure for Insolube Ash Estimation

After completing total ash estimation, treat the material in the crucible with 25 ml of the dilute hydrochloric acid (5 N) and boil it on burner for 10 min. Allow to cool and filter through a whatman filter paper No. 42 of its equivalent. Wash the filter paper with water until the washings are free from the acid and return it to the crucible. Keep the crucible in an electric air oven maintained at 135° ± 2°C for about three hours. Ignite it in a muffle furnace at 600° ± 20°C for one hour. Cool the crucible in a desiccator andweigh. Ignite the crucible again in the muffle furnace for 30 min, cool and weigh. Repeat this process till the difference in weight between two successive weighings is less than one milligram. Record the lowest weight.

Acid insoluble ash (on moisture free basis) percent by weight

$$= \frac{100(W_2 - W)}{(W_1 - W)} g/100g$$

Where,

W_1 = The lowest weight in gram of the Crucible with the acid insoluble ash.

W = Weight in gram of the empty Crucible

W_2 = Weight in gram of the Crucible with the dried material taken for the test.

Ash in Sugars and Sugar Products

(Method of AOAC, 1980)

Method I

Heat sample of appropiate weight for product being examined (usually 5-10g) in 50-100 ml platinum dish at 100°C until water is expelled; add few drops of pure olive oil and heat slowly over flame or under IR lamp until swelling stops. Place dish in furnace at about 525°C and leave until white ash is obtained. Moisten ash with water, dry on steam bath and then on hot plate, and again ash at 525°C to constant weight.

Method II

Carbonize sample of appropriate weight for product being examined (usually 5-10 g) in 50-100 ml platinum dish at about 525°C and treat charred mass with hot water to dissolve soluble salts. (In case of low-purity products, addition of few drops of pure olive oil, above may be desirable). Filter through ashless paper, ignite paper and residue to white ash and filtrate of soluble salts, evaporate to dryness, and ignite at about 525°C to constant weight.

Sulphated Ash

Weigh 5 g sample into 50-100 ml platinum dish, add 5 ml 10 percent (by weight) sulphuric acid, heat on hot plate until sample is well carbonized, and then ash in furnace at about 550°C, cool, add 2-3 ml 10 percent sulphuric acid, evaporate on steam bath, dry on hot plate, and again Ignite at 550°C to constant weight. Express result as percent sulphated ash.

References

AOAC, (1980). *Official Methods of Analysis of the Associatioin of Official Agricultural Chemists,* 10 th edn., AOAC Benjamin Frankin Station. Washington, DC, P 508.

IS: 2025-1979, (BIS) Indian Standards Institution, *Specification for Compounded Feeds for Cattle,* Third revision.

Paliwal, V.K., Yadav, K.R. and Krishna, G. (1981). Note on proximate nutrient composition of Agro-Industrial byproducts of Haryana State. *Indian J. Animal Sci.* 51: 1173-1176.

Chapter - 14

Wet Chemical Digestion of Biological Materials for Mineral Analysis

Introduction

Wet ashing is suitable for the determination of Ca, Cu, Fe, Mg, Mn, K, Na, Se and Zn in biological samples and may be applicable to the determination of other elements as well.

The organic matter of the sample is oxidized with concentrated nitric acid and perchloric acids. The acids are partially removed by volatilization and the solube mineral constituents remain dissolved in nitric acid. Any silica present is dehydrated and made insoluble.

Equipments

1. *Fume hood. Constructed for safe exhaustion of perchloric acid fumes.*
2. *Hot plate of Micro digestion bench (Thermostatically controlled).*
3. *Micro digestion flask (Pyrex).*
4. *Volumetric flask (Pyrex) 100 ml capacity.*
5. *Glass funnel 1.5 cm diameter.*

Reagents

1. *Digestion acid : Add 1 volume perchloric acid (60 to 62 percent perchloric acid) to 4 volume nitric acid (69 to 71 percent HNO_3).*
2. *Nitric acid 69 to 71 percent.*

Procedure

1. Weigh about 1 g sample (ground to pass a 1 mm sieve) into a 250 ml capacity micro-kjeldahl flask and add 20 ml digestion acid about 3 glass beads. Fix the flask in a clamp, keep it as such for overnight.
2. When the initial reaction subsided, increase the temperature of hot plate or micro-digestion bench slowly to 180° to 200°C.
3. Continue the digestion at this temperature with occasional swirling until there are no visible particles and the digestion acid is quite clear. If the solution darkens when the volume is reduced, remove the kjeldahl flask from the heating source, add 1 or 2 ml nitric acid and continue the digestion.
4. Allow the temperature to rise of the heating source to 240°C and evaporate the digestion acid until dense white fumes are formed within the digestion flask.
5. After completing the digestion, the flask is removed from the heating source. Filter the content of flask through acid washed filter paper in a 100 ml capacity volumetric flask using deionised water.
6. At the end, suitable aliquot of digested material may be transferred into washed polyethylene bottles and allowed to keep in a dust proof glass chamber.

Precautions

1. *Always add the nitric acid to tissue sample before adding perchloric acid. Perchloric acid can react explosively with untreated organic materials.*
2. *Be sure all organic material is destroyed before allowing the nitric acid to completely evaporate.*
3. *Because of potential contamination from the reagents used it is advisable to use a reagent blank prepared using the procedure described above but excluding the tissue sample.*
4. *For the determination of calcium and magnesium, the final dilution should contain 1 percent (W/V) Lanthanum solution of EDTA or Oxine (7-hydroxychinolin).* ***The oxine is the best amongst all the chelating agents.***
5. *Always use deionised or glass distilled water in the processing of sample.*
6. *The working place should be dust proof.*
7. *Nitric acid and perchloric acid should be distilled, using glass distillation assembly on oil bath (Linseed oil or Till oil).*

Reference

Krishna, G. (1973) Lic. Agric. (Ph.D.) thesis *"Infusion of volatile fatty acids and use of radio isotopes (^{14}C-VFA, ^{51}Cr-EDTA, ^{198}Au) in nutritional and biochemical studies related to the energy metabolism in sheep"*. Agricultural University of Norway Ås-NLH, Norway.

Krishna, G., Paliwal, V.K., Yadav, K.R. and Khirwar, S.S. (1981). Trace elements in Agro-Industrial byproducts and Wastes of Haryana State. *Indian J. Dairy Sci.,* 34: 336-338.

Krishna, G., Paliwal V.K., Yadav, K.R. and Khirwar, S.S. (1981). Note on alkaline earth metals in Agro-Industrial byproducts and Wastes of Haryana State. *Indian J. Anim. Sci.* 51: 170-72.

Chapter - 15

Nitrogen Free Extract in Feeds and Fodders

NFE Calculation

Introduction

As per statement of Dr. Henneberg of Weende Experiment Station (Göttingen, Germany) the carbohydrates are divided into two groups; crude fiber and nitrogen free extract. The nitrogen free extract, which comprises the sugars, starch and a large part of the material classed as hemicellulose, is determined by difference. It is represented by the figure obtained when the sum of the water, ash, protein, fat and crude fiber of a feed is subtracted from 100. Since the figure is determined by difference instead of directly, it includes the cumulative errors of the other determinations and thus is not an exact value.

Calculation

NFE (per cent) on as fed basis = DM (per cent) - (ash per cent) + crude fiber (per cent) + ether extract (per cent) + protein (per cent).

Example : Chemical composition of barseem hay (*Medicago sative*) on as fed basis:

Drymatter	=89.800	Percent on as feed basis
Ash	=13.410	
Crude fiber	=24.320	
Ether Extract	=1.275	
Protein	=17.03	

NFE, percent on as fed basis

$$= 89.80 - (13.410 + 24.320 + 1.275 + 17.03) = 33.765$$

Reference

Krishna, G. and Günther, K.D. (1987). Nutrient Composition and Amino acid content of some Agro-Industrial byproducts and wastes used as livestock feeds. *Z. Landwirtschalftliche Forschung*. 40: 277-280.

Maynard, L.A. and J.K. Loosli, (1969). *Animal Nutrition*, 6th edn., p. 77. New York: Mc Graw-Hill Book Company.

Paliwal, V.K., Yadav, K.R. and Krishna, G. (1981). Note on proximate nutrient composition of Agro-Industrial Byproducts of Haryana State. *Indian J. Anmal Sci.* 51: 1173-76.

Tewatia, B.S. and Krishna, G. (1991). Fodder tree leaves as Animal Feed IV. Proximate Composition, major and minor minerals, Carotene and Tocopherol in fodder tree leaves of arid and semiarid zones. *The J. of the Remount and Veterinary Corps*. 30: 177-183.

Chapter - 16

Determination of Food Carbohydrates

Limitation of Weende Method

The partition of carbohydrate into fiber (CF) and nitrogen free extract (NFE) is presumed to represent a separation of less digestible starch and sugars. *However, in 20 to 30 percent feeds listed by Morrison, the NFE is less digestible than the CF. This comes about for several reasons, the most important of which is the CF method (successive boiling with dilute sulphuric acid and sodium hydroxide) does not recover all the fiber and large portions of fibrous constituents are extracted into the NFE.* The most important of these fractions are lignin and hemicellulose are dissolved by both acid and alkali. The basic error of the NFE concept is the assumption that if constituents are soluble they are digestible. *Lignin, the rigid component of wood, not only is indigestible but lowers the digestibility of substances with which it is associated.*

Another portion of the indigestible part of NFE arises from an artifact in the calculation of faecal NFE, where it is presumed that faecal nitrogen is protein (N x 6.25). *Actually, 80-90 percent faecal nitrogen is NPN and is composed of bacterial residue in which the ratio of organic matter to nitrogen is about 1:4. Thus, part of the faecal NFE arises by an underestimation of the organic matter associated with faecal nitrogen.*

Various Systems of Partitioning Dry Matter of Forages

1. ***Organic Matter System***
   (a) Determine dry matter and ash
   (b) Organic matter = dry matter - ash
2. ***Weende Proximate System***
   (a) Determine dry matter, ash, crude fiber, crude protein and ether extract.
   (b) Nitrogen free extract = dry matter - (ash + crude fiber + ether extract + crude protein).
3. ***Crampton and Maynard System***
   (a) Determine dry matter, ash, ether extract, crude protein, lignin and cellulose.
   (b) Other carbohydrate = dry matter - (ash + ether extract + crude protein + lignin + cellulose.)
4. ***Van Soest System***
   (a) Determine cell walls (neutral detergent fiber) and dry matter.
   (b) Cell contents (neutral detergent solubles) = dry matter-cell walls.

The neutral detergent fiber (NDF) is representative of the fibrous cell wall constituents and contains lignin, cellulose, hemicellulose and some fiber bound protein. That part of the sample not appearing as residue is termed neutral detergent solubles, represent the cellular contents and contains lipids, sugars, organic acids, non-protein nitrogen, pectins, soluble protein and other water soluble matter. *Crude fiber contains most of the cellulose and only part of the lignin, so that ADF values are about 30 percent higher than those for crude fiber in the same feeds.*

The neutral detergent fiber differs from the previously developed acid detergent fiber, it represents the cellulose and lignin portion of the cell wall of plants. The ADF analysis will be required for evaluating the quality of fiber for ruminants and other fiber utilizing herbivores. For non-ruminants with little fiber utilizing capacity, the neutral detergent fiber will be the only fiber value required. The different steps of Van Soest analysis have been demonstrated in Fig. 1.

Classification I

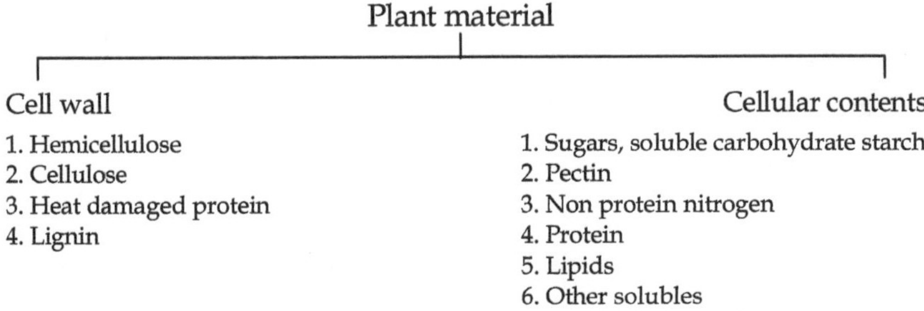

Source : USDA, Agriculture Handbook, No. 379.

Van Soest System of Partitioning Forages

Classification II

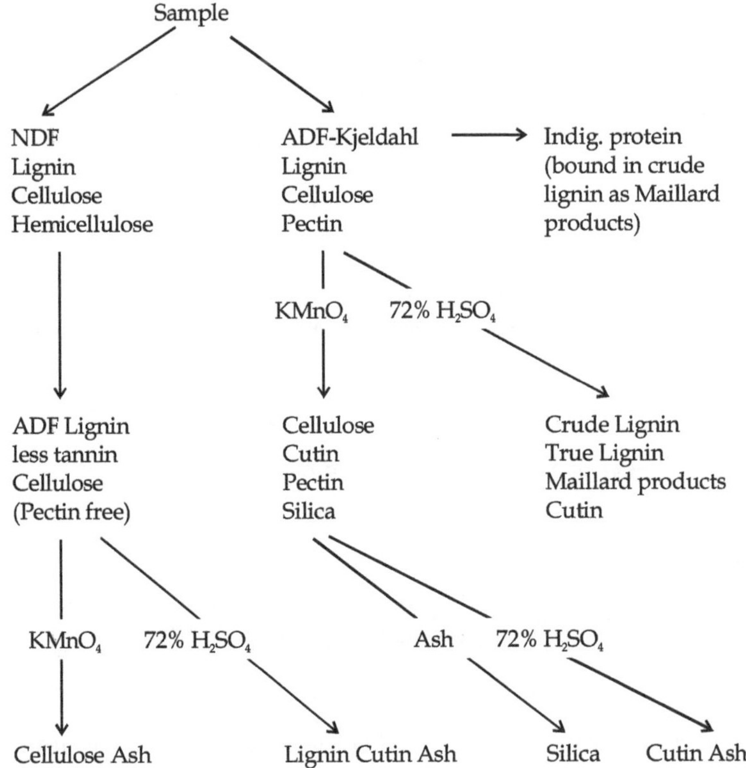

Fig. 1 : Sequences of analytical treatments of feed samples subjected to the detergent system: pretreatment with neutral detergent dissolve tannins, pectins and opaline silica that would otherwise contribute to acid-detergent fiber; permanganate removes tannins but not cutin.

Source : Nutrition Research Techniques for Domestic and Wild Animals, Inst. of Animal Nutrition, Agricultural University of Norway, Ås-NLH, Norway (Year 1972)

Classification III

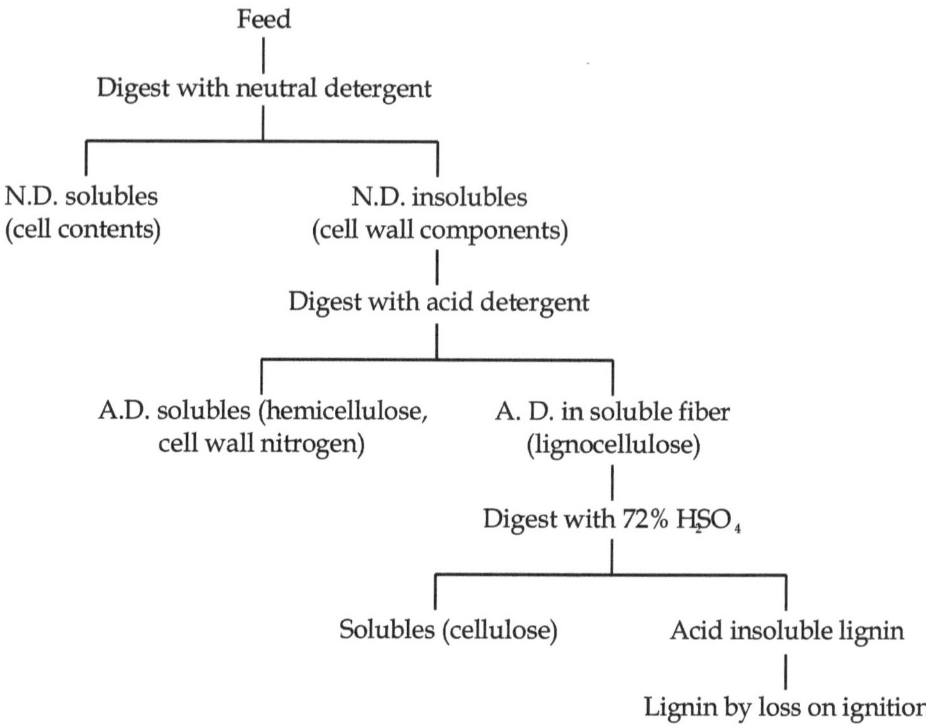

Source : Nutrition Research Techniques for Domestic and Wild Animals, Instt. of Animal Nutrition, Agricultural University of Norway, Ås-NLH, Norway.

Fonnesbeck and Harris System of Analysis

Classification IV

1. Cell contents percent = 100 percent – cell walls percent.
2. Cellulose percent = cell walls percent – (hemicellulose percent +lignin percent +acid insoluble ash percent).
3. Soluble ash percent = ash percent – acid insoluble ash percent.
4. Soluble carbohydrate percent = cell contents percent – (protein percent +ether extract percent + soluble ash percent.)

Source : Nutrition Research Techniques for Domestic and Wild Animals, Instt. of Animal Nutrition, Agricultural University of Norway, Ås-NLH, Norway (1972).

Classification V

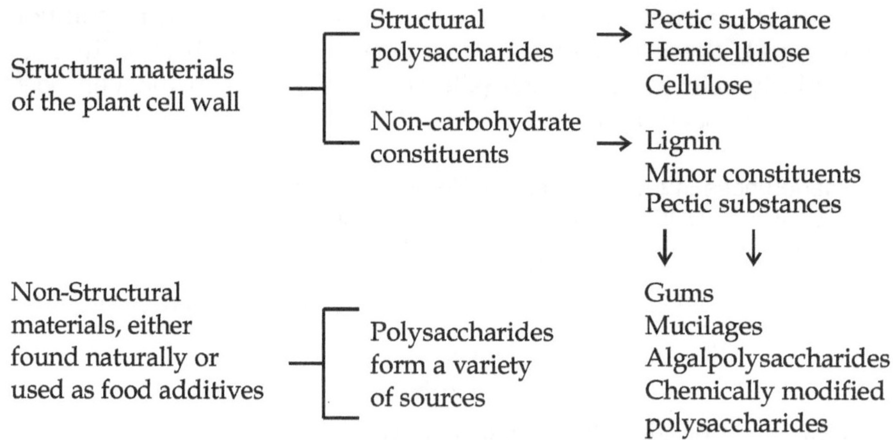

Source : Nutrition Research Techniques for Domestic and Wild Animals, Instt. of Animal Nutrition, Agricultural University of Norway, Ås-NLH, Norway (1972).

Improvement Over Van Soest System of Analysis

Van Soest's procedure was developed to analyse forages, however, extreme filtering difficulties are encountered when attempting to analyse feeds, protein supplements of mixed diets.

Background

Fonnesbeck and Harris have developed a cell wall procedure that more accurately partitions the cell wall constituents and may be used to analyse all types of feeds. The cell contents include nutritive matter that is digestible by enzymes secreted by the digestive system or is otherwise soluble enough for absorption. This includes soluble carbohydrates, protein, lipids. (ether extract) and soluble ash.

The plant cell wall constituents (cell wall) include, partially nutritive matter, cell wall carbohydrates. cellulose and hemicellulose, and are digested only by enzymes produced by micro organism within in the digestive tract. The nutritive value and digestibility of cellulose and hemicellulose may not differ enough to warrant their separation for most animals and the cell wall carbohydrate can be combined and reported as holocellulose. The non-nutritive matter includes lignin and acid insoluble ash (mostly silica). These constituents have no known nutritive value of animals. This system requires analyses for dry matter, ash, protein, ether extract, cell walls, lignin and acid insoluble ash. If it is desired to partition the cell wall carbohydrate into cellulose and hemicellulose, the hemicellulose analysis is also necessary.

Deviations from Van Soest Method of Analysis

1. Cell wall is determined at pH 3 in a citrate buffered detergent solution. At this pH, there is a greater recovery of cell wall constituents, particularly acid insoluble ash (silica). Interferences in the Van Soest method have been demonstrated in Table 1.

Table 1 : Interferences in the estimation of Hemicellulose as the difference between neutral detergent fiber (NDF) and acid detergent fiber (ADF)

Fraction	Recovery in		Influence on
	NDF	ADF	Hemicellulose Estimate
Cell wall protein	Recovered	Largely dissolved	Increase
Biogenic silica	Considerable solution	Quantitative recovery	Decrease
Pectin	Dissolved	Partial Precipitation	Decrease
Tannin	Dissolved	Precipitation as protein complex	Decrease

2. A pepsin digestion of this cell wall sample followed by detergent extraction removes 90 to 98 percent of the protein. Less than 1 percent protein of a sample containing 10 percent protein would be retained in the cell wall residue.

3. *In Van Soest's analysis, cellulose is determined as the difference between acid detergent fiber and acid detergent lignin or as the organic residue from the determination of permanganate lignin (Van Soest, 1967). Hemicellulose is calculated as the difference between cell wall constituents and acid detergent fiber (Keystal, 1969). Fonnesbeck and Harris (1971) separated the cellulose and hemicellulose of the cell wall with a hemicellulose and lignin analyses.*

4. Lignin values determined directly on the cell wall residue or on a hemicellulose extracted cell wall residue are considerably higher than acid detergent lignin values. Subsequent investigations showed that the acid detergent solution was dissolving part of the lignin. With the improvements in the cell wall analysis, the acid detergent preparation is considered unnecessary.

5. The techniques of the 72 percent sulphuric acid lignin method by Fonnesbeck and Harris (1970) make it unnecessary to add asbestos to the crucible to aid in filtering. Therefore, the ash remaining after the

lignin determination is entirely from the original sample and can be reported as acid insoluble ash or the acid insoluble ash can be extracted with 48 percent hydrobromic acid for a presumptive analysis for silica.

A. Cell Contents

Principle

The more readily utilizable nutrients are enclosed by the cell wall and can be grouped as cell contents. These include the protein, soluble carbohydrate, soluble minerals and lipids. A high percentage of cell contents is a good index of high nutritive value of a feed. The cell content is determined as the difference between the percent cell walls and 100 percent .

Calculation

Cell contents (percent) on dry basis = 100 percent – Cell walls (percent) on dry basis.

Example

If the percent cell walls on the dry basis is 49.8 percent then cell contents (percent) on dry basis = 100 - 49.8 = 50.2 percent cell contents.

B. Cell Wall (Neutral Detergent Fiber)

Reagents

1. Neutral detergent solution:

Distilled water	1 litre
Sodium lauryl sulphate USP	30 g
Disodium ethylene diaminetetra acetate (EDTA), dihydrate crystal, (Reagent grade)	18.61 g
Sodium borate decahydrate, (Reagent grade)	6.81 g
Disodium hydrogen phosphate, anhydrous, (Reagent grade)	4.56 g
2-ethoxy ethanol (ethylene glycol monoethyl ether) [Purified grade]	10 ml

Put EDTA and Na_2B_4O7. 10 H_2O together in a large beaker, add some distilled water, and heat until dissolved then add to solution containing sodium lauryl sulphate and 2-ethoxyethanol (ethylene glycol monoethyl ether). Put Na_2 HPO_4 in beaker, add some distilled water, and heat until dissolved, then add to solution containing other ingredients. Check pH to range 6.9 to 7.1. If solution is properly made, pH adjustment will rarely be required.

2. Decalin, decahydronaphthalene, (Reagent grade).
3. Acetone, (Reagent grade).
4. Sodium sulphite, (Reagent grade).

Proceture

1. Weigh by difference approximately 1.0 g sample that has been ground to pass through a 0.1 cm sieve and place the sample in Berzelius beaker for refluxing.
2. Add, in order, 100 ml cold (room temperature) neutral detergent solution, 2 ml decalin and 0.5 g sodium sulphite with a calibrated scoop. Heat to boiling in 5 to 10 min. Reduce heat as boiling begins, to avoid foaming. Adjust boiling to an even level and reflux for 60 min, timed from onset of boiling.
3. Place previously weighed crucibles on filtering apparatus. Swirl beaker to suspend solids and fill crucible. Do not admit vacuum at first, increase it only as more force is needed. Rinse sample into crucible with a minimum of hot (80°C) water. Remove vacuum, break up material and fill crucible with hot water. Filter liquid and repeat washing procedure.
4. Wash twice with acetone in same manner and suck dry later, dry crucibles at 105°C overnight and weigh.
5. Report yield of recovered neutral detergent fiber as cell walls (NDF)

Calculation

Name of sample : Rice polish

(NDF) Cell walls percent on dry matter basis

$$= \frac{\text{Wt. of crucible and cell walls} - \text{Wt. of crucible}}{\text{Wt. of sample on dry matter basis}} \times 100\text{g}$$

Example

1. Weight of crucible 22.172 g
2. Weight of crucible and cell walls 22.670 g
3. Weight of sample on dry matter basis 1 g

Cell wall percent on dry matter basis $= \frac{22.670 - 22.172}{1} \times 100$

Result : 49.8% cell wall (49.8 g per 100g dry matter)

Modified Neutral Detergent Fiber Method

(Method of Robertson and Van Soest, 1977)

The original neutral detergent fiber (NDF) was developed by Goering and Van Soest (1970), for the purpose of determining the indigestible component of forages. The method measures, in essence, total cell wall material. In some cases it may underestimate total dietary fiber because of a loss of water soluble polysaccharides (Robertson,1980).

Because of the high starch content of human foods in comparison to forages on which the method was tested, an overestimation of cell wall content occures with the NDF method due to starch remaining in the residue. A modified procedure was developed by Robertson and Van Soest (1977) in which a detergent stable bacterial alpha amylase is used to hydrolyse the starches. The amylase is derived from *Bacillus subtilus*.

Schaller (1978) used a hog-pancreas enzyme, this procedure requires separate treatment with enzyme at pH 4.5 and filtration after detergent extraction.

The various steps of this method are

Air dried or fresh sample
(0.5 - 1 g)
↓
Boil under reflux with buffered SLS solution containing
borate, phosphate and EDTA
(30 min.)
↓
Add 2 ml amylase and reflux for another 30 min.
↓
Filter, wash with hot water and acetone
↓
Dry and weigh
↓
Ignite at 550°C
↓
Reweigh
↓
Neutral detergent fiber (loss in weight after ignition), (NDF)

Acid Detergent Fiber (ADF)

Principle

The acid detergent fiber procedure provides a rapid method for lignocellulose determination in feedstuffs. The residue also includes silica. The difference between the cell walls and acid detergent fiber is an estimate of hemicellulose;

however, this difference does include some protein attached to cell walls. The acid detergent fiber is used as a preparatory step for lignin determination. Hemicellulose can be estimated from the difference between cell wall constituents and acid detergent fiber.

Cellulose = ADF - ADL

Hemicellulose = NDF - ADF

Equipment

Same as used with cell wall (neutral detergent fiber) analysis procedure as mentioned above.

Reagent

1. *Acid detergent solution. Sulphuric acid, Reagent grade standardized to 1 N. This is achieved by adding 49.04 g (correct for assay) sulphuric acid within each litre of distilled water. For 18 l of solution if requires 882.72 g of H_2SO_4. Add 20 g of cetyle trimethylammonium bromide (CTAB), technical grade to one litre of 1 N H_2SO_4 solution, or 360 g per 18 l. Stir to facilitate solution.*
2. *Decalin, technical grade decahydronaphthalene.*
3. *Acetone, Reagent grade.*
4. *Hexane, Reagent grade.*

Procedure

1. Weigh by difference approximately 1 g of sample into a beaker or container suitable for refluxing.
2. Add 100 ml cold (room temperature) acid detergent solution and 2 ml decahydronaphthalene. Heat to boiling in 5 to 10 min. Reduce heat to avoid foaming as boiling begins. Reflux 60 min from onset of boiling, adjusting boiling to a slow, even level.
3. Filter on a previously weighed crucible, which is set on the filtering apparatus, using light suction. Break up the filtered material with a rod and wash twice with hot water (90° to 100°C). Rinse sides of the crucible in the same manner.
4. Repeat washing with acetone until it removes no more colour. breaking up all lumps so that the solvent comes into contact with all particles of fiber.
5. Wash with hexane: Hexane should be added while crucible still contains some acetone (Hexane can be omitted if lumping is not a problem). Suck the acid detergent fiber free of hexane and dry at 105°C for 8 h or overnight, cool in a desiccator to room temperature and weigh.

Calculation

Acid detergent fiber percent on dry matter basis.

$$= \frac{(\text{Wt. of crucible} + \text{fiber} - \text{empty weight of crucible})}{\text{Wt. of sample on dry matter basis}} \times 100$$

Example

ADF (acid detergent fiber)

1. Empty weight of crucible = 22.933 g
2. Weight of crucible + ADF = 23.136
3. Weight of sample = 1 g

ADF = $\frac{(23.136 - 22.933)}{1} \times 100$

ADF = 20.3 g/100 g

Acid Detergent Lignin (ADL)

Principle

The acid detergent lignin (ADL) procedure utilized the acid detergent fiber procedure as a preparatory step. The detergent removes the protein and other acid soluble material which would interfere with the lignin determination. The principle of the procedure is that acid detergent fiber residue is primarily lignocellulose of which the cellulose is dissolved by 72 percent sulphuric acid solution. The remaining residue consists of lignin and acid insoluble ash, however, with sample containing large amounts of cutin, this is also measured as part of the lignin.

Equipment

1. *All equipment required for determination of cell walls as mentioned above.*
2. *Glass tray.*
3. *Muffle furnace, temperature controlled at 500°C.*

Reagents

Sulphuric acid, 72 percent by weight. Calculate the number of grams of acid and water needed in one litre of solution by:

$$\frac{100 \times 98.08 \times 12\,\text{moles}}{H_2SO_4\ \text{assay (percent)}} = \text{g acid needed}$$

Weight of one litre of 72 percent H_2SO_4

(1000 x 1.634) – g acid = g water needed

Take calculated amount of water into one litre volumetric flask (with a bulb in the neck) and add the calculated amount of sulphuric acid slowly with occasional swirling.

Precautions

Flask must be cooled in water bath (sink) in order to add the required weight of sulphuric acid. Cool to 20°C and check if volume is correct. If volume is too small, take out about 1.5 ml and add 2.5 ml water. Repeat, if necessary. If volume is too large, take out 5 ml and add 4.45 ml H_2SO_4. Meniscus should be within a 0.5 cm of calibration mark at 20°C.

Procedure

1. The first step is to prepare acid detergent fiber as prescribed previously.
2. Place the crucibles in the glass tray. Have one end of the tray 2 cm higher so acid will drain away from the crucibles.
3. Cover the contents of the crucible with cooled (5°C) 72 percent H_2SO_4 and stir with a glass rod to a smooth paste, breaking all lumps. Fill crucible half way with acid and stir. Let glass rod remain in crucible. Refill with 72 percent sulphuric acid and stir at hourly intervals as acid drains away. Crucibles do not need to be kept full at all times. Three additions suffice.
4. Keep crucibles at 20°C to 23°C.
5. After three hours, filter off as much acid as possible with vacuum. Rinse the residue once with 72 percent acid and filter it off.
6. Wash contents with hot water (85°C to 95°C) until free from acid. Rinse and remove stirring rod.
7. Dry crucible overnight at 100°C and weigh.
8. Ignite crucible in a muffle furnace at 500°C for three hours. Cool to 250°C and transfer to a desiccator. Cool to room temperature and weigh.

Calculation

Lignin (%) on 100 percent dry matter basis

$$= \frac{(\text{Wt. of crucible and lignin} - \text{Wt. of crucible and ash})}{\text{Wt. of sample on dry matter basis}} \times 100$$

Example

Name of sample: Timothy hay

1. Weight of sample on dry matter basis = 1.913 g

2. Weight of crucible and lignin = 18.1742 g
3. Weight of crucible and ash = 18.1047 g

$$\text{Lignin percent} = \frac{18.1742 - 18.1047}{1.913} \times 100$$

$$= 3.633 \text{ g/100 g}$$

Permanganate Lignin, Cellulose and Silica (Insoluble Ash)

Principle

An indirect method, for lignin utilizing permanganate allows the determination of cellulose and insoluble ash in the same sample. The insoluble ash is an estimate of silica content, which in many grasses is a primary factor in reducing digestibility. The permanganate lignin method is an alternate procedure to the 72 percent sulphuric acid method; each has its own advantages. The choice of methods will depend on materials analysed and on the purpose for which the values are to be used.

Advantage of the Permanganate Method Over the 72 percent Acid Method

1. It is a shorter procedure.
2. The permanganate reagents are much less corrosive and require no standardization.
3. Values are less affected by heat damage of artifacts and are closer to a true lignin figure.

Disadvantage of the permanganate Method over the 72 percent Acid Method

1. The cutin which is important in many seed hulls, is not measured. A variation of the analysis of seed hulls is to prepare the permanganate cellulose and treat with 72 percent sulphuric acid and asbestos for three hours.
2. The disadvantage of the permanganate method is that large particles are poorly penetrated by the reagent and yield low values. Consequently material high in water content must be partially dried and ground through a 0.1 cm sieve, and the method is not applicable to fresh faeces and forages, which have been ground in a meat grinder. *Because of higher sensitivity to heat damage, 72 percent acid method is preferred for assaying artifact lignin.*

Theory of the Method

Interfering matter fiber removed by preparing acid-detergent, which is chiefly composed of lignin, cellulose and insoluble minerals. Lignin is oxidized with an excess of acetic acid buffered potassium permanganate solution, containing trivalent iron and monovalent silver as catalysts. Deposited manganese and iron oxides are dissolved with an alcoholic solution of oxalic acid, hydrochloric acids leaving cellulose and insoluble minerals. Lignin is measured as the weight lost by these treatments, while cellulose is determined as the weight loss upon ashing. The ash residue is mainly silica and much of the non-silica matter can be removed by leaching with concentrated hydrobromic acid.

Equipment

Same as for acid detergent lignin is mentioned above.

Reagents

1. *Saturated potassium permanganate. Dissolve 50 g potassium permanganate and 0.05 g silver sulphuric in one litre distilled water. Keep out of direct sunlight. Add silver sulphate to dehalogenate the reagent.*
2. *Lignin buffer solution. For one litre, dissolve 6 g ferric nitrate non-ahydrate* [$Fe(NO_3)_3 \cdot 9H_2O$] *and 0.15 g silver nitrate in 100 ml distilled water. Combine with 500 ml glacial acetic acid and 5g potassium acetate (Reagent grade). Add 400 ml tertiary butyl alcohol (Reagent grade) and mix. For 12 litre, use the following amount of chemicals.*

Ferric nitrate non-ahydrate	= *72 g*
Silver nitrate	= *1.8 g*
Acetic acid	= *6.0 l*
Potassium acetate	= *60 g*
b-butyl alcohol	= *4.8 l*
Distilled water	= *1.2 l*

3. *Combined permanganate solution: Combine and mix saturated potassium permanganate and the lignin buffer solution in the ratio of 2:1 by volume before use. Unused mixed solution may be kept about a week in a refrigerator in the absence of light. Solution is usable if it is purple in colour and contains no precipitate.*
4. *Demineralizing solution: For 1 l, dissolve 50 g oxalic acid dihydrate in 700 ml 95 percent ethyl alcohol. Add 50 ml concentrated (approximately 12 N) hydrochloric acid and 250 ml distilled water and mix. For 18 l use the following amount of chemicals:*

Oxalic acid	= *900 g*
95% ethanol	= *12.6 l*

Conc. hydrochloric acid = *900 ml*
Distilled water = *4.5 l*

5. *Ethyl alcohol (80 percent). For one l mix 155 ml distilled water and 845 ml 95 percent ethyl alcohol. For 18l, mix 2.8l distilled water and 15.2l 95 percent ethyl alcohol.*
6. *Hydrobromic acid (Reagent grade).*

Procedure

1. The residue from the acid detergent fiber determination may be used (use original weight of samples for calculation).
2. Weigh approximately 1 g sample that has been ground through 1 mm sieve. If sample contains over 15 percent lignin, use 0.5 g
3. Place crucible in a muffle at 500°C for an hour or longer. Cool in desiccator to room temperature and weigh.
4. Prepare acid detergent fiber according to the procedure mentioned previously.
5. Place crucibles containing the acid detergent fiber in a shallow enameled tray containing approximately 1 cm deep cold water. Fiber in crucibles should not be wet.
6. Combine and mix saturated potassium permanganate and buffer solution 2:1 by volume and add approximately 25 ml of the crucibles. Do not overfill. Adjust level of water in pan to reduce flow of solution out of crucibles. Place a short glass rod in each crucible to stir contents, to break lumps and to draw permanganate solution up on sides of crucibles to wet all particles.
7. Allow crucibles to stand 90 ± 10 min. at temperature of 20° to 25°C adding more mixed permanganate solution if necessary. Purple colour must be present at all times.
8. Remove crucibles to filtering apparatus and filter off visible liquid. Do not wash. Place in a clean enamel tray, and fill crucibles not more than half full with demineralizing solution. After about five minutes, filter off visible liquid and refill halfway with demineralizing solution. Care must be taken to avoid spillage by foaming. Repeat the demineralizing solution treatment a third time if the filtrate from the second treatment is very brown. Rinse down the sides of the crucibles with a fine stream of demineralizing solution from a squeeze bottle. Treat until fiber is white. Total time required is 20 to 30 min.
9. Fill and thoroughly wash crucible and contents with 80 percent ethyl alcohol, filter off liquid and repeat washing two times. Wash and filter in similar manner using acetone.

10. *Lignin content :* Dry at 105°C overnight, cool in desiccator and weigh. Calculate lignin content as loss in weight from acid-detergent fiber.
11. *Cellulose content :* Ash at 500°C for three hours, cool in a desiccator and weigh. Loss in weight equals cellulose.
12. *Silica content :* A presumptive analysis for silica may be obtained by leaching contents of crucibles under S.No. (11) with concentrated hydrobromic acid (48%) until no further colour is removed. Wash sample with acetone (Use no water), and filter. Ash at 500°C for three hours. cool in a desiccator and weigh (this step is not necessary if residual ash is less than 2 percent of the original sample).

Precautions

Crucibles containing fiber of a high lignin content will require more permanganate solution: however, avoid additions of more solution than is necessary. Appearance of a yellow or brown colour indicates exhaustion of permanganate. If crucible is full, filter off solution on a vacuum and add more reagent. A yellow colour persisting after treatment of fiber with demineralizing solution indicates incomplete removal of lignin content. This will occur only in materials of a very high lignin content. The cutin material present in seed coates and other plant parts is not oxidized by permanganate and thus is neither determined as lignin nor bleached with the treatment. Seed coats will appear as coloured flakes among white cellulose particles and should not be confused with incomplete oxidation.

Excessive flow of permanganate solution through the crucibles should be avoided with samples of low lignin content, particularly in the case of immature grasses. In this method a single addition of permanganate solution suffices. Fiber from immature grasses is very rapidly delignified and there is danger in these materials of loss of cellulose carbohydrates if there is too much flow. Reduction in flow is accomplished by adjusting tray water level to near the brim of crucibles. These precautions are not needed with the demineralizing solution.

Calculation

1. Lignin percent on dry matter basis

$$= \frac{\text{Wt. acid detergent fiber} - \text{Wt. permanganate fiber residue}}{\text{Wt. of sample on dry matter basis taken for ADF analysis}} \times 100$$

2. Cellulose/percent on dry matter basis

   Wt. of crucible and permanganate fiber residue:

$$= \frac{\text{Wt. of crucible and ash}}{\text{Wt. of smple on dry matter basis taken for ADF analysis}} \times 100$$

3. Silica percent on dry matter basis

$$\frac{\text{Wt. of ash after hydrogen bromide washing}}{\text{Wt.of sample on dry matter basis taken for ADF analysis}} \times 100$$

Results: Expressed as g/100g

Example

Name fo sample : Rice polish

(a) **Lignin percent on dry matter basis**

(i) Weight of acid detergent fiber = 23.136 g

(ii) Weight of permanganate fiber residue = 23.117 g

(iii) Weight of dried sample = 1 g

Lignin percent $= \frac{23.136 - 23.117}{1} \times 100$

= 1.9 percent lignin, g/100g

(b) **Cellulose percent on dry matter basis**

(i) Weight of permanganate fiber residue = 23.117 g

(ii) Weight of crucible and ash = 22.991 g

(iii) Weight of dried sample = 1 g

Cellulose percent $= \frac{23.117 - 22.991}{1} \times 100$

= 12.6 percent cellulose g/100g

(c) **Silica percent on dry matte basis**

(i) Weight of empty crucible = 23.933 g

(ii) Weight of crucible + ash after hydrogen bromide washing = 22.959 g

(iii) Weight of dried sample = 1 g

Silica percent $= \frac{22.959 - 22.933}{1} \times 100$

= 2.6 percent silica, g/100g

Estimation of Unavailable Carbohydrates or Dietary Fiber in Foods (Method Southgate, 1969)

Southgate recommended the use of amyloglucosidase at 37°C for 18 h to remove starches from food samples. In this procedure using hydrolytic techniques unavailable carbohydrates are measured by the liberation of sugar components. The method gives values for two types of non-cellulose polysaccharides: those that are water-soluble and hydrolysable with dilute acid, and the cellulose and other associated non-cellulose pentosans and lignin.

The outline of Southgate's fractionation method is given in Chart 1.

Chart 1 : Southgate's Fractionation Method

Part - A

(Air dried sample, fresh or freeze dried)

↓

Extract with hot 85% V/V methanol at least four times

↓

Extract residue with diethyl ether, dry and grind.

↓

Weigh residue and take a portion (0.1 - 0.5 g)

↓

Incubate with takadiastase (amyloglucosidase) pH 4.5 - 5 (37°C 18 h)

↓

Add 4 volumes ethanol, centrifuge (or filter)

Part - B

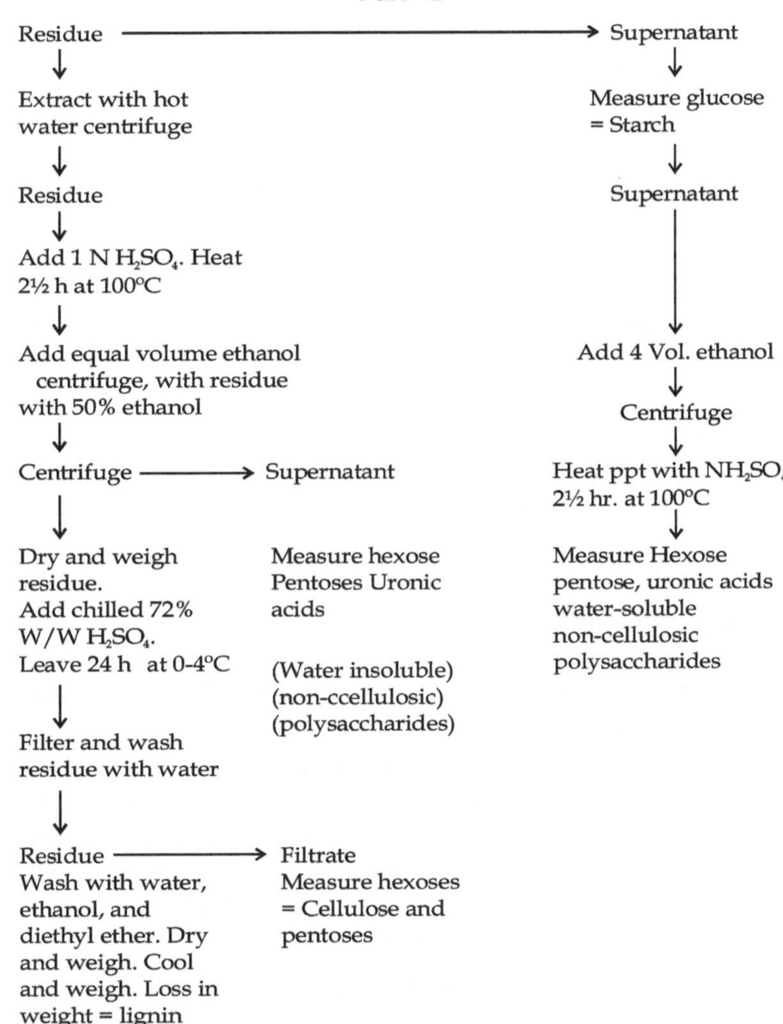

Procedure of the Southgate's Fractionation Method

1. Preparation of the sample.
2. Extraction of free sugars and preparation of the residue insoluble in 85% V/V methanol.
3. Enzymatic hydrolysis of starch.
4. Extraction of water-soluble material.
5. Hydrolysis with dilute acid.
6. Extraction of cellulose.

Preparation of Sample

The sample for analysis should be homogenous and representative one. Heating can often lead to the formation of condensation products between phenolic constituents and protein, which analyse as lignin. When it is necessary to dry a food. freeze-drying is the method of choice. Most fresh foods can be extracted directly with 85% (V/V) methanol. We should homogenize the sample only after freeze-drying to avoid enzymatic modifications that may occur when the cells are disrupted.

Extraction of Free Sugars and Preparation of a Residue Insoluble in 85% (V/V) Methanol.

Reagent

85% (V/V aqueous methanol)

Procedure

Weigh out duplicate portions of between 3 and 5 g (dry weight or equivalent) into weighed 100 ml beakers and add 25 ml 85% (V/V) methanol. Stir with a glass rod while bringing the mixture to the boil on an electric hot-plate. Filter hot through a whatman 541 paper (if sugars are to be measured in the sample, the filtration is made into a 100 ml volumetric flask). Repeat this process with 3 further portions of aqueous methanol, allowing the filter to drain between successive extractions. In the second and subsequent extractions it is essential to stir the mixture continuously while it is being heated to avoid losses through "bumping". Then extract the residue in the beaker and on the filter in a similar way with three portions of diethy ether and discard the extracts.

Allow the residue to dry in air and return to the original beaker. Heat the beaker and contents at 98-100°C for 10 min. in an air oven to remove residual solvent, allow to cool in air overnight and then reweigh. The residue should then be finely ground and stored in an air tight container.

☞ **Notes**

1. *If a fresh sample is being extracted, adjust the concentration of methanol added initially so that the first extraction is made at 85% (V/V).*
2. *This can be carried out in a fume cupboard but in practice the amount of solvent released are quite small. When using diethyl ether it is essential to ensure that spark-free apparatus is used.*
3. *The residue should only be returned to the beaker when it is dry and crumbles easily. Scrap the filter paper gently with a spatula to ensure quantitative transfer.*

Calculation : The residue insoluble in 85% (V/V) methanol is expressed as a proportion of the original sample. Fractionation of polysaccharides in the residue insoluble in 85% (V/V) methanol.

Enzymatic Hydrolysis of Starch

Reagents

(i) *2M acetate buffer pH 4.6*

(ii) *Takadiastase. Shake 10 g with 100 ml. Centrifuge and use supernatant.*

Procedure: Weigh out duplicate portions of about 200-300 mg (ideally containing approximately 100 mg starch) into a clean dry 50 ml centrifuge tube. Add 4 ml of hot water and stir with a glass rod. Place the tubes in a boiling water bath for 10 minutes to gelatinize the starch in the sample, cool and then add 0.2 ml of 2M acetate buffer (pH 4.6) followed by 1 ml of 10% Takadiastase, Mix the contents of the tube with the rod and "police down" any particles above the level of the liquid. Add a few drops of toluene and incubate at 37°C overnight.

The next morning add 4 volumes of ethanol (20 ml), performing the addition in two stages, stirring the mixture thoroughly after the first addition and finally rinsing the rod with the last drop of the ethanol. Leave the mixture for about 10 min. allow the precipitate to form then centrifuge for 10 min. 2500 rpm. Pour off the supernatant carefully into a volumetric flask (100 ml if the sample contains appreciable amount of starch, 50 ml if very low). Wash the residue by resuspending it in 10 ml of 80% (V/V) ehhanol and recentrifuge. Pour off the supernatant and combine it with the previous supernatant.

Make up the combine supernatants to volume, and label these as S (Starch) extracts. Glucose is measured in these extracts.

Extraction of Water-Soluble Material

Heat the tubes containing the residue after treatment with Takadiastase in a boiling water bath to drive off the ethanol. (Addition of a few ml of water at this stage is useful). When the tubes are free of ethanol, add 100 ml of hot (near boiling) water and stir with a glass rod. Leave the tubes in the water bath for 20 min, then centrifuge and pour off the supernatant. Repeat the extraction and combine the supernatants.

When the supernatants are cool, add 4 volumes of ethanol and centrifuge. Wash the precipitate by resuspension in 80% (V/V) ethanol and centrifuge. Resuspend the residue in 10 ml of N H_2SO_4 and heat in a boiling water bath for 2.5 h. Dilute the hydrolysates to volume and measure monosaccharides and uronic acids. Label the extracts W (Water extract).

☞ **Note**

Benzoic acid is added to the extracts as a preservative at this stage and all subsequent stages.

Hydrolysis with dilute acid

Suspend the residue after water extraction in the centrifuge tube with 10 ml of N H_2SO_4, cover the tube with a marble or perforated polythene and heat the tube in a boiling water-bath for 2.5 h. Mix the contents of the tube after 1h (if particles of the residues have been carried up the wall of the tube it may be necessary to rinse them back with additional acid. Allow the tubes and contents to cool, add an equal volume of ethanol and then centrifuge or filter the contents.

Centrifugation: Pour the supernatant carefully into a volumetric flask and wash the resuspension in 50% (V/V) ethanol and recentrifuge. Repeat this washing procedure and combine the supernatants. Finally wash the residue in the same way with ethanol and diethyl ether and allow the residue to dry in air.

Filteration: Filter the hydrolysate through a weighed sintered glass filter crucible (porosity 1). Wash the residue in the filter thoroughly with 50% (V/V) ethanol and transfer the aqueous alcoholic filtrate to a volumetric flask. Finally wash the residue with ethanol and diethyl ether and suck the crucible dry. Heat the crucible for 10 min. at 96-100°C, cool and weigh. Dilute the aqueous supernatant or filtrate to volume and measure hexoses, pentoses and uronic acids.

☞ **Notes**

1. *It is extremely difficult to filter at this stage, centrifugation is the only practical procedure. It is more time consuming.*
2. *The size of sintered glass filter crucible depends on the size of particles of sample being analysed.*

Extraction of Cellulose

Reagents

72 percent (W/W) sulphuric acid.

Procedure

Add chilled 72 percent (W/W) sulphuric acid to the dry residue (either in a centrifuge tube or on the sintered glass crucible) after dilute hydrolysis and stir gently. Stand the sintered crucibles in small beakers during this procedure. Leave the residue in content with the acid for a least 24 h at 0-4°C, stirring the mixture at intervals during the first few hours.

At the conclusion of this period, either filter the mixture through a sintered glass crucible as described above or rinse the exterior of the crucible into the beaker and wash the residue in the filter thoroughly with water. Dilute the aqueous filtrates to volume and measure hexoses, pentoses and uronic acids.

Wash the residue on the filter with ethanol followed by diethyl ether. Heat the crucible in an oven and reweigh. The gain in weight is taken lignin.

Limitations: This system has the benefit of recovering the pectins in the non-cellulosic polysaccharide fraction. However, the system is not favourable to rapid analysis and the precision of the chemical methods may not justify the time and labour required.

Total sugars in Molasses
(Method of AOAC, 1979)
Reagents

1. Fehlings's solution (Soxhlet modification)

   (a) Dissolve 34.639 g of copper sulphate $5H_2O$ in water and make up to 500 ml. Filter (b) Dissolve 173 g of potassium sodium tartrate $4H_2O$ and 50 g sodium hydroxide in water, dilute to 500 ml, stand for two days and filter through prepared asbestos.

2. Invert Sugar Standards. *Prepare stock solution by adding 5 ml of hydrochloric acid (Sp. gravity 1.18) to 9.5 g of sucrose in solution and dilute to around 100 ml. After storing for two days at room temperature, dilute to one. Prepare working solutions (5 mg/ml) by pipetting 100 ml of the stock solution into a 200 ml volumetric flask and neutralizing with 20 percent sodium hydroxide using phenolphthalein as indicator. Dilute to mark, and mix.*

3. *Hydrochloric acid (Sp. gravity 1.18)*

4. *Hydrochloric acid (0.5 N)*

5. *Sodium hydroxide (20%)*

6. *Phenolphthalein indicator (1% solution in alcohol)*

7. *Methylene blue indicator (1% aqueous solution).*

Apparatus

1. Electirc heater
2. Conical flask, 300 ml

Method

Sample preparation: For dried molasses, take an 8 g sample and shake with water, (250 ml preheated to 60°C) in a 500 ml volumetric flask for 30 min. Allow to cool then dilute to volume. Filter, discarding first 25 ml of filtrate. For liquids, dissolve 8 g and make up to 500 ml. Carry out an acid hydrolysis on 100 ml of the filtrate by adding 5 ml of hydrochloric acid (Sp. gravity 1.18) allowing to stand for 24 h. Neutralize with sodium hydroxide (20%) using phenolphthalein as indicator and then dilute to 200 ml.

Standardization of Soxhlet Solution

Pipette 10 ml of Soxhlet solutions (a) and (b) a conical flask, mix and add 30 ml of water. Add from a burette a volume of working standard that is almost sufficient to reduce the copper in the Soxhlet solution. Bring to boiling and continue boiling for two minutes. Add four drops of methylene blue and rapidly, complete the titration, while still boiling, until a bright orange colour is resumed. Repeat several times and determine the volume of solution required to completely reduce 20 ml of Soxhlet solution.

Titration of Sample

First, carry out an approximate titration: Pipette 10 ml of solution (a) and (b) into a flask add a 10 ml aliquot of the sample solution. Add 40 ml of water and bring to boil. If blue colour persist titrate with working standard solution and calculate the approximate sugar content of the sample.

Table 2 : Sample Volumes Used in Soxhlet Titration

ml H_2O	ml Sample	Sample aliquot, g	Total sugar as invert, %
40	10	0.08	73
35	15	0.12	82-58
30	20	0.16	61-41
25	25	0.20	49-35
20	30	0.14	41-29

Source : AOAC, 1970

To determine accurately the sugar content, pipette 10 ml of Soxhlet solution (a) and (b) into a flask and add an aliquot of the sample solution. The volume of sample used will depend on the sugar content of the sample.

Add water as indicated in Table 16.2, mix and boil. During boiling add a quantity of working standard from a burette so that the titration is nearly complete. Add methylene blue and complete the titration. Calculate % Sugar (as invert) by the formula.

% Sugar = $(F - M) \times 1 \times 100/W$, where F is the volume of standard needed to reduce 20 ml of Soxhlet solution. M is the volume of standard sugar solution required to complete the back titration, 1 is the weight of invert sugar in 1 ml of working standard an W is weight of sample in aliquot used.

References

AOAC, (1970). Official Methods of analysis of the Association of Official Agricultural Chemists. 10th Edn. AOAC Benjamin Franklin Station, Washington, D.C. pp. 540.

Fonnesbeck, P.V. and L.E. Harris, (1970). *Proc. Amer. Soc. Animal Sci. Western Sec.,* 21: 153.

_______, (1971). *Proc Amer. Soc. Animal Sci. Western Sec.,* 22: 77.

Goerring, H.K. and P.J. Van Soest, (1970). *Forage fiber analyses (apparatus, reagents, procedures and some applications).* ARS U.S. Dept. Agr. Handbook, No. 379, Superintendent of Documents, U.S., Government Printing Office, Washington , D.C., 20402.

Krishna, G. (1983). Note on nutritive value of paddy straw ensiled with some Agro-Industrial byproducts and its effect on the growth of calves. *Tropical and Animal Science Res.* 1: 194.

Krishna, G. (1982). Nutritional evaluation of a new maintenance ration fodder for feeding adult buffaloes. *I. World Review of Animal Production* 18: 29-37.

Robertson, J.B. and Van Soest, P.J. (1977). *J. Anim. Sci.* 45: 254.

Schaller. D.R. (1978) *Am. J. Clin. Nutr.,* 31: 599.

Southgate, D.A. (1969). *J. Sci. Fd. Agric.,* 20: 331.

Tewatia, B.S. and Krishna, G. (1991). Fodder tree leaves as Animal Feed II. Cell Wall Contents and *in vitro* dry matter digestibility of some tree leaves and shrubs in Arid and Semi arid zones. *The J. of the Remount and Vety. Corps.* 30: 35-43.

Van Soest , P.J. (1963). *J. Assoc. Off. Agr. Chem.,* 46: 829.

________, (1967). *J. Animal Sci.,* 26: 119.

Van Soest, P.J. and R.H. Wine, (1968). *J. Assoc. Off Agr. Chem.,* 51: 780.

Chapter - 17

Lignin and Acid Insoluble Ash by Fonnesbeck and Harris Method

Lignin and Acid Insoluble Ash

Principle

The residue remaining from the hemicellulose determination is digested with 72 percent sulphuric acid at room temperature. The lignin and acid insoluble ash are retained in the filter crucible while the digested carbohydrate passes through. The lignin is separated from acid insoluble ash by ashing the residue.

Equipment

1. *Acid digestion apparatus. A glass tray about 18 cm x 30 cm, 4 cm deep will hold twelve, 100 ml Griffen beakers. Another tray of the same size can be inverted over the beaker.*
2. *Filter crucibles. Same as described for cell wall determination.*
3. *Filtering apparatus. Same as described for cell wall determination.*

Chemicals

1. *Sulphuric acid (72%) : Standardize Reagent grade H_2SO_4 to specific gravity of 1.634 at 20°C.*
2. *Bromocresol green indicator solution : Dissolve 0.1 gram bromocresol green in 5 ml of dilute NH_4OH and dilute to 250 ml with water.*

Procedure

1. Place the weighed crucible containing the residue from the cell wall or hemicellulose analysis (Fonnesbeck and Harris method) in a 100 ml Griffen beaker containing 50 ml 72 percent H_2So_4. Allow the acid to filter up through the filter disc and wet the residue. Do not stir the sample residue at any time. Let the crucible stand for three hours. If the sample residue is not wet with acid within 15 minutes, add 72 percent sulphuric acid with a polyethylene squeeze bottle to wet the remaining particles. Let the crucible stand for three hours.
2. Transfer the crucible to the crucible holder of the filtering apparatus with forcep and filter off the acid with low suction. When acid has drained off, rinse down the inside of the crucible with 72 percent sulphuric acid. Allow the acid to empty between each rinsing.
3. Rinse the residue first wtih a few drops of near-boiling water with the suction on, then rinse freely with hot water until free of acid. After the rinse water drains off colourless, the residue can be broken up with a glass stirring rod so that a more complete rinsing can be accomplished. Rinse off ouside of crucible also. Test for removal of acid by adding a drop of indicator solution to the rinse water in the crucible. **A blue colour indicate satisfactory removal of acid.**
4. Dry the residue at 105°C, cool in a desiccator and weigh.
5. Ash the residue at 500°C, cool and weigh.

Calculation

Lignin percent on dry matter basis

$$= \frac{(\text{Wt. of residue before ashing} - \text{Wt. of residue after ashing})}{\text{Wt. of sample on dry matter basis}} \times 100$$

Acid insoluble ash percent on dry matter basis

$$= \frac{(\text{Wt. of residue after ashing} - \text{Wt. of empty crucible})}{\text{Wt. of sample on dry matter basis}} \times 100$$

Results

Expressed as g/100g

Reference

Tewatia, B.S. and Krishna, G. (1991). Fodder tree leaves as Animal Feed II Cell Wall contents and *in vitro* dry matter digestibility of some tree leaves and shrubs in Arid and Semi Arid Zones. *The J. of the Remount and Vety. Corps.* 30: 35-43.

Van Soest P.J. (1963). *J. Assoc. off. Agr. Chem.*, 46: 829.

Chapter - 18

Hemicellulose in Plant Cell Walls by Fonnesbeck and Harris Method

Hemicellulose Estimation

Principle

The residue from the cell walls determination is extracted with boiling 8 percent sulphuric acid for one hour to hydrolyse the hemicellulose without dissolving cellulose, lignin or acid insoluble ash.

Equipment

1. Refluxing apparatus.
2. *Filtering apparatus*: Same as described for cell wall determination
3. *Filtering crucibles*: Same as described for cell wall determination.

Reagents

1. **Sulphuric acid (8%) :** Standardize Reagent grade sulphuric acid to specific gravity of 1.052 at 20°C.
2. **Bromocresol green indicator solution:** Same as used for lignin determination.

Procedure

1. Add 75 ml 8 percent sulphuric acid to a Berzelius beaker. Hook the spout of the percolating tube over the edge of the crucible containing

the cell wall residue and lower the crucible into the beaker as shown in Fig. 1.

2. Place the beaker on the refluxing apparatus heater, cover with the condenser, and percolate boiling acid through the residue for one hour.
3. Remove the crucible, place on filtering apparatus and rinse freely with hot water to remove all acid. Rinse down inside and outside of crucible. Test completions of rinsing with a drop of the indicator solution (Yellow at pH 3.8, blue at pH 5.4).
4. Dry at 105°C, cool in a desiccator and weigh.

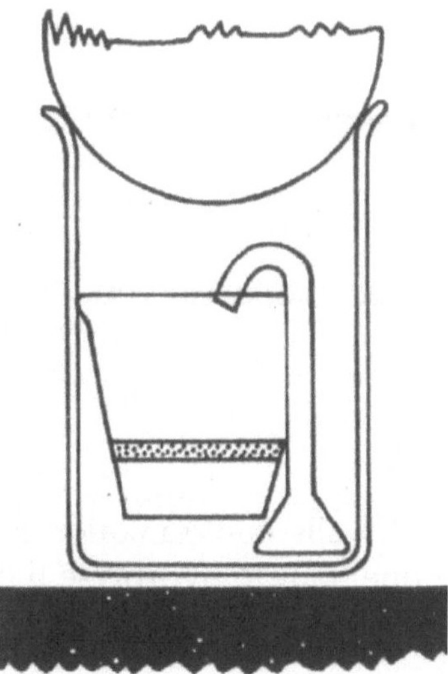

Fig. 1 : Apparatus for estimating Hemicellulose by Fonnesbeck and Harris method.

Calculation

Hemicellulose percent on dry matter basis

$$= \frac{(\text{Wt. cell wall residue} - \text{Wt. extracted cell wall residue})}{\text{Wt. of sample on dry matter basis}} \times 100$$

Result : Expressed as g/100 g.

References

Fonnesbeck, P.V. and L.E. Harris, (1970). *Proc. Amer. Soc. Animal Sci., Western Sec.*, 21:153

________, (1971). *Proc. Amer. Soc. Animal Sci. Western Sec.*, 22:77.

Chapter - 19

Cellulose and Lignin by Crampton and Maynard Method

Estimation of Cellulose in Feeds and Fodders

Principle

The feed well ground is digested with acetic acid which dissolves all other constituents like protein, disaccharides, fatty acids, etc., and cellulose and mineral contents are unaffected. The residue is made acid and alcohol free by washings. Alcohol removes water, benzene removes pigments and fat and at the end the sample is dried and ashed. The difference between the dried weight before ashing and weight after ashing gives cellulose content of the feed sample.

Reagents

1. *Glacial acetic acid, AR quality*
2. *Concentrated nitric acid, AR quality*
3. *Acid washed asbestos*

Equipment

1. *Filteration flask*
2. *Erlenmeyer flask 150 ml capacity*
3. *Gooch crucible*

Procedure

1. Weigh accurately 1-2 g of dried material in 150 ml capacity Erlenmeyer flask.
2. Add 12.5 ml of glacial acetic acid and 1.5 ml of concentrated nitric acid.
3. Place the flask on water bath for 20 min.
4. Filter through a gooch crucible with asbestos pad.
5. Wash with hot water, alcohol, benzene and alcohol one after another.
6. Dry at 100° C and weigh.
7. Ash the contents of the crucible in muffle furnace at 550°C for half an hour.
8. Weigh again.
9. Difference between dry weight and ashed weight is cellulose.

Calculation

Cellulose percent on dry matter basis (g/100g)

$$= \frac{(\text{Wt. of crucible} + \text{asbestos} + \text{material before ashing}) - (\text{Wt. of crucible and contents after ashing})}{\text{Wt. of material on dry matter basis}} \times 100\text{g}$$

Example

1. Weight of crucible + asbestos + material before ashing = 20.4460 g
2. Weight of crucible + asbestos + material after ashing = 20.0165 g
3. Weight of material on dry matter basis = 1.7837 g

Cellulose percent on dry matter basis $= \frac{20.4460 - 20.0165}{1.7837} \times 100$

= 24.08 percent.

Result: Expressed as g/100g

Estimation of Lignin in Feeds and Fodders

Reagents

1. *2 percent solution of pepsin in N/10 HCI.*
2. *40 percent formaldehyde.*
3. *72 percent sulphuric acid.*
4. *Chloroform and acetic acid (1:6 mixture).*

Procedure

Place the oven dried, ether extracted residue from a 1 g sample of feed or faeces in a 50 ml glass stoppered Erlenmeyer and add 40 ml of 2 percent solution of pepsin in N/10 HCI. Digest for 12 h at 40°C shaking frequently, especially during the first 4 or 5 hours.

Recover the non-digested residue by filteration through the bolting silk and wash successively with hot water, hot alcohol, hot benzene, hot alcohol and ether. Transfer the washed residue to a 100 ml beaker and remove the last traces of ether with mild heat. Moisten the residue with 4 ml of 40 percent formaldehyde. Then add 4 ml of 72 percent sulphuric acid, and allow it to penetrate the sample (2 min). Add 6 ml of concentrated sulphuric acid and stir vigorously with a glass rod to aid in solution of the sample which should be complete in 10 to 15 min. Partially immerse the beaker in a cold water bath, if necessary. to prevent the temperature from rising above 70°C. When dissolved, stir in 35 ml of a granulating reagent consisting of a 1:6 mixture (by volume) of chloroform and acetic acid, and then pour the whole into 500 ml distilled water in a 800 ml beaker. Boil gently until the chloroform has been driven off (15 min.), after which the solution should be clear and the lignin settle down in granular form. Filter on a Gooch crucible with suction. Wash in not less than 200 ml of 5 percent HCl. Dry at 110°C and determine lignin by calculating loss in ignition.

Example

Name of sample : *Gram husk.*

1. Weight of dried material taken = 1 g
2. Weight of crucible + material before ashing = 20.486 g
3. Weight of crucible + material after ashing = 20.363 g
4. Loss in weight of material = 0.123g

$$\text{Lignin percent on dry matter basis} = \frac{0.123 \times 100}{1} = 12.3\% \text{ lignin.}$$

Result: Expressd as g/100 g.

Reference

Crampton. E.W. and L.A. Maynard, (1938). *J. Nutr.*, 15: pp. 383-95.

Chapter - 20

Soluble Carbohydrate and Structural Carbohydrate Pentosan and Hexosan by Deriaz Method

Pentosan and Hexosan Estimation

Principle

Dried milled samples are extracted successively with diethyl ether, 0.5 percent ammonium oxalate solution, NH_2SO_4 and 72 percent sulphuric acid. Soluble carbohydrate in the ammonium oxalate extract determined with anthrone and hydrolysed pentosans and hexosans in the combined N H_2SO_4. Seventy two percent sulphuric acid extract are determined with aniline acetate and chromotropic acid respectively. The method gives a maximum variation of 4 percent from the mean of duplicates with each carbohydrate component. The residual material is ashed to obtain crude lignin and a nitrogen correction applied.

Soluble carbohydrate - this group, which includes sugars, oligosaccharides, and the fructosans of grasses, provides a source of nutrients readily available to livestock.

The soluble carbohydrates of grass and of lucerne have been determined by successive extractions with aqueous alcohol and with hot water, and a method for the determination of glucose, fructose, sucrose and fructosans in the two extracts from grass has been worked out by De Man and De Hens (1949).

Structural Carbohydrate

The remaining carbohydrates, which comprise the plant cell wall, are the β-1, 4-glucan cellulose, the hemicellulose, which include other polymeric sugars and possible combinations of these with glucronic acid, and pectin (polygalacturonic acid). The structrual carbohydrates contain glucose, xylose, arabinose and galactose, together with mannose in lucerne. the structrual carbohydrate need not be divided into fractions based on arbitrary solubility properties, if they are expressed as pentosan and hexosan, and this expression is used in the present work. Anthrone reagent may be used to determine pentoses or hexoses separately, but there is interference when mixture of these sugars are determined. *An orcinol reagent is used for the simultaneous determination of pentose and hexose in bacterial cell hydrolysate, but the method requires careful control of time and temperature of heating.*

Reagents

1. *Anthrone reagent: Add 760 ml of conc. sulphuric acid (Analar) to 330 ml of water, cool to room temperature and make up to one litre at 20°C with water. Dissolve 1 g of thiourea and 1 g of anthrone successively in this solution and store the reagent in the refrigerator.*
2. *Tracey's reagent (modified): Add 16 ml of colourless aniline to 100 ml of glacial acetic acid and stir. Add 24 ml of water and 5 ml of 5 percent aqueous oxalic acid (The reagent is most satisfactory if prepared immediately before use).*
3. *Chromotropic acid: Add 395 ml of conc.* H_2SO_4 *(Analar) to 130 ml of water, cool and dilute to 500 ml with water (this gives 15 M* H_2SO_4*). Dissolve 0.5g of chromotropic acid sodium salt (Analytical reagent grade for fomaldehyde determination) 5 ml of water, and add 250 ml of 15 M* H_2SO_4 *(Although the reagent is most satisfactory when fresh, it may be stored in a refrigerator for one or two weeks).*
4. NH_2SO_4.
5. *72 percent W/W sulphuric acid: Add 326 ml of conc. sulphuric acid to water to make 500 ml of solution.*
6. *Silicone solution (Dissolve 20g of silicone Fluid Antifoam) "A" in 1 l of carbon tetrachloride.*

Solution (Standards)

1. Glucose solution containing 0.200 g of glucose per litre.
2. Pentose solution (0.100 g/l) containing 0.070 g of xylose and 0.030g of arabinose per litre.

3. Hexose solution (of 0.200g/l) containing 0.180 g of glucose and 0.020 g galactose per litre. The standards are prepared weekly and are stored in a refrigerator.

Procedure

Dry a sample of the cut herbage in a forced-draught oven at 100°C for 8 to 12 hours and grind in a laboratory mill to pass a 0.8 mm sieve. Dry approximately 1 g of ground herbage in a 2 x 5 cm glass tube at 100°C for three hours. Weight to the nearest milligram and transfer the sample to a folded 12.5 cm Whatman No. 54 (hardened) filter paper and reweigh the tube. Extract the sample with diethyl ether in a Soxhlet extractor, for 72 h, remove it from the extractor and let it air dry. Brush the sample from the filter paper into a 500 ml flask. Add 150 ml of 0.5 percent ammonium oxalate solution and 6 drops (more if necessary) of silicone solution to suppress frothing, and boil under reflux for two hours. Allow the solution to cool. Add approximately 1 g of ashed celite 545 (John Mannvile) filter aid and transfer the solution to a 250 ml centrifuge tube. Rinse flask with about 25 ml of water and transfer the washing to the centrifuge tube. Centrifuge the solution for 5-10 min at 2200 rpm (1925 g) and carefully decant the supernatant into a litre standard flask. Add about 100 ml of water to the residue, stir and centrifuge again. Add the supernatant to the standard flask the solution up to volume with water and filter, about 30 ml through a 15 cm Whatman No. 44 filter paper, use the filtrate (solution A) for determination of soluble carbohydrate.

Transfer the residue from the centrifuge tube into flask with 67 ml of N H_2SO_4 used in three or four portions. Add approximately 3 drops of silicone solution and boil under reflux for one hour. Allow to cool, transfer the solution to a 250 ml centrifuge tube with 67 ml of water in several portions, and centrifuge. Transfer the supernatant to flask. Wash the residue with 10 ml of water, centrifuge and add the supernatant to flask. Set aside flask with contents. Wash the residue with about 100 ml of acetone, centrifuge and discard the acetone layer.

Allow the residue to dry overnight at about 40°C in an oven, with the centrifuge tube placed on its side. Break the residue into a powder with a spatula and remove the last traces of solvent at 100°C for 15 min. Allow to cool to room temperature. Add 12 ml of 72 percent sulphuric acid mix thoroughly with a glass rod until the mixture is entirely free from lumps, and set aside for 4 h at room temperature (20°C) with occasional stirring. With 105 ml of water, used in three or four portions, wash the material in the centrifuge tube into flask. Add approximately 6 drops of silicone solution and boil the liquid under reflux for two hours. Allow to cool and filter the solution through a sintered glass crucible (porocity 1) with the miniumum suction necessary in order to obtain a clear filtrate. Wash the residue with about 150 ml of water. Transfer the combined filtrate and washings to a one litre standard flask, make up to volume and use this solution (solution B) for determination of the structural carbohydrates. Wash the residue with about 150 ml each of acetone and diethyl ether. Dry the crucible to constant weight at 100°C, ignite at 450°C and reweigh.

Run a separate portion of the orignial herbage through the stages described to the point of filtration of the acid insoluble residue. Then isolate the residue by centrifugation, wash successively with water and acetone, dry and determine the nitrogen content by the Kjeldahl method.

Colorimetric Determination

1. Soluble carbohydrate

Pipette 2 ml of the test solution A in duplicate, 2 ml of glucose standard in triplicate, and 2 ml of water (as blank) into 2.54 x 15.24 cm boiling tubes. Add 10 ml of anthrone reagent slowly to each tube, with cooling in a beaker of tap water. Cover the boiling tubes and heat on the water bath at 100°C for 20 min. Cool in tap water for 10 min. and measure the colours (which are stable) at 625 mμ against the reagent blank in a 1 cm cell with a spectrophotometer.

2. Structural carbohydrate - Pentosan

Dilute 5 ml of the test solution B with an equal volume of water. Pipette 2 ml of the diluted test solution in duplicate, 2 ml of the pentose standard in triplicate and 2 ml of water (as blank) into 2.54 x 15.24 cm boiling tubes. Add 6 ml of Tracey's reagent to each boiling tube. Ignore any colouration which may appear immediately. Keep the tubes overnight at room temperature. Measure the colours (which are stable) at 472 mμ against the reagent blank as above.

3. Structural carbohydrate - Hexosan

Measure 2 ml of the test solution B in duplicate, 2 ml of the hexose standard and 2 ml of water (as blank) into 2.54 x 15.24 cm boiling tubes. Add 10 ml of chromotropic acid reagent to each boiling tube and cover them. Heat on the water bath at 100°C for 30 min, cool in tap water and measure the colours (which are stable) at 570 mμ.

Calculation

1. Soluble carbohydrate

Colour intensities for glucose solution up to 0.3 g/l are linearly related to concentration, so that the concentration of a test solution is calculated by relating its optical density directly to that of the standard. The results are expressed as percent glucose of the sample dry matter; no allowance is made for the presence in the original herbage of some glucose and fructose partially in the anhydrous form.

2. Pentosan

The concentration of pentose in the diluted test solution B is calculated by directly relating the optical density of the developed colouration to that of the standard, since there is a linear relationship between optical density and pentose concentration up to 0.120g/l. The pentosan content is obtained by multiplying the apparent pentose content of the herbage dry matter by 0.88.

3. Hexosan

Klein and Weissman (1953) showed that optical density is directly proportional to glucose concentration up to 0.3 g/l . The calculated (apparent) hexose content of the herbage is multiplied by 0.90 to obtain the hexosan content.

References

AOAC, (1970). Association of Official Analytical Chemists. 11th edn., Washington, D.C

De Man, T.J. and J.D. De Hens, (1949). *Trav., Chim., Pays - Bas,* 68:43.

Deriaz, R.E. (1961). *J. Sci, Food Agric.,* 12:152-160.

Klein, B. and M. Weissman, (1953). *Analyt. Chem.* 25:771.

Chapter - 21

Oxalic Acid in Biological Materials

Oxalic Acid Estimation

Method I

Reagents

1. *20% sodium carbonate.*
2. *Conc. hydrochloric acid.*
3. *4% sodium hydroxide*
4. *10% calcium chloride*
5. *Ammonium hydroxide*
6. *Potassium permanganate (0.05 N)*

Procedure

Take 2-5 g of powdered sample in a beaker without spout, and add 40 ml of water and boil for half an hour. In case of faeces, add 40 ml of 4 percent NaOH instead of 40 ml of water to form silicates. Now boil, for half an hour with cold water flask over the beaker, then add 10 ml of 20 percent sodium carbonate solution and boil for another half an hour. During these two cooking processes, the following changes take place.

(a) The cellular tissues are completely broken down.

(b) Fatty matters are saponified.

(c) All insoluble oxalate salts are converted into soluble sodium oxalate.

The liquid extract is then filtered and residue is washed with hot water till does not show any alkaline reaction. The combined filtrate and wash water is then concentrated to a small volume and allowed to cool. In the cold solution with constant stirring, HCI (1:1) is added drop by drop till the final acid concentration after the neutralization of the alkali becomes approximately 1 percent. At this stage a heavy precipitate of extraneous matter appears which is allowed to flocculate. The extract is then carefully filtered in 250 ml flask and the volume is made up to the mark. The organic matter is allowed to settle in the flask by keeping it overnight or so, and the supernatant is filtered through a dry filter paper in a dry beaker. An aliquot of this filtrate is taken in a 400 ml beaker, diluted with water to 200 ml and then made just ammoniacal and reacidified with acetic acid. In the cold medium 10 ml of a 10 percent solution of calcium chloride is added and mixture is stirred well to induce the precipitate of calcium oxalate to appear. The precipitate is allowed to settle overnight. The clear supernatant liquid is carefully decanted off through Whatman filter paper No. 42 leaving as much of the precipitate as possible undisturbed. The precipitate is then dissolved in hydrochloric acid (1 : 1) after allowing a few ml of the acid to pass through the filter paper and collecting it in the beaker containing the precipitate from hydrochloric acid solution, oxalic acid is reprecipitated by adjusting the pH by ammonium hydroxide solution. The contents are then boiled, allowed to settle overnight and oxalic acid is estimated as usual by titrating against $KMnO_4$ solution (0.05 N). *One ml of 0.05 N permanganate solution is equivalent to 0.00225 g anhydrous oxalic acid.*

Estimation of oxalic acid in cattle faeces

Since cattle faeces contain relatively large amount of silica it is necessary that this should be removed before oxalic acid is precipitated by calcium chloride. The sample of faeces is first cooked in 40 ml of 1 percent solution of caustic soda for half an hour. The rest of the procedure is as usual.

Method II

Determination of Water Soluble Oxalates

Two grams dried material is taken in 250 ml volumetric flask containing 250 ml of distilled water. The contents are digested for one hour in boiling water bath, cooled, made to volume and filtered. Two 50 ml aliquots are taken in beakers and to each are added 20 ml of 6 NVHCI. The mixture is evaporated to about one half of its volume and filtered. The precipitate is washed several times with warm distilled water.

To the filtrate (about 125 ml) 3-4 drops of methyl red indicator is added followed by concentrated ammonia till the solution turns faint yellow. It is then heated to 90°-100°C, allowed to cool and filtered to remove precipitate containing ferrous ion. The filtrate is brought to boiling, 10 ml of 5 percent calcium chloride is added with constant stirring and is allowed to stand overnight. It is filtered through Whatman filter paper No. 44. The precipitate is washed with distilled water till free of calcium ions. The precipitate is transferred to the original beaker by washing with distilled water, and sulphuric acid (1:4) is added till the precipitate is completely dissolved. The contents are brought to near boiling and titrated against 0.05 N potassium permanganate to near end point, when the filter paper is also added to the solution, stirred thoroughly and titration is completed. A blank is also run along with the test sample. From the amount of potassium permanganate used, the contents of the unknown sample are calculated.

Total Oxalates. In a 250 ml volumetric flask containg 190 ml of distilled water and 10 ml of 6 NHCI, 2 g of the plant material is placed. The mixture is digested for one hour on boiling water bath, cooled, diluted to volume and filtered. The rest of the procedure is the same as for the estimation of water soluble oxalates.

Recovery Tests. Recovery tests are performed by taking different strengths of oxalic acid (AR) solution. A mean recovery of 95.02 ± 0.46 percent should be obtained in 5 determinations.

Calculation: The amount of bound oxalate (total water-soluble oxalate) represents the fraction present mainly as calcium oxalate. Assuming that the oxalic acid forms insoluble oxalates only with calcium on stoichiometric basis, 126 g of oxalic acid should combine with 40 g of calcium or for every 3.15 g (126/40) of oxalic acid, 1 g of calcium will be bound as oxalate.

References

Abeza, R. H. J. T. Blake, and E.J. Fisher, (1968). *J. Assoc. Off. Agric. Chem.*, 51: 963.

AOAC, (1970). Association of Official Analytical Chemists, 11 th edn., Washington. D.C.

Moir, K.W. (1953). *Qd. J Agric, Sci.*, 10: 1.

Krishna, G. (1980). A note on tannins and Oxalic acid content of Agro-Industrial byproducts and wastes. *Agriculture Agro-Industries Journal*, 13: 7-8.

Chapter - 22

Tannic Acid in Feeds and Fodders

Tannic Acid Estimation

Introduction

Substances found in many plants are generally related to one of the phenols, pyrogallol or catechol. Tannins are solids, usually extracted by hot water insoluble in ether, chloroform, carbon disulphide, benzene; soluble in alcohol ether mixture, alcohol, water and in ethyl acetate, possessing a bitter astringent taste.

Tannic acid is Pentadigalloyl glucose, on hydrolysis yields digallic acid and glucose. Tannins are water soluble glucosides of polydepsides, polymeric ester of gallic acid. It is hydrolysed enzymatically and some efforts have, therefore, been made to preserve tannic, if it is to exert its activity in the duodenum. On the basis of physical or chemical principles which they employ, the methods of tannin analysis can be grouped as follows.

1. Precipitation by inorganic reagents, e.g. copper acetate salts of aluminium, zinc, lead and copper.
2. Precipitation by organic reagents, e.g., hide powder, cincohonine, gelatin and formaldehyde.

3. Formation of coloured products, e.g., alkaline phosphotungstate phosphomolybdate (Folin-Denis), ferric chloride, acid vanillin, diazotized p-nitroaniline and nitrous acid.

4. Oxidation with acid permanganate of ferricyanide on a volumetric basis.

Method I

Reagents

1. *Oxalic acid solution = 0.1 N, 1 ml = 0.006235g quercitannic acid or 0.0008 g Q_2 absorbed.*

2. *Potassium permanganate solution: Dissolve 1.333 g $KMnO_4$ in one litre water and standardize against oxalic acid.*

3. *Indigo solution. Dissolve 6 g sodium indigotin disulphonate in 500 ml water by heating, cool and add 50 ml sulphuric acid, dilute to one litre and filter.*

Procedure

Extract 2 g sample for 20 h with anhydrous ether. Boil residue for two hours with 300 ml water, cool, dilute to 500 ml and filter. Measure 25 ml of this infusion into two litre procelain dish, add 20 ml of the indigo solution and 750 ml water. Add standard $KMnO_4$ solution, 1 ml at a time until blue colour changes to green then add few drops at a time until colour becomes golden yellow. Similarly. titrate mixture of 20 ml of the indigo solution and 750 ml of water. Multiply difference between two titration by desired factor to obtain quercitannic acid or oxygen absorbed.

Method II

A Colorimetric Method for the Determination of Tannins in Tea

Löwenthal's volumetric permanganate method, after some modification, has been adopted as an official method for estimating tannins in coffee, tea, spices, condiments and wines. Horowitz (1955) used gelation in the determination of tannins in tea and coffee, to separate the tannins from other oxidizable substances present in the solution. Indigo carmine is used as indicator, and the permanganate is added with constant shaking of the titrant solution until a green colour is reached. The titration is then continued dropwise to a golden yellow end point.

Barua and Roberts (1940) criticized the Löwenthal method because of the error involved in the arbitrary end point. The detection of the end point needs considerable judgement on the part of the operator and the result is affected to a considerable extent by the time taken for the titration and by the vigour of the shaking. Replicate analyses often differ by 0.3 ml or more and variation between results obtained by different operators may amount to 1 ml. These authors further found that the method become completely unreliable for oxidized tannins. For this titration a different end point was used, owing to decrease in the rate of oxidation. The method thus gave eroneous results for manufactured (black) tea.

The Folin-Denis method is official for tannins in distilled liquors (Horowitz, 1955). It cannot , however, be applied directly to the determination of tannin in tea. In the present work, the Folin-Denis method has been modified so as to be applicable to tea.

Reagents

All solutions were prepared from analytical grade reagents Aqueous solutions were prepared with distilled water.

Folin-Denis Reagent: To 50 ml of water add 100g of sodium tungstae hydrated (Na_2WO_4. $2H_2O$), 20g of phosphomolybdic acid and 50 ml of conc. phosphoric acid. Reflux for two hours and dilute the solution to one litre.

Saturated Sodium Carbonate Solution

To each 100 ml of water used, add 35 g of anhydrous sodium carbonate, dissovle at 70-80°C and allow to cool overnight. Treat the supersaturated solution with crystals of Na_2CO_3. 10 H_2O and after the crystalization is complete filter the mother liquor through glass.

Standard Tannic Acid Solution Dissolve exactly 100 mg of tannic acid in one litre of water. Prepare fresh solution for each determination.

Gelatine Solution: Soak 2.5 g of gelatine in saturated sodium chloride solution for one hour, then warm until the gelatine dissolves, cool and dilute to 1000 ml with saturated sodium chloride solution.

Acid Sodium Chloride Solution: Add 25 ml of concentrated sulphuric acid to 375 ml of saturated sodium chloride solution.

Calibration curve: Pipette 0 to 10 ml aliquots (in appropriate steps) of the standard tannic acid solution into 100 ml standard flasks containing 75 ml of water. Add 5 ml of Folin-Denis reagent and 10 ml of sodium carbonate solution and dilute to the mark with water. Mix well and determine the absorbance at 760 nm after 30 min. Plot absorbance against mg of tannic acid taken.

Determination of Tannin Content: Apply the calibration curve procedure to the tea infusion and the corresponding "non-tannin" solution. The "non-tanin" value is subtracted from the tea infusion value to obtain the true tannin content.

Preparation of Tea Infusion: Boil 5 g of tea (made or dried green leaf) with 400 ml of water for one hour, cool and make up to 500 ml in a standard flask. Use a suitable aliquot, say 0.2 ml of this infusion for the determination.

Preparation of "Non-Tannin" Solution: The separation into tannins and non-tannins is usually effected with gelatine, as in the Löwenthal procedure. Mix 100 ml of tea infusion with 50 ml of gelatine solution. 100 ml of acid sodium chloride solution and 20 g of Kaolin powder. Shake the mixture for several minutes, allowing to settle, and filter. The filtrate is almost free from tannins.

Some non-tannin filtrate is evaporated to dryness and the residue extracted with methanol; the extract is subjected to two-dimensional chromatography with n-butanol-acetic acid-water (4:1:5) in the first direction and 2 percent acetic acid in the second, followed by identification by dip reagent (2 g of ferric chloride + 2g of potassium ferricyanide + 1400 ml of water) and small amounts of catechin and traces of theogallin and chlorogenic acids were found. Use 1 ml aliquot of this solution for the determination. (It was found experimentally that the non-tannin solution gave a linear relationship of absorbance to concentration only when the volume of non-tannin solution is above 0.5 ml)

Calculation : If the absorbance for the 0.2 ml of tea infusion corresponds to x mg of tannic acid, then 5 g of tea contains the equivalent of 2500 x mg of tannic acid. and tea contains 50 x percent of tannin plus non-tannin. Similarly, if the 1 ml of non-tannin solution gives an absorbance corresponding to y mg of tannic acid. the non-tannin content of the tea is 10 y percent. The tannin content is, therefore, (50x-10y).

References

AOAC, (1970). Association of Official Analytical Chemists, 11th edn., Washington, D.C

Bajaj, K.L. and A.K. Sharma, (1970). *Mikrochimica Acta*, pp. 322-325

Barua, D.N. and E.A.H. Roberts, (1940). *Biochem. J.*, 34: 1524.

Horowitz, W., (1955). *Official Methods of Analysis, AOAC*, p. 144.

Krishna, G. (1980). A note on tannins and oxalic acid content of Agro-Industrial byproducts and wastes. *Agriculture Agro Industries Journal*. 13: 7-8.

Chapter - 23

Cyanides in Plants

Cyanides Estimation

Principle

Cyanide is distilled from chloroform and water soultion into KOH solution, forming potassium cyanide. KCN is titrated with silver nitrate; 2 KCN + $AgNO_3$ = KCN. AgCN + KNO_3. An excess of $AgNO_3$ produces insoluble AgCN, which is the end point of titration.

Ag $(CN)_2K$ + $AgNO_3$ = 2AgCN + KNO_3

Equipment

1. *Kjeldahl distillation apparatus (macro).*
2. *5 ml burette (micro).*

Reagents

1. *2% KOH solution : Dissolve 2g of KOH in 100 ml H_2O.*
2. *Chloroform : Spectra-analysed. Fisher certificate, ACS or equivalent.*
3. *Potassium iodide.*
4. *Potassium chloride : Recrystallize three times with water, dry at 105°C, and then heat at about 500°C to constant weight.*

5. *Potassium chromate solution: Five percent solution of* K_2CrO_4 *in water.*

6. *Silver nitrate solution (0.1 N): Dissolve slightly more than theoretical quantity of* $AgNO_3$ *(equivalent weight - 169.89) in halogen-free water and dilute to required volume. Thoroughly clean glassware, avoid contact with dust, and keep prepared solution in amber glass stoppered bottles away from light. Standardize as follow: Weigh accurately sufficient quantity of KCI to yield titration of approx. 40 ml (about 0.3 g for 0.1 N solution) and transfer to 250 ml glass stoppered Erlenmeyer flask with 40 ml* H_2O*. Add 1 ml of 5 percent potassium chromate solution and titrate with* $AgNO_3$ *solution until appearance of first precipitable pale red-brown colour. Subtract from titration, millilitres of the* $AgNO_3$ *solution required to produce end point colour in 75 ml water containing 1 ml of* K_2CrO_4 *solution. Calculate normality of* $AgNO_3$ *solution.*

Procedure

Cut sample of forage into 0.6 cm length. Mix well, place 8 g sample in 800 ml kjeldahl flask. Add about 200 ml distilled water and 5 ml chloroform. Steam distill into a 100 ml test tube containing 5 ml 2 percent KOH, with the adaptor end of the condenser below the surface of the KOH solution. Distill over 60 to 70 ml and transfer to 600 ml beaker. Add enough water to make 300 ml. Add a few crystals of potassium iodide and titrate to faint opalescence with the silver nitrate solution. A drop of the silver salt in excess will produce a permanent turbidity, owing to the following reaction:

$$Ag(CN)_2K + AgNO_3 = 2\,AgCN + KNO_3.$$

The insoluble AgCN formed (in making this titration, it is advantageous to have beaker over black surface). From millilitres 0.1 N $AgNO_3$ used to calculate percent Cyanides, reaction is represented by following equation:

$$2\,NaCN + AgNO_3 = NaCN.\,AgCN + NaNO_3$$

Hence, 1 ml 0.1 N $AgNO_3$ = 0.005204 g Cyanides

Calculation

Cyanide (mg per kg) on dry matter basis

$$= \frac{52 \text{ ml } AgNO_3 \times N\, AgNO_3 \times 1000}{\text{Wt. of sample on dry matter basis}}$$

where, N denotes normality.

References

Boyd, F. T., O.S. AA, Modt, G. Bohstedt and E. Truog, (1938). *J. Am. Soc. Agronomy*, 30: 569.

Boyd, F.T. and E. Truog, (1955). *Determination of cyanide in grass and plants*. Jersey J. August Issue.

Scott, W.W., (1939). *Standard methods of chemical analysis*, Vol. 1, 5th edn., D.Van. Nostrand Company, Inc., New York.

Chapter - 24

Nitrates and Nitrites in Forages

Nitrates and Nitrites Estimation

Nitrates and nitrites are known to have injurious effects on animals when excess amounts are ingested. Nitrites are much more toxic but nitrates are reduced to nitrites by bacterial action in the digestive tract

Nitrites (NO_2) are rarely found in plants in appreciable amounts except under very unusual conditions such as severe disease infections; therefore, the results are usually reported in terms of nitrates (NO_3). The usual method is to determine the total nitrate and nitrite in terms of nitrate. However, the method can also be used to determine the nitrite content of a feed separately if a nitrite problem is suspected.

Principle

Nitrate is reduced to nitrite by zinc and manganese (11) sulphate. The reaction then consists of diazotisation of sulphanilic acid by the nitrite ion and subsequent coupling with 1-naph-thylamine to form a red dye. The reaction is optimum in the pH range of 1.7 to 3.0 interferring iron is complexed with citrate. Copper from 0.2 to 1.0 ppm aids the reaction but over 1.2 ppm, it interferes.

Equipment

1. Spectronic "20", Spectrophotometer or equivalent.
2. Centrifuge.

Reagents

1. *Standard nitrate solution: Dissolve 1.37 gram of sodium nitrate in 1 litre of water for a stock solution of 0.1 percent nitrate (1000 micrograms per ml)*
2. *20 percent acetic acid with 0.2 ppm copper: To 200 ml of acetic acid, add 5 ml of $CuSO_4$ Solution (0.1572g of $CuSO_4.5H_2O$ per litre) and dilute to 1000 ml.*
3. *Powder mixture (Bray's indicator) : Hundred grams of barium sulphate (dried at 105°C), 10 g of manganese (11) sulphate monohydrate, 2g of finely powdered zinc. 75 g of powdered citric acid, 4 g of sulphanilic acid, and 2 g of naphthylamine. Grind any coarse material to a fine powder. Mix the manganese (11) sulphate, powdered zinc, sulphanilic acid and 1-naphthylamine separately with portions of barium sulphate.Then mix thoroughly all ingredients including the barium sulphate and citric acid. Use extreme care to have room, table top, and equipment free of nitrate and nitrite. Store the powder in a blackened bottle, since light affects 1-naphthylamine. the reagent is stable for many months in a bottlle painted on the outside with black paint. If the determination of nitrite in the presence of nitrate is desired, make up a separate powder mixture that does not contain the powdered zinc and manganese (11) sulphate.*
4. *Hydrochloric acid (0.1 N): Mix 8.18 ml of 37 to 38 percent HCI per litre of water. Exact standardization is not necessary.*
5. *Activated charcoal: Merck No. 18351 activated charcoal N.F. powder.*

Sampling of Feeds

The nitrate content of plants or feeds from different parts of field, stack or silo often varies extremely. For example, the nitrate content of plants in a field vary between: different plant species, different stages of plant growth, different parts of a plant. different areas in a field, different times of a day and different days as climatic conditions vary. Nitrate content of feeds in stacks and silos vary because of the above factors and because of differences in how the hay or silage is handled in the field (including the loss of nitrate by leaching from rain) ; and losses and movement of nitrates during fermentation in the silo.

Therefore, at any one sampling time it is desirable to obtain separate samples from different places in the field, stack or silo and analyse each sample separately; for plants growing in the field, samples should be collected and tested at different times.

Nitrates many be lost from moist plant or silage samples between the time the sample is collected and time it is analysed if the sample are not handled properly. Such losses may be due to enzymatic or microbiological reduction of nitrates in the moist sample or to volatilization of nitrogen gases or acids during drying. Therefore, either the moist plant or feed samples should be frozen as soon as possible after they are collected and kept frozen until they are analysed, or plant samples (but not silage samples) may be dried immediately in an oven with an adequate ventilation at 60°C.

Procedure

1. Weigh by difference approximately 1 g of air dry plant material or 3 to 5 g of moist sample. The sample should contain 1 to 8 mg nitrate to be within the range of the standard curve. Place the sample in a 125 ml glass stoppered Erlenmeyer flask.
2. Add 100 ml of 0.1 N HCl. Stopper the flask and shake the sample until all parts of the sample are wetted. Let the sample stand with occasional shaking for one hour to extract nitrate. If the extract is strongly coloured, decolourize it by adding about 1g of activated charcoal to the extract in the Erlenmeyer flask and shake well. Filter the extract through filter paper.
3. Pipette 1 ml of the extract and 9 ml of the 20 percent acetic acid solution to a glass stoppered centrifuge tube. Add about 0.5 g of the Bray's indicator powder with a small measuring scoop. Stopper and shake each tube for 1 min. Keep away the solution from strong light.
4. Place the tubes in the centrifuge tube holder and centrifuge for 5 min. at 3000 or until the supernatant liquid is clear. Remove any film on top and pour the clear red solution into a spectrophotometer cuvette.
5. Observe the optical density at 520 mμ. Set the instrument at 100 percent transmittancy, with a blank solution that has been treated exactly as the sample solutions.
6. Compare the observations to a standard nitrate curve ranging from 0 to 10 micrograms nitrate per ml of solution in the cuvette. (Make the standard curve by diluting 0, 2, 5 and 10 ml aliquots of the standard nitrate solution to 100 ml in volumetric flasks witih water). Transfer 1 ml of the diluted solution to centrifuge tubes and continue the procedure as mentioned above. The solution in the cuvettes will contain 0, 1, 2, 5 and 10 micrograms nitrate per ml. The remaining solution in the 100 ml volumetric flasks may be transferred to polyethylene bottle and stored for several months and reused as needed.

7. When nitrites are to be determined in the presence of nitrates, follow the same procedure remembering to use the powder mixture that does not contain powdered zinc or manganese (11) sulphate.

Calculation

1. To determine the nitrate plus nitrite contents, the powder mixture containing zinc and manganese sulphate is used and all nitrates are reduced to nitrites. The result is the total of nitrate and nitrite in terms of nitrite when the standard curve is used.

   Total nitrate percent on dry matter basis

$$= \frac{\text{Conc. of nitrate in final solution in } \mu g / ml \times 1000 \times 100}{\text{Wt. of sample in grams} \times 1{,}000{,}000 \text{ on dry matter basis}}$$

$$= \frac{NO_3 \text{ microgram / ml from curve}}{\text{gram sample} \times 10 \text{ on dry matter basis}}$$

2. To determine only nitrite in the presence of nitrate, the zinc and manganese sulphate are omitted from the powder mixture.

   The nitrite percent on dry matter basis

$$= \frac{\text{Conc. of nitrite in final solution in } \mu g \text{ per ml} \times 1000 \times 100}{\text{Wt. of sample in grams} \times 1{,}000{,}000 \text{ on dry matter basis}}$$

$$= \frac{NO_3 \text{ microgram / ml from curve}}{(g) \text{ sample} \times 10 \text{ on dry matter basis}}$$

References

Hanway, J.J. J.B Herric, T.L. Willrich, P.C. Bennett, and J.T. McCall, (1963). The nitrate problem, Special Report No.34 Iowa State University Ames.

Nelson. J.L., L.T. Kurtz, and , R.H. Bray, (1954). Analytical Chemisty. 26: 1081.

Rider B.F. and M.G Mellon, (1946). Industrial Engineering Chemistry. Analytical Edition. 18: 96.

Wolley, J.T. Hicks, G.P. and Hageman, R.H. (1960). *Agr. Food Chem.*, 8: 481.

Chapter - 25

Aflatoxin in Feeds

Aflatoxin Estimation

Introduction

Aflatoxins are a group of highly subsituted coumarine, of which aflatoxin B_1 and G_1 are most highly hepatotoxic (toxic to liver) to animals. The toxins are produced by some strains of *Aspergillus flavus* and other species of Aspergillus which develop in many food stuffs, particularly groundnuts. cottonseed, and their cake and flour. Protein concentrates meant for babies as well as adult are now a day made from groundnut flour and the cakes are used as feed for poultry and livestock. It has been found that even fodgrains such as maize, rice and wheat are attacked by the fungus producing the toxins.

The presenceof compounds related to aflatoxins has been demonstrated in the milk of animals fed on feeds containing aflatoxin.

A method of aflatoxin analysis is outlined below which is suitable for materials such as groundnut meal. coconut meal and plam kernel meal.

Reagents

1. *Chloroform (Reagent grade)*
2. *Diethyl ether (Reagent grade)*
3. *Chloroform/methanol mixture (95:5 V/V)*

4. *Celite diatomaceous-earth*
5. *Kieselgel "G" (Merck).*
6. *Qualitative standard - Helps to distinguish aflatoxin spots from other fluorescent spots which may be present. A goundnut meal containing aflatoxins B_1 obtainable from the Tropical Products Institute, London, can be used for this purpose.*

Apparatus

1. Thin layer chromatography plates, 20 x 20 cm.
2. U.V. lamp. peak emission at 365 mμ.
3. Bottles wide mouth, 250 ml.
4. Micropipettes.
5. Shaking device.

Method

Weigh 10 ml of material into a wide mouth bottle and thoroughly mix in 10 ml of water. (If high fat material is used, a prior Soxhlet extraction with petroleum ether will be necessary). Add 100 ml of chloroform, stopper with a chloroform resistant cork and shake for 30 min. Filter the extract through "Celite", take 20 ml of filtrate and make up to 25 ml (solution A). Take another 20 ml of filtrate and concentrate to 5 ml (solution B).

Prepare thin layer plates by shaking Kieselgel "G" (100/g) with water (220 ml) for 20 min. and applying the mixture to the plates with a suitable apparatus to a depth of 508 micron. Leave for one hour, then dry at 100°C . Spot 10 and 20 μl of solution B and 5 and 10 μl of solution A onto a plate, together with a qualitative standard spot, in a line 2 cm from the bottom of the plate and at least 2 cm in from each side. Carry out the spot application in subdued light.

Develop the plate in diethyl ether to a height of 12 cm. Allow to dry in subdued light then redevelop the plate in chloroform methanol (95/5, V/V) to a height of 10 cm from the baseline. Examine the plate in a dark room, 30 cm from the UV source. The presence of a blue flourescent spot at Rf 0.5 to 0.55 indicates aflatoxin B (check that the standard spot also lies in this range). The presence of a second spot of Rf 0.45 to 5 indicates aflatoxin G. The toxicity level of a sample can then be classified in terms of aflatoxin B_1 and G_1 as given in Table 1.

Table 1 : Detection Parameters of Aflatoxins Toxicity

Volume applied (µl)	Conc. of aflatoxins (µg/kg) No fluorescence	fluorescence	Toxicity level of fluorescence observed
5µl (Soln. A)	< 1000	> 1000	Very high
10µl (Soln. A)	< 500	500-1000	High
10µl (Soln. B)	<100	100-500	Medium
20µl (Soln. B)	< 50	50-100	Low

Latest Aflatoxin Tests

(Method of Wilcox. 1983, Kansas State University, USA)

Aflatoxin, which have become a major concern of the feed industry, can be detected at levels of 10-15 ppb using a test requiring 5-15 min per sample. The method decribed here was developed by Kansas State University grain scientists. This test is not quantitative, but appears to be a fast way to determine the presence of aflatoxins.

Procedure

1. Place a 100 g sample of the material to be tested in an ordinary kitchen blender alongwith, 300 ml of the extraction solvent (seven parts methanol-three parts water). Run the blender 1 to 3 min at high speed for extraction. A longer grinding may be necessary for some blender or for extractions at levels near 15-20 ppb.

2. Allow the material in the blender to sit until a layer of noncloudy liquid forms on the surface. Filtration through a muslin cloth using vacuum can also be used if available to speed up separation (see modification described later on). Remove 80 to 150 ml of the liquid and place it in a 500 ml separatory funnel (See Modification 2 if it applies).

3. Add 30 ml benzene to the separatory funnel. Shake the funnel about 30 seconds and add 200 ml water. Allow time for separation and discard lower layer.

4. Place the upper layer into a beaker or vial and evaporate to total dryness (or see Modification 3). Resuspend in 0.5 ml Benzene. Spot a small amount (50 microlitres) on No. 4 Whatman filter paper. Allow the spot to dry and place it under a long-wave UV-light.

5. If the filter paper does not contain a blue fluorescent colour, then the sample contains no aflatoxin otherwise the sample is likely to contain aflatoxin.

Caution

Feeds containing ethoxyquin will give the characteristic blue fluorescence of aflatoxin on filter paper. For these feeds the benzene fraction should be applied directly on a thin layer chromatography plate with a standard and then developed to determine if the sample contains aflatoxin.

Modification one

Certain grain fractions (white corn and oats) in some cases are difficult to separate from the extracting solvent. Step 2 can be modified to overcome this problem by vacuum filtration of the blended material through muslin with a Buchner funnel. This filtering takes about one minute and produces a longer amount of extraction solvent. This modification may be used in all cases if a vacuum system is available since it results in more solvent and does so in a shorter period of time.

Modification two

If the product to be tested has a high fat content or a large amount of fat soluble pigment. a hexane wash may be used immediately after step 2. This may be accomplished by adding 50 ml hexane or skelly solve 'F' to the separatory funnel. This combination of extracting solvent and hexane is shaken vigorously, with venting, for about 30 seconds. After shaking, the addition of 50 to 100 ml of water usually gives a rapid separation. Drain off and save the lower layer and discard the upper layer. The part saved is then used in part 3.

Modification three

Most samples tested contain compounds other than aflatoxin that will be in the benzene fraction. In certain cases these compounds will produce a fluorescence of their own or will partially mark the fluorescence of the aflatoxin. To prevent this problem collect the benzene layer into a 50 ml beaker containing approximately 10 g of anhydrous sodium sulphate and 5g of green basic cupric carbonate. Swirl gently and filter through the procelain filter into a 50 ml Erlenmeyer flask and evaporate to dryness. Resuspend in 0.5 ml benzene and follow step 4 to the procedure.

Presence of aflatoxin should be verified by thin layer chromatography and appropriate standards. Confirmation and rough quantification may be carried out by using ready-made TLC plates silica gel G-HR (Brinkmann Instr.). Occassionally, when sample containing low levels of toxin (15 ppb) are tested, the light blue fluorescence is masked by traces of yellow pigments that may remain. In such cases. TLC appears to be the best procedure to follow to confirm the results.

Rapid Screening Methods for Aflatoxin in Corn by Kansas State University Test

(Method of Wilcox, 1983)

Reagents

1. *Toluene or benzene.*
2. *Methanol-water solution (80: 20, V/V)*
3. *Salt solution*

   600 g Nacl, 600 g Zinc acetate and 15 ml of glacial acetic acid dissolved in 4 l distilled water.
4. *Hexane : Acetone solution (80: 20, V/V).*

Equipment

1. *Waring blender (An explosion proof model perferred).*
2. *Vacuum sources (Aspirator on water line or vacuum pump).*
3. *Minicolumn. Keep minicolumns dry and out of light.*
4. *Holaday minicolumns may be made with glass tubing.*
5. *5 mm internal diameter and 160 mm long with 15 mm florisil (100-200 mesh) on bottom and 15 mm of neutral alumina. (100-200 mesh activity IV or E. Merck Activity 1) dry at 100°C for 2 h then add 15 percent distilled water by weight. Mix well, let stand at least 2 hour immediately above, held in place with 4 to 6 mm of paper pulp packing at bottom of florisil and at top of alumina.*

   Another minicolumn that may be used and considered to give more distinct band and more sensitivity is the CPC column.
6. *Test tubes with screw of watertight plastic caps.*
7. *Graduated cylinder, 25 ml or 10 ml and a 100 ml.*
8. *Pipettes (1 ml and mechanical device to draw up fluid). Do not pipette solvents by mouth. Shorter pipettes are easier to handle than long. Automatic pipette device will speed up dispensing of salt solution and toluene.*
9. *Glass fiber filter, 12 cm.*
10. *Filter paper, such as whatman 2 V or 114 plated, 18.5 cm. but size is not critical.*
11. *Funnels to fit filters listed above.*
12. *Blacklight.*

Procedure

1. Grind sample finely enough to pass through a No. 20 mesh screen.
2. Blend 100 g of finely ground sample with 200 ml of methanol-water solution for 1 min. at high speed in a blender (any size sample may be used as long as the ratio of sample weight to solvent volume remains the same; 50g is often used).
3. Fold fast filtering paper into a funnel and filter 10 ml of sample into a culture tube fitted with a plastic lined screw cap or rubber stopper. Tubes can be calibrated for 10 ml and marked with taps.
4. Add 10 ml of salt solution to test tube and shake vigorously for 5 to 10 min.
5. Filter 15 ml of contents through a glass filter fiber into a second culture tube.
6. Add 3 ml of toluene to solution, close tube and shake vigorously for 10 seconds, If problem with emulsion, shake less vigorously.
7. Let layers separate and pipette (use bulb or mechanical device on pipette, do not aspirate by mouth) 1 ml of upper layer toluene into the top of a minicolumn. Be sure not to pipette material from lower level.
8. After the toluene has been pulled through the minicolumn by vacuum, add 5 ml of the hexane-acetone washing solution to the top of the minicolumn and pull through. Evacuate column for an additional 2 min or until all of the washing solution evaporated from the mincolumn. Do not use top high a vacuum, as part of the column packing may be disrupted. Also, too high a vacuum may diffuse the fluorescent zone and increase differently in reading the minicolumn. if no vacuum is available, the column may be drained by gravity which will increase the time by 20 to 30 min.
9. Observe the minicolumn under long wave ultraviolet light. Use a high intensity light. A high intensity light is very important in the detection of borderline sample.
10. A blue fluorescent band appearing in the centre of the column, below the interface of the florisil and alumina, indicates at least 4 ppb of aflatoxin.

The amount of liquid from the toluene layer determines the detection limit of the method and can be used to design a “go” or “no go” system at various approximate levels as indicated as follows: 2 ml, 2 ppb: 1 ml 4 ppb; 0.5 ml , ppb; 0.2 ml, 20 ppb; and 0.1, 40 ppb. Keep in mind that these are approximate levels, instead of adding 0.1 or 0.2 ml directly to column it may be advisable to dilute to 1 ml with toluene and then add 1 ml of dilution. This is more accurate and will give a more uniform zone. Alternatively, add 1 ml of hexane-acetone washing solution before the 0.1 or 0.2 ml of the toluene extract is added to the column.

Method Recommended by JAOAC, 58, 163 (1975), Tropical Products Instt. Report G. 70 (1972), Official Methods of Analysis of AOAC, 13th Edn. (1980)

Processing of Sample

First mix the sample homogeneously and powder it through Wiley ball mill or any other appropriate mill (or Appropriate quantity) is taken into 500 ml conical flask and 25 ml water, 25 g diatomaceous earth (celite) and 150 ml chloroform are added to it. The flask is tightly closed with rubber cork covered with aluminium foil to prevent contact of rubber with chloroform. The contents of the flask are shaken on a wrist action shaker for 30 min. to extract. The contents are transferred to a buchner funnel precoated with about 5 mm layer of diatomaceous earth and filtered using light vacuum.

Removal of Interfering Substances

The chromatographic column consists of a glass tube 22 x 300 mm with a glass stopper at the bottom.

A small plug of glass wool is loosely packed at the bottom of the column and is covered with 5 g anhydrous sodium sulphate. Chloroform is added until the column is about half full when 10g of silica gel has settled, 15 g anhydrous sodium sulphate made as slurry in chloroform is added to the column. As soon as the chloroform is drained off to the top of the sodium sulphate layer, 50 ml of the sample extract to be chromatographed is added to the column. the chloroform is drained off and the column is washed, at a maximum rate, first with 150 ml hexane followed by 150 ml anhydrous diethyl ether. Finally the aflatoxins are eluted from the column with 150 ml Chloroform-methanol (97:3 V/V) mixture. The fraction is collected from the time the chloroform methanol is added until the flow stops. The elute is evaporated by warming on water bath under a stream of nitrogen. It is desirable to carry out the evaporation in a hood. The residue dissolved in a known volume of chloroform (0.2 or 1.0 ml) is ready for TLC.

TLC Method

The standard solutions containing quantites of aflatoxin B_1 are spotted along with the sample extracts on a TLC plate. The plates are developed ascendingly by dipping them in a chromatographic tank containing chloroform-acetone solvent mixture (95: 5) to a depth of not more that 1 cm.

It is necessary to saturate the tank with the solvent before use. The solvent front is allowed to reach 10 to 12 cm height. This would take about 30 min at 27°C. After development, the plates are dried in horizontal position and viewed under long wave UV lamp in a dark room or in a cabinet.

Spot sample aliquots on TLC plate. Alslo spot 10 mg of aflatoxin B_1 standard. Develop in chromatographic chamber containg 100 ml chlorform-acetone (95:5). Mark the position of the spots on TLC plate and scan the plate with densitometer. After exciting with 365 nm source, emission is measured at 420 nm. The area of the peaks are calculated.

Calculations

$$\text{Aflatoxin } \mu g/kg = \frac{(B x y x S x V)}{(Z \times W)}$$

B = Average of aflatoxin B_1 sample in aliquots

Y = Concentration of aflatoxin B_1 standard (µg/ml)

S = µl aflatoxin B_1 standard spotted

V = Final dilution of sample extracted (µl)

Z = Average are aflatoxin B_1 peaks in standard aliquots

X = µl sample extract spotted

W = g sample represented in final extract

Qualitative Method

This method consists of comparing the intensity of the fluorescent spots of the sample with the corresponding spots of the aflatoxin pure standard. A visual aflatoxin standard of 05 µg/ml concentration is used.

Extracted sample is diluted to 0.5 ml of suitable volume in benzene-acetonitrile (98:2 V/V) or chloroform. In subdued light, quickly spot on TLC plate 3 levels (5, 70 10 µl) of sample extract and 3 levels of aflatoxin standard to cover a range of 2 to 15 mg/spot. Develop the plate to a height of 12 to 14 cm in suitable solvent. After development the plate is dried in the dark. Under long wave UV compare the fluorescence intensities of the sample spot with those of the standard spots and determine which of the sample spots matches one of the standards. If the sample spot intensity is found to be between those of 2 standard spots, the actual intensity should be estimated. If spots of the smallest quantity of sample are too intense to match standards, the sample should be diluted and rechromatographed. *Estimates should never be made by extrapolation from the series of standard spots.*

Calculations

Calculate concentration of aflatoxin B_1 in µg/kg = $\frac{S \times Y \times V}{X \times W}$

where

S = µl aflatoxin standard which matches the unknown

Y = Concentration of aflatoxin B_1 standard µg/ml

V = µl of final dilution of sample extract

X = µl of sample extract spotted giving fluorescent intensity equivalent to S (B_1 standard).

W = gram of sample contained in final extract.

Spectrophotometric Method

The presence or absence of blue fluorescent spot corresponding to aflatoxin B_1 at Rf 0.50 to 0.55 and greenish blue fluorescent spot corresponding to aflatoxin G at Rf 0.45 is observed in UV light. The Rf values are checked with the standard aflatoxin run along with the sample extracts.

The area covering the spots or bands the marked by a sharp needle under the UV light and the silica gel covering each spot is scraped carefully with a blad and collected individually in clean, dry test tubes. The aflatoxins are extracted with 2 ml cold methanol for 3 min. and filtered through glass sinter. It is washed three times with methanol and combined filtrate is made up to 5 ml. The aflatoxin content is measured and determind by measuring the absorbance at 360 nm in quartz cell. For routine estimations, a standard curve for aflatoxin B_1 from 5 to10 µg is used. The amount of aflatoxin present in the sample extract is computed from the standard curve.

Calculations

The aflatoxin content (µg/kg or ppb) is calculated using the formula.

$$\frac{S \times V \times 5}{A \times W} \times 1000.$$

where

W = Weight in g of original sample

V = µl of sample prepared for TLC.

A = µl of sample extract spotted.

S = µl of aflatoxin calculated from the standard curve.

☞ **Note**

Aflatoxin B_1 is a ***potent carcinogen****. Dry crystalline toxin must be handled in hood using face masks and gloves because it is electrostatic in nature. Aflatoxin must be destroyed by sodium hypochlorite before discarding.*

Permissible Limit of Aflatoxin in Poultry Feeds

The research work conducted at Indian and Foreign laboratories concludes that a 0.4 ppm. level of aflatoxin B_1 is the limit which causes no adverse effects on producion performance of broilers. *A study conducted at IVRI/CARI (India) envisages that dietary aflatoxin at and above 0.3 ppm level leads to immuno supperssion in broilers. The research work conducted with chicks other than broilers indicate that White Leghorn. White Leghorn x Rhode Island Red, New Hampshire and Rhode Island Red chicks can tolerate dietary levels of aflatoxin B_1 ranging from 0.15 to 0.20 ppm. Several reports are available in the literature to show that even higher levels of the toxin in the diet are tolerated by different types of chicks.*

BIS Recommendation

As per Indian standard, Poultry Feeds - Specification (Fourth Revised publication IS 1374: 1992 BIS 1992) *the aflatoxin content B_1 of the poultry feed shall not exceed 500 mcg/Kg (500ppb) at the time of manufacture. It shall be tested by the manufacturer in accordance with the test method prescribed in IS 13427 : 1992 and declared on the label. Sampling of the poultry feed for estimation of aflatoxin content shall be done in accordance with IS 13426: 1992. Manufactures are required to test the aflatoxin B_1 content and declare it on the label and the instructions should be meticulously* followed.

The founder Director, Prof. Dr. B. Panda of CARI, Izatnagar, Bareilly (U.P.), India has reported following tolerance limit of dietary aflatoxin in poultry:

White Leghorm chicks	150 ppb
Pure bred broiler chicks	200 ppb
Cross bred broiler chicks	400 ppb
Quail starter chicks	300 ppb
Guinea fowl kitts	1500 ppb

Prof. Dr. B. Panda mentioned that about 50% sample of maize analysed by CARI, Izatnagar (U.P.) have been found to be positive for aflatoxin. Thus, our county has to face aflatoxin problem. At the same time, there is no need to create a scare among the farmers because the aflatioxin tolerance level is much higher than normally found in the feed.

References

JAOAC, (1975). 58: 163.

Jones, B.D. (1972). *Methods of aflatoxin analysis Report* No. G. 97.

Official Methods of Analysis of AOAC, 13th Edn., (1980).

Wilcox. R.A. (1983). Feedstuffs (Ref. issue) pp. 117.

Chapter - 26

Thioglucoside in Rapeseed Meal

Thioglucoside Estimation

The method described here gives an approximate thioglucoside and isothiocyanates contents in rapeseed meal.

Reagents and Apparatus

1. *Barium chloride (5% solution)*
2. *Volumetric flask, 600 ml*
3. *Steam bath*

Method

To 10 g meal (defatted by soxhlet extraction) add 250 ml distilled water, hydrolyse at 54°C for one hour and then boil for two hours, keeping volume constant. Filter, retaining filtrate and wash residue three times with 50 ml hot water. Add washings to initial filtrate and make up volume to 600 ml. Precipitate barium sulphate by heating and adding excess barium chloride solution. Leave on a steam bath for a few hours and then filter. Ash in muffle furnace and then weigh precipitate.

Calculate approximate thioglucoside content as:

$$\text{Percent thioglucoside} = \frac{(\text{M.Wt. thioglucoside}) \times (\text{Wt. of } BaSO_4)}{(\text{M.Wt. } BaSO_4)(\text{Sample Wt.})} \times 100$$

Reference

McGhee, J.E. L.O. Kirk and G.C. Mustakas, (1965). *J. Am. Oil. Chem. Soc.* 42: 889-91.

□□□

Chapter - 27

Free Gossypol in Cottonseed Meal

Gossypol Estimation

Two procedure are described for the determination of free gosssypol . The first for normal meals and the second for meals which have been chemically treated and so contain dianilinogossypol.

Reagents

1. *Aqueous acetone: 7 parts acetone, 3 parts distilled water (V/V).*
2. *Aqueous acetone-aniline solution: To 700 ml acetone and 300 ml distilled water, add 0.5 ml redistilled aniline. Prepare solution daily.*
3. *Aqueous isopropyl alcohol solution: 8 parts isopropyl alcohol. 2 parts distilled water (V/V).*
4. *Aniline Distill reagent grade aniline over a small quantity of zinc, dust discarding the first and last 10 percent of the distillate. Store refrigerated in a brown glass stoppered bottle. Solution is stable for several months.*
5. *Standard gossypol solution (a) Dissolve 25 mg of pure gossypol in anline free acetone and transfer to a 250 ml volumetric flask using 100 ml of acetone. Add 75 ml of distilled water, dilute to volume with acetone and mix. (b) Take 50 ml solution (a) add 100 ml pure acetone, 60 ml of distilled water, mix and*

dilute to 250 ml with pure acetone. Solution (b) contains 0.02 mg gossypol/ mg and is stable for 24 h in darkness.

Apparatus

1. Mechanical shaker
2. Spectrophotometer
3. Conical flasks, 250 ml.
4. Volumetric flasks, 25 and 250 ml.
5. Water bath (boiling)

Method

Grind sample to pass 1 mm sieve taking care not to overheat. Take approximately 1 g of the sample and add 25 ml of pure acetone. Stir for a few minutes, filter, and divide the filtrate into two. To one portion add a pellet of sodium hydroxide and heat in a water bath for few minutes. A deep orange red colour in the tube containing sodium hydroxide indicates the presence of dianilinogossypol and procedure (2) described below should be used. A light yellow extract which does not change colour with sodium hydroxide indicates that the cottonseed meal is untreated and procedure (1) described below should be used.

Procedure 1

Weigh 0.5 to 1 g of sample, depending on expected gossypol contents, into a conical flask and add glass beads. Pipette into it 50 ml of aqueous acetone solution, stopper the flask and shake for one hour. Filter, discarding the first few millilitres of filtrate and then pipette out duplicate aliquots into 250 ml volumetric flasks. (Take aliquots from 2 to 10 ml. again depending on expected gossypol content). Dilute one of the aliquots to volume with aqueous isopropyl alcohol (solution A). While to the other aliquot (solution B) add 2 ml redistilled aniline and heat in a boiling water bath for 30 minutes together with a reagent blank containing 2 ml of aniline and a volume of aqueous acetone solution equal to the sample aliquot. Remove solution B and the blank, add sufficient aqueous isopropyl alcohol to effect homogeneous solution and cool to room temperature in a water bath. Dilute to volume with aqueous isopropyl alcohol.

Read samples at 400 mμ. Set instrument to zero absorbance with aqueous isopropyl alcohol and determine absorbance of solution A and reagent blank.

If the reagent blank is below 0.022 absorbance, proceed as below, otherwise repeat the analysis using freshly distilled aniline. Determine the absorbance of solution (B) with the reagent blank set at 0 absorbance. Calculate the corrected absorbance of the sample aliquot: Corrected absorbance: (Absorbance solution B, Absorbance solution A.) Determine the mg free gossypol present in the sample solution using the calibration curve.

Procedure 2

Weigh out 1 g of sample into a conical flask, add 50 ml aqueous acetone and shake and filter as above. Pipette duplicate aliquots of the filtrate (from 2 to 5 ml depending on expected free gossypol level) into 250 ml volumetric flasks. Dilute one of the aliquots to volume (solution A) with aqueous isopropyl alcohol and leave for at least 30 min before reading on the spectrophotometer. Treat the other aliquot (Solution B) as in procedure-I, determine absorbance of solutions (A) and (B) as before and calculate the apparent content of gossypol in both solution A and B using the calibration curve.

Preparation of Calibration Curve

Pipette duplicate 1, 2, 3, 4, 5, 7, 8 and 10 ml aliquots of the 0.02 mg/ml gossypol standard into 25 ml volumetic flasks. Dilute one set (Solution A) to volume with aqueous isopropyl alcohol and determine absorbances as described previously. To the other set (Solution B) add 2 ml of redistilled aniline and proceed as described previously. Prepare, one reagent blank, using 2 ml aniline and 10 ml of aqueous acetone, heated together with the standards. Determine absorbances as in Procedure 1 and calculate the corrected optical density for each standard solution.

Corrected absorbance = (absorbance solution B - absorbance solution A). Plot the standard curve, plotting corrected absorbance against gossypol conc. in the 25 ml volume:

Calculate free gossypol percent in normal meals as:

$$\text{Free gossypol percent} = \frac{5G}{WV}$$

where,

G = Graph reading

W = Sample weight

V = Aliquot volume used

For chemically treated meals:

$$\text{Free gossypol percent} = \frac{5(BA)}{WV}$$

where

A = mg apparent free gossypol in sample aliquot (A)
B = mg apparent free gossypol in sample aliquot (B)
W = sample weight
V = aliquot volume used.

Reference

Amercian Oil Chemists Society, (1972). Official and tentative methods, 3rd edn., Method Ba 7-58.

Chapter - 28

Desoxyribonucleic Acid and Ribonucleic Acid in Animal Tissue

DNA and RNA Estimation

Isolation of RNA from Rat Liver

(Method of Schmidt and Thannhauser, 1945)

Principle

Most of the RNA (ribouncleic acid) of cells is found in the nucleoli and microsomes.These fractions of cells may be isolated by differential centrifugation of cellular homogenates and thus provide an enriched starting material for RNA extraction. Such methods require high speed centrifugation. An alternate procedure used in the present method is to disrupt the whole cells by homogenization and isolate the nucleic acid of entire homogenate. This procedure consists of the following sequential steps.

(a) Precipitation of all macromolecules (Proteins and nucleic acids) with cold trichloroacetic acid (TCA) to free the preparation of small molecules.

(b) Extraction of the precipitate with acetone and ether to remove lipid materials and excess TCA.

(c) Extraction of the lipid-free precipitate with salt solution to dissolve the nucleic acid.

(d) Final precipitation of the nucleic acid by alcohol precipitation.

This method is effective for nucleic acids in general. With certain tissues having a high RNA/DNA ratio (e.g. rat liver) a relatively pure preparation of RNA may be obtained.

Apparatus

1. Waring blender
2. Clincial centrifuge

Reagents

1. *Cold 30 percent trichloroacetic acid (w/v)*
2. *Acetone*
3. *Ether*
4. *10 percent NaCl (w/v)*
5. *Ethanol*

Procedure

One large (200g) rat is decapitated: the liver is removed and quickly cooled in an ice bath before weighing to the nearest gram. The liver then is homogenized with 5 volume of ice cold distilled water in an ice-cold waring blender. The homogenate is quickly collected and cold 30 percent TCA is added until a final concentration of 15 percent TCA is obtained. After standing for 20 min. in the cold (0-2°C), the precipitate is collected by centrifugation in the cold room and washed by suspension and centrifugation in 3 ml of acetone (twice), 3 ml of acetone-ether (50/50, once), and finally 3 ml of ether (once). The later two washings may be conducted at room temperature. The dry powder is then suspended in a volume of 10 percent NaCl equal to twice the volume of the powder and placed in a boiling water bath for one hour (The test tube containing the mixture is covered with aluminium foil and from time to time during the heating period distilled water is added to replace that which has evaporated). The remaining precipitate then is removed by centrifugation of the cooled extract; 2 volume of absolute ethanol is slowly added to the supernatant solution. After cooling the suspension in an ice bath for five minutes, the precipitated RNA is collected by centrifugation. washed once with ethanol and then ether, dried, weighed, and stored in a stoppered bottle for further processing.

Characterization of RNA

Principle

RNA is readily hydrolysed to nucleotides by treatment with mild alkali. This case of alkaline hydrolysis of RNA apparently is due to the presence of free 2′ hydroxyl of ribose which allow the formation of an intermediate 2′, 3′

phospho- diester nucleotide which subsequently breaks down to a mixture of 2′ and 3′ nucleotides.

The desoxyribose in DNA lacks a 2′ hydroxyl group and, therefore, is incapable of forming such an intermediate. DNA is relatively stable to mild alkaline treatment. Acidification of the preparation after alkali treatment will precipitate DNA. The nucleotides released by alkaline hydrolysis of RNA may be readily identified by comparision with known nucleotides by paper electrophoresis. At pH 3.5 the overall net charges on the four RNA nucleotides are quite distinctly different. This can be seen from Table 1.

Table 1 : Values of Ionizable Groups of Nucleotides

Acid type	NH_3	First OH	Primary Phosphate	Secondray Phosphate
Adenylic acid	3.7	—	0.9	6.0
Guanylic acid	2.3	9.7	0.7	5.9
Cytidylic acid	4.3	13.2	0.8	6.0
Uridylic acid	—	9.4	1.0	5.9

Since the extent of movement of similar molecule in an electric field is largely a function of the overall net charge of the molecules, paper electrophoresis at pH 3.5 serves as a ready means of separation and identification of the nucleotides in question.

The quantity of RNA and DNA present in a given sample can be determined by measurement of the ribose and desoxyribose content of the sample; the RNA and DNA content of the original sample may be calculated from the ribose and desoxyribose determination. *Mejbaum's quantitative procedure for pentoses, often called the orcinol determination, may be applied to the nucleotides released by alkaline hydrolysis for the quantitative determination of RNA. The quantitative diphenylamine reaction which is specific for desoxyribose may be applied to the DNA precipitated from acidified alkaline hydrolysates for the quantitative determination of DNA.*

Apparatus

1. Paper electrophoresis apparatus
2. UV lamp

Reagents

1. *0.5 N KOH*
2. *1.0 N KOH*
3. *20 percent perchloric acid*
4. *2 N HCl*

5. *10 percent TCA (trichloroacetic acid)*
6. *0.02 M citrate buffer pH 3.5*
7. *1 percent starch solution*
8. *0.01N I_2 0.01 N KI*
9. *0.02 M Na citrate or 0.05 M NH_4 formate (pH 3.5)*
10. *1 percent orcinol in 0.1 percent $FeCl_3$ dissolved in conc. HCl freshly prepard DNA standard-DNA (1 mg/ml) dissolved in 10 percent TCA by heating to 90°C for 15 min.*
11. *Ribose standard (10 μg/ml)*
12. *Diphenylamine ragent freshly prepared.*

Procedure

The material obtained from rat liver is dissolved in sufficient 0.5 N KOH to give a concentration of 100 mg RNA/5 ml. This solution is stored at room temperature for 24-48 h. One half of the solution is then cooled in ice and titrated to pH 1-2 with 20 percent $HClO_4$ (a few drops of $HClO_4$) ml of original KOH solution). The precipitated $KClO_4$ and DNA and/or protein are removed by centrifugation. The supernatant is adjusted to approximately pH 3.5 with 1 N KOH. Any additional precipitate formed is removed by centrifugation, the supernatant then is used for the electrophoresis separation as described below:

The remaining one-half of the alkaline hydrolysate is cooled and acidified to pH 1-2 with 2 N HCl and any precipitate (protein and DNA) is collected by centrifugation and saved for DNA analysis. The supernatant is saved for the pentose determination.

It is possible that no precipitate will form, indicating that the preparation is relatively free of DNA and protein. In this case, the acidified solution is used directly for the diphenylamine assay below:

It is precipitate (Protein and DNA) obtained above, as given is suspended in 1 ml 10 percent TCA and the DNA present is hydrolysed by heating the suspension at 90°C for 15 min. The remaining precipitate (protein) is removed by centrifugation and discarded. The supernatant is saved for the diphenlylamine assay as follows:

Electrophoresis

The exact instructions for operation of the electrophoresis unit depend on the design of the unit to be used. However, in general, the following criteria must be met:

1. Sufficient RNA hydrolysate and separate nucleotides must be placed on the paper (s) to allow ready location of the material with a U.V. light.
2. A control containing a spot of 1 percent starch solution is run with the other materials. Subsequent location of the starch by spraying with 0.01 N I_2, 0.01 N KI determines the extent of solvent migration during the separation. Appropriate corrections are then made.
3. The paper (s) saturated with appropriate buffer (0.02 M citrate-citric acid or 0.05 M ammonium formate formic acid at pH 3.5) and maintained in state where water is not lost from the paper. This may either be in a box saturated with water vapour or in a bath of CCI_4.
4. The material moving further in any given direction is assigned a relative mobility of 1.0. The relative mobilities of all other material are determined with respect to the furthest moving material and are recorded as decimal fractions (e.g., 0.75 and 0.63)

Quantitative Estimation of RNA-Orcinol Test

Various aliquots (0.05 0.1 and 0.5ml) of the HCl acidified hydrolysate, ribose standards (1 to 3 ml), and a water blank are made upto 5 ml (with water); 5 ml of orcinol reagent are added with mixing; and the tubes are heated in boiling water bath for 20 min. After cooling, the optical densities at 625mμ are determined.

Quantitative Estimation of DNA - Diphenylamine Test

Aliquot (0.1, 0.5 and 1 ml, if possible) of the HCl acidified supernatant and of the TCA hydrolysed precipitate, 0.4 and 0.8 ml aliquots of the DNA standard and a water blank are all made up to 3 ml (with water); 6 ml of the diphenylamine reagent are added to each tube with mixing; and the tubes are heated in a boiling water bath for 10 min. After cooling, the optical densities at 600 mμ are determined. In all cases, the water blank is set at zero optical density units.

Results

The Rf's (relative to the fastest moving component of the 4 nucleotides) are determined after correcting for fluid migration as exemplified by the starch control. The compounds released from the RNA by alkaline hydrolysis are compared with the relative Rf's of the known nucleotides to confirm the identity of the original sample.

The quantity of RNA and DNA in the original sample is calculated from the optical density data. Determination of the exact value for RNA content will require calculation of the percent pentose in a 1:1:1:1 mixture of nucleotides. The results obtained by this colorimetric method are compared with the results of the electrophoretic separation.

Reference

Schmidt, G. and S. J. Thannhauser, (1945). *J. Biol. Chem.*, 161: 83.

Chapter - 29

Non Esterified Fatty Acid Concentrations in Plasma

NEFA Estimation

Principle

(Method of Patterson 1963)

The albumin bound long-chain fatty acids of plasma are usually referred to as unesterified or non-esterified fatty acids (NEFA) to distinguish them from the long-chain fatty acids present in the esterified form in neutral fats and phospholipid. In the case of ruminant plasma, it is also important to distinguish these "free fatty acids" from the small molecular weight steam volatile fatty acids of dietary origin which are found in the free state as the carboxylate ion.

Basically, the method of Dole (1959a) has been used to estimate plasma NEFA employed by Annison (1960), which is to evaporate the heptane extract of plasma to dryness before titration. This is conveniently done in a stream of nitrogen on a warm hot plate rather than by evaporation in vacua. In place of the 0.05 M- phosphate buffer (pH 6.0) of Annison or the 0.02 N-H_2SO_4 used by Dole (1956a), in the present method 0.02 N-HCI is used as an extraction medium. This is preferred because owing to its volatility, it is less likely to cause serious accidental contamination of the supernatant heptane layer.

Reagents

1. *Extraction solution*
   Iso-propanol: n heptane: 1.0 N HCl 40: 10: 1 (v/v)

2. *Standard solution*
   Dissolve 0.25642 g palmitic acid in 100 ml n-heptane, then dilute 10 ml aliquot upto 100 ml with n-heptane
3. *0.01 N alcoholic NaOH*
   Dissolve 4g NaOH in 100 ml alcohol, then dilute 1 ml of this solution upto 100 ml.
4. *Ethanolic Nile blue solution (0.02 percent)*
5. *HCl (1 N)*
   Dissolve 88.45 ml HCl (< 35%) in one litre distilled water
6. *n-heptane*
7. *Ethanol*

Procedure

Deliver 2 ml plasma and 10 ml extraction mixture into a 30 ml stoppered test tube. The initial extraction is carried out by vigorous mixing for 30 seconds. After leaving for 5 min., 4 ml distilled water and 6 ml heptane are added and the fatty acids are redistributed to the upper heptane layer by shaking for 60 seconds (Approximately 82.5 percent of the NEFA fraction is extracted in this way). The upper layer is separated rapidly and completely on standing. After 30 min, there is no difficulty in removing a 5 ml aliquot of the heptane layer which is evaportated to dryness in a 25 ml conical flask under nitrogen on a warm hot plate. Control extractions are carried out at the same time, 2 ml water replacing the plasma samples in the above procedure. Replicate standards are also prepared following the control procedure but using tubes in which 2 ml of a 1 m-molar heptane solution of recrystallized plamitic acid is used. Thus pure palmitic acid and plasma NEFA are extracted at the same time under identical conditions.

The residues obtained from blank, standard and plasma extracts are dissolved in 2.5 ml warm 95 percent ethanol (redistilled from calcium oxide) and titrated with approximately 0.01 N-NaOH using 0.5 ml 0.02 percent ethanolic Nile Blue solution as indicator (in a stream of nitrogen). *A Conway micro-burette is convenient for these titrations.* The blue to red end-point is observed to span the addition of less than 2 μl 0.01 N-NaOH.

Result

The concentration of NEFA in plasma is computed from the ratio of the sample to standard titrations (allowance being made for blank titrations) and is expressed as microequivalents/litre calculated as palmitate.

NEFA, micro equivalent/litre

$$= \frac{\text{Titre value with sample - Titre value with blank}}{\text{Titre value with standard - Titre value with blank}} \times 100$$

Reference

Patterson. D.S.P. (1963). *Res. in Vety. Sci.,* 4: 230-37.

Chapter - 30

Enzymatic Determination of Polyunsaturated Fatty Acids

PUFA Estimation

(Method of Joseph Mac Gee, 1959)

Principle

A simple and rapid enzymatic method for the quantitative estimation of total cis-methylene- interrupted polyenoic acids has been devised. *Linoleic, linolenic and arachidonic acids, the more common acids of this group were used to calibrate the method.* The potassium salts of the fatty acids are oxidised by atmospheric oxygen in the presence of the enzyme lipo-oxidase, and the absorption of the conjugated diene hydroperoxide is measured at 234 mμ. As little as 5 μg of linoleic acid can be quantitatively measured with good accuracy and precision. The total content of polyunsaturated fatty acids containing the cismethylene-interrupted diene structure of fats, oils, hydrogenated oils, fatty acids, esters blood plasma, microorganisms and plant seeds has been measured directly by this method.

Reagents

1. Potassium Borate Buffer 1.0 M, pH 9.0

Dissolve 61.9 g of boric acid and 25.0 g of potassium hydroxide in about 800 ml of distilled water by stirring while heating on a steam bath. After complete solution, allow the solution to cool to room temperature with stirring. Adjust the pH of the solution to 9.0 by addition of 1 N potassium hydroxide or 1 N hydrochloric acid as required. Adjust the volume of the solution to 1 litre by adding distilled water.

0.2 M. pH 9.0 Transfer 200 ml of the 1 M buffer to a 1 litre volumetric flask, and dilute to volume with distilled water.

2. Lipo-oxidase

Dissolve 10 mg of lipo-oxidase in 10 ml of ice cold 0.02 M buffer.

3. Dilute Solution

Mix 2 ml of the stock solution with 8 ml of ice-cold 0.2 M buffer.

4. Boiled Dilute Solution

Transfer 5 ml of the dilute solution to a test tube and hold in a boiling water bath for 5 min.

Because the activity of the enzyme may vary from batch to batch, each bottle of enzyme must be tested before use.

Processing of Sample for Free Fatty Acids

The polyunsaturated fatty acid content of free fatty acids is determined after solution of the acids in 0.2 M buffer. This is most conveniently done by adding one fifth of the final volume of 1 M buffer to the sample, mixing well, and diluting with distilled water to volume-yielding a solution in 0.2 M buffer.

Processing of Sample of Fatty Acids Esters

Esters must first be saponified. Saponify a sample containing 0.5 mg of polyunsaturated fatty acids by mixing it in a 200 ml volumetric flask with 1 ml of 0.5 N alcoholic potassium hydroxide, and holding in the dark for at least 4 h. After saponification, add 20 ml of the 1.0 M buffer, 1 ml of 0.5 N hydrochloric acid, and water to the 100 ml mark.

Procedure

Place 3 ml aliquots of fatty acid esters in each of two 1 cm quartz cuvettes for the Beckman DU spectrophotometer. To the first cuvette, add 0.10 ml of the boiled dilute lipo-oxidase and mix. Use this cuvette to zero the instrument at 234 mμ. Add 0.10 ml of the dilute lipo-oxidase (unboiled) to the second cuvette. mix, and note the time. Place the second cuvette in the instrument and take readings of the absorbance of the second cuvette against the first cuvette as a blank at 1 min. intervals. The absorbance should increase to a maximum level in the second cuvette in less than 5 min. If not, either more concentrated preparations of dilute solution and boiled dilute solution must be prepared and tested to yield the necessary rate, of a more active supply of lipo-oxidase is necessary.

The enzyme and solutions must be stored in a freezer. The solutions can be thawed by placing them in a water bath at room temperature, but they should be held in an ice and water bath as soon as they are completely thawed. The stock solution, dilute solution and boiled solution used after storage for several months without noticeable deterioration.

Sample Solution

Prepare a solution in the 0.2 M buffer such that each 3ml contains between 5 and 25 μg of the free polyunsaturated fatty acids.

In each of the two test tubes, place 2 ml of the sample solution. To the first tube (the blank) add 0.10 ml of the boiled dilute enzyme solution and mix. To the second tube (the sample) add 0.10 ml of the unboiled dilute enzyme solution and mix. Allow the contents of the tube to stand to room temperature for 30 min, then transfer to 1 cm quartz cuvettes and place in the Beckman DU spectrophotometer. Set the instrument at zero with the blank Sample and measure the absorbance of the reacted sample solution at 234 mμ. Calculate the polyunsaturated fatty acid content from the following fomula:

$$\%\,\text{PUFA} = \frac{\text{A} \times 3964}{\text{W}}$$

where,

A = difference in absorbance between the blank and sample

W = total micrograms of sample in 3.0 ml of sample solution.

Source of Factor

$$3964 = \frac{3.1}{3.0} \times \frac{1000}{78.2} \text{ x } 100 \text{ x } 3$$

where

$\frac{3.1}{3.0}$ = dilution factor, 3 ml of sample plus 0.1 ml of enzyme

78.2 = specific extinction coefficient (absorbance of 1 g of PUFA per litre in 1 cm light path at 234 mμ)

1000 = Conversion from grams per litre to micrograms per ml

100 = Conversion to percentage

3 = Volume of sample

Reference

Joseph, Mac Gee, (1959). *Analytical Chem.* 31: 298.

Chapter - 31

Total Lipids in Serum or Plasma

Total Lipids Estimation

(Method of Bloor, 1928 Modified by Folch *et al.*, 1957)

Gravimetric Method — Principle

Total lipids in plasma consist of neutral fats, phospholipids, chloesterol esters and free cholesterol. Minor components include non-esterified fatty acids (NEFA), phosphatides and sphingo myelin. Total lipids in serum or plasma are extracted using ethyl alcohol and petroleum ether, separated and weighed after drying at 105°C.

Procedure

Pipette 5 ml serum in a separating funnel, add 5 ml ethyl alcohol and 12.5 ml pertroleum ether. Shake the contents of funnel two times for 3 min. atleast. Keep the contents of funnel as such for one hour. Transfer the contents of funnel in the moisture cup, dry and weigh. Calculate the result by difference method using the following formula.

Total lipids

$$= \frac{\text{g(wt.of lipid in moisture cup)} \times 12.5 \times 100}{5 \times 5}$$

= g lipids x 50

Colorimetric Method

(Method of Zollner and Kirsch, 1962)

Principle

When heated with concentrated sulphhuric acid in the presence of phosphoric acid and vanillin, lipids form a pink coloured complex, the intensity of which is proportional to the lipid concentration. the colour is measured between 510 and 550 nm.

Reagents

1. *Standard (1000 mg total lipid/100ml)*
2. *Total lipid reagent (11.8 M phosphoric acid: 13 m M Vanillin)*
3. *Sulphuric acid concentrated (AR)*

Procedure

Wavelength: 510-550 nm (Hg 546 nm): Glasss cuvette 1 cm light path.

Temperature: 100°C and 20-25°C. Measure against blank.

Set-I : Pipette Into Dry Test Tubes

	Blank	Standard	Sample
Standard sol.	—	0.05 ml	—
Serum	—	—	0.05 ml
Sulphuric acid	—	2.00 ml	2.00 ml

Mix thoroughly. Plug test tubes with cotton wool and stand in boiling water bath for 10 min. Cool in a cold water bath.

Set-II : Pipette Into Dry Test Tubes

	Blank	Standard	Sample
From above mixture.	—	0.10 ml	0.10 ml
Sulphuric acid	0.10 ml	—	—
Total lipid reagent	2.50 ml	2.50 ml	2.50 ml

Mix thoroughly and allow to stand at room temperature for 30 min. Measure density of sample (E sample) and standard (E standard) against the blank within 30 min.

Calculation

Upto a lipid content of 4000 mg per 100 ml serum, the optical density is proportional to the lipid concentration. The calculation of total lipid content is based on the standard which is treated in the same way as the unknown sample.

$$\frac{\text{Esample}}{\text{Estandard}} \times 1000 = \text{mg total lipid/100 ml serum}$$

☞ Notes

1. *With values of over 4000 mg total lipid/100 ml serum. dilute only 0.1 ml sample with 0.9 ml physiological saline and repeat the determination using 0.05 ml of this solution (Result x 10).*
2. *Both lipid reagent and sulphuric acid are very viscous and should therefore be pipetted into the bottom of the test tube. Always mix the solutions thoroughly.*
3. *Fill cuvettes carefully, as trapped air bubbles escape very slowly. Fats and detergents interfere with this determination.*
4. *Assay kit based on this method may be procured from the following organisation.*

The Boehringer Corporation (London) Ltd. Bilton House. Uxbridge Road, London, W 5 2 TZ, London.

Annexure 1 : Mean Values For Plasma Lipids (Human Subjects)

Particulars	mg%
Totat lipids	700 ± 200
Phospholipids	200 ±100
Neutral fat	150 ±60
Free fatty acids	50 ±30
Cholesterol esters	150 ±100
Free cholesterol	30 ±100

References

Bloor. W.R. (1928). *J. Biol. Chem.* 77: 53.

Folch,. J.M. Less. and Stanley. G.H., Solan (1957). *J. Biol. Chem.,* 226: 497.

Zollner, N. and Kirsch. K. (1962). *Z. ges. exp. Med.* 135: 545.

Chapter - 32

Lipase in Serum

Lipase Estimation

Introduction

(Titrimetric Method of Cherry and crandall, 1932 Modified by Tietz and Fiereck, 1966).

In 1932, Cherry and Crandall employed olive oil as the substrate for pancreatic and serum lipase (LPS. Triacylglycerol lipase) determinations. In subsequent years this method was improved (Tietz *et al.,* 1959; Tietz and Fereck, 1966: Tietz. 1972), reducing the original 24 h, period to 6 h and finally to 3 h.

Principle

This procedure is based on the hydrolysis of triglycerides in olive oil into fatty acids, diglycerides and to some small extent into monoglycerides and glycerol.

$$\text{Olive oil} \xrightarrow{\text{Lipase}} \text{Fatty acids + Diglycerides}$$

The amount of fatty acids formed, under the specific conditions of the test, is a measure of lipase activity in the sample. The fatty acids formed are determinad by titration with sodium hydroxide.

Materials

1. Waterbath or incubator set at 37°C
2. Test tubes, with rubber stoppers
3. Flasks, Elenmeyer 50 ml
4. Pipettes, 1 ml Ostwald -Folin
   1 ml and 10 ml volumetric
   5 ml and 10 ml serological
5. Burette, 10 ml or 25 ml, graduated in 0.05 ml or 0.1 ml (Alternately, a 5 ml Mohr pipette graduated in 0.1 ml may be used for titration).

Reagents

1. *Gum Acacia (5 percent): Suspend 5 g of gum acacia in 100 ml of warm water containing 0.2 g sodium benzoate. Mix well and let stand overnight.*
2. *Olive oil emulsion: Homogenize (preferablry in a blender) a mixture of equal parts of pure olive oil and 5 percent suspension of gum acacia containing 0.2 percent sodium benzoate. Keep in refrigerator when not in use.*
3. *Buffer solution: Dissolve 4.7 g of anhydrous disodium phosphate (Na_2HPO_4) and 1.4 g of monopotassium phosphate (KH_2PO_4) in water, dilute to 100 ml and mix. Add sodium Azide (0.1%) as preservative.*
4. *Thymolphthalein indicator solution*
   0.9% Thymolphthalein (w/v) in ethanol.
5. *Sodium hydroxide (0.05N NaOH). Dilute 5 ml of 1 N sodium hydroxide to 100 ml with distilled water.*

Procedure

Place 3 ml distilled water and 1 ml of serum into each of two tubes or flasks. Place one tube (control) into boiling water for five minutes and cool. Add 0.5 ml of buffer solution and 2 ml of olive oil emulsion to both tubes, shake well and incubate at 37° C for 24h . Then add 3 ml of 95 percent alcohol and 2 drops of thymolphthalein indicator solution and mix. Titrate each tube with 0.05 N sodium hydroxide until the appearance of a permanent pink colour (pH 10).

Calculation

(ml) Titre value (NaOH) for unknown (ml) NaOH used for control = unit lipase activity per ml of serum.

☞ Notes

1. *If sodium hydroxide solution used has a normality other than 0.050 N, calculate lipase activity as follow:*

$$\begin{pmatrix} ml\, of\; NaOH\; needed\; to \\ neutralize\; fatty\; acids\; formed \end{pmatrix} \times (Normality\; of\; NaOH)$$

2. *It is advisable to use Sigma assay kit No. 800 for the estimation of serum lipase activity and could be procured from M/S Sigma Chemical Company. P.O. Box 14508, Saint Louis, Missouri 631778 USA.*

References

Cherry, I.S. and L.A. Crandall, K. (1932). *Am. J. Physiol.,* 100: 266.

Tietz, N.W., T. Borden and J.D., Stepleton, (1959). *Am. J. Clin. Pathol.,* 31: 148.

Tietz. N.W. and E.A. Fiereck, (1966). *Clin, Chem. Acta.,* 13: 352.

Tietz. N.W. (1972). Measurement of lipase activity in serum. In standard methods of clinical chemistry, pp. 19 Vol. 7, Ed. by . G.R. Cooper. New York: Academic Press.

Chapter - 33

Blood Lipid Components

Blood Cholesterol Estimation

Blood Cholesterol

(Colorimetric Method of Lieberman, 1885: Burchard 1889 Modified by Watson, 1960).

Introduction

According to Liebermann-Burchard reaction, treatment of chloesterol with acetic anhydride and concentrated sulphuric acid in a water-free environment, polymerized unsaturated hydrocarbon with an intense blue-green colour are produced. The values for cholesterol esters may be calculated by deducting free cholesterol from total cholesterol.

Principle

With acetic anhydride and concentrated sulphuric acid, cholesterol forms bluish green compounds. Their intensity is proportional to the cholesterol concentration and can be measured at 560-580 nm. It is not neccessary to deproteinize the serum.

Reagents

1. *Cholesterol Standard, 400 mg / 100 ml acetic acid : Cholesterol must be recrystallized several times from methanol and dried well. Commercial*

preparations may contain upto 20% impurities, 400 mg of the dried cholesterol is dissolved in 100 ml of glacial acetic acid. Stable indefinitely.

A. Cholesterol Reagent : 5.6 g 2, 5-dimethyl benzene- sulphonic acid dihydrate is dissolved in glacial acetic acid and the volume is made upto 100ml, 300ml of acetic anhydride and 100 ml of glacial acetic acid are added. This reagent can be preserved several months at room temperature in tightly closed containers.

2. *Sulphuric Acid, Concentrated : Dissolve into well-filled and well closed 5 ml bottles. Reseal immediately after use.*

Procedure

Mixture (test tubes in water bath at 25°C)	**T**	**RB**	**S**
Cholesterol reagent, ml	1.0	1.0	1.0
Serum, ml	0.02	—	—
Dimineralized water, ml	—	0.02	—
Standard, ml	—	—	0.02

T - Testing
RB - Reagent blank
S - Standard
A - Reading of Spectrophotometer

Add the sulphuric acid to each test tube individually and shake until the precipitate is redissolved. Between 10 and 20 min, after the addition of sulphuric acid, read at 560-680 nm against distilled water. Use a flow cuvet; the solution is viscous and the cuvet should be rinsed with acetic acid or cholesterol reagents.

Calculation

$$\text{mg cholesterol/100 ml} = \frac{A(T) - A(RB)}{A(S) - A(RB)} \times 400$$

☞ Notes

1. *Use only thoroughly clean and well dried glass ware since even trace amounts of moisture interfere with the reaction.*
2. *Haemolysed serum should not be used.*
3. *Serum or plasma collected with the use of heparin is recommended. The use of oxalate, citrate, flouride and EDTA results in slightly lower cholesterol values.*
4. *Total serum choloesterol is stable for at least 7 days stored at room temperature and presumably longer when refrigerated.*

Enzymatic Determination of Total Serum Cholesterol and HDL Cholesterol

(Method of Allain *et al.*, 1974)

Introduction

Cholesterol is a steroid widely distributed throughout the body and serves as a precursor of other steroids, bile acids, sex hormones and adrenocortical hormones. The determination of serum cholesterol in one of the most frequently performed tests in the clinical laboratory, since elevated levels have been regarded as indicators of predisposition to coronary artery disease. Cholesterol and other lipids are present in blood in the form of lipoproteins, and recently diagnostic significance has been attached to the cholesterol concentrations associated with the major serum lipoprotein fractions. Levels of high density lipoproteins (HDL) cholesterol are considered to be inversely related to the incidence of coronary artery disease. The lipoporteins are distinguished according to their density and size and may be separated by ultracentrifugation, electrophoresis or selective precipitation with divalent cations and polyanions. These characteristics are elaborated in Table 1.

Table 1 : Characteristics of Lipoprotein

Characteristics	Lipoprotein (high density lipoprotein)	Lipoprotein (low density lipoprotein)	Lipoprotein (very low density lipoprotein)
Sp. gravity (g/ml)	1.210-1.063	1.063-1.006	< 1.006
Molecular or particle size	70-100 A	100-300 A	2000A
Protein	49%	32%	2-13%
Triglyceride	7%	7%	64-80%
Cholesterol	17%	34%	8-13%
Phospholipids	27%	25%	6-15%
Cholesterol Phospholipids	0.6	1.4	1.4

Principle

Cholesterol Measurement

Cholesterol esters are hydrolysed to free cholesterol and fatty acids by cholesterol esterase. The free cholesterol is then oxidized by cholesterol oxidase to cholest-4-en-3-one, with the simultaneous production of hydrogen peroxide. The latter reacts with 4-aminoantipyrine and phenol in the presence of peroxidase to yield a quinoeimine dye which has a maximum absorbance at 500 nm.

$$\text{Cholesterol Esters} \xrightarrow[\text{Esterase}]{\text{Cholesterol}} \text{cholesterol and fatty acids}$$

$$\text{Cholesterol} + O_2 \xrightarrow[\text{Oxidase}]{\text{Cholesterol}} \text{cholest-4en-3-one} + H_2O_2$$

$$2H_2O_2 + 4\ \text{Aminoantipyrine} + \text{phenol} \xrightarrow[\text{Quinoeimine Dye} + 4H_2O]{\text{Peroxidase}}$$

The amount of colour produced is directly proportional to the concentration of total or HDL cholesterol in the sample.

HDL Cholesterol Separation

Serum low density and very low density lipoproteins are selectively precipitated by Mg^{++} phosphotungstate and removed by centrifugation. The chloesterol associated with the soluble HDL fraction is measured using the enzymatic procedure described below.

HDL and Total Cholesterol Assay

Sigma Assay Kit No. 350-HDL can be procured from Sigma Chemical Company, P.O. Box 14508. Saint Louis Missouri, 63178 USA, for the assay of HDL and total cholesterol.

Cholesterol Ester in Serum of Plasma

(Colorimetric method of Leffler, 1959; Zak *et al.*, 1954 and Watson. 1960).

Principle

Serum total cholesterol is determined as per method of Lieberman, 1885; Burchard, 1889 modified by Watson, 1960. Free cholesterol is extracted with isopropyl alcohol, then precipitated with digitonin solution. The precipitate is washed, redissolved and the free cholesterol estimated.

Reagents

1. *As mentioned at "A" under blood cholesterol. (See cholesterol Reagent)*
2. *Digitonin-isopropanol solution, 0.25 g/100 ml*
   250 mg Digitonin is dissolved in 100 ml isopropanol
3. *Isopropanol.*

Procedure

Precipitation with Digitonin

Mixture	T	TB
Serum plasma, ml.....	0.1	0.1
Isopropanol, ml......	—	—
Digitonin isopropanol solution, ml...	1.0	—

1. Allow to stand 10 min. and then centrifuge.
2. Discard the clear supernatant.
3. Forcefully blow in 5 ml of acetone so as to resuspend the residue and then agitate with a glass rod.
4. Centrifuge, decant the supernatant, and dry in a vacuum.

Dry residuse	++	++
Cholesterol reagent, ml	2.5	2.5

Stir the precipitate with a glass rod and then centrifuge.

Measurement

Mixture	T	TB	RB	S
Supernatant, ml	1.0	1.0	—	—
Cholesterol reagent, ml	—	—	1.0	1.0
Standard solution, ml	—	—	—	0.02
Glacial acetic acid, ml	—	—	0.02	—
Place in a water bath at room temperature for five minutes				
Conc. sulphuric acid, ml	0.2	0.2	0.2	0.2

Add the sulphuric acid to each test tube with vigorous shaking until the precipitate is dissolved.

Read the absorbance after 10-20 min. between 560 and 580 nm against water.

Calculation

(a) **Free cholesterol**

$$\text{mg}/100\ \text{ml} = \frac{A(T) - A(TB)}{A(S) - A(RB)} \times 197$$

(b) **Ester cholesterol**

Ester cholesterol = Total cholesterol – Free cholesterol

Lipoproteins in Serum

(Turbidimetric Method of Burstein and Samaille, 1959; Hartmann *et al.*, 1962)

Principle

The β-lipoproteins of human serum are selectively precipitated by heparin in the presence of calcium chloride at reduced ionic strength. The content of β-lipoproteins in non-lipemic serum can easily be evaluated by measurement of the absorbance (turbidity) in the long wavelength range before and after the addition of calcium chloride.

Reagents

1. *Calcium chloride solution, 25 mM*

   Dissolve 368 mg of calcium chloride in demineralized water and the volume is made upto 100 ml. It should be kept frozen.

2. *Sodium chloride heparin solution*

   1 ml 1 percent heparin solution and 4 ml of physiological sodium chloride solution are mixed and kept frozen.

Procedure

Mixture	B	T
Calcium chloride, ml	1.0	1.0
Distiled water, ml	0.02	—
Heparin solution, ml	—	0.02
Serum, ml	0.02	0.02

Allow to stand 5 min. at room temperature. Measure the absorbance between 640-650 nm against distilled water.

Calculation

1. Turbidity of the serum

   $$A = B \times \frac{BV}{TV}$$

   $B = B \times 52$

2. β-lipoprotein content

   $A = (T\text{-}B) \times 52$

   Normal values

   i. Turbidity 0-0.1

   ii. β-lipoproteins 4-10

☞ Notes

1. *Test should always be performed on fasting serum.*
2. *Plasma cannot be used.*
3. *The determination must be carried out during the day on which the blood is collected.*

Neutral fat (Triglycerides) and Glycerol in Serum
(Manual Triglyceride Method of Laurell, 1968)

Introduction

Approximately 100 g of exogenous glycerides are absorbed by the intestinal mucosa daily transported as chylomicrons into the blood stream. Tryglycerides, accumulated in adipose tissue in fatty acids and free glycerol. The free glycerol in serum is said to be derived largely from fatty tissues and its respective concentration serves as does the concentration of the fatty acids as a useful index for the extent of lipolysis.

Principle

Triglyceride is measured after hydrolysis by estimating its glycerol content. The commonest procedure involves oxidation of glycerol to formaldehyde which is measured colorimetrically with chromotropic acid. The lipid extract of serum must therefore be freed from other sources of glycerol, in particular phospholipid, and from glucose which on oxidation can also yield formaldehyde. Silicic acid is used to absorb these interfering substances from isopropyl ether solution. The isopropanol extract of serum, after adsorption by the zeolite mixture, may conveniently be used for a combined automated procedure for both cholesterol and triglyceride.

Reagent

1. *Silicic acid (100 mesh) : Activate by heating at 120°C for two hours. Store for up to two weeks in a tightly stoppered tube.*
2. *Extraction mixture : Distilled isopropyl ether is stored over KOH pellets at 4°C. Mix 95 ml with 5 ml of absolute ethanol. Prepare each day this mixture so as to get accurate results.*
3. *Potassium hydroxide (33 percent)*
   Dissolve 33 g of KOH per 100 ml in water.
4. *Alcoholic potassium hydroxide*
   Mix 1 ml of 33 g per cent KOH with 19 ml of absolute ethanol.
5. *Sulphuric acid (0.6 N). Slowly pour 17 ml of concentrated sulphuric acid into water and make up to one litre.*
6. *Potassium metaperiodate (0.02 M)*
   Dissolve 42 mg/10 ml in water
7. *Sodium arsenite (0.2 M)*
   Disslove 260 mg/10 ml in water

8. *Chromotropic acid*

   Cautiously add 300 ml of concentrated sulphuric acid to 150 ml of water. Dissolve 1 g of chromotropic acid which should be colourless in 100 ml of water. Add the sulphuric acid solution slowly to the chromotropic acid solution and store at 4° C in a brown bottle. Discard as soon as the colour of the reagent deepens, or it blank values increase.

9. *Triglyceride stock standard*

   Recrystalize tripalmitin three times from hot ethanol. The material should give a single spot on thin layer chromatography on silicic acid in heptane-ethyl ether-acetic acid 84:15:1. Dissolve 200 mg of tripalmitin in 100 ml of isopropylether.

10. *Triglyceride working standard*

    Dilute 1 ml of stock standard to 50 ml in extraction mixture.

Procedure

Test : Place approximately 0.5 g of silicic acid in the tube; it may be measured with sufficient accuracy using a suitable spatula. Add 1 ml of extraction mixture, followed by 0.1 ml of serum. Then add 5 ml of extraction mixture, put stopper firmly and shake vigorously for 30 s, then intermittently for 30 min. A vortex mixer may be used or several tubes may simultaneously be shaken in a suitable rack. Centrifuge briefly or allow the tubes to stand for one hour.

Standard

Mix 0.5 gram of silicic acid, 1 ml of extraction mixture, 0.1 ml of water and 5 ml of working triglyceride standard.

Blank

Mix 0.5 g of silicic acid, 0.1 ml of water and 6 ml of extraction mixture.

Colour Development

Pipette 4 ml of supernatant from each tube into a similar stoppered tube, taking care not to carry over adsorbent. Add 0.6 ml of alcoholic potassium hydroxide, mix and heat in a water bath at 55°C for 15 min. to saponify the triglyceride. After the tubes have cooled, add 1.5 ml of 0.6 N sulphuric acid, stopper, mix and allow the phases to separate completely. Remove and discard the upper organic layer completely with a fine Pasteur pipette connected to a water pump. Pipette 0.5 ml of the sulphuric acid solution, containing the glycerol into clean 10 ml stoppered tubes. Add 0.2 ml of periodate solution and mix briefly. After 10 min add 0.2 ml of arsenite solution. mix, stopper and heat in a boiling water bath for 30 min. protect the tubes from bright light while they are hot.

After cooling, read the optical densities in a spectrophotometer at 570 nm.

$$\text{Serum triglyceride (mg/100 ml)} = \frac{T - B}{S - B} \times \frac{100}{0.1} \times 0.2$$

where

T - Testing

B - Blank

S - Standard

Reference

Allain. C.A., L.S. Poon, C.S.Chan. W. Richmond and P.C. Fu. (1974). *Clin. Chem.* 20: 470.

Burchard, H. (1869). Inang, Diss. Rostock University, Germany.

Burstein. M., and J. Samaille, (1959). *Ann. Biol. Clin.* 17: 23.

Hartmann. G., G. Cruex, L.K. Widmer and H. Saaub, (1962). *Helve. Med. Acta.* 29: 515.

Laurell S. (1966). *Scand. J. Lab. Clin. Invert.* 12: 66.

Leffler. H.H. (1959). *Amer. J. Clin. Path.* 31: 310.

Liebermann, C. (1885). *Ber dtsch. Chem. Ges.*, 5: 637.

Zak. B., *et al.* (1954). *J. Clin. Path.*, 24: 1307.

Chapter - 34

Glucose in Blood

Blood Glucose Estimation

(Method of Froesch and Renold, 1956; Froesch *et al.*, 1957)
Enzymatic with Glucose-oxidase / Peroxidase

Introduction

Glucose oxidase enzyme specific for the oxidation of glucose, was discovered in a fungus preparation by Müller in 1928. This enzyme is present in bacteria and in moulds such as (*Pencillium notatum*), which promotes the oxidation of glucose (β-ring form) to gluconic acid with the production of an equivalent amount of hydrogen peroxide. Normal values for whole blood glucose oxidase are 60 to 90 mg/100 ml. Results by the enzyme methods are lower than by the best "true sugar" reduction methods largely because of their specificity, but inhibition of glucose oxidase by uric acid may be a contributory factor. *In suspected cases of diabetes, values below 120 mg per 100 ml call for further investigation, for example, by glucose tolerance test. Due to the presence of glycolytic enzymes in red cells, blood must be collected into an antiglycolytic/anti-coagulant preservative, if there is to be a delay of more than 1 to 2 h. in processing or estimation. A fluoride/oxalate mixture, containing 2 mg of fluoride per ml of blood, is suitable and the glucose content will then remain unchanged for upto 3 days at 4°C.*

Principle

The following reactions take place in the estimatioin of glucose with glucose oxidase and peroxidase:

1. $\text{Glucose} + H_2O + O_2 \xrightarrow{\text{Glucose Oxidase}} H_2O_2 + \text{Gluconic acid}$
2. $H_2O_2 + DH_2 \xrightarrow{\text{Peroxidase}} 2H_2O + D$

The glucose is first oxidized by glucose oxidase producing gluconolactone and hydrogen peroxide. The peroxidase transfers hydrogen from a hydrogen donor (DH_2) to the peroxide producing water. The reduced colourless indicator (DH_2), e.g. O-dianisidine hydrochloride, is hereby transformed into a dyestuff D. Maximal colour intensity of the indicator is developed on acidification. The absorbance is directly proportional to the amount to glucose oxidized if glucose oxidase, peroxidase and the hydrogen donor are present in excess. The determination of glucose in whole blood requires preliminary deproteinization but in determination in plasma, serum, CSF or urine this step may be omitted.

Reagents

1. *Perchloric acid. 0.33 N (3.3 g/100 ml)*

   2.85 ml 70% perchloric acid are diluted to 100 ml of dimineralized water. It can be kept indefinitely.

2. *Potassium phosphate solution, 0.6 M*

   Dissolve 104.5 g of dipotassium monohydrogen phosphate dissolved in distilled water and diluted to one litre. It can be kept indefinitely.

3. *Sulphuric acid, 9.3 N (36%)*

   64 ml of concentrated sulphuric acid is added to 36 ml of water and brought to 100 ml. It is stable indefinitely.

4. *Glucose standard (100 mg/100 ml)*

   Dissolve 1 g of glucose in one litre cold saturated benzoic acid solution. It is stable indefinitely but should be allowed to stand at least two hours before use.

5. *Tris buffer, 100 mM. pH 7.5*

6. *Glucose reagents*

   Each portion of chromogen and glucostat x 4 is dissolved in a mixture of 100 ml of dimineralized water and 100 ml of glycerol. The solution is preserved frozen in full 50 ml polyethylene bottles, but it can also be kept at 4°C for a few weeks. The appearance of a reddish yellow colour does not disturb the determination. However, the absorbance of the blank should not exceed 0.10. It should be kept in the dark.

7. *Working solution*
   Mix equal parts of Tris buffer and glucose reagent. It should be prepared fresh daily.

Procedure for Blood

Deliver 0.02 ml of blood (capillary or venous blood) of standard with a heamoglobin pipette directly into 0.2 ml of perchloric acid and the pipette is washed out. Add 0.2 ml of potassium phosphate solution and centrifuge.

Mixture (test tube)	**T**	**RB**	**S**
Working solution, ml	1.0	1.0	1.0
Supernatant, ml	1.0	—	—
Dimineralised water, ml	—	0.1	—
Standard, ml	—	—	0.1

Incubate for 30 min. at room temperature or 20 min. at 37°C

Sulphuric acid, ml	1.0	1.0	1.0

The absorbance is read against water within 5 to 30 min, after the addition of sulphuric acid using a wavelength between 510 to 560 nm. The colour is stable.

Calculation

$$\text{mg Glucose } /100 \text{ ml} = \frac{A(T) - A(RB)}{A(S) - A(RB)} \times 100$$

Procedure for Serum, Plasma, Cerebral Spinal Fluid

Mixture	**T**	**RB**	**S**
Working solution, ml	1	1	1
Serum, plasma urine, CSF, ml	0.02	—	—
Dimineralized water, ml	—	0.02	—
Standard solution, ml	—	—	0.02

Inclubate for 30 min. at room temperature or 20 min. at 27°C.

Sulphuric acid, ml	1.0	1.0	1.0

The absorbance is read against water at a wavelength between 510 and 560 nm within 5 to 30 min. after the addition of sulphuric acid. The colour is stable.

Calculation

$$\text{mg Glucose/ 100 ml} = \frac{A(T) - A(RB)}{A(S) - A(RB)} \times 100$$

☞ Notes

1. *The use of Tris buffer makes the method absolutely specific for glucose (Muller, 1928; Keilin and Hartree, 1948). Glycosidases, such as maltase. lactase, saccharase which may be contaminants of the enzyme mixture. are so strongly inhibited by tris that their hydrolytic effects must be taken into account only when disaccharides are present in very high concentration.*

2. *In place at 20 μl even 10 μl of plasma can be used. With glucose concentrations above 400 mg/100 ml. only 10 μl should be added, and the result is to be multiplied by 2.*

3. *This is the best available method for glucose estimation in blood samples and most of the advanced laboratories follow this method.*

Blood Sugar Determination

(Colorimetric Method of Hultman, 1959)

Principle

The principle of the blood sugar determination according to Hultman (1959) is based on the condensation of glucose with o-toluidine in glacial acetic acid. This reaction leads to the formation of the equilibrium mixture of glycosylamine and the corresponding Schiff base.

The blue-green colour of the reaction mixture follows Beer's law over a wide range of concentration and the intensity of it is a measure of the glucose concentration and can be determined colorimetrically at 630 nm.

The reaction is dependent on temparature and time by standardizing these to 100°C and 5 min. respectively, reproducible results will be obtained. By adding thiourea as a stabilizer to the reagent Hyvarinen and NiKKila (1962) eliminated interference by possible contaminants. Due to this, a stable reagent is obtained with a blank reading of practically zero and accordingly a stable colour of the final reaction mixture.

The colour formed is stable for 20 min. after which a slow decrease in optical density of approximately 2.5% per 30 min. occurs.

When the water content of the reaction mixture is less then 10%, it has been demonstrated that colour development is only slightly influenced by fluctuations in the time factor and there is a linear relationship between optical density and glucose concentration over a wide range of values.

Although with a o-toluidine method the isomers galactose and lactose are also determined with a o-toluidine method, this is not considered as a disadvantage, as these sugars are practically never present in blood in interfering quantities. Naturally, in patients with galactosaemia and in galactose interfering tolerance tests, this glucose determination cannot be applied.

Reagents

1. *Glucose reagent*
   Composition

o-Toluidine	*10% (w/v)*
Glacial acetic acid thiourea	*0.15%*

   If refrigerated at (0-4°C) the reagent can be kept for a longer period

2. *Glucose standard*
   Composition

Glucose	*exactly 5.56 mmol/1 (100.0 mg/100ml)*
benzoic acid	*0.2%*

3. *Trichloroacetic acid solution 5%*
   Composition

Trichloroacetic acid	*5% (w/v)*

Procedure

Pipette into 2 centrifuge tubes	**Test**	**Standard**
Trichloroacetic acid solution 5%	1 ml	1 ml
Blood	1.1 ml	
Glucose standard	—	0.1 ml
Mix well		
Centrifuge the test solution for 5 min.		
Pipette into 2 test tubes		
Glucose reagent	5 ml	5 ml
Clear supernatant solution (test)	0.5 ml	—
Diluted glucose standard	—	0.5 ml
Mix well		
Place both tubes in a boiling water bath for exactly 5 min. Immediately cool the tubes down to room temperature in running water. Measure the O.D. of both solutions against aqua dest as a blank at 630 nm. within 20 min.	A(T)	A(S)

Calculation

Calculate the blood glucose content from the formula:

$$= \frac{A(T)}{A(S)} \times 5.56$$

= m mol glucose/litre blood

$$= \frac{A(T)}{A(S)} \times 100$$

= mg glucose/100 ml

Procedure for Glucose Content in Serum, Plasma, Urine or Cerebrospinal Fluid

Dilute the urine 1:10 with physiological saline or aqua dest. It is not necessary to dilute serum, plasma or cerebrospinal fluid.

Pipette into 2 test tubes	Test	Standard
Glucose reagent	5 ml	5 ml
Sample	0.1 ml	—
Glucose standard	—	0.1 ml
Mix well		
Place both tubes in a boiling water bath for exactly 5 min. Immediately cool the tubes down to room temperature in running water. Measure the optical densitiesof both solutions against aqua dest as a blank at 630 nm. within 20 min.	A(T)	A(S)

Calculation

Calculate the glucose content in the sample from the formula:

$$= \frac{A(T)}{A(S)} \times 5.56$$

= m mol glucose /litre sample

$$= \frac{A(T)}{A(S)} \times 100$$

= g glucose/100ml

Normal value

In fasting blood : 3.3-5.0 m mol/1 (60-90 mg/100 ml)

In cerebrospinal fluid : 2.5-4.1 m mol/1 (45-75 mg/100 ml)

In serum : 3.3-6.1 m mol/1 (60-110 mg/100 ml)

☞ Notes

1. *For whole blood the test can be carried out as a micro determination using 0.2 ml of the clear supernatant and 2 ml Glucose Reagent.*
2. *When examining serum, plasma, urine or cerebrospinal fluid deproteinization can be omitted.*
3. *In urinary analyses, the sample should be diluted 1:10 with aqua dest or physiol saline and the results are multiplied by a factor 10.*
4. *With optical density values of over 0.8, the sample should be diluted with glacial acetic acid, aqua dest or physiological saline and the dilution factor is taken into account.*
5. *It is advisable to close the test tubes with parafilm or a glass bead to avoid evaporation.*
6. *Using a freshly prepared glucose reagent, in general, higher optical density values will be measured than using older reagents. However, this decrease in optical density does not influence the results, as each serum and standard solution is measured against a blank.*

Glucose Tolerance Test

1. *Offer no breakfast.*
2. *Collect sample of blood just before test for qualitative sugar.*
3. *Collect sample of blood just before taking glucose for quantitative sugar (control value).*
4. *Take 50-100 g of glucose in glass of water. Note time.*
5. *Collect sample of blood 30 min, 1 and 1.5 hrs after taking sugar.*
6. *Collect urine at approximately the same time intervals for qualitative sugar.*

References

Froesch, E.R. Reardon, and A.E. Renold, (1957). *J. Lab. Clin. Med.*, 50: 918.

Froesch, E.R. and A.E. Renold, (1956). *Diabetes* 5: 1.

Hultman, E. (1959). *Nature* 183: 108.

Hyvarinen, A. And E.A. Nikkila, (1962). *Clin, Chem Acta*, 7: 140.

Keilin D. and E.F. Hartree, (1948). *Biochem. J.*, 42: 221.

Muller, D. (1928). *Biochem. J.*, 199: 136.

Chapter - 35

Regulations for Radioisotope Work in the Laboratory

Regulations for Radioisotope Work

The term "laboratory" refers to the room in the building specifically equipped for the chemical manipulation of radioisotope. The word "shall" is used to indicate procedure which are mandatory.

1. No unnessary materials are to be brought into the laboratory. Eating drinking, smoking and the using cosmetic in the laboratory are specifically forbidden.
2. Pipetting or the performance of any similar operation by mouth suction is prohibited.
3. Laboratory protective clothing (gloves, smocks, etc.) shall be left in the laboratory; gloves shall be removed before using the counting equipment.
4. Before leaving the laboratory, the hands shall be washed first, then checked with a beta-gamma survey meter. Contamination remaining after thorough washing shall be reported to the instructor.
5. If, in the course of work, personal contamination is suspected, a survey with a suitable instrument shall be made immediately, to be followed by the required cleansing. Routine precautionary surveys should be made at intervals.
6. No person shall work with active materials while having abrasions in the skin on the hands without using rubber gloves.

7. Active liquid wastes shall be poured into labelled beakers provided. they shall never be dumped into a standard drain. Active solid wastes and contaminated materials shall be placed in containers labelled "Radioactive waste".

8. Good housekeeping shall be maintained at all times. Spillage should be prevented, but in the event of such an accident the following procedure shall be used:

   (a) The liquid shall be blotted up with kleenex. Wear rubber gloves.

   (b) All disposable materials contaminated by the spill and cleaning shall be placed in a radioactive trash can.

   (c) Mark the area of the spill and the type of radioactivity (e.g., I^{131}).

9. In general, active materials and contaminated materials are to be retained within the laboratory and at specific points within the laboratory. Expect for properly enclosed samples being taken to special purpose rooms, no transfer of activity shall be made without specific instructions from an instructor.

10. No person shall work in the laboratory without wearing together two pocket ionization chambers. The readings must be recorded at the end of each laboratory period.

11. All wounds, spills or other emergencies shall be reported to the instructor immediately.

12. Always work over a spill tray and in a ventilated enclosure [except with small (< 1 m Ci) quantities of ^{3}H, ^{35}S or ^{14}C compounds an involatile form in solution.]

13. Always label containers of radioactive material clearly indicating nuclide, total activity, compound, specific activity, date and the level of radiation at the surface of the container.

14. Never use ordinary handkerchiefs; use paper tissues and dispose of the them as active waste.

15. Never work with cuts or breaks in the skin unprotected, pariticularly on the hands or forearms.

16. In the event of a spill, it is essential to minimize the spread of contamination:

   (a) Cordon off the suspected area of contamination.

   (b) Ascertain, if possible, the type of contamination, i.e., the nuclides (s) involved (as if may be necessary to use breathing apparatus, protective clothing or other equipment).

(c) Determine the area of contamination by monitoring after taking the necessary precautions.

(d) Starting from the outer edge, decontaminate the area in convenient sectors by wiping and scrubbing.

(e) Before moving on, ensure that a sector is clean by monitoring.

17. Dispose of all radioactive waste according to statutory requirements. Short lived radionuclides, for example, ^{32}P may stored with suitable sheilding and left to decay: After 4 half lives less than 10 percent of the original activity remains, after 7 half lives < 1 percent; after 10 half lives < 0.1 percent. For longer lived radionuclides, for example, ^{3}H, this is impracticable and alternative arrangements should be made.

18. The international Commission on Radiological Protection (ICRP) recommends that occupational exposure should not exceed 10 percent of the occupational exposure levels.

19. To minimize the dose to the extremities. tongs or other remote handling equipment should be used where appropriate.

Units and Conversion Factors

Atomic

Mass of ^{12}C atom	=	Exactly 12 amu
1 atomic mass unit (amu)	=	1.661×10^{-24} g
Proton charge	=	4.803×10^{-10} esu
Proton rest mass (Mp)	=	1.007277 amu
Proton rest mass (Mp)	=	1.6725×10^{-24} g
Neutron rest mass (Mn)	=	1.6748×10^{-24} g
Mass of hydrogen atom (MH)	=	1.007825 amu
Mass of hydrogen atom (MH)	=	1.6734×10^{-24} g

Energy

1 electron volt (eV)	=	1.6020×10^{-12} erg
1 million electron volts (MeV)	=	10^{6} eV
1 horse power	=	746 W
1 atomic mass unit (amu)	=	9.31×10^{2} MeV
1 MeV	=	1.07×10^{-3} amu
1 Erg	=	6.71×10^{2} amu
1 Calorie	=	2.81×10^{10} amu
	=	2.62×10^{13} Mev
	=	4.18×10^{7} ergs

Radiation

Planck's constant (h)	=	6.6256×10^{-27} erg-s
Speed of light in vacuum	=	2.9979×10^{10} cm/s

Radioactivity

1 Curie (Ci)	=	3.7×10^{10} dps
1 millicurie (mCi)	=	10^{-3} curie, 3.7×10^{7} dps
1 microcurie (μ ci)	=	10^{-6} Curies
	=	3.7×10^{4} dps
1 rutherford (rd)	=	1×10^{6} dps
	=	6×10^{7} dpm
	=	1/37 millicurie
1 millirutherford (mrd)	=	10^{-3} rutherfords = 10^{3} dps
1 microrutherford (μ rd)	=	10^{-6} rutherfords = 1 dps

Radiation Dose

1 roentgen (r)	=	1 esu/cc of standard air
	=	2.083×10^{9} ion pairs/cc of standard air
	=	1.61×10^{12} ion pairs/g standard air
	=	6.77×10^{4} MeV/cc of standard air
	=	5.24×10^{7} MeV/g of standard air
	=	83.8 erg/g air
1 milliroentgen	=	10^{-3} roentgens
1 rad	=	100 ergs/g
1 rep	=	84 ergs/s in air
	=	93 ergs/g in water or tissue.

Natural Logarithms

ln 10 x 7	=	2.30258
	=	2.71828

Nomenculature Related with Structure of Simple Atom

Isotope

These are atoms of the same chemical element, but having atomic weights differing from each other by small whole numbers. Actually it is the mass numbers which differ by small whole numbers. Atomic masses are specified in term of the atomic mass unit, which is 1/12 of the mass of an atom of ${}^{12}_{6}C$. According to Avogadro's hypothesis, one gram-atomic weight of any element contains 6.02252×10^{23} atoms. This, then, is the number of atoms in 12 g of ${}^{12}C$, one twelfth of one atom would weigh.

$$\frac{1}{12}\times\frac{12g}{6.02252\times10^{23}}=1.66044\times10^{-24}g$$

which is the value of one atomic mass unit.

Isobars

These are atoms having the same number of mass particles, but different numbers of protons and neutrons, and hence different atomic numbers.

Istones

These are atoms having the same number of nuclear neutrons, they have both different mass numbers and different atomic numbers.

This may be summarized as below:

Atomic number: number of protons in nucleus— symbol Z.

Neutron number: number of neutrons in nucleus—symbol N.

Mass number: number of mass particles in nucleus— symbol A.

$A = Z + N$

Neutron excess : Excess of neutron number over proton number = (N-Z)

For $^{2}_{1}H$ and $^{3}_{2}He$ there is no neutron excess, but a deficit; in each case

$N -- Z = -1$.

For elements of atomic number 1 to 20, one isotope has $N - Z = 0$, or $N = Z$. After helium all elements have atleast one isotope for which N--Z is greater than 0.

The symbol used for a particular nuclear species or nuclide is

$^{A}_{Z}$chemical symbol, e.g., $^{23}_{11}Na$

Isotope atoms have same Zs, different A's, and hence different N's:

$^{35}_{17}Cl, ^{37}_{17}Cl$

Isobar atoms have same A's, different Z's, and hence different N's:

$^{64}_{28}Ni, ^{64}_{30}Zn$

Isotone atoms have same N's, different Z's, and different A's:

$^{40}_{18}A, ^{41}_{19}K, ^{42}_{20}Ca$

Isomer atoms have same Z's and same A's, but different energy states in the nucleus.

Diameters of nuclei range from 10^{-12} to 10^{-13}cm.

Units of Activity

In 1923, Marie and Pierre Curie (France) discovered polonium and radium. Subsequently later on P. Curie (France) found that the rays emanating from radium consisted of two kinds of very different penetrating power and deviated in different directions in a magnetic field. These rays later became known as alpha (α) and beta (β) rays.

The amount of a radioactive nuclide is specified in terms of its disintegration rate, or its activity. the unit of activity is the Curie (Ci), which is 3.7×10^{10} *disintegrations per seconds (d/s)*. The millicurie (MCi) and the microcurie (μCi) are disintegration rates one thousandth and one millionth respectively of the curie.

1 Kilocurie	=	3.7×10^{13} d/s
1 Curie	=	3.7×10^{10} d/s
1 millicurie	=	3.7×10^{7} d/s
1 microcurie	=	3.7×10^{4} d/s
1 nanocurie	=	3.7×10 d/s
1 picocurie	=	3.7×10^{-2}

SI Unit of Radioactivity

The unit of radioacitivity in the international system of units (SI) is the becquerel, which is equal to one nuclear transformation per second. It is expected that this unit will come into wide spread use over next few years.

Conversion Table

Table 1 provide to convert curie activities to becquerels.

Table 1 : Conversion Table

μCi mCi Ci	kBq MBq GBq	μCi mCi Ci	MBq GBq TBq
0.1	3.7	30	1.11
0.2	7.4	40	1.48
0.25	9.25	50	1.85
0.3	11.1	60	2.22
0.4	14.8	70	2.59

0.5	18.5	80	2.96
1	37	90	3.33
2	74	100	3.70
2.5	92.5	125	4.62
3	111	150	5.55
4	148	200	7.40
5	185	250	9.25
6	222	300	11.1
7	259	400	14.8
8	296	500	18.5
9	333	600	22.2
10	370	700	25.9
12	444	750	27.7
15	555	800	29.6
20	740	900	33.3
25	925	1000	37.0

kBQ = kilobecquerels = 10^3 Bq
MBq = megabecquerels = 10^6 Bq
GBq = gigabecquerels = 10^9 Bq
TBq = terabecquerels = 10^{12} Bq

Expression of Data

The results of radioactive determinants are expressed in different ways depending on the nature of the experiment and of the counting equipment used.This should however, be presented unambiguously with sufficient information to permit intercomparisons to be made between different laboratories. In general, one of the following ways of recording the results of experiments with radioisotopes might be used:

1. Percentage Recovery (percent of dose)

The total radioactivity of the sample studied is expressed as a percentage of that of the whole of the compound administered (a drug. foodstuff, fertilizer material, etc.).

2. Specific Activity

The specific activity of a radioactive preparation is the amount of radioactive isotope per unit amount of material. In biological investigations, the specific activity of a tissue or of a compound isolate from a tissue may be recorded in any one of the following ways:

As a count rate (counts/min., for example) or a disintegration rate (in μ Ci, for example):

(a) measured at infinite thickness.

(b) per unit weight of material.

(c) per mole of millimole of compound

(d) per unit weight of the element concerned or of an inorganic compound derived from it.

3. Relative Specific Activity

In some investigations it is required to compare the result from two or more separate but similar experiments, e.g., experiments on a number of different animals. Often this can best be done by measuring the relative specific activity in each experiment, i.e., the ratio of two specific activities determined in the same experiment.

The approximate administered dose in an isotope experiment should be stated in terms of both radioactivity and mass. This enables the reader to judge whether there might be radiation effect or mass effect and also gives a lead as to the amounts of activity that might be required for similar experiments.

Chapter - 36

Common Terms Used in Nuclear Research Work

Activation : The process of causing a substance to become artificially radioactive by subjecting it to bombardment by neutrons or other particles.

Activation Analysis : Any analytical procedure permitting the detection and measurement of trace quantities of elements following their exposure to a flux of neutrons.

Activity : The strength of a radioactive source. In absolute units, it relates to the number of radioactive atoms decaying per unit of time. It is also a synonym for radioactivity. Absolute activity is usually expressed in curies or millicuries.

Alpha Particle : A particle which is identical to the helium nucleus, consisting of two protons and two neutrons. It carries a positive charge of 2.

Alpha Rays: A stream of helium nuclei. The helium nucleus has a mass number of 4 and an atomic number of 2. If consists of two protons and two neutrons.

Angstrom : A unit of length equal to 10^{-8} cm.

Anion : A negatively charged ion.

Annihilation Radiation : The radiation produced by the reaction between a particle and an anti-particle resulting in the annihilation of both. The radiation is electromagnetic possessing a total energy equivalent to the masses of the particle annihilated.

Barn : A unit of area used for expressing the area of nuclear cross sections. 1 barn = 10^{-24} cm^2.

Beta Emitter : Any radioactive nuclide that decays by beta decay with the emission of a beta particle.

Biological Half Life : The time required for one-half of an administered substance to be excreted from the body or from an organ or section of living tissue.

Bombardment : The act of subjecting a substance to a flux of neutrons or other high energy particles.

Carrier : Stable atoms which are mixed with radioactive atoms of the same element (i.e., same atomic number) in the same chemical form for the purpose of carrying out a chemical process.

Cyclotron : A circular magnetic resonant accelerator.

Deuterium : An isotope of hydrogen having one proton and one neutron in the nucleus. *It is often called heavy hydrogen.*

Disintegration : A spontaneous, radioactive transformation of one species of nucleus into a nucleus of a different type, usually accompanied by the emission of radiation.

Dose : The amount of ionizing radiation energy absorbed per unit mass of irradiated material at a specific location, such as a part of the human body. Measured in reps, rems and rads.

Effective Half Life : The half life of a radioisotope in a biological system as a result of the combined effects of the biological half life and the radiological half life.

Fallout : Debris (radioactive material) that resettles to earth after a nuclear explosion. It descends to earth within 24 h near the site of the detonation and in an area extending for some distance (often hundreds of miles), depending on meteorological conditions and the yield of the detonation. The other form, called "worldwide fallout", consists of lighter particles which ascend into the upper troposphere and stratosphere and are distributed over a wide area of the earth by atmospheric circulation. They then are brought to earth, mainly by rain and snow, over periods ranging from months to years.

Fluorescence : The extranuclear emission of photons caused by excitation of an atom.

Half Life : The time required for one-half of a given number of radioactive atoms to undergo decay. Symbol t ½.

Heavy Water : Water in which the hydrogen has been replaced by deuterium. Thus, its formula is D_2O. Its density is greater than that of water . Density = 1.076 g/ml at 20°C.

Lambda : A unit of volume. Synonym for microlitre.

Mean Life : The average life of a radioactive atom. Symbol = γ . It is equal to the reciprocal of the decay constant. $\gamma = 1/\lambda$

Nuclear Reactor : A device for supporting a self-sustained nuclear chain reaction under controlled conditions.

Phosphor : A material, such as zinc sulphide, which gives off visible light when struck by nuclear radiation. The inside face of a television picture tube is coated with phosphor.

Photomultiplier Tube : A phototube of exceptionally high sensitivity, the electron or electrons released at the photocathode initiating a cascade from one dynode to another with a resultant amplification of a as high as 10^9.

Radioisotope : Synonym for radioactive isotope. Any isotope which is unstable, thus undergoing decay with the emission of a characteristic radiation.

REP : Abbreviation for Roentgen Equivalent Physical.

Roentgen : The quantity of gamma radiation such that the associated corpuscular emission per 0.001293 g of air (i.e., 1 ml at 0°C and 760 mm) produces in air, ions carrying 1 electostatic unit of quantity of electricity of either sign.

Roentgen Equivalent Man (REM) : The quantitiy of radiation which when absorbed by man produces in effect equivalent to the absorption of one roentgen of X or gamma radiation.

Roentgen Equivalent Physical (REP) : The amount of ionizing radiation which is capable of producing 1.615×10^{12} ion pairs per gram of tissue or that amount which will be absorbed by tissue to the extent of 93 ergs per gram. This unit is used in particular to measure beta radiation.

Roentgen Rays : Synonym for X-rays.

Rutherford : A unit of decay rate defined as the amount of substance undergoing 10^6 disintegrations per second.

Scintillation : The flash of light produced in a phosphor by radiation.

Stable Isotope : An isotope which is not radioactive. Examples are the heavy isotopes of nitrogen, N^{15}, O^{18} and C^{13}.

Generally, in the experiments with human subjects radioactive isotopes are not usually employed because fo the harmful effect of radiation released within the body. *Stable isotopes are quite harmless. This is expressd on a percentage basis, as isotopic atom percent. This is a specific isotope content (isotopic atoms per 100 atoms to total material). The atom percent excess means the excess abundance of the isotope over its normal occurrence, expressed as a percentage. Suppose a sample* C^{13} *has been enriched to contain, say, 82%* C^{13}*, we say it has* $82 - 1 = 81$ *atom percent excess* C^{13}.

Tracer : An isotopic tracer is an isotope used to tag or follow a chemical reaction or process such that its location and concenration can later be determined.

Tritium : A hydrogen isotope of mass three. its nucleus contains one proton and two neutrons.

Wavelength : Distance between any two similar points of two consecutive waves.

X-rays : Electromagnetic radiation in the region below 100 angstroms.

Chapter - 37

Radioactivity Measuring Instruments

Ionization Chambers for Gases

Generally these type of instruments are known as dose-rate meter (e.g., the so called "cutie-pie"). Radiation intensity (i.e., a constant stream of particles or photons) gives rise to a continuous series of pulses, and if these are allowed to merge, they form a weak electric current, which may be amplified and registered by an electronic circuit. The final scale reading will then be a measure of the energy dissipated in the following chamber per unit of time by the ionizing particles or photons. In gas-flow counters, the radioactive samples are placed inside the detector which will be transfused by a gas at atmospheric pressure. This instrument counts particles of low energy, such as the β particles from ^{14}C, effectively (Window-less counting).

Geiger-Müller (G.M) Counter

This instrument is used for activity of solids. Generally each β or γ -ray entering the counter is measured separately. Geiger Müller counter detectors (G.M tubes) operate at "plateau". G.M tubes operate at a reduced gas pressure (about one-tenth atmosphere), containing a certain amount of "quenching" gas. Energetic β or e particles and or X-photons emitted by radioactive liquids may be counted with a thin glass wall "dip-counter" G.M tube which is immersed in the liquid or with a specially designed liquid detector that consists of a cylindrical glass container around the G.M tube. *G.M counters are used mostly to measure the activity of β-particles.* In the case of γ-rays they are not very effective. (1-3 percent efficiency), since most of the photons will penetrate the gas without any interaction.

Solid Scintillation Counters

These instruments are particularly suited for the detection of gamma-rays and X-ray becaues of the high stopping power of the solid. When a gamma-photon interacts with a crystal, e.g., of thallium-activated Na I, at least one fast electron is liberated and a constant fraction of the electron's kinetic energy is spent on excitation of orbital electrons in atoms of the crystal. On de-excitation these give rise to the emission of a light flash consisting of a number of photons. The number of light photons will be proportional to the energy dissipated in the crystal by the gamma-photon. The radiation coming from the sample strikes a crystal of sodium iodide containing traces of thallium iodide. *Recently, special plastic scintillators (as well as anthracene and naphthalene) which have a much higher efficiency then Na crystals have been devised for use in solid scintillation counting equipment.*

Liquid Scintillation Counters

These instrument is used for the counting of very low-energy beta particles such as H^3 (0.018 MeV) and C^{14} (0.155 MeV). A method of detection called "liquid scintillation counting" is often employed. Usually, the sample to be counted is placed in solution with the scintillator so that each radioactive atom or molecule is surrounded by molecules of the scintillator. By this method absorption is reduced, and hence counting yield increases. In this scintillator system, solvent like toluene or dioxane is used and a solute which is the actual scintillator. The solvent absorbs the energy and transfers it to the solute, which then emits the light flash. Usually a secondary solute which acts as a wavelength shifter is added; i.e., it increases the wavelength of the light flash emitted to one for which the photomultiplier tube is more sensitive, thus increasing the counting yield.

One of the most popular primary solutes is 2, 5-diphenyl oxazole (PPO), which combines a high solubility with a high fluorescence quantum efficiency. The PPO fluorescence spectrum has a mean wavelength of about 3, 700 Å, while the 311 cathodes of the photomultipliers originally used for liquid scintillation counting had a peak response at about 4,300 Å wavelength. This spectral mismatch led to the introduction of a secondary fluorescent solute (Z) such as 1, 4-di-2-(5 phenyloxazolyl) - benzene (POPOP), which has a mean fluorescence wavelength of about 4,300 Å and a high fluorescence quantum efficiency.

Birks (1964) has recommended the following composition of scintillator solution:

Toluene containing 4 g/l PPO, to which 0.1 g/l POPOP may be added as a secondary solute if required.

Corbett *et al.*, (1971) have recommended the following formula of scintillation fluid

POPOP	*0.01 percent*
PPO	*0.4 percent*
Carbosil	*3.4 percent*
Toluene	*100 ml*

Krishna and Ekern (1974 a, b) used scintillation fluid containing 8 g PPO toluence, however they advised to use methyl cellosolve to bring the solution in a single phase. A more efficient water miscible scintillator for the counting of aqueous solutions is 1, 4-dioxan containing 50g/l naphthalene and 7 g/l PPO, to which 0.05 g POPOP may be added as a wavelength shifter.

Generally the results are expressed in disintegrations per minute. one micro curie = 2.220×10^6 DPM. The counting efficiency may be estimated by the following formula:

$$\text{Efficiency} = \frac{\text{The observed counts per minute}}{\text{DPM}}$$

Quench Correction

Beside from impurity quenching, which causes a reduction in the scintillation efficiency by competition with event in the normal scintillation process, the additioin of higly coloured or opaque materials to the scintillated solution is deleterious. These adsorb some of the scintillation light output before it reaches the photomultiplier, thereby reducing the output pulse amplitude. One approach is to bleach the specimen, before incorporation, by treatment with hydrogen peroxide, chlorine, charcoal etc, but it is essential to ensure that no volatile radioactive products are lost. If the specimen to be assayed is highly coloured or opaque, the concentration added to the scintillation solution should be kept as small as possible. Secondary solutes, such as POPOP, can be advantageous in such circumstances, by shifting the spectrum of the scintillation emission to a region in which the specimen is more transparent.

Method of Quench Correction

Internal Standard Calibration: The specimen of unknown activity A is counted (net count rate =C). It is then recounted (net count rate = C + Cs) after the addition of a known activity (As) of a non quenching standard (e.g., toluene labelled with tritium or 14 carbon). The channel counting efficiency

E = Cs/As, and the unknown activity A = C/E = C As/Cs. This may be simplified as given below:

$$\frac{\text{(CPM of sample + added isotope)} - \text{(CPM of sample)}}{\text{DPM of added isotope}}$$

$$\text{DPM of sample} = \frac{\text{CPM of sample}}{\text{efficiency}}$$

External Standard Calibration : A series of sample of known activity A, with various quenching factors, is counted (net count rate = EA) and then recounted (net count rate= EA + CE) after bringing an external gamma-ray source into a well defined position near the sample. A calibration curve is thus obtained of the beta channel counting efficiency E versus the external count rate CE. Using this calibration curve E for an unknown sample can now be determined from the observed CE. The calibration is only valid for specimens of the same basic scintillator composition, scintillator volume, vial dimensions and beta emitter, observed with identical instrument settings. A change in any of these parameters necessitates a new calibration.

Channels-ratio Method

The counting channel is split into a lower part a and an upper part b. the effect of quenching is to increase the net count rate Ca, in channel a, and to decrease the net count rate C_{b}, in channel b. The channels ratio (C_b/C_a) is thus a measure of Q, and since it depends only on the shape of the beta spectrum, it is independent of the sample activity. From a series of measurements of samples of known activity A with different quenching factors, a calibration curve of channel counting efficiency.

$E = \frac{C_a + C_b}{A}$ versus channels ratio (C_b/ C_a) is obtained.

External Standard Channel-ratio Method

This combines the two previous methods. Three channels are used, one set for the beta-emitter to be assayed and the other two to determine the channels ratio (C_b/C_a), for the external standard. A set of samples of known activity are used to obtain calibration curve of beta channel counting efficiency E versus external standard channels ratio (CE_b/CE_a).

Among all the methods, internal standard calibration technique is the most accurate one and is usually followed in the majority of laboratories.

Chromatogram Scanners

This apparatus is used for detecting radioactive spots separated on chromatograms by the use of proportional or G.M. counters.

Chapter - 38

General Use of Tracer Techniques in Nutritional Biochemistry Studies

We may study the nutrient metabolism in a better way as explained in the following summarized form in Table 1.

Table 1 : Nutrient Metabolism

Radionuclide or lablelled compound	*Determinations*
^{15}N	1. *Rate of ammonia production in rumen*
	2. *Rate of incorporation of N compounds into microbial protein*
	3. *Overall conversion of NPN to tissue or milk protein*
^{14}C	1. *Rate of hydrolysis of C-containing NPN*
	2. *Turnover and entry rate of amino acids and volatile fatty acids*
	3. *Estimates of protein synthesis*
^{13}C	1. *Estimates of microbial protein synthesis*
	2. *Estimates of microbial contribution to synthesis of milk*
^{51} *Cr EDTA*	1. *Indicator to study digesta flow rates, dilution rate and extent of absorption of amino acids.*

	2. Rumen water volume
^{51}Cr- labelled erythrocytes	*Erythrocyte volume*
^{59}Fe-labelled erythrocytes	*Plasma volume*
*RISA**	
^{42}K	*Potassium space*
^{22}Na, ^{24}Na	*Sodium space*
Tritiated water	*Total body water*
*RISA**	*Cardiac function, coronary circulation*
^{131}I-Diodrast	*Kidney function*
^{131}I-Hippuran	
^{131}I-Rose Bengal	*Liver function*
^{125}I-Rose Bengal	
^{198} Au-colloidal	*Organ blood flow (liver, lungs and heart)*
	Rate of passage of DM in ruminants
*RIFA***	*Pancreatic acid intestinal function (fat absorption)*
^{131}I. ^{125}I.^{131}I Triiodothyronine and Thyroxine	*Thyroid function*
^{47}Ca. ^{18}F, ^{85}Sr	*Bone*
^{59}Fe	*Bone marrow*
^{137} mBa, RIFA, RISA ^{99} Tc	*Heart*
^{131}IOr ^{125}I labelled Diodrast or Hippuran	*Kidney*
^{197} Hg or ^{203} Hg- labelled Neohydrin	
^{131}I-labelled serum albumin aggregates	
Colloidal ^{198}Au	*Liver*
^{131}I or ^{125}I-labelled Rose Bengal	
^{131}I-labelled serum albumin aggregates	*Lungs*
^{75}Se-methionine	*Pancreas*
RISA ,^{51} Cr-labelled erythrocytes	*Placenta*
^{131}I-labelled serum albumin aggregates, colloidal, ^{198}Au, ^{51} Cr-labelled denaturated erythrocytes, ^{197} Hg or ^{203} Hg-BMHP	*Spleen*
^{131}I. ^{125}I. ^{132} I	*Thyroid*
Acetic acid-1- ^{14}C. sodium salt, n-Butyric acid-1- ^{14}C, sodium salt Propionic acid-1-^{14}C, sodium salt	*Rumen volatile fatty acids net entry or production rate*
^{14}C-urea	*Urea entry rates in ruminants*

* Radioiodinated serum albumin (RISA)

** Radioiodinated fatty acids (RIFA)

Important Information Related to Radio-Active Nuclides

The data related to radio active nuclides are presented in Table 2 given below:

Table 2 : Physical Data for a Number of Radioactive Nuclides

Element	Atomic Number Z	Mass Number A	Half life	Radiation
Antimony	51	122	2.8 d	β, e.c.
		124	60.4 d	β, γ
Argon	18	37	35.1 d	e.c.
Arsenic	33	72	26hr	β^+, e.c., γ
		74	18d	$\beta^-\beta^+$, e.c., γ
		76	26.5 hr	β^-, γ
Barium	56	131	12.0d	e.c.l, γ
		133	7.2 y	e.c., γ
Beryllium	4	7	53 d	e.c., γ
Calcium	20	45	165d	β^-
		47	4.5 d	β^-, γ
Carbon	6	11	20 min	β^+
		14	5730 y	β^-
Cerium	58	141	32.5d	β^-, γ
Cesium	55	131	9.7 d	e.c.
		134	2.05 y	β^-, γ
Chromium	24	51	27.8d	e.c., γ
Cobalt	27	56	77 d	β^+, e.c., γ
		57	270 d	e.c., γ
		58	71 d	β^+, e.c., γ
		60	5.27 y	β^-, γ
Copper	29	64	12.8 h	β^-, β^+,e.c.
		67	58.5 h	β, γ
Fluorine	9	18	110 min	β^+,e.c.
Gold	79	198	2.7 d	β, γ
		199	3.15 d	β, γ
Iodine	53	123	13.0 h	e.c., γ
		124	4 d	β^+, e.c., γ
		125	60 d	e.c., γ
		126	13d	β^-, β^+,e.c., γ
		130	12.3 h	β^-, γ
		131	8.04d	β^+, γ
		132	2.26 h	β^-, γ

contd.....

Iron	26	52	8.2 h	β^+, e.c., γ
		55	2.6 y	e.c.
		59	45 d	β^-, γ
Manganese	25	52	5.7 d	β^+, e.c., γ
		54	303 d	e.c., γ
Molybdenum	42	99	66.7 h	β^-, γ
Nitrogen	7	13	10 min.	β^+
Oxygen	8	15	2.5 min	β^+
Phosphorus	15	32	14.2 d	β^-
		33	25 d	β^-
Selenium	34	75	120 d	e.c., γ
Sodium	11	22	2.6 y	β^+, e.c., γ
		24	15.0 y	β^-, γ
Strontium	38	85	64 d	e.c., γ
		87 m	2.8 h	IT. γ
		89	52 d	β^-
Sulphur	16	35	87.9 d	β^-
Technecium	43	99m	6.04 h	IT, γ
Thallium	81	204	3.8 h	β^-,e.c.
Vanadium	23	48	16.2 d	β^+, e.c., γ
Zinc	30	65	2.45 d	β^+, m,e.c., γ

Chapter - 39

Isotope Dilution Technique

For the first time, isotope dilution analysis was introduced by Hevesy and Hafer in 1934, but it was not until 1940, the usefulness of isotope dilution technique was revived by Rittenberg and Foster (1940). There are three general types of isotope dilution methods. These are (a) direct (b) inverse and (c) double isotope dilution. In general isotope dilution methods may be used for the following type of studies.

(a) In isolation purification and identification of unknown intermediate in a chain of metabolic reactions.

(b) To obtain evidence of synthesis (incorporation), and precursor-product relationships between known compounds.

(c) As an analytical tool in the assay of known compounds. In isotope dilution techniques, the labelled intermediate, which is being diluted by unlabelled carrier, is a known compound.

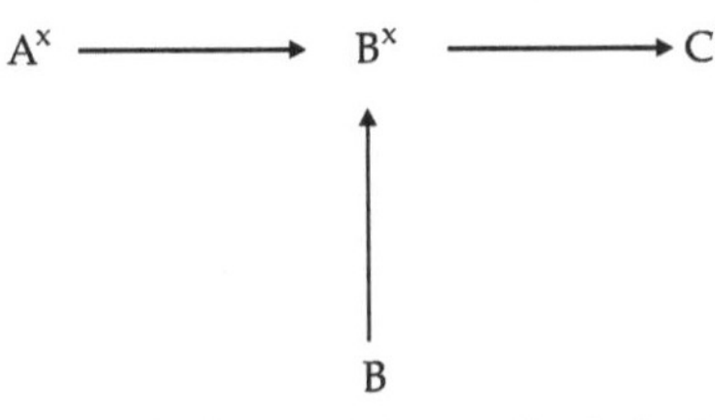

In reaction A $\rightarrow$ C, compound B is an intermediate. The reaction went on with labelled A and labelled C is obtained. When reaction is complete, unlabelled carrier B comes in reaction. If B occures as an intermediate in the reaction, the carrier B molecules will mix with the labelled B molecules and thus pick up the label.

Estimation of Net Entry Rate, Effective Production Rate of VFA, Turnover Rate, Turnover Time, Pool Size and Exchange Rate of VFA

(a) Continuous Infusion Technique

This technique based on the measurement of plateau specific radioactivity has been adopted by various worbers to measure the production of volatile fatty acids (Bergman *et al.,* 1965, Leng and Leonard 1965; Leng and Brett, 1966; Gray *et al.* 1966: Weller *et al.,* 1967; Leng *et al.,* 1968; Weston and Hogan 1968).

Leng (1969) pointed out that in continuous infusions of ^{14}C labelled acids the transfer of labelled carbon out of the pool and back to it result in higher specific radioactivity of the acids at the plateau specific radioactivey rather when it is not operative. Esdale *et al.,* (1968) obtained steady-state conditions after two hours of continuous infusion of ^{14}C labelled acids in the rumen. It has been reported that considerable interconversion of VFA apparently occur in the rumen (Bergman *et al.,* 1965). According to Leng *et al.* (1968) steady state condition is reached after 3 hour of continuous infusion of ^{14}C labelled acids in the rumen.

(b) Single Injection Technique

This technique follow the first order kinetics. isotope is injected into rumen fluid and the exponential decline in specific radioactivity of the acid is followed for some time. This technique has been adopted by various workers to measure volatile fatty acid production (Gray *et al.,* 1960; Knox *et al.,* 1967; Jayasuriya and Hungate, 1959). Steele *et al.,* (1956 and Leng *et al.,* (1965) pointed out that single isotope injection technique does not take into account the interconversion between acids.

Semilogarithmic relation is fitted between Log^{10} specific activity (μci/gac) and sampling hours.

SRt = Ae^{-} mt

SRt = Specific radioactivity (mμ/m mole)

mt = Rate constant (min^{-} 1)

The pool size (p. m mole) and entry rate (E, m mole/min.) are then determined by the following equations.

$$p = \frac{\text{injected dose}}{\text{A(Sp.activityat"O"hour.)}}$$

$$E = p \times mt$$

The term pool means the compartment (s) of tracee which compose a biologically distinguishable entity and pool size means the total mass of tracee distributed through all compartments within the biological system.

Other Parameters of Kinetics

Turnover Rate and Turnover Time

The term turnover means. "the process of loss and replacement of tracee in a given compartment (or pool) and turnover rate means. "the fraction of tracee present in a given compartment renewed per unit time". In this experiment turnover time has been defined as, "the time required for an amount of tracee equivalent to that in the compartment to be transfered into and out of the compartment"and is thus the reciprocal of turnover rate.

Turnover rate

$$= \frac{\text{Log (Sp.activity at "O" hr and specific activity at "t" hour)}}{t}$$

Turnover time = 1 ÷ turnover rate

Exchange Rate or Flux

In this experiment the flux has been defined as "the rate (mass/unit time) at which all tracee enter and leaves a compartment which is in steady state. Actually in general it may be divided in two.

Irreversible Loss Rate

This is "a fractional flux rate equal to that fraction of the flux of tracee (mass/unit time) which leaves the compartment and does not return to it during the experimental period."

Recycling Rate

This is "a fractional flux rate equal to that fraction of the flux of tracee (mass/unit time) which leaves the compartment and returns to it during the experimental period."

Flux or exchange rate = Pool size × turnover rate.

Units of Expressioin of Kinetic Parameters

Trait	Unit
1. Turnover rate	m M/min./g acid
2. Turnover time	min.
3. Flux or exchange rate	m M/min.
4. Pool size	mole/1
5. Net entry or production rate	mole/day
6. Effective production rate	mole/day

The net entry rate or production rate of acetic acid, propionic acid and butyric acid may be calculated by the formula of Leng (1969).

VFA Net Entry Rate or Production Rate

1. Yac = -- 0.475 + 0.0461 Xac
2. Y Prop = + 0.134 + 0.0344 Xprop
3. Y but = + 0.033+0.0453 X but

VFA Effective Production Rate

1. Yac = -- 0.410 + 0.0400 Xac
2. Y Prop = + 0.134 + 0.0344 Xprop
3. Y but = + 0.020 +0.0280 Xbut

where, Y = Production (m mole/min.)

X = Concentration (m mole/litre)

The calculation of calorific value of daily VFA produced from DOM intake (g/day) is made by applying the formula proposed by Leng and Murray (1972).

Y(kcal) = 89.5 + 2.30 X

where, Y = VFA production (kcal/day)

X = DOM intake (g/day)

The correction of VFA net entry rate or production rate to effective production rate is made by using the factors suggested by Leng (1969).

1. Effective production rate of acetate = Net entry rate of acetate × 0.864.
2. Effective production rate of propionate = Net entry rate of propionate × 1.0.
3. Effective production rate of butyrate = Net entry rate of butyrate × 0.618

Calculation of Various Parameters of Kinetics

(Method of Knox *et al.*, 1967)

Dose of isotope depends upon :

(a) Size of animal

(b) How rapidly the material is metabolized or turned over.

(c) Specific activity of the injected compound.

(d) Efficiency and background activity of assay equipment.

Example : Calculation of amount of ^{14}C-acetate to be added to the rumen.

(a) 75 kg sheep x 10kg rumen contents/100 kg sheep = 7.5 kg rumen contents.

(b) S.A. of ^{14}C-acetate = 59 m Ci/mM.

(c) Rumen fluid has about 70 mEq acetate per litre.

(d) Rumen contents are about 80 percent liquid.

(e) You need about 100 x more activity than your background activity.

(f) Scintillation counters are about 80 percent efficient for ^{14}C.

(g) **Calculations**

7.5 kg rumen contents x 80 percent fluid = 6 kg liquid or six litre silica gel columns will separate about one ml (equivalent) of rumen fluid.

Each ml of rumen fluid contains about 0.07 mM acetate, it should count about 10^4 CPM (assume background = 100 CPM.)

Therefore :

(10^4 CPM/ml rumen (fluid) x 6 l rumen fluid

= 6 x 10^7 CPM per animal.

$$\frac{6\times10^7\,\text{CPM}}{0.8\,\text{CPM / DPM}} = 7.5\times10^7\,\text{DPM.}$$

$$7.5\times10^7\ \text{DPM}\times4.55\times10^7\ \frac{\mu\text{ci}}{\text{DPM}} = 34\ \mu\text{Ci}$$

$34\,\mu ci \div 59\times 10^3\ \mu ci/mM = 1/2\times 10^{-3}$ mM (add to rumen)

Check

$0.5\times 10^{-3}mM\times 59\ \mu Ci/mM = 34\ \mu Ci/animal$

$34\,\mu ci/6\times 10^3$ ml of rumen fluid $=10^{-2}\ \mu Ci/ml\times 1$ ml

for assay $= 5\times 10^{-3}\ \mu Ci$

$10^{-2}\ \mu ci\times 2.22\times 10^6\ DPM/\mu Ci$

$=2.22\times 10^4\ DPM\times 0.8\ CPM/DPM = 9\times 10^3$

Source : **Krishna *et al.*, 1974a,b,c**

Calculation of Pool Size

Turnover rate and turnover time : With a single injection experiment these calculations are rather simple.

(a) Pool size = $\frac{\text{amount of radioactivity in } \mu\text{Ci}}{\text{zero time concentration of radioactivity}}$

Example

Inject 60 μCi ^{14}C-acetate, zero time specific activity =0.15 μCi/mM acetate. Thus

60 μCi /0.15 μCi/mM = 400 mM acetate =Pool size. This would be equivalent to = 67 mEq/l

(b) Turnover rate is calculated from the slope of this decay curve. If the change in specific activity is semilogarithmic then the best fitting line can be statistically calculated using the method of least squares. The equation is:

Y = a +bx, where a = specific activity at time zero and b = slope of the line or the fraction of the pool turning over per unit time.

(c) Flux is calculated by multiplying the pool size and the turnover rate. This is the total amont of material passing through the pool per unit time.

(d) Turnover time is 1 ÷ turnover rate.

Source : Krishna *et al.,* 1974a,b,c

Rates of Production of Volatile Fatty Acids in the Rumen (Method of Weller *et al.*1967)

Total VFA production (moles/day)

$$= \frac{\text{Rate of infusion of}^{14}\text{C}(\mu\text{Ci / day})}{^{14}\text{C in total VFA}(\mu\text{Ci / mole})}$$

VFA pool = Rumen volume × concentration of VFA in rumen liquor.

Infusion

(12 h ; 735 ml containing 0.0262 μCi/ml)

with ^{14}C distribution, total quantity 19.2570 moles/day

0.0102 μCi/ml infusate as acetic acid (39 percent)

0.0114 μCi/ml infusate as propionic acid (43 percent)

0.00456 μCi/ml infusate as butyric acid (18 percent).

^{14}C Concentration in Composite Sample of Rumen Fluid

Total VFA = 0.00777 μCi/m mole total VFA

Individual acids = 0.00444 μCi/m mole acetic acid

= 0.0187 μCi/m mole propionic acid

= 0.0098 μCi/ml mole butyric acid

Therefore,

Production of total VFA $= \frac{735 \times 0.0262}{7.77}$

= 2.48 moles/12 h

Production of Individual Acids

Acetic $= \frac{735 \times 0.0102}{4.44}$ = 1.69 moles/ 12 h = 68 percent.

Propionic $= \frac{735 \times 0.0114}{18.7}$ = 0.45 mole/ 12 h = 18 percent

Butyric $= \frac{735 \times 0.00456}{9.8}$ = 0.34 mole/ 12 h = 14 percent

Total 2.48 mole/12h

Rumen Acids during VFA Infusion

Infusion, 100 μCi/hour, molar proportions of VFA in the rumen: acetic (A) 68 percent, propionic (P) 19 percent, butyric (B) 13 percent.

A 29 μCi/g atom C = 58 μCi/mole A = 38.8 μCi/mole toal VFA

P 652 μCi/g atom C =1956 μCi/mole P = 372 μCi/mole total VFA

B 31 μCi/g atom C = 24 μCi/mole B = 14 μCi/mole total VFA

Total 424.8 μCi/mole total VFA

Therefore production of VFA $= \frac{100 \times 24}{424.8} = 5.7$ moles/24 h.

References

Krishna, G. & Ekern, A. (1974a). Volatile fatty acid metabolism in sheep I. Volatile fatty acid production and availability of energy by using Isotope Dilution Technique. *Z. Tierphysiologie Tierernährung* und *Futtermittelkunde*. 33: 275-280.

Krishna, G. Ekern A. (1974b). Volatile fatty acid metabolism in sheep II. Studies on the kinetics of volatile fatty acid tool as determined by Isotope dilution technique. *Z. Tierphysiologie Tierernährung* und *Futtermittelkde*. 33: 281-284.

Krishna, G. & Ekern, A. (1974c). Volatile fatty acid metabolism in sheep III. Effect of intraruminal infusion of volatile fatty acid on the utilization of nutrients and some biochemical constituents, rectal temperature and pulse rate. *Z. Tierphysiologie Tierernährung* und *Futtermittelkunde*. 33: 323-328.

Chapter - 40

Production and Kinetics of Volatile Fatty Acids

Isotope Dilution Technique

(Based on research conducted by Author at Agricultural University of Norway, Ås-NLH, Norway)

Studies on Volatile Fatty Acids Production and Kinetics of VFA Pool as Determined by Using "Isotope Dilution Technique"

(Method of Krishna and Ekern, 1974a,b and c)

Details of Experiment

Materials

(i) **Animals :** Two fistulated sheep of Dala × Texel breed weighing about 72 and 76 kg are selected.

(ii) **Experimental Diet :**

Basal Diet : Two experimental sheep are maintained on 1.1 kg early cut timothy hay per day. The ration is divided in four equal parts and offered four times a day during the preliminary period of about twenty days. One day before infusion of labelled VFA, the sheep are fed regularly at one hour interval (1.1 kg hay divided in equal parts) to help in increasing the mixing rate of rumen ingesta. The animals are given water adlibitum but they are not allowed to drink water during infusion. Digestible energy and metabolizable energy (ME) of the basal diet is determined by conducting a separate metabolism trial on the same sheep.

(iii) **Dosage of ^{14}C- Labelled Acids:**

Infusion of Individual ^{14}C- Labelled Acids

Name	Dose	Infusion rate
1. Acetic acid-1-^{14}C Na salt	40 μCi	0.1904 μCi/min.
2. Propionic acid-1-^{14}C Na salt	30 μCi	0.1428 μCi/min.
3. n-Butyric acid-1-^{14}C Na salt	25 μCi	0.1190 μCi/min.

Infusion of VFA Mixture ^{14}C-Labelled Acids

Name	Dose	Infusion rate
1. Acetic acid-1-^{14}C Na salt	25 μCi	
2. Propionic acid-1-^{14}C Na salt	15 μCi	0.238 μCi/min.
3. n-Butyric acid-1-^{14}C Na salt	10 μCi	

The above labelled acids are dissolved in 500 ml distilled water and 0.1 mole of VFA per 500 ml as carrier is added. The infusion of this solution is started at 07.45 hours and finished at 11.15 hours.

(iv) Method of Infusion: Acetic acid-1-^{14}C, propionic acid-1-^{14}C, n-Butyric acid-1-^{14}C (sodium salt) are procured from the Radiochemical centre, Amersham (Buckinghamshire). England Single isotope injection method followed by (Gray *et al.,* 1960; Knox *et al.,* 1967 Jayasuriya and Hungate, 1959, Sheppared *et al.,*1959) is adopted to study the daily VFA production rete and parameters of kinetics of the VFA pool. ^{14}C labelled acids are infused for 210 min at constant infusion rate of 2.38 ml/min.

(v) Sampling of Rumen Liquor: Homogeneous rumen samples are drawn from different parts of rumen by suction, using plastic tube about 30 mm in diameter, with several 9 mm holes in the lower two inch portion. Precautions are taken to minimize contact with the rumen wall. The timing for aliquoting the rumen liquor are 1, 2, 3, 4, 5, 6, 7, 8, 9, 13, 17, 21, 22, 23 and 24 h after infusion. The rumen samples are preserved with thymol 10 percent (W/V) dissolved in isopropanol and stored at -20°C.

(vi) Chemical Analysis

(a) *Distilling of Rumen Samples and Processing for Counting Specific Activity:* 10 ml. of rumen liquor and 2 ml of saturated magnesium sulphate solution (2.5 percent by volume of concentrated sulphuric acid) is distilled by Markham (1942) distillation unit method developed by McAnally (1944), followed by Annison (1954) and Kromann *et al.,* (1967) in their studies. About 120 ml of distillate collected, and titrated with N/100KOH in the presence of phenolphthalein. Little excess of alkali is added after titration. The volume of this distillate is reduced to 5 ml by drying in vacuum drying oven at 40°C. Immediately after drying is complete, the reduced volume of distillate is transferred to a test tube by adding 15 ml of isopropanol and 1.4 N sulphuric acid (40 : 1) V/V, which is then shaken for about 30 seconds. One ml of this colourless solution is taken in a scintillation vial, five ml phosphor solution containing 8 g PPO/1 toluene and five ml methyl cellosove (Ethylene-glycol) monomethyl ether, Dowanol EM. 2- methoxyethanol. BP 124-26°C, FP 106°F is added. The contents of the vial is shaken for 30 seconds so as to obtain single phase system. The specific activity is measured by Tricarb packard liquid scintillation spectrometer. Model 3310, using window 50-100 and gain 20 percent at +5°C. For quench correction, internal. standard method is used, where ^{14}C toluence is used as an internal standard. The specific activity of internal standard is 4.17 $\times 10^5$ dpm per ml 0.05 ml is added in each sample give activity. 20850 dpm. The counting efficiency is 65-72 percent. The net to cpm observation is divided by counting efficiency to convert it into dpm. The values of dpm are converted into µCi by using the factor (1 µCi =2220000 dpm or 1 µCi = 2220 dpm).

(b) *Measurement of Activity in Volatile Fatty Acid Fractions:* Celite column of Wiseman and Irvin (1957) is used for partitioning the volatile fatty acids. Two grams of rumen liquor and 0.5 ml of 0.6 NH_2SO_4 are mixed thoroughly with cap material and put on the top of column. PA_1,PA_3,PA_{15},PA_{35},PA_{50} is used to elute VFAs fractions from the column.

The chronolgy of events of elution from the column is in the order-valeric, butyric, propionic and acetic. Complete extraction of each acid from the column is judged by the movement of blue bands from the top to the bottom. Eluate are collected in 100 ml conical flasks, little excess of N/100 KOH (prepared in methanol and isopropanol 50 : 50) is added. The contents of the flask are reduced to 5 ml after drying in vacuum drying oven. This dried eluate is processed in the same way as mentioned for counting by liquid scintillation spectrometer except 10 ml aliquot is taken instead of 1 ml, thus the counting vials contained 10 ml sample + 5 ml methyl cellosolve + 5 ml phosphor solution (8 g PPO/l toluene). The setting of the instrument is window 50-1000 and gain 25 percent.

(c) *Gas-liquid Partition Chromatography of Volatile Fatty Acids:* Method of James and Martin (1951) developed by Annison (1954) and Bernard *et al.,* (1968) with latest modifications made at the Agricultural University of Norway, Krishna and Ekern (1974a,b and c) is used to measure the quantity of each acid. Ten millilitres rumen liquor mixed with 0.5 ml of 50 percent formic acid, is centrifuged for fifteen minutes at 2,000 rpm.

Five ml of supernatant is taken for quantitative estimation of VFA. Gas chromatograph Model 810 with FID attached with micro recorder equipped with Model, 228 disc chart integrator is used. An aliquot of 0.9 μl CRL is injected directly into the column (8 ft x 2 mm) packed with chromosorb W 80-100 mesh washed with HCI (10 percent SP 1200,1 percent phosphoric acid) impregnated with 20 percent carbowax 20 M.

Basis of the Calculation of Results

Estimation of Rumen Water Volume

Author advise to follow the method of Weston and Hogan (1967) modified by Krishna and Ekern, 1976 for estimating rumen water volume and this procedure is given in detail under the separate. Chapter 41 of this compendium.

Calculation of net entry rate, effective production rate of VFA, turnover rate, turnover time, pool size and exchange rate of VFA.

It is advisable to follow the method of Knox *et al.* (1967) and Weller *et al.*, (1962, 1967 and 1969) so as to calculate the data related to this aspect of study. Krishna and Ekern (1974 a, b) followed the same principles of calculation while studying volatile fatty acid metabolism and rumen water volume in adult sheep at the Agricultural University of Norway, Ås - NLH Norway.

References

Krishna, G. and Ekern, A. (1974). Estimation of rumen water volume, rate of flow of water and rumen dry matter turnover time by using 51Cr-EDTA. *Indian Vety. J.* 53: 265-270.

Krishna, G. (1973). Lic Agric (Ph.D Thesis), "Infusion of Volatile fatty acids and use of radio isotopes (14C-VFA, 51Cr-EDTA, 198Au) in nutritional and biochemical studies related to the energy metabolism in sheep. Agricultural University of Norway, Ås-NLH. Norway.

Chapter - 41

Estimation of Rumen Water Volume, Rate of Flow of Water and Average Rumen Dry Matter Turnover Time

Rumen Water Volume Estimation

(Method of Hyden 1955a,b)

I. Use of Polyethylene Glycol (PEG)

These compounds are manufactured through the reaction of ethylene oxide with water, ethylene glycol or diethylene glycol to furnish functional groups (in this case hydroxyl) for the propagation of the reaction. The process results in a mixture of diols of different chain lengths, in which the numbers of molecules of various sizes are presumed to be represented by Poisson's distribution (Shaffer, Critchfield and Nair, 1950b). Polyethylene glycols 200, 300, 400 and 600 are fluids: compounds 1,000, 1,500, 4000, 6000 and 1,0000 are solids of increasing firmness. PEG compounds of molecular weight above 1000 are not absorbed from the gastrointestinal tract of the rat and man.

Polyethylene glycol has been used frequently as a water soluble marker in studies of absorption in man and animals (Sperber *et al.*, 1953; Hyden, 1955a,b; Corbett *et al.*, 1956; Gray *et al.*, 1960; Weller *et al.*, 1962; Ulyatt, 1964a,b; Walker and Hawley, 1965; Tulloh *et al.*, 1965; Sinha *et al.*, 1970; Nagel and Piatkowshi, 1972).

Disadvantage of PEG Method

The recovery of PEG in faeces is only 94.8 percent. It has been observed that PEG associates itself with the liquid phase and not the solid phase of digesta (Hyden, 1955a,b; Corbett, Greenhalgh, Gwyn and Walker; 1958; Corbett *et al.*, 1959; Sinha *et al.*, 1970). The lack of specific, sensitive and accurate method for the analysis of PEG has been seen as a serious limitation in its use as a reference substance.

II. Complex of ^{51}Cr with Ethylene Diamine Tetra -Acetic Acid ^{51}Cr-EDTA (Method of Krishna and Ekern, 1976)

This has been used by many workers to estimate rumen water volume and rate of flow of water from reticulo-rumen (Dowens and McDonald, 1964; Hogan, 1964; Weston and Hogan.1967; Warner and Stacy, 1968a, b; Klooster *et al.*, 1970; Hecker. 1971). When it is not desirable to take the use of radioactive indicator then stable Cr-EDTA can be used. Binnerts *et al.*, (1968) used stable complex in digestion experiments with ruminants using the method for estimation by Atomic absorption. Krishna and Ekern (1976) used ^{51}Cr-EDTA based method for estimation of rumen water volume at the Agricultural University of Norway, Ås-NLH-Norway in his Ph.D. research programme.

Hypothesis

Hyden's calculations for the estimation of rumen water volume based on the assumptions:

1. *The volume of water in the rumen remains constant during the experiment.*
2. *The rate of flow of water into and out of rumen is continuous and constant.*
3. *The marker used should not be taken up or absorbed, produced or destroyed to any significant degree by micro organisms or by other parts of the contents in the gut.*
4. *Assuming that the volume and the flow rate remain unchanged during the experiment the concentration (Y) time (X) curve will follow a standard general linear regression equation.*

   $Y = a + bx$, where 'a' is constant and 'b' is slope of curve.

   Thus, The Semilogarithmic Graph will give a Straight Line.

Choice of Method

In a comparative study of use of PEG and ^{51}Cr-EDTA. Downes and McDonald. (1964) gave the evidences in the favour of use of ^{51}Cr-EDTA to estimate rumen water volume and rate of flow of water. *Till and Downes (1965) reported that PEG labelled with ^{3}H or ^{14}C may be used successfully to estimate rumen water volume, rate of flow of water from rumen.*

Animals and Diets

Two fistulated male sheep of indigenous (Norwegian) breed weighing about 72 and 76 kg are selected. Experimental sheep are offered one kg timothy hay (divided in four equal parts) four times daily at 08.00, 12.00, 16.00 and 19.00 hours. About 15 g mineral mixture and salt are given daily. During the experimental period, animals are housed individually in metabolism cages, each of which has sufficient space for free movement. Each unit has sufficient space for free movement. Each unit should have an extendable metal floor equipped with devices for the quantitative separation of urine and faeces. Animals are given water twice a day.

Procurement of Tracer Compound and Dosage including Method of infusion

^{51}Cr-EDTA may be obtained from the Radiochemical centre. Amersham, Buckinghamshire, England. On the day of infusion, about 800 g timothy hay is offered early in the morning at 07.00 hours. Rest of 200 g hay is offered after thirteen hours of infusion. No water is given during 13 h after infusion of ^{51}Cr-EDTA to avoid the effect of feeding and drinking on the outflow of rumen water. After four hours of feeding hay, 100 μCi of ^{51}Cr-EDTA (diluted in 200 ml distilled water) is infused in the different part of rumen through fistula using a syringe attached with reservoir and pulsating rubber bulb. Whole of the radioactive solution is infused in about fifteen minutes. Rumen contents are thoroughly mixed with the help of thin wooden rod.

Method of Sampling : Measurements and Analysis

(i) Sampling of Rumen liquor; Rumen Contents, Faeces and Urine: Homogeneous rumen samples are drawn from different parts of rumen by suction, using plastic tube about 30 mm in diameter: with several 9 mm holes in the lower two inch portion. Precautions are taken to minimize contact with the rumen wall. The rumen samples are taken at 1, 2, 3, 4, 5, 6, 7, 8, 9, 13, 17, 21, 22, 23 and 24 h after infusion radioactive ^{51}Cr-EDTA in the rumen., Thymol in isopropanol (10 percent W/V) is used to prevent the activity of paunch micro-organism of rumen liquor. The urine and faeces sample are collected for four days regularly after infusion. On the day of infusion, an representative sample of rumen content is taken for dry matter estimation.

(ii) *Measurement of Specific Activity in Rumen Liquor, Urine and Faeces Samples:* The activity in rumen liquor, faeces and urine samples is counted by Nuclear Enterprises International Series Solid Scintillation Spectro photo meter (Edinburgh, U.K.) having a well counter consisting sodium Iodide thallium activated crystal of $1 \times 3/4'' \times 2''$ size. A particular point in the form of the use for Sodium Iodide over anthracene for gamma ray detection is the much greater density of the sodium iodide. The purpose of a well counter is to improve the counting geometry to obtain a higher counting efficiency. Five ml of rumen liquor is taken in screw capped polythene test tubes for the measurement of activity. Similarly an aliquot of urine sample is taken in a polythene screw capped test tube. Five ml of distilled water is added and faeces is mixed thoroughly by stirring. A standard of 0.5 μCi, ^{51}-Cr-EDTA is added in the blank sample of rumen liquor, faeces and urine so as to convert the cpm reading into microcuri. Different counting method is adopted to measure the activity. The apparatus is set at 1,000 V, gain 512, DL=0.8 E level 2.40, E =1.50. The results are not corrected for their decay in activity since the samples are immediately processed for the measurement of activity and *half life of* ^{51}*Cr-EDTA is only 27.8 days.*

Basis for the Calculation of Results: During the present investigation, technique adopted by Hyden (1961 a) is followed to estimate rumen water volume and rate of flow of water from rumen. A straight line is fitted by least square regression analysis method between the natural logarithm (log 10) of marker concentration and sampling hours (upto 13 h only). It is notworthy that visible activity in rumen samples is present upto 13 h only, therefore calculations are based on 13h study only in this experiment. In the semilogarithmic regression equation:

$$Y = a + bx$$

where constant "a" represents the "O" hour concentration of marker and "b" represents slope of the curve for turnover rate of the marker.

Rumen water volume (V) is calculated from the relationship.

$$V = \frac{p}{C^a - C^b}$$

Where p is the amount of marker administered and C^a and C^b are marker concentations in the rumen before and after dosing.

Calculation of Rate of Flow of Water from Rumen

Weston and Hogan's Formula (1967)

$$F = \frac{0.693\,V}{t^{1/2}\,(\text{half time of mar ker})}$$

Note: In isotope dilution technique, half-life of the marker is also used to calculate turnover time. The half life is approximately 0.693 of the cycle time (Hungate, 1966). Sperber *et al.,* (1953) reported a cycle time of 13 h in cattle.

Klooster and Roger's Formula (1970)

$$F = 2.3 \times b \times R.V.$$

Calculation of Total Rumen Dry-Matter Content

An approximate total rumen dry matter (DM) content is estimated from the relationship.

$$\frac{\text{DM percent}}{\text{Water percent}} = \frac{\text{Total rumen DM (g)}}{\text{Rumen water volume (ml)}}$$

Calculation of average dry matter turnover time in days (Z) in Rumen only (Hungate 1968).

$$Z = \frac{A}{B \times C}$$

where, A = Dry matter in rumen, kg

B = Percent digestion of rumen contents

C = Daily intake, kg

Cycle time or turnover time is defined by Hungate (1966) as the length of time required for the consumption of an amount of food that is equal to that represented in the rumen. According to this definition, turnover time represents the average time that particles of digesta remain in the rumen.

Practical Application in Research Work

Krishna and Ekern (1976) of Agricultural University, NORWAY have used ^{51}Cr-EDTA for estimating rumen water volume, rate of flow of water and rumen dry matter turnover time in adult sheep. They obtained reproducible results and advise to use ^{51}Cr-EDTA in the above mentioned area of research. These parameters are required in connection with the study of different kinetics norms viz., pool size, turnover time, turnover rate, volatile fatty acid production rate and microbial protein production rate, etc.

Reference

Krishna, G. & Ekern, A. (1974). Estimation of rumen water volume, rate of flow of water and rumen dry matter turnover time by using ^{51}Cr-EDTAS. *Indian Vety. J.* 53: 265-270.

Chapter - 42

Estimating Rate of Passage of Hay Using Marker ^{198}Au (Radiogold) in Sheep

Rate of Passage of Hay

Extent of Passage

(Method of Krishna and Ekern, 1974D)

Definition of Terms

The term extent of passage is used to describe how far a given ingested material travelled or was allowed to pass. The point at which undigested residue of the food comes to or has passed through the alimentary tract may be found by the use of markers without disturbing the subject. In some conditions of digestive system malfunction or disorder , the food residue may be blocked at point along with digestive tract.

Transit Time

This is the time it takes the digesta of a meal to pass through the alimentary tract or segments of it. This time also represents the retention time in the tract or the particular segment. A simple way of calculating it is by recording the time of first or last appearance of the marked residue of a meal. Other more useful methods for calculating retention time include "mean retention time" (Castle 1956a), "mean time" (Blaxter *et al.,* 1956) and "turnover time" (Hungate, 1968).

Rate of Passage

According to Balch (1961), the rate of passage is the rate at which undigested residues from a given meal pass a given point in the gut, or are eliminated in the faeces. In contrast, the rate of flow of digesta expresses the rate at which the mixture of undigested residues from previous meals passes a given point in the gut or is eliminated in the faeces.

Rate of Flow

This denotes any quantity of digesta (as weight or proportion) that travels a distance in a given time (e.g.,g/cm/h).

Rate of Transport

This denotes the distance (in length or proportion of length) travelled by the digesta of a meal through the alimentary tract or segments of it in a given time.

Digesta

Food and ingested material subjected to digestion within the digestive tract. Technically, it would include secretions and extractions (mucosal cells) from digestive organs.

External Indicator

An indicator or a marker which is added to the diet or taken orally, e.g., chromic oxide.

Internal Indicator

An indicator or a marker which occurs naturally in the diet, e.g., lignin.

Tracers in the Rate of Passage Study

Garner *et al.,* (1960) used ^{144}Ce as a marker in digestibility, and observed that equilibrium was reached after 5 or 6 days in cows given ^{144}Ce twice daily. Francois *et al.,* (1968) used ^{144}Ce for the measurement of rate of passage in sheep and rat. At the University of Wyoming, Laramie, Gibbs and Rice (1969) used strontium 85 microspheres for the study of rate of passage of alfalfa hay and low and high moisture alfalfa silage, William and George (1971) used ^{51}Cr in a study of food passage in the white tailed deer.

Bris *et al.,* (1967) demonstrated the use of radioactive ^{198}Au to study the passage of ingesta in Cattle and Sheep administered orally. They have recommended the use of ^{198}Au for the measurement of rate of passage in ruminants, on *the basis that this radio-isotope is harmless to the digestive tract, its half life (64.8 h) is long enough to process the samples for the measurement of* activity very small amount of ^{198}Au can be detected in the presence of large amounts of ingesta *the country animals administered ^{198}Au may not be used for human consumption and the ^{198}Au is β and γ emitting isotope so it must be handled with appropriate caution.*

Krishna and Ekern (1974) of Agricultural University of Norway, compared stained hay method as well as Radiogold ^{198}Au in adult sheep for measuring rate of passage of hay at two levels of feeding. *They have concluded that the use of radiogold is more accurate as compared to stained hay method for measuring rate of passage.*

Method of Krishna and Ekern (1974) for Measuring Rate of Passage of Hay at Two Levels of Feeding

Animals and Experimental Diets

Select two sheep of any breed. During restricted feeding period, 800 g timothy hay (chaffed coarsely) divided in three equal parts is fed three times a day to both the sheep for ten days regularly. During *ad-libitum* feeding, about 1 kg timothy hay (chaffed coarsely) is offered in the morning and 0.8 kg hay is given later on as and when the manger is found empty. Both the sheep are given free access to clean water supply.

Method of Dosing of Radiogold ^{198}Au

Radiogold (^{198}Au) containing sterile colloidal gold about 3.5 mg/ml, could be obtained from Institute for Atomenergi, Kjeller-Norway. Since the half-life of this tagged compound is only 64.8 h, precautions are taken to calculate the actual activity at the time of dosing by applying respective decay corrections using decay-chart. The required amount of dose is absorbed on cotton placed inside an empty gelatine capsuls and capsule is wrapped by a thin layer of absorbant cotton to prevent the fall out. All 11.30h gelatine capsule previously standardized containing 6 and 7 μCi are administered orally to sheep I and II simultaneously during restricted feeding. While in the case of *ad-libitum* feeding the dose of ^{198}Au administered is 80 μCi and 70 μCi to make the counting more visible.

Aliquoting of Excreta Samples

The samples of faeces are collected at 6, 8, 9, 10, 11, 12, 13, 21, 22, 23, 24, 25, 26, 27, 28,29, 30, 31, 32, 33, 34, 35, 42, 44, 46, and 48 h after administering radiogold by mouth. Simultaneously, later on faecal samples are also collected at 6 h. interval for next three days and at 12 h interval for next three days. Urine samples are also collected for four days after dosing radiogold to check up if any activity is excreted through urine.

Method of Measurement of Specific Activity in Faeces and Urine Samples

Immediately after collection, the faeces samples are mixed thoroughly in the mixer. One gram of faeces and 5 ml distilled water are taken in screw caped polythene test tube. The specific activity is counted by nuclear enterprises International series solid scintillation spectrometer (Edinburgh, UK) having a well counter consisting Sodium Iodide Thallium activated crystal of size. The activity in each sample is counted for 30 min. in a similar way, blank samples of faeces are taken to obtain the values of background count. Standard of 0.025 and 0.050 μCi is also prepared and activity is measured in cpm.

An aliquot of five ml urine out of daily collected sample is taken in a screw caped polythene test tube for the measurement of activity. For comparing net cpm count, blank sample of urine is also taken.

Final results are expressed as μCi of radiogold excreted per gram of wet faeces, using the figures of standard.

Calculation of Turnover Time of Dry Matter Content of Digestive Tract Using Stained Particle

Simple linear regression equation is fitted between the values of stained particles as percent of total excreted (Y) and time required (X).

Turnover time is calculated by the following relation:

$$\frac{1}{\text{Value of constant "b"}}$$

= where "b" indicate slope of curve which mean turnover rate.

References

Krishna, G. and Ekern, A. (1974d). Level of feeding and rate of passage of hay as measured by stained hay method and using Radiogold in Sheep. *Acta Agriculture Scandinavica.* 24: 211-216.

Krishna, G. (1973). Lic Agric. (Ph.D.) thesis with title "Infusion of Volatile fatty acids and use of radio isotopes (^{14}C-VFA, ^{51}Cr-EDTA, ^{198}Au) in nutritional and biochemical studies related to the energy metabolism in sheep, Agricultural University of Norway, Ås-NLH, Norway.

Chapter - 43

Effect of Hormones on Fat Synthesis Through ^{14}C Labelled Acetate in Chicken Adiopose Tissue

Fat Synthesis

Investigation of the effect of Various Hormones on Fat Synthesis from ^{14}C Labelled Acetate in Chicken Adipose Tissue

(Method of OMea and Leveille, 1968, Folch, Less and Solane Stanley, 1957 and Vaughan, 1961)

Reagents

1. *Krebs-Ringer calcium-free bicarbonate buffer 7.4*
   100 parts 0.154M NaCI (0.9001 g in 100ml)
   4 parts 0.154M KCI (0.0459 g in 4 ml)
   1 part 0.154M $MgSO_4$ *(0.0380 g in 1 ml)*
   (3 parts 0.110M $CaCI_2$*)*
   21 parts 0.100M $NaHCO_3$ *buffered to 7.41 by bubbling through* CO_2
2. *25 percent KOH*
3. *2N* H_2SO_4
4. ^{14}C *labelled acetate*
5. *Insulin, thyroxine, somatotropin, cortisone*
   Reagents for Fat Extraction

(i) *0.9 percent sodium chloride*
(ii) *2:1 chloroform/methanol*
(iii) *3:48:47 chloroform/methanol/saline*

Procedure for Incubation

1. Add 3 ml of Kreb Ringer to each of 12 labelled flasks.
2. Add hormones in duplicate to 8 of these flask as follows:

Insulin	0.5 mg
Thyroxin	20 μg
Somatotropin	2 mg
Cortisone	1 mg

3. Place in shaking water bath at 38°C for temperature and chemical equilibration.
4. Remove adipose tissue from clavicluo-coracoid region (between neck and sternum) of freshly killed chicken and divide among flasks in pieces weighing about 200 mg.
5. Fill flasks with 95:5 O_2/CO_2 atmosphere.
6. Prepare 2 blanks by adding KoH and H_2SO_4.
7. At known times, add 1.0 μCi of substrate to each flask by mean of syringe and needle through stopper.
8. After 30 min. remove blank flasks to freezer.
9. Incubate 10 remaining flasks for 2 h and then add 0.1 ml KOH through stopper onto filter paper and similarly 0.5 ml H_2SO_4 into body of the flask. This stops the reaction and liberates CO_2 from the medium which is then absorbed by the KOH.
10. Continue shaking for half an hour to ensure complete liberation of CO_2 and place in freezer for 10 min.
11. Remove glass container from stopper, dry outside with a clean filter paper and place in a liquid scintillation vial-within a paper fold to dry.
12. Lay 2 cm square of 4 thickness of folded dried filter paper flat on base of vial and add 10ml toluene liquid scintillation fluid, rinsing inside of glass container.
13. Measure activity of samples by liquid scintillation counting to determine CO_2 produced.

Fat-extraction

14. Rinse tissue three times with 0.9 percent NaCI and weigh.
15. Add 20 ml chloroform/methanol mixture to each flask to extract fat, return flasks to shaker and leave for about 6 h or overnight. Discard de-fatted tissue.
16. Add 4 ml of 0.9 percent sodium chloride (1/5 of volume to flasks, shaker vigorously, and allow to stand untill extract becomes clear).
17. Non lipid radioactivity settles into the upper water/methanol/salt phase which is removed by suction and discarded.
18. Repeat 16 and 17
19. Wash the remaining surface with chloroform/methanol/saline to remove traces of water phase.
20. Pour remaining chloroform into weighed metal trays and evaporate. Re-weigh.
21. If fat is sufficiently pale for colour quenching to be negligible, dissolve fat residue in 10 ml toluene scintillation fluid and transfer to counting vial, otherwise burn fat in oxygen, dissolve CO_2 liberated in ethanolamine and use this solution.
22. Count activity of fat in liquid scintillation spectrometer to determine extent of lipogenesis.

Chapter - 44

Estimation of Trace Minerals in Tissues by Neutron Activation Analysis

Neutron Activation Analysis

(Method of Saryre, 1963 and IAEA, 1969)

Introduction

This technique helps in detection of very small amount of stable elements in fairly large quantitites of extraneous matter. Trace elements like zinc, copper, molybdenum and arsenic which exist in minute amounts in certain organs or tissues. For example, to detect the amount of copper present in one gram of tissue. using 1 mg of thin copper foil as control. Normal copper contains 69 percent ^{63}Cu and 31 percent ^{65}Cu. The (n,r) reactions on these two stable isotope produce ^{64}Cu and ^{66}Cu respectively. The half life of ^{64}Cu is 12.8 h and that of ^{66}Cu is five minutes. Therefore the latter can be ignored, if more than that an hour elapses between the end of the irradiation and the measurement. The specific activity of the unknown separate is compared with that of the known standard separate, and the content of Cu in the original tissue sample is thereby calculated.

Reagents

1. *Nitric acid (24N, 16N and 1N)*
2. *Na_2SO_3 15 percent W/V*
3. *KSCN 20 percent W/V*
4. *$Fe(NO_3)_2$ 10 percent W/V*
5. *CH_3CO_2H 18N*
6. *Ammonia 15N*

7. *Ammonia 2N*
8. *$NH_4H_2PO_4$ 10 percent W/V*
9. *Salicylaldoxime in C_2H_5OH*
10. *Acetone*
11. *SO_2 saturated water*
12. *Cu carrier (20 mg cu/ml): 6.28 g Cu $(CH_3CO_2)_2$. H_2O in 100 ml water.*

Procedure

Take about 0.05 g of tissue and 1 µg of copper standard sealed in polythene. Activate for 13 h.

1. In a fume chamber, transfer tissue and standard to 50 ml centrifuge tubes, and add 10 drops of 24N HNO_3. Boil until tissue has dissolved, and add 10 mg of copper (0.5 ml of copper carrier). Make up to 4 ml with water, add 1 ml of Na_2SO_3 and 1 ml of KSCN. Boil, and spin down CuSCN when it has settled, reject supernatant and wash precipitate with hot water saturated with SO_2.
2. Dissovle precipitate in 0.5 ml of hot 16N HNO_3; add 5 drops of Fe $(NO_3)_3$ and 1 drop of $NH_4H_2PO_4$ then 15N NH_3 till dark brown. Boil, spin down Fe $(OH)_3$ precipitate and wash it once with 2N (NH_3).
3. Combine supernatant and washings in a fresh tube. and acidify with CH_3CO_2H till pale blue. Then add 0.5 ml of 16 N HNO_3, 1 ml of Na_2SO_3 and 1 ml of KSCN; boil and spin down CuSCN. Pour away supernatant and wash precipitate with hot water saturated with SO_3.
4. Dissolve precipitate in 0.5 ml of 16N HNO_3; and 15N NH_3 until solution is deep blue, add CH_3 CO_2H until it is pale blue. Add 3 ml of salicylaldoxine, and boil for three minutes. Spin down precipitate and wash it twice with water and once with acetone.
5. Slurry precipitate with acetone onto a weighed aluminium counting tray, dry under a lamp, and count with an end-window G.M counter. Correct counts for decay and self-absorption, and check the half life of the separated copper-64. The chemical steps take about 2 h for eight samples. The chemical yield is about 75 percent.

Calculation

$$\mu g \text{ Cu in sample} = \frac{\text{Cpm sample}}{\text{Cpm standard}} \times \frac{\text{Weight standard Cu - salicylaldoxime}}{\text{Weight sample Cu - salicylaldoxime}}$$

Range and Accuracy

0.05-08 µg of Cu is a convenient range for determination within an accuracy of 5 percent.

Chapter - 45

Techniques of Microbial Protein Biosynthesis in the Rumen

Rumen Microbial Protein Biosynthesis

(Method of Phillipson et. al., 1961, Black , 1968; Pilgrim *et al.*, 1970; Nolan *et al.*, 1972; Beever *et al.*, 1974 and Smith *et al.*, 1977)

Introduction

Smith 1979 who separated mixed rumen bacteria at different times after adding tracer doses of ^{15}N-urea into the rumen of steers, maintained protein high and urea-high rations. N components of the bacteria were separated after acid hydrolysis and relative ^{15}N abundances determined. From this and other data it was concluded that the probable sequence of events following ammonia capture is as follows. Much of the ammonia entering the cell is initially captured in the form of amide groups of glutamine and/ or asparagine. These groups are used for the subsequent amination of α ketoglutarate to glutamate possibly by direct incorporation (Erfle, Sauer and Mahadevan, 1977).

Smith (1969) and Ellis and Pfander (1965) used nucleic acid and McDonald (1954) and Ely *et al.,* (1967) used difference in solubility of zein and microbial protein in ethanol. Blackburn and Hobson (1950) used a method based on solubility differences between casein and microbial protein. McDonald and Hall (1957) used organic phosphorus content in casein to estimate the extent of conversion of casein to microbial protein some workers (Ely *et al.,* 1967; McDonald, 1954 and Temier-Kucharski and Gausseres, 1965) determined microbial protein in rumen digesta by difference in lysine content between microbial and dietary proteins. Some workers (Conrad *et al.*, 1967; Walker and Nader, 1968) have studied microbial protein synthesis in the rumen employing the rate of incorporation of ^{35}S in microbial cells. Others (el Shazly and Hungate, 1966; Weller *et al.*, 1962) *have studied microbial growth with diaminopimelic acid. (DAPA) as a marker since it has been found in bacterial protein but not in protozoal and dietary protein. Previous studies have indicated that aminoethyl phosphonic (AEP) acid is in protozoal protein but not in bacterial or dietary protein (Abou Akkada et al., 1968; Horiguchi and Kandatsu, 1960 and lbrahim et al., 1970).*

Method Using ^{35}S

(Method of Henderickx *et al.*, 1972)

This method was developed by above workers at the Department of Nutrition and Hygiene, faculty of Agricultural Sciences, University of Ghent, Belgium. In this technique tracer $^{35}S_4^2$ is used. It is based on the constant N/S ratio in the microbial protein. The method is applied using rumen contents incubated *in vitro*. From a control incubation made under such conditions that presumably only microbial synthesis could take place, the ratio ^{35}S/mg protein N synthesized is calculated. In other incubation units loaded with the same rumen fluid, the change in total protein is chemically determined, the ^{35}S/N is determined after an incubation of six hours and from these figures the feed protein is broken down and the microbial protein synthesized are calculated. *However the procedure is technically rather simple, it could not be applied in vivo because of the following reasons:*

1. *It is impossible to establish the standard ratio ^{35}S/g protein N synthesized in the same rumen fluid, i.e., in the same animal at the same time.*
2. *Changing the method from a comparative set up to an absolute measurement by determining size and rate of dilution of the SO_4^2 pool is difficult. The incorporation of SO_4^2 into sulphur amino acids is a multiplied reaction, each at its own rate. Not all the SO_4^2 disappearing is recovered in the sulphur amino acids (Müller and Von Erichsen, 1952; Landis 1963). The pool is not constant because the amount of sulphate or compounds metabolized into sulphate of feeds is variable (Muller and Von Erichsen, 1952). Also supply from saliva or other secretions cannot be excluded.*
3. *The possible adaptation of some organisms and the influence of sulphate, sulphide, methionine and cystine on the incorporation of sulphur into proteins as described by Halverson and Co-workers (1968) makes the method not a simple as it was orginally thought. Despite these difficulties the method seems to have been applied in vivo by Roberts and Muller (1969), although no technical details are given.*

Walker and Nader (1968) improved the ^{35}S method for the measurement of microbial synthesis in whole rumen contents incubated with Na ^{35}S in a completely closed *in vitro* system. The $^{35}S^{-2}$ is used for labelling the sulphide pool, and the incorporation of the label into microbial cells is calculated from the size and rate of dilution of the pool together with the radioactivity measured in the microbial cells and the N/S ratio of microbial protein. The calculation of the $^{35}S/N$ ratio in the protein fraction precipitated with trichloroacetic acid gives an estimate of the amount of protein synthesized. In some cases methionine and cystine is separated and their specific radioactivities is determined (Panic *et al.*, 1968).

The results are expressed as given below:

***In Vitro* Studies Parameters**	**Units**
1. Protein incorporated ^{35}S	μCi/g precipitated N
2. Cystine	μCi/ mgS
3. Methionine	μCi/mg
4. Urease	mg NH3-N/100g contents per minute

Method Using ^{14}C

The scientists may study the research papers-published by (Gray *et al.*,1966, 1967., Weller *et al.*, 1967. Leng and Brett. 1966. Leng *et al.* 1968) for estimating microbial protein synthesis. In the case of high energy diets, technique suggested by whitelaw *et al.*, (1970) may be followed.

Later on Henderickx *et al.* (1970) have suggested to use stoichiometric reactions for estimating protein synthesis using VFA production data (^{14}C labelled volatile fatty acids). *On an average, microbial protein synthesis is 2.5-2.8 g N/ mole VFA. About 5.5 to 6.6g protein is synthesized per mole ATP.*

Estimating protein synthesis from the flow of RNA (^{14}C labelled)

Smith (1969) reviewed several of the published methods and assuming the proportion of RNA-N in total N in sheep bacteria to be 7.6 percent (McAllan and Smith, 1973).

DNA reflects the number of micro-organisms present whereas RNA is associated more closely with protein synthesis. From the ratio of RNA/ total N in rumen micro-organisms and in rumen digesta of a calf it is estimated that 70 percent of the total non-ammonia N is microbial.

According to El-Shazly and Abou Akkada (1972) microbial protein synthesis from ammonia-N is affected by many factors which are given below:

(i) *Sources of N intake, i.e., protein or non protein.*

(ii) *Type of protein, i.e., easily degradable or not so easily degraded.*

(iii) Level and source of energy.

(iv) C/N ratio

(v) Dilution rate

(vi) Mineral balance, and

(vii) Growth factors (known and unknown)

On an average rumen microbial dry matter contains 10.72 percent nitrogen (83.5 percent being protein N), 46.16 percent carbon, 6.32 percent hydrogen and 30.66 percent oxygen. The amino nitrogen is 75 percent of the total nitrogen in mixed organisms for the rumen. Nucleic acid nittogen may account for the 14-19 percent of total nitrogen in rumen microbes. Most of this is RNA since DNA accounts for 2.2-4.1 percent of total nitrogen. *The ratio of RNA: DNA in bacteria is 4:1, RNA and DNA may be estimated by the method of Mc Allan and Smith (1969). We may use labelled diaminopimelic acid (DAPA) content as marker and this may be estimated by the method of Mason (1969) and this is found only in bacteria. While in the case of protozoa aminophosphonic acid is present which may be estimated by the method of Horiguchi and Kandatsu (1960).*

It is advisable to follow the method of Beever *et al.,* (1974) for estimating dietary and microbial protein in duodenal digesta of ruminants. Potential value of gastro intestinal re-entrant cannulae for studying digestive processes in the sheep has been demonstrated by various workers. However, the cannulae have a wider usage, since they have been used successfully for preparing duodenal (Ash, 1961 a and b), ileal (Goodall and Kay, 1962), cannulated re-entrant fistula in sheep.

Chapter - 46

Technique of Separation of Bacteria and Protozoa from Rumen Contents

(Method of Ibrahim *et al.*, 1970)

Method I

Rumen fluid is collected from whole digesta by squeezing through two layers of cheese cloth into a warmed Dewar flask. Protozoa are harvested by gravimetric technique. One litre of strained rumen fluid is diluted one to one (V/V)with an acetate-phosphate buffer ($NaC_2H_3O_3$. 2.15 g; KH_2PO_4 0.35g; K_2HPO_4 1.00g; NaCI 5g; $MgSO_4$ 0.12g made) upto one litre with distilled water), bubbled with carbon dioxide, and incubated in a 3 litre separatory funnel at 39 to 40°C for one hour. Protozoal fractions at the bottom of the separatory funnel are diluted with one to one (V/V) acetate phosphate buffer and incubated for one hour more. The protozoal fraction is transferred to 200 ml centrifuge tubes and repeatedly washed with acetate phosphate buffer, centrifuged at 200 × g and examined microscopically for contamination with bacteria and food debris.

Protozoal residue is transferred and spread on glass plates and is then dried at 39°C in a forced air drying oven, and dry weight is recorded. The bacterial fraction is obtained by differential centrifugation. One litre of strained rumen is centrifuged at 100 × g for 10 min. to remove protozoa and food debris, then the supernatant recentrifuged at 50,000 × g for 20 min. in 50 ml centrifuge tubes. The bacterial fraction is resuspended and washed with acetate-phosphate buffer and recentrifuged three times. The bacterial fraction is transferred and spread on glass plates to dry at 39ºC in forced air oven, and dry weight is determined.

Method II

(Method of Blackburn and Hobson, 1960)

A sample of rumen fluid (100 ml) is strained through two thickness of surgical gauze to give liquid F_1. The coarse debris thus removed is resuspended in 0.85 percent (W/V) NaCI solution saturated with chloroform, diluted to 100 ml and strained again (Liquid F_2). The debris is squeezed each time to remove as much liquid as possible. Liquid F_3 consisted of 10 ml portions of F_1 and F_2. A 10 ml portion of F_3 is centrifuged at 114 g for five minutes and the deposit (a) washed in saline. The supernatant liquid and washings are then recentrifuged at 19,000 g for 20 minutes and the deposit (b) washed once in saline. Liquid F_3 is called the whole fraction, deposit (a) protozoal fraction (b) the bacterial fraction, and the remaining supernatant liquid and washings the clear fluid fraction F_1 clarified by centrifuging at 19,000 g is used to determine levels of protein and non-protein nitrogen (NPN) in the rumen fluid. Compared with F_1 the the clear fluid fraction had an identical ratio of protein N to NPN and there seems to be no loss of ammonia or changes in constituents due to washing. Protein nitrogen is precipitated by TCA in a final concentration of 0.36 N and precipitate washed once. Non-ammonia, non-protein nitrogen (NANPN) is obtained by difference between NPN and ammonia nitrogen.

Chapter - 47

Method for Estimation of Rumen Microbial Nitrogen

Rumen Microbial Nitrogen Estimation

(Method of Schultz and Schultz, 1969)

Method I

The perchloric acid method entailed repeated washings with 0.9 percent in distilled water solution, centrifugation at 22,000 × g, and resuspension in distilled water before dry matter determination. The samples are then made 0.4N perchloric acid to release soluble materials and the acid precipitate residue washed once with 0.4N perchloric acid.

Method II

The tungstic acid (TA) procedure consisted of adding 5 ml of 1.07N sulphuric acid and 5ml of 10 percent sodium tungstate to each 20 ml aliquot and mixing thoroughly. After standing a minimum of 4 h, the mixture is centrifuged at 2,000 × g for 20 min. and the precipitate is washed twice in a solution of four volumes of water plus one volume each of the sulphuric acid and sodium tungstate solution.

Method III

In a separatory funnel (SF) technique, the rumen fluid is diluted 1:1 (V/V) with a pH 7 buffer solution, and incubated for one hour ar 39°C in a

Bunsen Valve- equipped separatory funnel The feed residue of free lower portions are withdrawn and dried at 39°C for analysis of the microbial cell mass.

After prepartion of samples by any of the above mentioned methods, dry matter, protein nitrogen and feed contamination are estimated by the crude fiber method mentioned in this compendium.

Technique for Studying Nitrogen Metabolism in Sheep using ^{15}N Labelled Isotope

Nolan *et al.*, (1972) have used ^{15}N-ammonium chloride (260 mg 95 percent enriched with ^{15}N in 100 ml water) and ^{14}C urea (50 µCi; 50 mg in saline), injected intraruminally and intravenously respectively, subsequently ^{15}N and ^{14}N labelled urea (217 mg of 97 percent) enriched and 50 µCi was injected intravenously. Following the injection of isotopes, samples of ruminal fluid and blood are taken at intervals over periods upto 24 h or 3 days. They collected urine samples from catheters in the bladder, faecal samples from the rectum over 24 h period.

The reader may consult the papers published by Mathison and Milligan (1971), Pilgrim *et al.*, (1970) for planning the experiment based on this technique.

Chapter - 48

Technique for the Measurement of the Rate of Production of Bacteria in the Rumen of Buffalo Calves

Bacteria Production Rate in Buffalo Calves

(Method of Singh *et al.*, 1974a)

Rumen liquor from the rumen of calves is drawn through specially built metallic probe covered with nylon mesh. Strained rumen liquor is collected in conical flask, saturated with CO_2 atmosphere to mantain anaerobic conditons. The samples of ruminal fluid are centrifuged at 200 g for 2 min. to remove protozoa and larger feed particles. Later on the bacterial cells are labelled either with ^{14}C or ^{35}S by incubating the sample containing rumen content at 39°C in the presence of CO_2. The incubating mixture contained 100 ml synthetic saliva (Mc Dougall, 1948), 1 g powdered starch or concentrate mixture and 100 ml freshly drawn centrifuged rumen liquor. To each flask is added 8 ml iso-osmotic saline containing either 400 µCi (^{4-14}C) DL- Leucine or 2 µCi (^{35}S) sodium sulphate. After 16 h incubation in a metabolic shaker, the bacteria are separated from the coarse feed particle small protozoa and large bacteria by centrifuging at 200 g for 2 min. To maintain anaerobic condition about 5 ml of liquid parafin is added in each centrifuge tube. The supernatant alongwith liquid paraffin is added in each centrifuged tube. The supernatant alongwith liquid paraffin is further centrifuged in super speed centrifuge at 15,000 g for 15 min. The pellet is washed three times with centrifuged rumen liquor (20,000 for fifteen minutes) under liquid paraffin to remove radioactivity. The sediment is suspended in 500 ml of centrifuged rumen liquor and an aliquot is taken for estimating the amount of radioactivity added. The bacterial suspension is injected into the rumen through the cannula in a single dose. The contents of the rumen are mixed simultaneously by hand.

Sampling and Processing of Bacterial Cells

Samples (35 ml) from the rumen are drawn at various time intervals upto 9-10 h from four different sites using specially built probes with a large number of holes drilled at the end and covered with fine nylon mesh. The rumen fluid samples are received in a cool vessel and are processed immediatley. The sample of the ruminal fluid are centrifuged at 20,000 g to separate protozoa and other larger feed particles. The supernatant is mixed with an equal volume of a detergent solution (iso-osmotic saline containing 0.5 g poly-oxyethylene - 23-lauryl ether/litre) and centrifuged at 15,000 g for 15 min. The supernatant is discarded. The layer of bacteria on the pellet is transferred to another centrifuge tube by mild shaking with the detergent solution and again centrifuged. The bacterial cells are drawn through a fine capillary and transferred to another centrifuge tube. After suspending in detergent saline, the sample are centrifuged twice more at 15,000 g for 15 min. By this process the bacterial samples are found to be free of protozoa and feed particles. The bacterial pellet is treated once with 10 percent trichloroacetic acid (TCA) and subsequently with ethanol, ethanol: ether (3:1) and ether is then dried, weighted and transferred into scintillation vials.

Measurement of Radioactivity

The bacterial pellet is dissolved in a soluene TM_{100}. The samples are counted for radioactivity in liquid scintillation. The scintillation fluid consist of 4 g PPO and 0.5 g dimethyl POPOP/litre toluene.

Chapter - 49

Technique for the Measurement of the Rate of Production of Protozoa in the Rumen of Buffalo Calves

Protozoa Production Rate in Buffalo Calves

Preparation of Labelled Protozoa

(Method of Singh *et al.*, 1974b)

Protozoa are separated from the rumen liquor by centrifugation at 100 g for two minutes under anaerobic conditions. The protozoa enriched fraction is incubated *in vitro* under CO_2 atmosphere at 39ºC in a metabolic shaker for about 12 h in the presence of (U-^{14}C) glucose. The CO_2 is constantly passed through the medium. Each incubation flask contained 175 ml of salt solution (K_2HPO_4, 0.15 percent; NaCI, 0.6 percent; MgSO4. $7H_2O$, 0.001 percent and $CaCI_2$. 0.001 percent). 75 ml centrifuged rumen liquor (23, 000 g for 30 min); cysteine hydrochloride 50 mg, sodium bicarbonate 1.25 g and starch 1.25 g. This medium is autoclaved at 121°C for 30 min. To each incubating flask, protozoa separated form 150 ml rumen liquor and 300 μCi of ^{14}C- glucose are added. At the end of the incubation period (12 h) the protozoa are separated from the incubation medium under a CO_2 atmosphere and a layer of liquid paraffin by centrifuging at 100 g for 2 min and subsequently washed three times with centrifuged rumen liquor (23,000 g supernatant). The washed protozoa preparation is resuspended in 250 ml centrifuged rumen liquor and a sample is taken for counting. The protozoa suspension is injected into rumen through the canula in a single dose.

Processing of Protozoa for Radioactivity Measurement

The protoza is separated by centrifuging at 100 g for 2 min. The sediment is suspended with iso-osmotic saline containing polyoxyethylene 23-lauryl ether (0.5 g/l) and is centrifugated at 100 g for two minutes. The layer of protozoa is taken out with a small syringe and is resuspended in iso-osmotic saline containing the detergent. The process is repeated three times to give a protozoa pellet practically free of feed contaminants. This pellet is treated with 10 percent TCA and washed with alcohol, alcohol: ether (3:1) and finally with ether or acetone. It is then dried at 60°C for 30 min and the samples are transferred after weighing into scintillation vials. The proceedure for measurement of the radioactivity is same as described in bacterial counting.

Chapter - 50

Studying Urea Kinetics Using ^{14}C-Labelled Urea in Ruminants

Urea Kinetics in Ruminants

(Method of Cocimano and Leng, 1966; Conrad, 1972; Varady & Harmeyer, 1972)

Hypothesis

The validity of measuring urea kinetics using a single dose of ^{14}C-urea and using urinary excretion as a sampling system is based on specific assumption:

1. There is a rapid equilibration of ^{14}C-urea with the endogenous urea pool following infusion. This pool is conceived to be a measure of all body compartments permeable to urea and in equilibrium with the plasma urea pool.
2. Experimental animals are metabolically maintained in a steady state during the test period and metabolic breakdown of urea is random.
3. Specific radioactivity for urinary urea is proportional to the dilution of replenishment and simultaneous depletion rate of the urea pool.
4. That the metabolic parameters of urea are correctly measured.

Calculation

Mathematical calculations are made as given below (Zilversmit, 1960).

1. Urea Pool Size

This is the total amount of urea present in the body. It can be calculated from the semilogarithmic plot of the specific activity of plasma urea versus time. Extrapolation of the linear part of the curve to zero time gives an estimate of the specific activity at this time.

$$\text{Urea pool size, g} = \frac{\text{injected dose}(\mu ci)}{SA_0(\mu ci/\text{g urea carbon})} \times 5$$

Where, SA_0 = equal specific radioactivity at zero time and 5 is a factor for conversion of urea grams carbon to grams urea.

2. Half Time

$$(t\,½) = \frac{ln_2}{k} = \frac{0.693}{k}$$

where k is the fractional turnover rate.

3. Urea entry rate or Flux Rate

$$E = \frac{P}{t_{½} \times 1.44}$$

$$= \frac{\text{pool, g}}{\text{turnover time}}$$

4. Plasma Urea Space (ml)

Space may be calculated in a similar way to the pool as

$$S_p = \frac{A_o}{H_o}$$

where,

Ao = total dose of activity injected (Dpm)

Ho = activity per ml of plasma water (Dpm/ml) at zero time

When ^{14}C urea is injected, 1.5 g of N-acetyl-4- aminoantipyrine (NAAP) are also adminstered to the animals. NAAP space is calculated giving an estimate of the empty body water space. By combining the two methods changes in the relation of urea space to NAAP space could be detected. NAAP is determined by the method of Brodie and Axelrod (1950).

5. Total Turnover (μ mol/min. kg)

It can be calculated from the slope of the semilogarithmic plot of the specific activity of plasma urea versus time.

$$= T_1 \, 2.303 \, \frac{\Delta \log S.Pu}{\Delta t.w}$$

where, $\Delta \log S = \log S_2 = \log S_1$

$S_1; S_2$ = Specific activities of urea (Dpm/ μ mol) in plasma at times t_1 & t_2

$\Delta t = t_2 - t_1$ (min)

W = Weight (kg)

Pu = urea pool (μmol)

6. Exogenous Turnover (μ mol/min. kg)

This is the excretion rate of urea by the kidneys. It can be calculated by

$$Tex = \frac{Cu - Fu}{W}$$

where Cu = urea concentration in urine (μ mol/ml)

Fu = urine flow (ml/min)

W = weight of the animal (kg)

7. Endogenous Turnover (μ mol/min. kg)

The endogenous turnover of urea can be calculated by substracting exogenous turnover from total turnover. This fraction is also known as degradatioin rate of urea within the body. Alternately, the difference between the entry rate and rate of excretion of urea in the urine is taken to indicate the quantity of urea degraded in the digestive tract.

Procedure

(Method of Varady and Harmeyer 1972)

The animals are equipped with Teflon jugular vein catheters. Urea metabolism is investigated by mean of a single injection of ^{14}C-labelled urea (sp. activity 70 Dpm/μmol). 50-100 μCi of label are used per experiment dissolved in a volume of 20 ml. Urine is collected and 15 blood samples are taken during a period of 10 h.

The reader may consult a very important research paper published by Cociman and Leng (1966), for calculating the dose of ^{14}C-labelled urea in sheep.

The radioactivity of urea is determined by liquid scintillation counter using phosphor solution consisting PPO 4 g, POPOP 0.2 g, Naphthalene 60 g, Methanol 100ml, ethylene glycol 20 ml and Dioxam to 1,000 ml (Bray, 1960).

Chapter - 51

Estimation of Endogenous Calcium and Phosphorus in Ruminants

Endogenous Calcium and Phosphorus in Ruminants

(Method of Visek *et al.*, 1953; Lueker and Lofgreen, 1961)

By using isotope dilution technique, It is possible to separate faecal calcium into endogenous and exogenous fractions. The true digestibility can be measured independently by making correction for faecal endogenous loss. The isotope dilution method described by Visek *et al.*, (1953) involves daily intravenous injection of ^{45}Ca for 15 days, followed by a collection of the serum and the faeces for 15 days. However, these numerous veinpunctures result in considerable discomfort to the animal. Lueker and Lofgreen (1961) modified this method in sheep by giving a single subcutaneous injection of ^{45}Ca, followed by a collection of blood and the faeces for 7 days only.

The endogenous faecal calcium and true digestibility of calcium is calculated by the formula of Lofgreen and Kleiber (1954) as given below:

$$\frac{\theta(t+x)}{\pi(t)} \times \text{daily faecal Ca(g)}$$

(t) = Specific activity of serum Ca at time t

θ (t +x) = Specific activity of faecal Ca at time t +x.

$$\frac{\theta(t+x)}{\pi(t)} = \text{Ratio of the faecal to serum activity}$$

x = Time lag in days when the maximum activity in serum is reflected as maximum activity in the faeces.

True digestibility of calcium

$$= \frac{\text{Calcium intake - (faecal calcium - endogenous calcium)}}{\text{Ca intake}}$$

☞ Note

All the figures of intake, faecal calcium and endogenous calcium should be in grams.

Technique for use in Buffalo Calves

1. Select two buffalo calves weighing 250 and 280 kg, respectively and feed daily a growth ration in 2 equal portions at 8.00 and 20 hours. Offer water *ad libitum* daily at 9.00 and 21.00 hours. The calves consumed the whole ration within one hour.
2. Inject 10 ml of solution $^{45}CaCl_2$ (specific activity 9.6 μCi/g Ca; adjusted to pH6 containing 10 μCi ^{45}Ca by subcutaneous route in the cervical region into each animal. To establish the time lag, when peak activity in the blood is reflected in the faeces, blood samples are drawn at intervals of 1/2, 1, 2, 4, 6 and 8 h after the injection on the first day at 8 and 20 h on the second and third day. Thereafter, up to 22 days after the injection, the blood samples are collected daily at 8.00 hours. For the first three days after the injection faecal samples are collected at every defaecation and thereafter a representative sample is taken daily at 8.00 h for 19 days from the faeces collected manually during the 24 period, One millilitre of the serum and 1 ml of the acid extract of faecal ash obtained in the above method is dried to a constant weight in stainless steel planchets under infrared lamp and activity is measured by an end-window Geiger Müller counter.

Chapter - 52

Incorporation of Radioactive Carbon from Oxalic Acid ^{14}C into Ruminal Microbial Constituents under *in vitro* system

Incorporation of Radioactive Carbon from Oxalic Acid in Rumen Microbes

Introduction

It is a well known fact that the soluble oxalates are broken down by rumen microbes from buffalo and cattle and one of the end product formed is bicarbonates.

The rumen microbes are obtained from a fistulated buffalo calf fed on wheat bhusa and sarson cake supplemented with 60 g potassium oxalate daily for about three months. Representative sample of rumen ingesta is drawn before feeding and mixed culture is prepared by the method as described Donefer *et al.,* (1960). Mixed culture and basal nutrient mixture (Quicke *et al.,* 1959) of pH 6.9 mixed in equal quantities. Fifty millilitres of this mixture are added into each incubation flask containing one gram of wheat straw, ground to 40 mesh as substrate. In the incubation flasks are added 35,100 and 550 mg oxalic acid in the form of potassium oxalate and 0.24 µCi sodium oxalate ^{14}C. Blank (containing no substrate, no oxalic acid added) and two controls, one having substrate but no added oxalic acid and the other containing the above plus radioactivity, are also run alongwith. All the incubation flasks are taken in duplicate. The flasks are incubated at 39°C for 24 h in an incubator and at the end of this period microbial activity is stopped by the addition of few drops of saturated solution of mercuric chloride.

Preparation of Oxalate- ^{14}C

Oxalate ^{14}C is prepared from formate 1-^{14}C obtained from Bhaba Atomic Research Centre, Trombay. Two µCi of formate ^{14}C is heated in the presence of one ml 1 percent NaOH solution at 300°C for three hours on oil bath.

$$2HCOONA \xrightarrow[\text{in the presence of NaOH}]{300^{\circ}\text{C for 3 hours}} \begin{array}{c} COONa \\ | \\ COONa \end{array} + H_2$$

Estimation of Titrable Alkalinity of Incubated Mixture

Ten millilitre of supernatant of incubated mixture is titrated against N/10 HCI using methyl red as an indicator. The end point is taken when yellow colour changed to rose pink. One ml of N/10 HCI is equivalent to 0.006 g HCO_3.

The reader should refer the research papers published by Morris and Garcia-Rivera (1955) and Watts (1957) for conducting studies on *in vitro* metabolism in detail.

Chapter - 53

Estimation of Radioactive ^{45}Calcium by Liquid Scintillation Counting

Radioactive ^{45}Calcium

Principle

Inorganic salts are relativity insoluble in aromatic solvents which has been detrimental to the estimation of ^{45}Calcium by scintillation counting. This technique inolves the counting of ^{45}Calcium as calcium 2-ethyl hexanoate in a solution of toluene phosphor; and the counting as calcium chloride in a tertiary mixture of absolute ethyl alcohol-hydrochloric acid-toluene-phosphor.

Reagents

1. *^{45}Calcium. A ^{45}Calcium solution supplied as calcium chloride in hydrochloric acid solution, is suitably diluted.*
2. *Calcium chloride, 0.045 N, is prepared by dissolving ACS grade calcium carbonate, dried to constant weight at 110°C, in 5 N hydrochloric acid.*
3. *Calcium acetate, citrate, lactate, acid phosphate, chloride and hydroxide.*
4. *Ammonium oxalate solution, 4 percent*
5. *2-Ethyl-hexanoic acid.*
6. *Toluene-diphenyloxazole solution, 2g of diphenyloxazole are dissolved in 500 ml of toluene.*

Extraction of Calcium from Biological Fluids

Into a 15 ml centrifuge tube are placed 2 ml of distilled water, 1 ml of 4 percent ammonium oxalate, and 1 to 2 ml of serum by pipette, and the solution is mixed by swirling. After at least 4 h at room temperature, the mixture is centrifuged at 15,000 to 2,000 rpm, for 10 min. The supernatant solution is decanted and the tubes are inverted on filter paper for at least 10 min; the lip of the tube is wiped dry with tissue and the precipitate is broken up by a stream of wash mixture (2 percent ammonia in equal parts of ethyl alcohol, ethyl ether and water), using a total volume of 4 ml. The mixture is again centrifuged for 10 min at 2,000 rpm, the supernatant solution is decanted and the tubes are drained for 10 min. The tubes containing the precipitate are dried in a boiling water bath or a constant temperature oven at 100°C for 10 to 30 min and 0.3 ml of concentrated hydrochloric acid is added to dissolve the precipitates. Solution may be hastened by placing the tube in boiling water for 30 seconds. Three millilitres of absolute ethyl alcohol, followed by 5 ml of 0.4/percent diphenyloxazole in toluene are added to each tube with careful mixing after each addition; the cloudy mixture is immediately decanted into a counting vial and drained for 30 to 60 s. To each tube is then added 1 ml of absolute ethyl alcohol, which is decanted again into the counting vial. The vials are stored at 0°C or below until counting.

Urine and Stool Digesta

Into a 50 ml centrifuge tube are pipetted 5 to 25 ml of the urine or stool digest (containing no more than 50 mg of calcium). Methyl red is added and the pH adjusted to just alkaline with 1 M ammonium hydroxide and 1N hydrochloric acid is necessary. To each tube is added 1 ml of 4 percent ammonium oxalate, the contents are mixed by swirling, and the mixture is kept at room temperature for at least 4 h. Therefore, the samples are treated like those of serum.

Standards

One millilitre aliquots from suitable dilutions of a ^{45}Calcium solution are pipetted into 15 ml centrifuge tubes containing 0.5 ml of 0.045N calcium chloride and 2 ml of distilled water; 1 ml of 4 percent ammonium oxalate is added with careful swirling. Therefore, the samples are treated like the serum samples.

☞ Note

This technique requires only a simple preliminary precipitation to concentrate the calcium and thereafter uses the high sensitivity, precision, and effciency of the liquid scintillation counting technique. The present procedure is of particular value in studies requiring the examination of large number of samples over a wide range of radioactive concentrations.

Chapter - 54

Determination of Digestibility with Cerium as an Inert Marker

Determination of Digestibility with Cerium

(Method of Olbrich *et al.*, 1971)

Jones and Ekman (1960) showed that ^{144}Ce is absorbed to a very small extent in the gut of the ruminant and suggested its use as a marker in digestibility trials. Huston and Ellis (1968) studied the affinity of radioactive cerium for feedstuffs and digesta particles *in vitro* experiments and found that cerium is rapidly absorbed onto and remained tenaciously bound to digesta particles. Ellis and Huston (1968) tested radioactive cerium as a particulate flow marker in sheep with favourable results.

Experimental Procedure

Three Holstein bulls weighing 315, 239 and 305 kg and one Holstein steer weighing 327 kg are used. Twice daily, at 9.00 am and 9.00 pm, they are fed 3.4 kg of a balanced ration, meeting NRC requirements for normal growth and maintenance.

Cerium is incorporated into the feed at a concentration of approximately 165 ppm by dissolving 294 g of ceric ammonium nitrate $(NH_2)_2 Ce (NO_3)_6$ in 11.35 litres of distilled water and thoroughly mixing this with 11.35 kg of alfalfa ground in a hammermill equipped with a 1.27 cm screen. The alfalfa cerium mixture is then dried for 2 days at 60°C and substituted for an equal amount of alfalfa meal in the complete ration.

The ration without cerium is fed to the animals for 2 weeks before starting the trial, and the ration containing cerium is fed for 4 days before faecal collection began. The animals are placed in digestion crates and given 2 days of adjustment before collection is started. After this period of adjustment, feed intake is measured and faeces are collected for a 6 day period (King *et al.*, 1960). During each of the 6 days of faecal sampling, samples are taken of the thoroughly mixed daily faecal composite just before the morning feeding. To test for diurinal excretion patterns of Cerium, grab samples of fresh faeces are also collected during days 3 and 4 at 12.00 noon, 3.00 pm, 6.00 pm and 9.00 pm or 3, 6, 9 and 12 h after 9.00 am feeding.

All feed and faecal samples are placed in dried, weighed glass plates immediately after collection, weighed and dried for 5 days at 60°C and then reweighed to determine dry matter percentages. The dried samples are ground in a stainless steel mill and 0.2 g sub-samples are placed in plastic vials for activation analysis.

The samples are processed for neutron activation analysis. These are irradiated for 20 min with thermal neutrons in the reactor at a flux of approximately $4x10^{13}$ *neutrons/cm*^{2}*/s. The samples are irradiated by use of a pneumatic tube system, with four faecal samples, one feed sample and one cerium standard placed in each rabbit.* After irradiation, the samples are allowed to decay for 7 days and then counted for 2 min in a well type 45 cc sodium iodide scintillation detector coupled to a 400 channel pulse height analyser calibrated at an energy of 0 to 0.5 MeV. Only those counts integrated under the ^{141}Ce, 0.145 MeV gamma-ray peak are recorded. Each sample's counts per minutes (CPM) is corrected for background. Dry matter digestibility is determined by standard indicator method using background corrected CPM of the cerium in the feed and faeces.

Proximate analysis is run on all feed and faecal samples as per methods compiled by author in this compendium and nutrient digestibility is determined using the cerium ratio technique.

Cerium has a considerably longer half life (32.5 days).

☞ Note

The data suggest that an accurate determination of dry matter digestibility using the cerium ratio technique could be obtained by faecal grab samples taken any day at any time after a 6-day cerium adjustment period.

Chapter - 55

Determination of Strontium-90 by An Ion Exchange Method

Strontium - 90 Determination

(Method of Bryant *et al., 1959)*

Strontium and barium are adsorbed on a cation-resin column, and after a suitable gowth period, yttrium-90, the daughter of strontium-90, is selectively eluted. The yttrium-90 is then adsorbed on and eluted from a second cation-resin column and counted. The radiochemical yield is greater than 97% gravimetric measurement of the recovery of strontium and yttrium carriers is not required. The method, with modifications, is applicable to samples that contain 100 mg of iron or uranium.

Apparatus

1. *Aluminium counting plates, 3¼ x 2½ x* $\frac{1}{16}$ *inch*
2. *Double-sided scotch tape.*
3. *Mylar film, 1.7 mg per sq cm.*
4. *Fritted-glass pressure filter, with a 25 to 30 ml reservoir and a drip tip, fine fritted disk,*
5. *Beta proportional counter, methane-flow, 2 inch diameter, 4.8 mg per sq cm, aluminium window.*
6. *Ion Exchange Column, Three types of columns are used. The first cation column is prepared by scaling a 12 cm length of glass tubing 18 mm inch inside*

diameter, to a 9 cm length of tubing 6 mm inside diameter fitted with a drip tip. The second cation column is prepared in a similar manner from a 9 cm length of tubing 5 mm inside diameter and a 15 ml centrifuge cone. The anion column is prepared by scaling a 40 ml, centrifuge cone to a 10 cm length of tubing 10 mm inside diameter fitted with a drip tip.

Reagents

1. *Sea sand, washed with concentrated hydrochloric acid and rinsed with water. Ammonium hydroxide solution, approximately 0.6 F NH_4 OH, prepared by saturating water with ammonium gas and diluting the saturated solution 1 to 25 with water.*
2. *Eluting reagents. A solution of 0.5F a-hydroxyisobutyric acid (Fair Mount Chemical Co.) made up to pH 3.55 with concentrated ammonium hydroxide.*
3. *A solution of 0.5 F a-hydroxyisobutyric acid made up to pH 6 with concentrated ammonium hydroxide.*
4. *Barium, lanthanum, strontium, the zirconium carrier solution, 2 mg of barium, 1 mg of lanthanum, 4 mg of strontium, 1 mg of zirconium per ml as nitrates in 1 F nitric acid.*
5. *Lanthanum carrier solution, 0.3 mg of lanthanum per ml added as nitrate to a 0.4 F hydrochloric acid solution.*
6. *Strontium carrier solution, 4 mg of strontium per ml as nitrate in water.*
7. *Barium, lanthanum, and zirconium carrier solution, 2 mg of barium, 1 mg of lanthanum, 1 mg of zirconium per ml as nitrates in 1 F nitric acid.*

Exchange Resin

AG 50 X-4, cation resin, 200 to 400 mesh, processed from Dowex 50X-4 by Bio-Rad Laboratories, 32nd and Griffin Ave., Richmond, Calif converted to the ammonium form by treatment with 6 F ammonium hydroxide, and washed with water, AG1X-8, anion resin, 100 to 200 mesh, chloride form, processed from Dowex 1X-8 by Bio-Rad Laboratories.

Preparation of Resin Columns

The tip of column is plugged with glass wool and a slurry of the resin is added. The resin, when settled, should extend to within about 2 cm of the shoulder. One to 2 cm of sand is added to prevent agitation of the resin. Just before use, the cation columns are washed with water and the anion columns are washed with concentrated hydrochloric acid.

Recommended Procedure

The basic procedure can be applied to samples which contain not more than about 1 mg of iron, 10 mg of uranium, or 10 mg of calcium. A supplementary procedure is used for removal of 100 mg amounts of iron and uranium.

Basic Procedure

Step 1: Add the sample to a 40 ml centrifuge cone which contains 1 ml of concentrated perchloric acid and 1 ml of the barium, lanthanum, strontium and zirconium carrier solution. Evaporate the solution to concentrated perchloric acid on a steam bath and add about 20 ml of water (the evaporation to perchloric acid ensures removal of iodine-131). Bubble in ammonia gas untill a flocculent precipitate forms, and continue bubbling for about 10 S. Digest the mixture on a steam bath for about 5 min.

Step 2A: For samples that contain less than about 1 mg of iron, 3 mg of uranium, or 10 mg of lanthanum. Transfer the contents of the centrifuge cone to a fritted-glass filter placed in position above the first cation-resin column. Apply air pressure to force the liquid through, the filter into the reservoir of the column. Rinse the centrifuge cone with 3 ml of the 0.6 F ammonium hydroxide solution and transfer to the filter. Use the liquid to wash the walls of the filter and then force the liquid through the filter. Repeat the wash at least once.

Step 2B: For samples that contain about 1 mg of iron, 3 to 10 mg of uranium, or 10 to 100 mg of lanthanum. Centrifuge the contents of the cone and decant the supernatant solution into a fritted-glass filter placed in position above the first cation resin column. Apply air pressure to force the liquid through the filter into the reservoir of the column. Dissolve the precipitate in the centrifuge cone with a minimum amount of perchloric acid, add 1 ml of the strontium carrier solution, and add water until the volume of the solution is about 10 ml. Reprecipitate the hydroxides with ammonium gas as described in Step 1. Transfer the contents of the centrifuge cone to the filter and force the liquid through the filter into the reservoir of the column.

Step 3: Remove the filter and apply air pressure to the cation column to force the liquid through the resin at about 1ml/per minute. Wash the resin with two 5 ml portions of water, the cation resins are never blown dry, remove pressure when the liquid surface reaches the sand.

Step 4: Wash the resin with 10 ml of 0.2 F perchloric acid. The acid is necessary for conversion of yttrium and lanthanide hydroxides on the resin column to a form in which they can be eluted.

Step 5: Force two 5 ml, portions of the pH 6 ammonium a-hydroxiso-butyrate solution through the resin column at about 1 ml/per minute. This solution strips yttrium, lanthanum, and other rare earth ions from the resin.

Step 6: Wash the resin immediately with 5 ml of water and record the time as the beginning of the growth period for yttrium-90. Cover the trip of the column with a rubber policeman, add about 1 ml of water to the reservoir, stopper the column, and set it aside.

Step 7: After 2 or more days remove the policeman and the stopper and allow the water in the reservoir to flow through the resin. Place the second cation column with a policeman covering the tip, in position under the first column. Put 3 ml of the lanthanum carrier solution in the reservoir of the second column (the hydrochloric acid in the lanthanum carrier solution is necessary to break up the yttrium a-hydroxyisobutyrate complexion). Add 5 ml of the pH 3.55 a-hydroxyisobutyric acid solution to the reservoir or the first column. Force the a-hydroxyisobutyric acid solution through the resin at about 1 ml per minute and collect the effluent in the reservoir of the second column. Record, as the end of the growth period and the begining of the decay period for yttrium-90, the time at which the elution is complete. The first column may be discarded at this point. If desired, a second sample of yttrium-90 may be obtained from this column. Wash the column with water and proceed as in Step 6.

Step 8: Stir the mixture in the reservoir of the second column, remove the policeman, and force the solution through the resin, Wash the column with 5 ml of water.

Step 9: Force 10 ml of 0.5 F ammonium perchlorate through the second column and test the last few drops of effluent with pH paper to determine whether the column has been completely converted to the ammonium form. If conversion is complete, the pH will be that of 0.5 F ammonium perchlorate (about 5); if incomplete, less than about 3. When the conversion is complete, wash the column with 5 ml of water.

Step 10: Prepare a counting plate for sample collectioin by sticking a 4.25 cm disk of No. 2 Whatman filter paper to an aluminium counting plate with double-sided Scotch tape. Place the counting plate on a hot plate position the second column so that its tip is about 0.5 inch above the centre of the paper. Add 4 ml of the pH 3.55 a-hydroxyisobutyric acid solution to the reservoir of the column and allow the liquid to pass through the resin onto the paper by force of gravity (about 2 drops per min). Adjust the temperature of the hot plate so that evaporation takes place smoothly (about 250°C). The Scotch tape and the filter paper will usually turn brown in the hour required for elution and evaporation.

Step 11: When the elution is complete, remove the aluminium plate, allow it to cool, and cover the filter paper with Mylar film.

Supplementary Procedure for Removal of Iron or Uranium

Step 1: Add the sample to a 40 ml centrifuge cone which contains 1 ml of the strontium carrier solution and 1 ml of concentrated perchloric acid. Evaporate to concentrated perchloric acid on the steam bath. Add 10 ml of concentrated hydrochloric acid and transfer the solution to the reservoir of the anion-resin column. Allow the solution to flow through the resin and drip into a receiver. Rinse the centrifuge cone and the sides of the reservoir with three 5 ml portions of concentrated hydrochloric acid. Allow each rinse to flow through the resin. Force the last drops of the final rinse from the rinse with air pressure. If the sample contains more than about 100 mg of iron or uranium, a larger anion-resin column and more hydrochloric acid are necessary.

Step 2: Add to the collected effluent 1 ml of barium, lanthanum, and zirconium carrier solution. Evaporate the concentrated perchloric acid and proceed as in Step 1 of the basic procedure.

Calculations

Calculate the strontium-90 disintegration rate in the original sample by the formula.

$$D(Sr^{90}) = A\ (\gamma^{90})\ (e^{y-1}\ e^{\lambda t}\ (1\text{-}e\text{-}\lambda T)\ \text{-}1$$

Where, D $(S\gamma^{90})$ is the disintegration rate of strontium-90, $A(Y^{90})$ is the measured activity of yttrium-90 at time t after separation of the yttrium from the strontium (steps 7), T is the time allowed for growth of the yttrium-90 (Steps 6 and 7), λ is the decay constant for yttrium-90 (half life 64.03 h).

□□□

Appendix

Approximate Dose of Radioisotopes

Procedure	Isotopes and compound	Approximate dose
Thyriod function		
Uptake and excretion	^{131}I-sodium iodide	0.1-1.0 μCi /kg
Red cell uptake (*in vitro*)	^{131}I-triiodothyronine	0.01 μCi ml blood
Conversion of iodide to thyroxine	^{131}I-sodium iodide	0.5-1.0 μCi /kg
Kidney function	^{131}I hippuric acid	0.4 μCi /kg
	^{131}I-Diodrast	0.4 μCi /kg
Liver function	^{131}I-rose Bengal	0.2 μCi /kg
Pernicious anemia	^{57}Co (or ^{60}Co) – Vit B12	0.01 μCi /kg
Haematology		
Cardiac output	^{131}I-serum albumin	0.2 – 0.3 μCi /kg
Blood volume	^{131}I-serum albumin	0.1 – 1.0 μCi /kg
Red cell mass and turnover	^{51}Cr- sodium chromate	1–3 μCi /kg
	^{51} Cr-glycine	2 μCi /kg
Myocardial blood flow	^{131} serum *albumin*	0.3 μCi /kg

Platelet turnover	^{35}S-sulphate	
R.B.Cs formation	^{59}Fe-Citrate	2 μCi /kg
Leukocyte studies	^{3}H-thymidine (*in vitro*)	2 μCi / ml (blood)
Globulin turnover	^{131}I-r-globulin	1 μCi /kg
Copper-ceruloplasmin	^{64}Cu and ^{64}Cu (ionic)	6 μCi /kg (^{67}Cu)
Myocardial circulation	^{131}I-serum albumin,	0.03 μCi /kg
	^{131}I-Diodrast	0.03 μCi /kg
Hypertension	^{24}Na	0.03 μCi /kg
Digestion studies		
Iron absorption	^{59}Fe-citrate	0.01 μCi /kg
Water absorption	^{3}H-water	–
Albumin secretion	^{131}I-serum albumin (Sheep)	5 μCi /kg
Fat absorption	^{131}I-oleic acid	0.3 μCi /kg
Phosphorus digestion	^{32}P-phosphate	10 μCi /kg
Calcium digestion	^{45}Ca-chloride	10 μCi /kg
Milk fever	^{45}Ca-chloride	10 μCi /kg
Acetonemia (ketosis)	^{14}C-organic compounds	10 μCi /kg
Rickets, ovine	^{32}P-^{45}Ca-inorganic	10 μCi /kg

Source : Kaneko, J.J. and Comelius, C.E. 1971 Clinical biochemistry of domestic animals. 2nd Edn. Academic. Press, New York, pp. 272.

Chapter - 56

Measuring Colour, Fluorescence, Polarisation and Spectrum of Particulate Matter

General Definitions

1. *Colour :* Colour is the name for all sensations arising from the activity of the retina of the eye and its nervous mechanisms, this activity being a specific response to radiant energy of certain wavelength and intensities. Colour is basically psychological and is not synonymous with wavelength.

2. *Lambert's law :* Which states that the proportion of radiant energy absorbed by a substance is independent of the intensity of the incident light.

3. *Beer's law :* Which states that the proportion light absorbed depends only on the total number of absorbing molecules through which it passes independently of their concentration.

4. *Extinction :* Extinction is the logarithmic ratio of the intensity of the incident light to that of the emergent light.

   $$E = \varepsilon cl = \text{Log}10 \frac{I10}{I}$$

   where molecule extinction coefficient = ε

intensity of the incident light = Io
intensity of the transmitted light = I
concentration of substance (mole/litre) thickness of solution (cm) = l

The amount of light absorbed will clearly be dependent upon the wavelength of light and consequently the so called constants will have differnt values with different wavelength of the light.

5. Extinction coefficient ($E^{1\%}_{1cm}$)

This is the value of log $\frac{I_0}{I}$ for a 1 cm path through a 1% solution of the substance. The formula mentioned under 4 (Extinction) is modified as below :

$$\text{Extinction coefficient} = E^{1\%}_{1cm} = \frac{A \times 1(cm) \times 1(\%)}{l \times c}$$

where

A = observed absorbance or optical density

l = cell length (cm)

c = concentration (%)

The term optical density refers to any extinction measured, irrespective of the concentration and light path.

Hence :

$$\text{optical density} = A = \log \frac{I_0}{I} \text{ and } \log T = 2\text{-}A$$

where

$$T = \%\ \text{transmission} = \frac{I}{I_0} \times 100$$

6. Molecular extinction coefficient, is the optical density when the layer of solution is 1 cm thick and the concentration of the absorbing substance is one g molecule per litre.

7. Specific extinction coefficient may be defined as the extinction coefficient per unit concentration. In medical biochemistry it is convenient to take 1mg/100 ml as the unit of concentration, although in other branches 1g/100ml may be used as the unit.

8. Transmission : This is defined as the ratio of the intensity of the transmitted to that of the incident light.

Thus :

$$T = \frac{I}{I_0} x 100 = \% \text{ transmission}$$

9. *Transmittance* may be defined as the ratio of the transmission of a cell containing the coloured solution to that of an identical cell containing water or a blank solution.

10. *Wavelength* (λ) the distance, measured along the line propagation, between two points which are in phase on adjacent waves. Wavelengths are usually expressed in tenth meters (10^{-10}m) or Ångstrom units (Å). The latter unit derives its name from the worker who introduced the wavelength scale in 1869. The international Ångstrom is now universally known as the Ångstrom (Å), since the length of the metre is known in terms of wavelength of the red cadmium line to an accuracy greater than one part in ten million, the Ångstrom is defined by international agreement in terms of the red cadmium line. Millimicron is a unit of length equal to one thousand[th] of a micron (μ), which in turn is equal to 10^{-6} metre. It is almost, but not exactly equal to 10 Ångstrom.

    Ångstrom is a unit of length equal to 1/6438.4696 of the wavelength of the red line of cadmium.

    1 Ångstrom = 0.1 millimicrons = 10^{-4} microns = 10^{-8} cm

Selection of proper wavelength : It is desirable to use the wavelength of maximum absorption for the test substance, since at that wavelength there is the greatest change in the transmittance for a given change in concentration. This is turn gives maximum sensitivity for quantitative determination of concentration. The first step in choosing the most suitable wavelength of the incident light. This is most accurately carried out in a spectro-photometer but for the present purpose the Photoelectric colorimeter may be used in the manner mentioned below :

Absorption characteristics of standard solution in the wavelength range of 400-650 millimicrons (4000-6500 Ångstrom units). Record the percent transmittancy of the standard solution from wavelength 400 mμ to 650 mμ at interval of 10mμ. A graphical plot of the absorption (decrease in transmittance) vis-a-vis the wavelength will be used to determine at what wavelength maximum absorption occurs.

Preparation of a Standard Curve

Using the appropriate wavelength, read and record each standard tube. Graphically plot % transmittance against concentration being certain that the units on the coordinates are uniform. A second plot on the same piece of graph paper is made using absorbance (opitical density = 2-log%T) versus concentration. The latter plot is a standard curve from which the concentration of unknown is determined.

Unknown Measurements

Read transmittance on a photoelectric colorimeter. From the absorbance determine the concentration of the solution from the standard curve.

If, with the unknown, one simultaneously analyses a solution of a known concentration close to that of the unknown (e.g., differing by not more than a factor of 2) and if their respective optical densitites are measured, the concentration of the unknown is given by the calculation.

We may work out our own factor using the following relationship between density of unknown and density of standard.

$$\text{Concentration of unknown} = \frac{\text{Density of unknown}}{\text{Density of standard}} \times \text{conc. of standard}$$

Selection of light filters : When a beam of white light is allowed to pass through a coloured solution, absorption will take place in a definite region or regions or spectrum. It is for this reason that the solution appears coloured. For example, a solution which absorbs most of red, orange yellow and green components of the incident light will appear blue to the eye, because this colour is predominantly transmitted. Similarly, a solution which absorbs most of the blue, green yellow component from white light will appear red. The proportion of the incident light absorbed by a coloured solution varied, then, with its wavelength: and the accuracy in the estimation of the concentration of a coloured solution can be achieved only if the photoelectric measurements are made with light of the most suitable wavelength.

Photocell

It is used as substitute for the eye in Photoelectric colorimeter. These are of two types:

1. *Photoemissive type*
2. *Barrier layer type*

When light strikes such a cell, there is a flow of electric current which is directly proportional to the light intensity. This current may be measured by micro-ameter, a galvanometer, or, in case of null point instruments, by a combination of variable resistance and galvanometer. Photoelectric cells, though not quite so sensitive as the eye in detecting visible light, as far superior to it in their ability to match or make quantitative estimations of light intensitites.

Advantage of Photoelectric Method over Usual Methods of Analysis

1. Subjective factor is eliminated, which is inherent in usual comparative measurements.
2. Photoelectric methods have more accuracy.
3. There is an extension of the range of colorimetric analysis to pale colours.
4. Determination could be done by Photoelectric colorimeter even in the presence of interferring colours.

Principles of Colorimetry

White light contains all wavelength. All coloured solutions absorb some of the light at certain wavelengths and transmit other wavelength. In passing a beam of light through a homogenous medium, a part is lost by reflection, another part absorbed by the medium and a third part will be transmitted. The proportions are independent of the intensity of the incident light. By keeping reflection constant, the following relationship applies.

I_0 = Intensity of incident light
I_A = Intensity of absorbed light
I_T = Intensity of transmitted light

Expressed as a fraction of incident intensity, these are designated *"absorbance"* and *"transmittance"* respectively. Thus, by definition, the transmittance of the absorbing medium is $T = \frac{I_T}{I_0}$ or is the ratio of the intensity of the transmitted to that of the incident light. There are two types of photoelectric photometers : those with one photoelectronic cell and those with two. When one cell is used, the machine is calibrated by determining the readings with known concentrations of the substance being studied. When two cells are used, a tube containing the substance in known concentration is compared with a tube containing an unknown concentration.

Single Cell Photoelectric Colorimetres

These instruments are relatively simple and are very suitable for routine colorimeter analyses. They have a light source comprising a tungsten filament supplied from a battery or constant voltage transformer designed to maintain a steady light output. A coloured light filter is used to allow only a narrow range of wavelengths to fall on the photocell; the instruments is then using approximately monochromatic light.

Filters may be of dyed gelatin or glass or may depend on multiple optical interference to produce monochromatic light. The chance red (640nm), green (530nm) and blue (480 nm) glass filters have been found suitable for most purposes. Alternatively, the Ilford bright spectrum series of gelatine filters offers a greater range of alternative wavelengths.

Light passing through the cuvette falls on the sensitive surface of a selenium photocell which generates a current proportional to the light intensity. The cell is connected to a galvanometer whose scale is graduated in optical density or transmission. An adjustment is provided either in the light path or in the galvanometer circuit to enable the optical density to be set at zero with the blank cuvette in place. The unknown coloured solution is compared, by inspection, with a series of colour standards representing the substance being determined in known graded concentrations. The concentration of the unknown solution is given by the concentration of the standard which it exactly matches. Example is DUBOSQ COLORIMETER (Bausch and Lomb).

Duboscq colorimeter is also known as Duboscq comparator. This instrument is extensively used for the colour comparisons. This instrument permits a comparison of two beams of light one of which has passed through a standard and the other through an unknown solution, the two beams being brought side by side in the eye piece, By means of a plunger and movable cup the depth of liquid through which the light passes may be varied until the intesnsities in the two fields are the same and the colours are said to match. When such adjustment has been made the depth of the fluid through which the light passes are inversely proportion to the concentration of the colour. A scale on the instrument gives a measure of the depth of fluid in each cup through which the light passes. Thus from the scale readings and strength of the standard solution the concentration in the unknwon may be calculated by the following formula.

$$\frac{\text{Reading of standard}}{\text{Reading of unknown}} = \frac{\text{Concentration of unknown}}{\text{Concentration of standard}}$$

when using a Duboscq comparator first focus the eyepiece until the line demarking the two fields stands out sharply, then adjust the instrument in front of a window or artificial light until the two fields are equally illuminated. The dull reflector is usually used instead of the mirror. Ordinarily, daylight or artificial "daylight" is used although filter are orginally furnished to give narrow spectral regions.

For checking the accuracy of readings, place the standard solution in both cups (filling the cups a little more than half full so that they will not overflow when the plungers are immersed) setting the right hand cup so that a convenient depth of liquid is obtained (usually 20mm) and then adjusting the left hand cup until the two field match. Readings should be made until variations not greater than 0.3 mm are obtained, and the depths of liquids in the two cups do not vary by more than 0.3 mm. The colour from the left hand now matches the colour produced by a depth of 20 mm in the right hand cup. When the suitable readings have been obtained remove the right hand cup (without disturbing the setting of the other), rinse the cup and plunger twice with portions of the unknown solution then introduce a portion of the unknown and compare it with the standard. In case the readings of the unknown is less than two-thirds or more than one and one-half times the reading of the standard, the determination should be repeated using enough of the solution being analysed to get a suitable depth of colour when the reagents are added.

When the determination is finished, rinse the plungers and cups by filling the cups half full of distilled water and immersing the plungers as in a determination. Care should be taken not to spill fluid on the reflector and not to chip the plungers.

Selection of Test Tubes

Test tube used in the Photoelectric colorimeter must be carefully selected. Those supplied with the instrument are to be preferred, but the analyst may select his own tubes in the following manner :

A series of best quality, thin wall, soft glass tubes 6″ x 5/8″ are thoroughly washed, and filled with distilled water. The outside of each tube is then carefully wiped with a cloth to remove finger marks, and the tube introduced into the light path. The instruments is adjusted to give a full scale deflection (zero reading on the logarithmic scale) as previously described. The test tube is marked with a diamond pencil so that it can always be used in the same position relative to the light path. Another test tube is now introduced into the path of light. If the light transmission is equal for the two tubes, the galvanometer reading will once more be zero. All the tubes found suitable must be marked to show the position in which they may used to give equal light transmission. On turning the tubes in the adaptor there should not be more than an insignificant change in light transmission as indicated by the galvanometer reading.

Cleaning of Test Tubes

It is obviously important in all optical measurements that all glass surfaces should be perfectly clean and free from dust. All dry surfaces should be cleaned with a soft dry clothes, while for dam surfaces, best quality chamois leather is recommended.

From time to time, glass cells or tubes to be used to hold the fluids under examination must be placed in chromic acid cleaning solution overnight. When required for use, they are rinsed first in tap water and then in distilled water. They are then allowed to drain on a pad of filter paper, and covered as a protection from dust. Tubes should be kept in the inverted form in beaker on a pad of filter paper and covered with petridish. The surfaces of tubes and glass cells should be polished with soft cloth before being placed in the instruments for reading. Care should be taken to hold the vessels in such a way that errors due to finger marks on the glass surface are avoided.

Detailed Procedure for Operating Photoelectric Colorimeter

1. Place the correct filter in the space provided between the source of light and adaptor.
2. Make sure that the galvanometer reads zero (lower scale). If it does not, make the necessary adjustment by means of the screw to be found infront of the scale.
3. Introduce water or blank solution into the test tube or glass cell and place in the adaptor.
4. Switch on the light.
5. Bring the galvanometer reading to zero on the logarithmic scale by rotating the knob below the photocell unit, the final adjustment being made with the variable resistance.
6. Substitute the test or standard solution for the water or blank.
7. Note the reading on the logarithmic reciprocal scale.
8. Replace the water or blank solution. The galvanometer should now return to zero. If it does not, read just and repeat the reading on the coloured solution.
9. It is important to remember that measurements of transmitted light are required, and it is essential to avoid cloudiness, turbidity and bubbles which absorb light. The solution must appear optically quite clear since the photoelectric cell is more sensititive than the eye to small changes in transmission.

Photometry

In relation to analytical chemistry, photometry refers to the measurement of the light transmitting power of a solution in order to determine the concentration of light absorbing substance present. Photometry can of course, employed to the transmission of energy in the ultraviolet and infrared regions of the radiant energy spectrum, as well as to the visible (coloured) spectrum.

Basically, in all such instruments, monochromatic light is passed through an absorbing column of coloured solution of a fixed depth. From the absorbing solution, the transmitted light is directed upon a photosensitive device which converts the radiant energy into electrical energy. The current produced under these conditions is measured by means of a sensitive galvanometer.

Photometric Instuments Possess the Following Advantages over Visual Colorimeters

1. They employ light which is essentially monochromatic. Beer's law is true only with monochromatic light. Measurement of colour in photometric instruments is, therefore, on a more reliable basis than in usual chemistry.
2. The "electric eye" is far more reliable than the human eye.
3. A "blank" is used which compensate for extraneous colour which may be present in a solution in which it is desired to make a colorimetric determination. This makes possible a more accurate determination and in certain cases permits carrying out determinations which would be impossible with visual colorimetry.

Principles of Operation of Photometer

Colour intensity as measured in photometers, involves not only the coloured product in the solution but also all of the molecules of the liquid through which the light passes. It is necessary, therefore, to adjust the instrument by means of a "blank". This blank is prepared by placing in the absorption tube (called a cuvette) all of the constituents of the unknown solution (solvents, reagent etc.) but under condition that will not permit the colour-reaction to take place.

The blank solution is used to set the galvanometer of the instrument at a fixed point (100 on a scale of 0 to 100, in most instruments). After adjusting the galvanometer, the cuvette containing the unknown is placed in the instrument. The unknown has a coloured in addition to the other ingredients producing its absorbance. The effect of the other ingredients was cancelled by setting the instrument on 100 with the blank cuvette in place. It follows that the reading of the galvanometer with unknown cuvette in place is a measure of the amount of colour present in the unknown. The greater the number of molecules or ions of coloured substance present, the greater is the absorption of light or, in other words, the more, the colour, the greater is the deflection of the galvanometer from the original (blank) setting. Thus, the concentration of coloured component present in a solution may be sensitively and accurately measured by a photometer.

Calculation of Results in Photometer

With all the photometers the general formulae for calculations are as follows :

$$\text{For blood} \frac{A_u}{A_s} \text{x mgs x} \frac{V_u}{V_s} \text{x} \frac{100}{\text{ml blood analysed}}$$

$$\text{For urine} \frac{A_u}{A_s} \text{x mgs x} \frac{V_u}{V_s} \text{x} \frac{\text{Vol. of urine voided in 24 hours}}{\text{ml of urine analysed}}$$

where A_u = log 100 - log of unknown reading = 2 – log u

A_s = log 100 - log of standard reading = 2 – log s

V_u = concentration (mg) in unknown sample

V_s = concentration (mg) in standard sample

The galvanometer scale on photometer is graduated from 100 to 0, which explains the above factors.

The above general formulae are the same as those used for usual colorimeter, except for the first factors. Logarithms must be used here because the transmittance of light through a coloured solution is actually measured by logarithmic, not linear values. From Beer's law it follows that light passing through an absorbing solution of a fixed depth suffers a logarithmic reduction in its intensity. Since in photometers, the depth of solution is fixed, we are concerned with measuring only the intensity of the transmitted light, logarithmic values are used in the first part of the general formulae.

Klett-Summerson Photoelectric Colorimeter

This instrument has two photocells. In operation, with a suitable filter in place, the reference solution contained in a test tube is placed in the path of light striking one of the two photocells, which are arranged in a potentiometric circuit so that the current from one cell is opposed to that from the other through a null-point instrument (low sensitivity galvanometer). With the photometer scale set at zero (corresponding to zero optical density) the current out put from the second photocell is adjusted so that it exactly balances that coming from the photocell which is subject to the light emerging from the solution. The scale in the Summerson instrument is graduated in units which are proportional to optical density ; the actual numerical values represent the optical density divided by two and with decimal point omitted. Thus a scale reading of 400 corresponds to an optical density of 0.800. Following formula is applicable.

$$\frac{100 \times D}{2} = R$$

We may use scale reading directly in the calculation work since it bears a constant relationship with optical density.

Operation of Klett-Summerson Photoelectric Photometre Before Turning the Photometer Lamp on

We should check that a light filter is in place in the space provided for it between the lamp housing and the instrument proper. Examine the pointer to make sure that it coincides exactly with the line on the blank pointer scale. If it does not, it should be adjusted by the instructor. The pointer should be at its proper setting before turning the lamp on.

To Use the Instrument

Place a clean photometer tube containing distilled water in the instrument. Turn the scale by means of the large knob on the front of the instrument until the scale reading is "0". Switch on the photometer lamp by means of the lamp switch located on the front of lamp housing. Switching the lamp on will in general cause the pointer to move somewhat away from the line on the pointer scale. Find the zero adjustment knob, which is located in the top of the photometer to the left of the test tube, and turn this knob one way or other until the pointer is brought back to the line on the pointer scale. This operation is called setting the zero.

Allow the lamp to "on" for a few minutes to permit the instrument to reach equilibrium. Again check the position of the pointer to be sure that it is on the line. If it is not, turn the zero adjustment knob carefully until the pointer is exactly on the line. The instrument is now ready for use.

To Read an Unknown Solution

Remove the distilled water tube and place the photometer tube containing the unknown solution in the instrument. The pointer will be deflected from its position at the zero line. Turn the scale knob until the pointer has been brought back exactly to the zero line. The reading on the scale at this point is the reading unknown solution. The concentration of the unknown solution is ordinarily then obtained from the scale reading (corrected for the reagent blank if necessary by multiplying the scale reading by the proper factor).

The light filters : The light filter is inserted in the filter holder and placed in the instrument in the space provided for it just in front of the lamp housing. The frame containing the filter should always be inserted with the round opening facing the operator. As mentioned above the photometer lamp should not be turned unless a filter is in place in the instrument.

The Zero adjustment knob : It cannot be too strongly emphasized that all the photometeric measurements with the instrument are based on the pointer being at its zero position when the distilled water tube or reagent blank tube is in the photometer and the photometer scale reads 0. This adjustment is made possible by the use of the zero adjustment knob.

The photometer tube : The smallest volume that can be safely read in a tube is a little under 5 ml. Bubbles formed on the sides of the tube in certain photometric procedures may be dislodged by tapping the tube smartly on a wooden block or table top. The tube should be seated firmly and as deeply as possible in the opening provided for it in the photometer. Always place the tube so that the orientation mark faces the operator.

The scale : It has been designed so that for the majority of the common photometric procedures and under certain specified conditions the scale reading is directly proportional to the concentration of the substance being determined. The scale reading is a measure of and is proportion to the optical density of the coloured solution as determined by the photoelectric cell, and since the optical density is theoretically proportional to the concentration of coloured substance (Beer's law), the scale readings are likewise proportional to the concentration under the same conditions. In reading the scale, note that it is logarithmically spaced and no linearly spaced. For good photometric measurments, readings should fall between approximately 150 and 400. Readings above 500 or 600 should not be used as a basis for calculating results, since such readings represent relatively dense solutions for which a small change in concentration produces an almost undetectable change in colour. From 0 to 100 other errors enter since transmission are over 90%.

Selection of Wavelength in Photometer

As the concentration of the material in solution is increased there is increased light absorption at all wavelengths at which any light is absorbed at all. This increase is usually greater per unit increment in concentration at certain wavelengths than at others. Hence, it can be readily seen that maximum sensitivity in a photometric method is obtained at the precise wavelength at which there is the most increase in absorbance per unit increase in concentration. For many compounds there is the wavelength of the "peak" of the absorption curve. Some substance display maximum sensitivity at some other point on the absorption curve.

The most ideal wavelength is the one at which at a given solution depth, shows agreement with Beer's law over as wide a range as possible of the concentration apt to be encountered in the analyses, and which also permits this range to be read within the most accurate region of the photometer scale. It has been experienced that maximum error involved in a photometric measurement increases greatly at transmittancies less than 20 per cent or more that 60 per cent. This corresponds to a range of absorbancies from 0.2 to 0.7. Thus, readings outside the range 20 to 60 per cent transmittancy represent solutions which are either too dark or too light for accurate photometry.

Spectrophotometry

It has a light source followed by a monochromator or filter. The incident beam of chosen wavelength, having an intensity of Io, enters the sample. Some of this light is absorbed and the transmitted beam, I, impinges on the photodetector. In more refined instruments, there is a reference beam which by passes the sample to provide double beaming for stability. The relationship between the beams is expressed by the well-known Beer's Law equation.

$$I = I_0 \exp - \varepsilon cl$$

I and I_0 have already been defined; ε is the molar absorbtivity; C is the concentration of the solute; and l is the length of the light path in the solution. The factor ε is a property of the compound which is constant for any given wavelength of the incident light, and l is set by the geometry of the cell used, so the relationship between the transmitted and incident beam is dependent upon c, the concentration of the compound. Since this is a logarithmic function, the basic relationship between concentration, c and Io/I is nolinear. Calculations with this basic equation are very awkward, so absorbance, defined as the log of Io/I is commonly used because it has linear relationship with concentration. In the regions of very low transmission (very high sample concentration), accuracy begins to suffer because of the asymptotic approach to zero per cent transmission. In the regions of high transmission (low sample concentration), accuracy begins to suffer again. *A spectrophotometer is designed to analyse samples over a relatively narrow range of concentrations. This range may be varied somewhat by charging the path length-higher concentrations may be brought into the region of accuracy by reducing the path length, and lower concentrations may be accomodated by increasing the path length. There is, however, a practical limit to the range expansion which may be accomplished by these means.*

Grating Spectrophotometers

These instruments are allied to photoelectric colorimeters. The major difference is in the method of producing monochromatic light. In place of coloured filters, a diffraction grating is fitted which disperse the white light into a continuous spectrum. By turning the wavelength adjustment, the grating is rotated and different parts of the spectrum allowed to fall on the photocell. The band of wavelengths used is similar to that passed by a good narrow-cut filter, but there is a tendency for the readings to be affected by stray light, i.e. light wavelength other than that selected penetrates the optics and falls on the selenium cell. This trouble may cause non-linearity in response.

Glass Prism Spectrophotometers

Such type of instruments are Beckman Model B or the unicam S.P. 600. Light from a tungsten filament is focused on the entrance slit., it then passes through the prism which forms an extended spectrum. Only the light which falls on the exit slit can traverse the cuvette and illuminate the photocell vacuum photocells are used; *they have the advantage that their response can be readily amplified, and it usual to provide alternative photocells, one sensitive to the shortwave length range of the instrument (360 to 625 nm), while the other is used for the longer wavelengths (600 to 1000 nm).*

Transmission measurements are made by resorting the amplified signal from the photocell to a circular calibrated slide-wire and obtaining a balance indicated by the reading of a small meter. With no light falling on the photocell the dark current adjustment is regulated to obtain balance. Then with the blank cuvette in place, the sensitivity of the spectrophotometer is altered until it balances at D = 0 (T = 100 per cent); this setting is often assisted by the provision of a "check" switch position, which automatically puts a resistance into the circuit equal to that of the slide-wire set at D = 0. The test solution is then substituted, and rebalancing with the slide-wire gives the optical density.

Quartz Spectrophotometers

The instrument of such type are Beckman, D.U.; Hilger-watts Uvispek S.P. 500. By replacing glass prism with quartz prisms it is possible to measure the test samples below 200 nm. An additional hydrogen discharge lamp with a quartz envelop is provided in such type of instruments. It has been observed that this source is rich in ultraviolet radiation.

Calibration of Wavelength Scale of Spectrophotometer

This can be easily done by taking advantage of the transmittancy curves of solution of acid base indicator such as methyl orange. It is known that the transmittancy curves for the different pH values for any particular dye all intersect at a point known as the isosbestic point, which has a value of 469 mμ for methyl orange. It is clear, therefore, that if an acidic and a basic solution made from equal volumes of the same stock solution of methyl orange are put in two cuvettes and the difference in their transmittancy (absorbancy) observed at different wavelengths then the difference in zero at only one wavelength, namely 469 mμ.

The Procedure is as follow

Prepare a stock solution of pure methyl orange by dissolving 0.0400 gram in water and diluting to 100 ml. Next prepare a buffer solution to pH 2.8 and a buffer solution of pH 4.8. Pipette 3 ml of the stock methyl orange solution into each of two 200 ml volumetric flasks and dilluted one to volume with pH 2.8 buffer and the other to volume with the pH 4.8 buffer. Mix and determine the absorbancies of 469 mμ. If the wavelength setting is accurate, the absorbancies will be identical. If they differ, the wavelength setting must be readjusted according to directions specific for each type of instrument.

Usually wavelength (λ) is expressed in one of the following forms :

nanometre (nm) = millimicron (mμ) = 10^{-6} mm

$$\text{Ångstrom}\,(\text{Å}) = 10^{-7}\ \text{mm} = \frac{\text{m}\mu}{10}$$

Ranges of wavelength measurements

1. *Ultra-violet* 185-400 nm Use UV spectrophotometer
2. *Visible* 400-760 nm Use absorptiometer with coloured filters. (Table 1)
3. *Infra-red* 0.76-15 nm Use infra-red spectrophotometer.

Table 1 : Filters for absorptiometry

Wavelength/nm	**Colour of filter**	**Colour observed**
400	Violet	Greenish yellow
425	Indigo-blue	Yellow
450	Blue	Orange
490	Blue-green	Red
510	Green	Purple
530	Yellow-green	Violet
550	Yellow	Indigo-blue
590	Orange	Blue
640	Red	Bluish-green
730	Deep red	green

Source : Pearson, D. 1973. *Laboratory techniques in food analysis*, Ist edn., Butterworths & Co. (Publishers) Ltd., England, pp 290.

Table 2 : Transmission regions of ilford spectrum filters

Number	Colour of filter	Peak Wavelength/nm	Tranmission region/nm
600	Spectrum deep violet	405	380-450
601	Spectrum violet	425	380-470
602	Spectrum blue	470	440-490
603	Spectrum blue green	490	470-520
604	Spectrum green	520	500-540
605	Spectrum yellow green	550	530-570
606	Spectrum yellow	580	560-610
607	Spectrum orange	600	575 onwards, with absorption increasing from 600.
608	Spectrum red	660	620 into infra-red
609	Spectrum deep red	690	650 into infra-red
621	Bright spectrum violet	445	340-515
622	Bright spectrum blue	470	375-530
623	Bright spectrum blue-green	490	460-545
624	Bright spectrum green	520	490-575
625	Brighter spectrum yellow-green	540	510-590
626	Bright spectrum yellow	575	545-620

Source : Pearson, D. 1973. *Laboratory techniques in Food analysis*, Ist edn., Butterworth & Co. (Publishers) Ltd. England, pp 291.

Make of Photoelectric Colorimeter and Spectrophotometer Used in the Different Laboratories of World

I. Photoelectric filter photometers

1. Coleman photoelectric colorimeter
2. Evelyn photoelectric colorimeter
3. Fisher clinical electrophotometer
4. Hellige "clinicol" colorimeter
5. Klett-Sumerson photoelectric colorimeter
6. Leitz-Rovy photometer
7. Lumetron colorimeter
8. Weston colorimeter

II. Spectrophotometers

1. Bausch and Lomb spectronic-20 colorimeter
2. Beckman Model B spectrophotometer

3. Beckman Model DU photoelectric spectrophotometer
4. Coleman Junior Spectrophotometer
5. Coleman Universal spectrophotometer

UV-VIS Spectrophotometer

The UV-VIS spectrophotometers give us information regarding the presence and nature of unsaturation in a given chemical particularly conjugated double bonds and aromatic rings. As solvents used in spectroscopic work must be free from such impurities contaning aromatic and conjugated double bond groups.

Infrared Spectrophotometer

In a well equiped quality control laboratory, *the infrared spectrophoto-meter is the instrument of first choice to analyse any unknown sample-organic or inorganic. The sample can be a solid, a liquid or a gas and it need not be soluble or vaporizable. An infrared spectrophotometer is an instrument which draws a spectrum showing the transmittance of a sample (ordinate) as a function of wavelength of frequency (abscissa, usually expressed as wavenumber). The location (wavenumber) of the absorption bands gives qualitative information about what the sample* is. Various functional groups (such as carbonyl, amine, hydroxyl etc.) have characteristic absorption frequencies and their presence can be established when these absorptions occur in the spectrum. *Different molecules have different absorption patterns and the molecules can be identified from their infrared spectra much like people can be identified from their fingerprints.*

These instruments plot the absorption curves of samples in the infrared in essentially the same manner that instruments such as the Beckmen DU.

The source of light is different, being a Globar (a bonded SiC rod) or a glower (a mixture of Zn, Th and Y oxides); the dispersing element of choice is rapidly becoming a grating, but if it is a prism, it must be made of a salt such as Nacl or KBr rather than of quartz; and the detector is usually a thermocouple. These differnces in the components of the infrared instrument from those of the visible ultraviolet apparatus are necessary because the lamps used as sources of visible and ultraviolet light are poor sources of infrared, and glass and even quartz are essentially opaque to the infrared. It should be noted, however, that infra-red spectrophotometry does not distinguish between optical isomers.

Infrared spectrophotometry can also be used for the quantitative determination of a single compound or a mixture of several compounds when each of the substances being determined possess a sharp peak that is not shared with any other substance that is present. For accurate work the infrared curve of a compound that is not itself a liquid is preferably obtained from a solution of the substance in an organic liquid that is transparent to infrared over the wavelength range being investigated. Common solvents are carbon disulfide and carbon tetrachloride. For most purposes water cannot be used as a solvent, but because of its opacity to the infrared and because it would dissolve the Nacl or KBr windows of the infrared tubes; the only exception is in working in the near-infrared (i.e., the wavelength proximate to the red portion of the visible spectrum), where aqueous solution can be analysed in tubes with AgCl windows. If a sample is insoluble in one of the usable solvents, its spectrum is obtained either in a mull with Nujol or a liquid fluorocarbon, or in a pellet made by mixing it with KBr and compressing the mixture.

There is one technique for obtaining infrared spectra that is in a class by itself. Attenuated total reflectance, or "ATR". This method is based on the fact that radiation, when totally internally reflected at the face of a high-index medium such as AgCl or "KRS-5" (thallium bromide-iodide), penetrates a few microns beyond the interface into the adjoining low-index material. By making use of this principle, it is possible with properly-designed and operated equipment to obtain directly spectra of the surfaces of materials such as rubber, plastics and foods. The resulting spectrum is not identical with the absorption spectrum of the sample, but proper adjustment of the equipment, it resembles the absorption spectrum closely enough to permit direct comparison. *Infrared spectroscopy has been used to identify chromatographic fractions.*

The manufactures of infrared spectrophotometers are Beckman Instruments, Inc., and Perkin-Elmer corporation. Barnes Engineering Co., Instrument Division. 30 Commerce Road, Stamford, Conn., and Wilks Scientific Corp., P.O. Box 441, South Norwalk, Conn., are suppliers of infrared equipment.

Fluorometry

Flourometry is extremely sensitive - it is capable of analysing compounds at concentrations as low as 1 part in 100 billion. This is approximately 10,000 fold lower than the extreme limit of spectrophotometry. We may measure wide range of concentrations of any given compound ; micrograms, tenths of micrograms, hudnredths of micrograms and thousandths of micrograms may all be analyzed in the same final volume of solution. On the lines of spectrophotometer construction, it has a light source and a filter or monochromator between the light source and the sample. The wavelength of the incident beam, Io entering the sample will very likely be the same as that which would be used for measuring the same sample in a spectrophotometer. The beam enters the sample; a portion is absorbed and a portion is transmitted. The transmitted beam is deliberately eliminated by black baffles. The absorbed light causes the sample to fluoresce, and this fluoresent light is emitted uniformly in all directions. A secondary filter or monochromator, chosen to absorb or stop light of the wavelength of the incident beam and transmit light of the wavelength of the admitted fluorescent light, is placed between the sample and detector. *In the case of fluorometry, concentration is directly proportional to fluorescence. If concentration is doubled, fluorescence is doubled, and so on.* The second point is that there would be virtually no limt to the range of concentrations that could be analysed fluorometrically. If sample concentrations are steadily decreased, fluorescence obviously goes down. If the fluorescence decreases below a level which may be accurately measured, such type of situation may be alleviated by either increasing the intensity of the exciting light or increasing the sensitivity of the detection system. Modern fluorometers utilize a photomultiplier tube (which is capable of measuring very small amounts of light) as the detection system. This fact, coupled with the ability to increase fluorescence by increasing the intensity of the incident light, permits fluorescence measurements from extremely low concentrations of sample.

For example, if a sample reads 100 fluorescence units (arbitrary units) with a relative instability in either beam of ± 0.1%, the blank can be ajdusted to zero fluorescence units ± 0.1%. Thus, the difference between blank and sample is 100±0.2%. Therefore, the uncertainty is 0.2% of the calculated sample concentration. This type of direct measurements permits accurate measurements of materials when transmission of the incident light is as high as 99.999%.

Arrangement is such that concentrations as low as a few parts per trillion can be measured, and this is many thousands of times greater sensitivity than is possible with the indirect measurements, required by spectrophotometry. At present in most of the fluorometers, the stability is generally held to within 0.5%.

In practice, a sample of known concentration is prepared (in the concentration range expected for the unknowns), placed in the instrument, and adjusted to give the desired reading. If a wide range of concentrations is expected and the instrument has repeatable sensitivity settings, several such samples (standards) should be prepared. Unknowns are then measured and calculated by simple ratio. For example, at a given sensitivity setting, a 1 μg sample may read 100 divisions; an unknown sample reading 50 divisions would then contain 0.5μg. Using a differnt setting, 3μg might read 100 divisions; an unknown sample reading 50 divisions would then contain 1.5 μg, and so on. Usually in the market, filter fluorometers and spectro-fluorometers. The make of fluorometry have filter (in which wavelenghts are selected by coloured filters, as used in the colorimeters) as sensitive and very nearly as versatile as the spectrofluorometer (which employs monochromators to select wavelengths, as used in spectrophotometers). This is in direct contrast to absorptiometry, where filter colorimeters are frequently less sensitive and commonly less widely applicable than spectrophotometers. For these and other reasons, the filter fluorometry remains a very useful instrument where many repetitive assays are performed and where spectra are not required. *Fluorescence may be affected by pH and temperature etc.*

Nephelometry

It is the device to measure the scattered light by particulate matter in suspension. It is commonly used for the detection and quantitation of unwanted particles or haze in liquids and is a valuable technique in certain types of quantitative chemical analysis, e.g., determination of sulphate. Modern fluorometers can be converted into extremely sensitive nephelometers by simply removing the secondary filter or adjusting the secondary monochromator to the same wavelength as the primary monochromator. *One of the important advantage is that traces of haze may be accurately measured in highly coloured fluids.*

Mass Spectrometry

This instrument is used for assay of stable isotope concentration, e.g. ^{15}N, ^{18}O. *The sample is converted to a gaseous form, the gas is ionized, and the ions are accelerated by an electric field. The stream of ions is then deflected by a mangnetic field, the angle of deflection varies with the weight of the ions, so that the heavier isotopic ions arrive at a differnt target than the lighter, normal ions.* At the target, the concentrations of the respective ions are measured and registered. Probably the greatest value of mass spectrometry to the food chemist is in the identification of gas chromatographic fractions. Teranishi et al (1963) used this apparatus in the analysis of hydrocarbons present in orange oil. This apparatus is manufactured by the Bendix corporation, Cincinnati Division, 3625 Hauek Road, Ohio, USA.

Nuclear Magnetic Resonance Apparatus

In NMR spectrometry, a liquid or a solution is placed in a strong magnetic field and irradiated with ratio frequency waves - the spectrum is a graph that records an increasing magnetic field along the abscissa and the corresponding intensity of energy absorption along the ordinate. The "chromophore" in proton NMR spectra is the proton, and such a spectrum of a compound will show signals for nothing but protons (not even deuterium or tritium) but it will show every proton in the molecule. The best NMR spectra are obtained on liquid samples, and solutions can be employed for solid compounds. *The primary use of NMR spectroscopy is as an aid in determining the structure of pure compounds, but it has been employed to estimate the total hydrogen content of a sample.* Manufacturer for NMR apparatus is M/S Varian Associates 611 Hensen Way, Palo Alto, Calif.

Nuclear Quadrupole Resonance spectrometers

The practical advantage of the nuclear quadrupole resonance spectrometer over the NMR apparatus, for those that can be detected by both, lies in the fact that the quadrupole instrument require no magnet and is consequently less expensive. It is however, applicable only to samples that contain at least one isotope whose nucleus has a quadrupole resonace (NQR) spectrometry does not require an added magnetic field as does NMR is because the frequencies at which NQR signals appear are fixed by the electronic structures of the bonds. *This instrument is used for the quantitative analysis of mixture of compounds particularly geometrical isomers such as the hexachlorocylohexanes (benzene hexachloride). This instrument is manufactured by Wilks Scientific Corporation, P.O. Box 441, South Norwalk, conn.*

Polarimeter

It is well known that a substance is said to be opticallly active if the plane of polarized light is rotated when passing through the substance. Ever since the discovery of this optical phenomenon. *Polarimetry has been used in analysis for the identification and determination of optically active substances and in stero-chemistry for the structural elucidation in organic and inorganic chemistry. In routine quality control work, purity of organic compounds such as Dextrose is determined by polarimetric analysis.* Polarimeters calibrated to read directly in terms of per cent sucrose when the rotation of a solution of 26 grams of sample in 100 ml is measured at 20° in a 200 mm tube, using sodium D light, are called Saccharimeters. The manufacturers of polarimeters are Cary Instruments, 2724 South Peck Road, Monrovia, Calif, USA O.C. Rudolph Sons, Inc., P.O. Box 446. Caldwell, N.J., USA Rudolph Instruments Engineering Co., Inc., 61 Stevens Ave., Little Falls, N.J.

Table 3 : Relationship between transmittance in % T and the absorbance (extinction or optical density)

% T	A	%T	A	%T	A	%T	A
100	0.000	75	0.125	50	0.301	25	0.602
99	0.004	74	0.131	49	0.310	24	0.620
98	0.009	73	0.137	48	0.319	23	0.638
97	0.013	72	0.143	47	0.328	22	0.658
96	0.018	71	0.149	46	0.337	21	0.678
95	0.022	70	0.155	45	0.347	20	0.699
94	0.027	69	0.161	44	0.357	19	0.721
93	0.032	68	0.168	43	0.367	18	0.745
92	0.036	67	0.174	42	0.377	17	0.770
91	0.041	66	0.171	41	0.387	16	0.796
90	0.046	65	0.187	40	0.398	15	0.824
89	0.051	64	0.194	39	0.409	14	0.854
88	0.056	63	0.201	38	0.420	13	0.886
87	0.061	62	0.208	37	0.432	12	0.921
86	0.066	61	0.215	36	0.444	11	0.959
85	0.071	60	0.222	35	0.456	10	1.000
84	0.076	59	0.229	34	0.469	9	1.046
83	0.081	58	0.237	33	0.482	8	1.097
82	0.086	57	0.244	32	0.495	7	1.155
81	0.092	56	0.252	31	0.509	6	1.222
80	0.097	55	0.260	30	0.523	5	1.301
79	0.102	54	0.268	29	0.538	4	1.398
78	0.108	53	0.276	28	0.552	3	1.523
77	0.114	52	0.284	27	0.569	2	1.699
76	0.119	51	0.292	26	0.585	1	2.000

References

Teranishi, R.T., Schultz, T.H., Mc Fadden, W.K., Lundin, R.B. and Black, D.R. (1963). *J. Food Sci.,* 26: 54.

Reference for Further Study

Bose, A.K. (1965). *Protein Nuclear Magnetic Resonance Spectroscopy in* : Freeman, S.K. (ed.) : Interpretive Spectroscopy New York : Reinhold Publishing Corp. pp. 212-13.

Brame, E.G. (1967). *Anal Chem.* 39: 918.

Clark, G.L. (1960). *The Encylopedia of Spectroscopy.* New York : Reinhold Publishing Corp. pp. 212-13.

Demico, J.N. (1966). J. Assoc. Offic. Anal Chemists, 49: 1027

Gilman, H. (ed.). (1947). *Organic Chemistry,* An Advanced Treatise, 2nd ed. New York : John Wiley & Sons, Inc. Chapter 4.

Gohlke, R.S. (1958). *Anal. Chem.*, 31: 535

Grasselli, J.G. and Snavely, M.K. (1962). *Applied spectrophotometry*. 16: 190.

Guilbault, George, G. (1967). *Fluorescence : theory, instrumentation and practice.* Marcel Dekker, Inc., New York, pp. 697.

Harrington, D.B. (1960). In : Clark, G.L. (ed.) : *The Encyclopedia of spectroscopy*, New York: Reinhold Publishing Corp. pp 630-43.

Leblane, R.B. (1960). Mass spectrometry. In : Clark, G. L. (ed.) : *The Encyclopedia spectroscopy.* New York : Reinhold Publishing Corp., pp 582-83.

Oser, B.L. (1954). *Hawk's physiological chemistry*, 14th edn., Mc Graw-Hill Book Co. London, pp 980-1016.

Parker, C.A. and Reis, W.T. (1964). *Absorption, fluorescence and polarographic methods*. pp 228-246. In. : J. Paul Cali (ed.). *Trace analysis of semiconductor materials.* Pergammon Press ; Inc., Oxford (England) pp 282.

Passwater, A.R. (1967). *Guide to fluorescence literature* ; Plenum Press, New York, pp 367.

Undenfriend, S. (1969). *Fluorescence assay in biology and medicine,* Academic Press, New York, Vol II. pp 660.

Vetkinson, J.H. (1960). *Anal. Chem.*, 32: 981.

White, C.E. and Argauer, R.J. (1970). *Fluorescence analysis : a practical approach.* Marcel Dekker, Inc. New York pp 389.

White, C.E. and Weissler, A. (1970). *Anal.Chem.*, 42 : 57R-76R.

Wootton, I.D.P. (1974). *Microanalysis in Medical biochemistry,* Edn., Churehill Livingstone, Edinburgh and London pp 10-17.

Chapter - 57

Gas Chromatography

Introduction

Chromatography was first employed by Ramsey (1905) to separate mixture of gases and vapours. These first experiments used selective adsorption on, or desorption from, solid absorbents such as active charcoals. The following year Tswett (1906) obtained discrete coloured bands of plant pigments on a chromatographic column. He coined the term "chromatography" (literally "colour writing") which is obviously a misnomer when used retrospectively. *Contribution of Martin and Synge (1941) in a study for which they were awarded the Nobel prize, and later James and Martin introduced gas-liquid chromatography in 1951 and 1952.*

Definition of Chromatography

Chromatography is the process by which a mixture is separated by ad- sorption or solution partition between two immiscible phases, wherein one is a mobile phase and the other one is stationary.

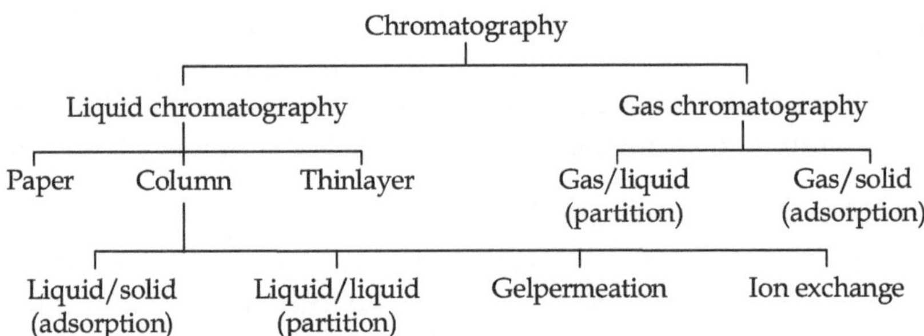

Gas chromatography is mainly aplicable to the analysis of relatively volatile, low molecular weight substances, whereas liquid chromatograph finds main application in the analysis of high molecular weight compounds.

Review of Chromatographic Technique

For the moving or mobile phase, only gas and liquid may be considered, while the stationary phase will be either liquid or solid. Therefore, there are four possible chromatographic methods.

Gas liquid]	Gas chromatography
Gas solid]	
Liquid-Liquid	Column, paper and partition
Liquid-solid	Chromatography and ion-exchange

Gas Chromatography can be Subdivided into

(a) *Gas solid chromatography (absorption gas chromatography)* : In this case the stationary phase is a solid material with surface active properties. The separating principle depends on the variation in the extent to which constituents of a mixture are absorbed on the adsorbant e.g., molecular sieve. The separation is obtained because of the different adsorption affinities which the column packing has towards the sample components. Molecular sieves (sodium or calcium aluminium silicates), silica gel (SiO_2). alumina (Al_2O_3) and charcoal; are among the most commonly used adsorbents in gas solid chromatography.

(b) *Gas liquid chromatography (partition gas chromatography)* : where the stationary phase is a liquid distributed on a solid support material. The separating principle depends on the difference in the partition coefficients between the liquid and gas phases of the constituents of a mixture. Those constituents which favour the gas phase move more quickly through the columns while those favouring the liquid phase are delayed.

In GLC the sample is separated by passing it in the gas phase, through a tube packed with an inert powder (called the support) on which is coated a film of an involatile liquid (the stationary phase). A stream of gas, called the carrier gas, is passed continuously through the tube, or column as it is called, and the separation of the sample components is achieved by a partition process involving the sample, the moving carrier gas and the stationary liquid phase.

Limitations of Gas Chromatography

The applicability of gas chromatography is normally limited to those substances which may be volatilised without decomposition. The technique may be extended to those materials which may be thermally decomposed in a reproducible manner (Pyrolysis), or can be converted by simple chemical reactions to form derivatives with the required properties.

Parts of a Gas Chromatograph

A standard gas chromatograph consists following parts :

1. Carrier gas cylinder
2. Flow controller and pressure regulator.
3. Injection port (Sample inlet).
4. Column
5. Detector (with necessary electronics).
6. Recorder.
7. Thermostate for injector column and detector.

The above parts are illustrate in Fig. 1

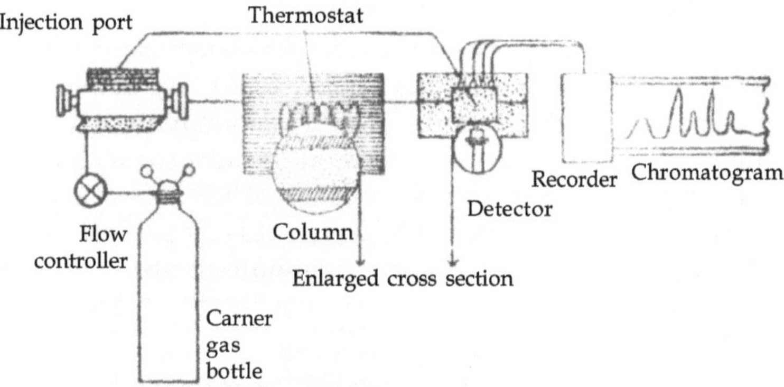

Fig. 1 : Schematic drawing of a gas chromatographic system. (*Coustesy:* Mc Nair H.M. and Boneth, E.J. 1969 *Basis gas chromatography*, 5th edn, Varian aerograph, Switzerland).

Working Principle

The carrier gas, normally N_2. Ar or He is taken through gas regularly to the column. An injection system at the column inlet allows the introduction of a sample. A detector is fitted to the outlet of the column which feeds an electrical signal to a strip chart recorder via the detector amplifier/supply.

The column is housed in an oven in which air is circulated over electrical heaters by a fan. The temperature of the oven is accurately controlled using a proportional temperature controller with a resistance thermometer sensing element.

Selection of Column Material

The success of any gas chromatographic analysis depends upon the separating ability of the column. *Column performance is dependent on several factors and is measured in terms of "efficiency" or number of theoretical plates and resolution factors.* A support material used in partition chromatography should be inert towards the sample. Commonly used support materials are firebrick and a diatomaceous earth called "Celite" supports must be carefully graded and greater efficiencies are achieved with narrow mesh ranges e.g., 80 to 100 or 100 to 120 BSS mesh. The mesh range must be consistent with the length of column and resistance to gas flow. The stationary phase must be non-volatile at all temperatures at which the column will be operated, and chosen for the selective retention characteristics of components in the sample.

Doelle (1969) compared 13 different column materials to find a suitable combination for the separation and determination of a micro quantities of formic, acetic, propionic, isobutyric, n-butyric, isovaleric, n-valeric, isocaproic, n-caproic and heptanoic acid. The results are mentioned in Table 1.

Table 1 : A survey of nine column materials for the separation and highest sensitivity of ten linear fatty acids

Substances	1. Formic acid 2. Acetic acid	1. Propionic acid 2. Isobutyric acid 3. n-butyric acid	1. Isovaleric acid 2. n-valeric acid 3. Isocaproic acid 4. n-caproic acid 5. n-heptanoic acid
20% carbowax 20 M	No separation	No separation	Low sensitivity
21% PEG-600	No separation	Low Sensitivity broad peaks	Low sensitivity
15% DEGS	No separation	No separation	As Carbowax
2% PEGA	Good separation	Low sensitivity	-
3-1% PEGA	Good separation	High sensitivity	-
20% DEGA	Retention time very close	Retention time very close	Good sensitivity
25% Carbowax 20 M	No separation	No separation	Low sensitivity
10% Carbowax 20 M	No separation	No separation	Low sensitivity
20% LAC-269 2%H3PO4	No separation	Close retention time	Good separation Good sensitivity

Table 2 : Common saturated and unsaturated fatty acids

Name	B.P. C°	M.P. C°
Saturated fatty acids		
Formic	100.8	8.6
Acetic	118.1	16.6
Propionic	114.1	-36.5
Butyric	163.5	-7.9
Palmitic	278.0	62.4
Stearic	291.0	69.3
Unsaturated fatty acids		
Acrylic	141.0	12.5
Oleic	286.0	14.0

Table 3 : Acids and their carbon atom

Acid	Carbon atom
Formic	C_1
Acetic	C_2
Propionic	C_3
Butyric	C_4
Valeric	C_5
Caproic	C_6
Oenanthic	C_7
Caprylic	C_8
Pelargonic	C_9
Myristic	$C_{14:0}$
Palmitic	$C_{16:0}$
Palmitoleic	$C_{16:1}$
Stearic	$C_{18:0}$
Oleic	$C_{18:1}$
Linoleic	$C_{18:2}$
Arachidic	$C_{20:0}$
Linolenic	$C_{18:3}$

Silanization

The adsorption effects which often cause pack tailing can be minimized if the celite is treated with a silating agent such as hexamethyldisilazine (HMDS) or dimethyldichlorosilane (DMCS) where the hydroxyl groups on the celite surface are modified.

It has been observed that dimethyldichlorosilane to be more effective for pretreating glass column than silylating agents which do not contain chlorosilanes. It is extremely important that the glass surface be inert, otherwise it is foolish to fill the column with an expensive silane treated support. We use SYLON-CT for column treatment, a solution of 5% dimethylchlorosilane in toluene for our convenience. Supleco, S.A. Switzerland, manufacture SYLON-CT under catalogue No. 3-3065.

Sample Modification

In some applications the sample itself can be modified in order to overcome tailing effects. Examples of this are the widely used techniques of converting fatty acids to their methyl esters, to avoid tailing due to hydrogen bound effects of the carboxyl group, and in steroid analysis the use of trimethyl silyl either derivatives of hydroxyl compounds.

Stationary Phase

The stationary phase must be involatile at all temperatures at which the column will be operated and chosen for the selective retention characteristics of components in the sample it will be used to separate. In general highly polar stationary phases are used to selectively retard polar compounds while non-polar stationary phases offer little selectivity and components tend to be eluted in order of boiling point. For analytical packed columns 1 to 10% W/W of stationary phase on the support is normally employed.

The Support

The support material is used to provide a supporting surface on which is coated the staionary phase film. The support should have a large surface area relative to its volume, it should be inert towards both stationary phase and sample and the particles should be of uniform size. The raw material for most gas chromatographic support is diatomite., also known as diatomaceous silica, diatomaceous earth, and the German word "Kieselguhr". Chromosorb is Johns Manville's registered trade mark for G.C. support material. The types of chromosorb are A, G, P, W and T. Each is available either untreated or treated and in variety of mesh ranges.

Table 4 : Chemical analysis of supports

Chemical components	Fire brick 022	Celite 545	Chromosorb P	Chromosorb W
SiO2	89.7	89.9	89.2	91.2
Al_2O_3	5.1	3.6	5.1	4.1
Fe_2O_3	1.55	1.65	1.50	1.15
TiO_2	0.30	0.30	0.30	0.25
CaO	1.30	1.75	0.90	0.40
MgO	0.90	0.70	1.00	0.65

Source : Blandenet, G., Robin, J. (1964). J. Gas Chromatograph, 2: 225.

Liquid Phase

1. Good absolute solvent for sample components - if solubility is low, components elute rapidly, and separation is poor.
2. Good differential solvent for sample components.
3. Nonvolatile-vapour pressure of 0.01 to 0.1 mm at operating temperature for reasonable column life.
4. Thermally stable - instability can be promoted by catalytic influence of the support as temperature increases.
5. Chemically inert toward the solutes of interest at the column temperature. For an efficient, normal separation, the liquid phase should be similar in chemical structure to the components of the mixture.

Example: Hydrocarbon compounds are best separated with a hydrocarbon solvent. Paraffins on squalene (a long chain hydrocarbon), polar compounds with a polar solvent., alcohols en Hallcomid (an amide).

Liquid Phase Classification

Class A (I)

FFAP, 20M-TPA, Carbowaxes, Ucons, Versamid 900, Hallcomid, Quadrol, Theed, diglycerol.

Class B (II)

XE-60, XF-1150, Amine 220.

Class C (III)

OV-17, all polyesters, dimethylsulphonate.

Class D (IV & V)

SE-30, SF-96, DC-200, OV-1, squalane.

Manufacture of the Column

1. The stationary phase is weighed out and dissolved in a suitable boiling solvents.
2. Support material, treated, screened as necessary, and is weighed out.
3. A mixture of (1) and (2) is made to produce a mobile slurry.
4. The solvent is evaporated while gently but continuously stirring and applying heat by a water bath. This step is continued until the odour of the solvent is no longer apparent.

5. Any residual solvent is removed by heating in a vacuum oven at a suitable temperature and full vacuum for two hours.
6. The impregnated powder is then packed into the column. Colums are often vibrated while packing is blown or sucked into position. The column is plugged at both ends with quartz wool. The evenness of packing is of prime importance in making an efficient column.
7. Column must be preheated or "aged" before use. This step is carried out by installing the column in the oven without connecting to the detector and purging the column with carrier gas for 24 hours at the maximum temperature at which the column is to be used. The conditioning process remove volatiles which could contaminate the detector, and provides a column which can be used for higher sensitivity work.

Operating Parameters

1. Carrier Gas Flow

The speed of analysis is proportional to the flow of the carrier gas. However, there are restrictions on the selection of this flow because every column has an optimum flow rate at which it will offer the best efficiency. It is note worthy that these flows are related to the cross sectional area of the column, indicating gas optimum linear gas velocity in a conventional column. Further, it is observed that the efficiency of a column falls off rapidly at flow rates below the optimum, because at these velocities, the cross diffusion effect becomes significant for flow rate exceeding the optimum the efficiency of the column falls off more slowly and in practice, this region is frequently used in order to length from the increased speed of analysis.

Column Temperature

Raising the temperature of the column will increase the speed of analysis without detracting from the efficiency of the column, but care must be taken not to lose the required separation of the sample. At a certain temperature a stationary phase will become volatile and vaporise (or bleed) from the column, and will be detected as a drift on the baseline. Detector contamination may occur, and any High background signal will detract from the accuracy of the analysis. The use of constant operating parameters of the temperature and flowrate for the column restricts the analysis of wide boiling range samples. Temperature programming is the controlled increase in the temperature of a column while a separation is in progress.

Detection System

Factors governing the choice of detectors are :

1. Sensitivity
2. Linearity
3. Specificity

Following types of detectors are used in Gas chromatograph

a. *Flame Ionization detector (F.I.D.)*
b. *Thermal conductivity (or Katharometer) detector (T.C.D.)*
c. *Electron capture detector (E.C.D)*
d. *Thermionic detector (TD or phosphorus detector)*
e. *Nitrogen detector*
f. *Flame photometric detector*

a. Flame ionization detector (F.I.D.)

The detector is used to measure an ionization current in a hydrogen flame. When an eluted substance is burned in the flame an increase in ionization current occurs, the signal is fed to an amplifier and then to the recorder. This is by far the most widely used detector, responding with high sensitivity to all organic compounds (with the exception of formaldehyde and formic acid). The sensitivity of the F.I.D. enables 10^{-9} g of many components to be detected, and the linear range of approximately 10^{7}g is much wider that obtained from other detectors. *The FID does not respond to inorganic gases or water.*

b. Thermal conductivity (or Katharometer) detector (T.C.D.)

The detector consists of electrically heated filaments arranged in a wheatstone Bridge circuit, with both a "reference" and "measuring" arm. When the composition of the gas in the measuring arm changes with the elution of a component, the filament temperature changes causing the bridge of produce an "out of balance" signal which is displaced on a recorder. The sensitivity varies depending on which carrier gas is used, but when using helium, 10^{-7}g of inorganic gases can be detected. The TC detector finds its greatest use in permanent gas and low sensitivity routine analyses.

c. Electron capture detector (E.C.D.)

The EC detector has both a high sensitivity and specificity to compounds containing electronegative atoms or groups e.g. halogens. The detector operates on the principle that the ionization current set up by a suitable radioactive source e.g. Ni^{63} or H^{3} is reduced when an electron capturing compound is introduced. *Great use is made of the EC Detector in the pesticide field as halogen containing compounds have a high electron affinity. Polychlorinated compounds such as DDT and aldrin can be detected at* 10^{-12}g levels. However, the linear range is limited, generally <5 x 10^2, but some workers have taken advantage of the high sensitivity by preparing electron capturing derivatives. An example of this is the preparation of halogenated silyl ether derivatives in steroid analysis.

d. Thermionic detector (TD or Phosphorus Detector)

The thermionic detector is highly selective towards phosphorus containing compounds. Similar in construction to the FID, an alkali metal halide salt electrode is used to "seed" the flame of the TD. Ionic dissociation of the salt is greatly increased when minute trace of organ phosphorus compounds are present resulting in an increase in ionization current. The life of the ions and the respective position of electrodes determine the selective properties of the detector. *10^{-10}g of organophosphorus pesticides is the detection limit of this detector, and the linear range is 10^3.*

e. Nitrogen detector

The nitrogen detector produces a selective response to organo-nitrogen compounds and its main use is in pesticide, herbicide and drug analyses. It is based on the alkali Flame ionization detector principle and used the well proven three electrode design. It has a detectability of 4 x 10^{-13}g N/sample with a linear range of 10^4. It is used with the standard ionization amplifiers.

f. Flame photometric detector

Developed specially for the determination of organo-phosphorus and organo-sulphur compounds. An important feature is the novel method of sample introduction to the detector to prevent extinction of the flame. Thus samples with a large solvent content, as is found in trace determination, can be readily analysed. It has a detectability of 8 x 10^{-13} g P/sample and 1 x 10^{-11} g per sample.

Column Performance

a. Column efficiency

The "efficieny" of a column is usually quoted as the number of theoretical plates per unit length. This number is determined from the spread of the peak as it passes through the column, and is measured by comparing the peak width "Y", with the peak retention time "X", and substituting in the formula.

$$n = 16 \left(\frac{x}{y}\right)^2$$

where n = number of theoretical plates per unit length
x = retention volume
y = peak width

b. Resolution factor or separation factor

It is defined as the separation of the peak maxima divided by the average peak width. Therefore, to increase the resolution factor, either the difference between retention volumes must be increased by changing column operating conditions, or a more efficient column must be prepared to obtain peaks of a smaller width.

Resolution Factor

$$= 2 \times \frac{\text{Difference between retention volume}}{\text{Sum of peak widths}}$$

$$= 2\,Y / (Ya + Yb)$$

where y = difference between retention volumes,

Ya = peak width of a peak a.

Yb = peak width of peak b.

Types of Column

Following types of columns are used in gas chromatography

a. Capillary column

b. Packed columns

a. Capillary columns

In this type of columns, stationary phase is coated directly on the inside of tubing approximately 0.25 mm in diameter. Generally very efficient columns are produced since the cross diffusion of the sample molecules is minimised by the narrow diameter. Capillary columns can not handle more than 0.010 µl, which has to be overcome by the use of inlet splitters. *Usually maximum number of theoretical plates are 300,000.*

Now-a-days, M/s Pye Unicam (Philips) have started manufacturing capillary columns under the proprietory names - Quartz WCOT, Glass. WCOT, Glass SCOT etc.

M/s Supelco, S.A., Switzerland, manufacture the following capillary columns for use in gas chromatography.

Capillary Columns

Name	Description	Temperature range
SP-2100	Methyl silicon fluid	0-280°C
SE-30	Methyl silicone gum	0.-280°C
SE-52	95-5 Methyl phenyl silicone	0-280°C
SE-54	94-5 Methyl phenyl silicone (1 % vinyl)	0-280°C
SP-2250	50-50 Methyl phenyl silicone	0-250°C
Carbowax 20 M	Polyethylene glycol (PEG) 20 M	70-220°C
SP-1000	PEG-20 M Nitroterephthalic acid	70-220°C

b. Packed columns

These are conventional one, and for analytical work 2 mm or 4 mm internal diameter tubing with lengths up to 20 m are used. *The expected efficiency for a packed column is 1800-2500 plates/meter. Maximum sample size vary from 1 to 1000 μl. Generally the number of theoretical plates (total) vary from 15,000 to 60,000. For preparative chromatography the internal diameter is 6 to 25 mm, and the packing material specification is changed to cope with increased loading.*

Column Rejuvenator

In spite of considerable improvement in silane treated solid supports during the past few years there often remains small amount of active sites which are responsible for peak tailing and sample loss. This is normally noticed when working with sample in the sub microgram range. Also, a column may develop active sites after prolonged use. We may improve results and salvage a deteriorating column by infection of 10 to 15 microlitres of REJUV-8 directly into the column. The silylating agent contains no chlorosilanes. REJUV-8 is packaged in septum sealed serum bottles.

Note : REJUV-8 is manufactured by Supelco, S.A., Switzerland.

Retention Time

The retetion time is that time from injection to the peak maxima. This property is characteristic of the sample and the liquid phase at a given temperature. With proper flow and temperature control, it can be reproduced to witihin 1% and used to identify each peak. Several compounds can have identical or close retention times, but each compound has only one retention time. This retention time is not influenced by the presence of other components. *In nutshell, retention time is the time a component is retained in the column.*

Retention Volume

It is the volume of carrier gas passed during the retention time. The area enclosed by a peak is indicative of the quantity of that component present, which is the basis of quantitative analysis. Uncorrected retention volume is that volume measured from point of injection to the peak maximum. It depends on the following factors :

1. *Column dimensions (length and diameter)*
2. *Liquid phase (type, amount)*
3. *Column temperature*
4. *Flow rate*
5. *Type of carrier case*
6. *Instrument dead volume*
7. *Pressure drop*

Amino Acids in Biological Materials by Gas Chromatography (Method of Cliffe *et al.*, 1973)

The possibility of determining amino acids by gas liquid chromatography of volatile derivatives is attractive because of the speed and sensitivity of the method. Methyl esters had earlier been found too volatile for convenient use (Lamkin and Gherke, 1965 Darbre and Blau, 1963). although Ragen and Black (1965) showed good graphical correlations between instrument response and quality of volatility of N-TFA methyl esters.

Apparatus

1. *Gas chromtographs with dual columns and dual flame ionization detectors.*
2. *The reservoir for methanolic hydrogen chloride (needed for the preparation of methyl esters) is constructed from a 250 ml round bottomed flask using Sovirel screw joints and Inter-flow stopcocks (see Fig. 2).*

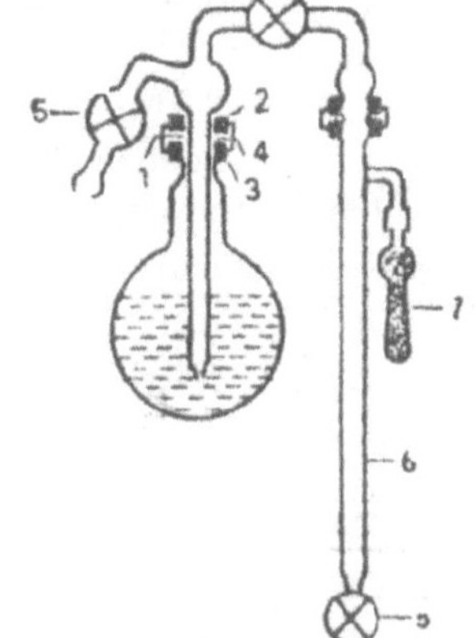

Fig. 2 : Dispenser for methanolic hydrogen chloride. (1 = PTFE-covered plastic washer, 2 = Threaded glass joints, 3 = threaded plastic nut, 4 = aluminium retaining ring, 5 = PTFE-keyed stopcocks, 6 = 25 ml burette, 7 = calcium chloride drying tube)

Reagents

1. *Methanol (Analytical grade) is redistilled from calcium hydride.*
2. *Trifluoroacetic anhydride distilled immediately before use.*
3. *Dichloromethane is distilled from anhydrous calcium sulphate and then stored over anhydrous calcium sulphate.*
4. *Methyl ethyl ketone (for the preparation of stationary phases is dried by distilling from $CaCl_2$).*
5. *Methanolic hydrogen chloride (generated from ammonium chloride and concentrated sulphuric acid) is prepared by passing the gas first through concentrated sulphuric acid (to ensure dryness) and then into the anhydrous methanol to a concentration 4m. After titration, the solution is adjusted by dilution to 4 M.*
6. *Methyl stearate.*
7. *Column material. A mixture of 46 per cent of XE-60 (Cyanoethyl, methyl, dimethyl silicone gum rubber), 27 pecent of MS-200 (Silicone oil) is dissolved in methyl ethyl ketone to give a total concentration of 1 percent. Fifty millilitres of the solution is added to 19.5 g of the solid support (Diatoport-S, 80-100 mesh) - Hewlett-Packard, Slough Bucks, and solvent is removed by distillation under vacuo at 40°C in a rotary evaporator, which is sialinised by the manufacturer. AW-DMCS chromosorb W, 80-100 mesh may be used as an alternative.*

Procedure

An aqueous solution containing approximately 0.5 μ mole of each amino acids is accurately measured into a Pyrex tube of 5 mm I.D. with a conical closed end. The sample is then dried in vacuo (0.1 to 1 mm Hg) over P_2O_5 and NaOH, with cautions heating by infra red lamp. One millilitre of the 4 M methanolic HCl is then added from the dispenser and the tube is drawn out in a flame to produce a constriction of about (a) 0.5 mm or (b) 3 mm in diameter. The tube is then cut at the narrowest point and inserted in a wider test tube partially immersed in an oil bath maintained at 65°C. This temperature is selected to reduce loss of solvent by evaporation. After 90 minutes the tube is withdrawn, the constriction is removed and the sample (now the methyl ester hydrochloride) is dried as before. The tube is again constricted, this time to about 1 mm and 200μl of 20 per cent trifluoroacetic anhydride and 1 per cent (W/V) methyl stearate internal standard in dichloromethane are added. The tube is then sealed and heated as before at 120°C for 20 minutes giving a solution of the N.TFA methyl esters of the amino acids.

An aliquot of the solution of derivatives of amino acids (10 μl) is placed on the precolumn, taking care to first dry the syringe by filling two or three times with anhydrous dichloromethane. The reagents are then removed by placing the precolumn in a stoppered ungreased B 19 test tube with a side arm and a ground glass tap through which it could be connected in rapid sequence to a filter pump (1 min.), an oil pump (3 min.) and finally a source of dry air, the tube meanwhile being immersed in ice-water. The precolumn is then rapidly pushed into the injection port of the gas chromatograph.

Attenuation is set at 20 x 10^2 (2 x 10^{-9} a.f.s.). Injection heaters are adjusted to the setting which gave 235°C at the injection point when the oven temperature is 90°C. Flow rate is 15 ml/min. of oxygen free nitrogen.

Temperature programming conditions are : intial temperature 90°C followed by 1°C/min. for 20 min., 3°C/min. for 7 min., hold for 22 min,, 6°C/min. for 12 min., hold for 6 min., 4°C/min. for 7 minutes final hold at 231°C.

Quantitative Estimation of Lower Volatile Fatty Acids in Biological Samples by Gas Liquid Chromatography

(Method of Baumgardt, 1964. Erwin *et al.*, 1961 and Simkins 1965)

Sample Preparation

Various procedures have been described in the literature for determining volatile fatty acids in silage extract, rumen fluid and plasma. Many of these procedures use a stem distillation step to obtain maximum amount of VFA but also to remove interfering peaks during GLC analysis (Mahadevan and Zieve, 1969., Perry *et al.,* 1970). The major short comings of these procedures are the lengthy steam distillation step and the use of 5 ml or more plasma, thus limiting the methods used with large animals. Recently a new micro method for measuring plasma VFA was described (Ramsey and Demigne, 1974). In this procedure, the VFA are extracted from 200 μl of plasma with 1 ml of ethanol in the presence of 20 μl of isobutyrate internal standard. After agitation and centrifugation, the supernatant liquid is transferred to a 4 ml flask and made alkaline with 20 μl of 0.2 M NaOH. It is then evaporated in an air current at 20°C. The dry residue is redissolved in 15 μl of water a few minutes before analysis just before injection on the columm, 5 μl of 25% (V/V) orthophosphoric acid is added. Recovery studies showed that the VFA are quantitatively extracted by ethanol.

It has been observed that the samples contain non-volatiles which will accumulate at the inlet of the column and, in time, cause the performance of the column to deteriorate. To avoid this problem, a replaceable glass lined inlet should be used in which the non volatiles will accumulate. The glass liner must be periodical replaced (daily with heavy usage). Samples containing non volatiles should not be be injected directly into the column as it will be very difficulty to remove the accumulation from the column. An alternative to use of a glass liner is to clean up the sample by steam distilling it according to the procedures of Ross and Kitts (1971).

Procedure A : Preparation of rumen fluid samples GLC analysis of VFA

1. Shake sample of strained rumen fluid. Pipette 5 ml into a centrifuge tube.
2. Add 1 ml 25% metaphosphoric acid
3. Mix thoroughly
4. Allow to stand for 30 minutes
5. Centrifuge at 2000 rpm (on an international centrifuge, size 2, model head 250 A) for 10 minutes
6. The supernatant liquid can be chromatographed without further preparation.

Procedure B : Preparation of blood plasma samples for GLC analysis of VFA

1. Pipette 8 ml of 0.2 N sulphuric acid into a 50 ml Erlenmeyer flask
2. Add 2 ml blood plasma, using an Ostwald Folin pipette. Mix the flask's contents by swirling and allow the mixture to stand for 10 minutes.
3. Add 2 ml of 10 per cent sodium tungstate (W/V) to the flask's content. The Erlenmeyer flask should be swirled gently during the addition of the sodium tungstate and should be swirled for 30 seconds after the tungstate has been added to ensure complete mixing.
4. After 10 minutes have elapsed, centrifuge the mixture at 5000 rpm for 10 minutes. Collect at least 7.5 ml of supernatant liquid in any suitable vessel.
5. Transfer 7.5 ml aliquot of the above liquid into a 6′ x 3/4″ test tube.
6. Make the liquid alkaline by adding 0.20 ml of 3 N NaOH.
7. Freeze the liquid in the test tube in a dry ice-ethanol mixture.
8. Place the test tube in a lyophilizer and freeze dry. When all the water has been removed from the sample, a fine white powder remains in the test tube.
9. Add 0.2 to 0.5 ml of metaphosphoric acid reagent (prepared by diluting 250 g of 36 per cent metaphosphoric acid to one litre with distilled water) to the test tube. This will dissolve the powder and the resulting solution is used directly for chromatographing the VFA's.

Procedure C : Preparation of silage samples for estimation of VFA

Water extracts of silage are prepared according to Wiseman and Irvin (1957) using only sufficient water to cover the silage to keep the VFA as concentrated as possible. The silage extract is acidified and centrifuged as in the procedure for rumen fluid and the supernatant liquid is used directly for G.L.C. analysis.

1. Depending on the material, weigh out 50 to 100 grams and transfer to a 4 ounce bottle or print mason jar, depending on sample size.
2. Unless otherwise specified, use distilled water to cover the tamped sample. Also, add a pinch of thymol as an antiseptic and secure cap. Note down the size of sample and the amount of water used.
3. Place in refrigerator in a corked bottle at 4°C and leave for 6-7 days.
4. Squeeze material from the jar through two layers of cheese cloth (or glass wool in a funnel). Centrifuge liquid at about 2000 rpm for five minutes. Place in capped tubes or bottles and store in cooler.
5. Into a 10 ml centrifuge tube, pipette 5 ml sample (from 4) and 1 ml 25% metaphosphoric acid.
6. Mix and allow to set for a minimum of 30 minutes.
7. The contents are centrifuged at 4000 rpm for 20-30 minutes. This supernatant liquid is used directly for the determination by GLC.

Silage sample's extract prepared in this manner is heavily ladened with nonvolatiles. To prevent extraneous peaks caused by the accumulation of nonvolatiles in the inlet, change the glass liner frequently and /or inject 2-3 injections of water after every 2-3 injections of sample.

Volatile Fatty Acids (VFA) Mixture Standard

Formula I

VFA	Rumen (mg/100 ml)	Blood (mg/100 ml)
Acetic	314.7	12.59
Propionic	99.3	3.97
Isobutyric	47.5	1.90
n-butyric	95.8	3.83
Isovaleric	43.1	1.72
n-valeric	47.0	1.88

The blood standard may be prepared from the rumen standard by a 1:25 dilution with water.

Formula II

VFA	milliequivalent per litre	per cent
Acetic acid	50	0.300
Propionic acid	20	0.148
Isobutyric	5	0.044
Butyric	20	0.176
Isovaleric	5	0.051
Valeric	5	0.051

Choice of Column Material and Column for VFA Analysis

A special type of column packing is required to elute and separate free carboxylic acids. If these special packing are not used, the peaks will tail badly due to the interaction of the acid and the chromatographic support. Generally these packagings have an acid incorporated into the stationary phase which deactivates the support and permits the acid to elute as a symmetrical peak. Terephthalic acid has been widely used for deactivation, but H_3PO_4 is even more effective. Metal chromatographic tubing can also cause tailing if it is not a high quality grade. If H_3PO_4 is incorporated into the packing, then almost any quality of tubing can be used as the H_3PO_4 deactivates not only the support, but also the tubing.

Column Material for Rumen Sample VFA (Author Experience)

I. 10% SP-1200/1% H_3PO_4 on 80/100 chromosorb W AW, 6 ft x 2 mm ID, Glass column, Col. Temp. : 130°C, Inlet Temp : 170°C, Detector Temp.: 175°C, Flow rate : 40 ml/min. Nitrogen, Sample size : 0.6 µl, Sens. : 10^{-11} x 8

   Availability Source : SUPELCO, SLAE, RTEDE, CELIGNY 3, 1299 CRANS, SWITZERLAND under Catalogue No. 1-1965.

II. Supelco, S.A. : Switzerland also manufacture column material under the proprietary name "Supelco 101" - Catalogue No. 02-213. *Experience of Author : Author of this compendium have tried both the materials and he got excellent separation of VFA peaks on the chromatogram. "Supelco 101" was tried in an Indian made Gas Chromatograph manufactured by Nucon Engineers under the conditions - nitrogen flow 20 kg/cm^2, hydrogen flow 1 kg/cm^2, injection temperature 220-230°C, sensitivity x 100, attenuator 128.*

Author carried out research at the world famous Prof. (Late) Dr. K. Breirem's Institute of Animal Nutrition, Agricultural University of Norway Ås-NLH, Norway, he found excellent separation of VFAS using column cited at S.No. I and II, recommend strongly for use in GLC.

At the Agricultural University of Norway Ås-NLH Norway, Krishna and Ekern (1974a,b,c) used above column material "Supelco 101" for quantitative estimation of volatile fatty acids in rumen liquor, they obtained excellent results of volatile fatty acids analysis as mentioned above.

In India M/S Universal Ferro and Allied Chemicals Ltd., Liberty building, Sir Thackersey Marg (New Marine Lines). Mumbai is authorised dealer for supplying Gas Chromatographic materials being manufactured by Supelco., S.A. Switzerland.

Column Material for Blood Sample VFA Estimation

10% SP-1200/1% H_3PO_4 on 80/100 Chromosorb WAW, 6ft. x 2 mm ID, Glass column, Col. Temp. : 125°C, Inlet Temp. : 170°C, detector temperature :175°C, Flow rate : 40 ml/min. Sample size : 0.6µl, Sens. : 10-12 8 x and 4 x (Note: This column material is also manufactured by Supleco, S.A. - Switzerland).

Ross and Kitts (1971) have developed improved method for the determination of volatile fatty acids in ruminant blood plasma. This method gives excellent results of VFA analysis. The column was 183 cm long by 0.64 cm outer diameter and the packing material was the same as that used by Baumgardt (1964) with a solid support of firebrick 60/80 mesh with neopenthylglycol succinate (20%). and 2% H3 PO4, the liquid phase. They analysed the processed plasma samples using GLC under the following conditions.

Air 283 ml/min., nitrogen 50 ml/min., hydrogen 60 ml/min., temperatures, columns 160°C, inlet 195°C, detector (dual flame ionization) 195°C. The electrometer input attenuator was set at (x 10) while the output attenuator varried from 1 to 16 x as required. The recorder was operated at 2.54 cm/min. at a fixed span of one millivolt per 25.4 cm of chart.

Calculations

The calculation of the contents of acid may be carried out according to Shelley *et al.* (1963). For each acid the relative (R) is calculated as below :

$$R\,(\text{acid}) = \frac{{}^{h}(\text{acid}).\ {}^{c}(\text{standard})}{{}^{c}(\text{acid}).\ {}^{h}(\text{standard})}$$

where C = Concentration in m mol/l or mEq/lit or per cent

h = peak height in mm or counts

Schmekel (1966) reported that calculations based on peak height only gave the best results. For narrowing peaks, the writer should be reduced to 4.2 mm/min.

Or we may write the above formula as concentration of acid (mEq/lit.) in the given sample will be.

$$= \frac{\text{peak height (counts) in unknown sample x mEq/lit. acid in standard}}{\text{peak height (counts) of standard}}$$

Example : Estimate concentration of lower volatile fatty acids in silage extract of sample A (apply VFA standard formula II)

VFA	Concent. in Std (mEq/lit)	Peak height (Counts)	Factor
Acetic acid	50	36	$\frac{50}{36}=1.39$
Propionic acid	20	15.5	$\frac{20}{15.5}=1.29$
Butyric acid	20	11.0	$\frac{20}{11.0}=1.82$

Concentration of VFA in silage extract will be

= Peak height (counts) x factor in silage extract

VFA	Peak height (counts)	Factor		Conc. (mEq/lit.) in silage extract
Acetic acid	15	1.39	=	20.85
Propionic acid	10	1.29	=	12.90
Butyric acid	1.5	1.82	=	2.73

☞ **Note**

Conc. (mEq/lit) may be converted into percent concentration by applying values of VFA standard formula II, respectively.

Quantitative Estimation of Fractions of Volatile Fatty Acids in Rumen Liquor by GLC (Method of Cottyn and Boucque, 1968)

Samples of rumen liquor are taken by suction through rumen fistula. After immediate pH determination and filteration through muslin cloth, a few drops of toluene is added to inhibit fermentation. The samples may be analysed immediately or stored in a freezer at -15°C. For the analysis, 5 ml of the strained rumen fluid is pipetted into a centrifuge tube, after which 1 ml of a 3 to 1 V/V solution of metaphosphoric acid and formic acid (25%) is added. The metaphosphoric acid precipitates the proteins which contaminate the column. After 30 minutes, the contents are centrifuged at 4000 rpm for 20 minute. The clear supernatant is ready for direct injection.

A stainless steel column (4 foot x 1/8 inch) packed with 20% Tween 80 on Diatoport W.A.W. 40 to 60 mesh is used. A temperature programmed cycle from 90 to 130°C., rising by 4°C per minute, is used. The injection block is maintained at 265°C to provide rapid vaporization of the injected fluid. Nitrogen is used as a carrier gas with a flow rate of 60 ml per minute. The hydrogen flow rate to the detector is 50 ml per minute, and the air flow is 380 ml per minute, Under these conditions, the analysis of a rumen fluid sample requires about 8 minutes from acetic to valeric acid.

Quantitative Estimation of Lower Volatile Fatty Acids in Rumen Liquor (Method of Schmekel, 1966)

Five ml rumen fluid and 2.5 ml 1 M H_2SO_4 are introduced into a test tube adapted to steam distillation. The tube is then lowered into a 2 litre steam generator filled with distilled water to three quarter of its volume. A piece of china, a few drops of concentrated NaOH and phenolphthalein are added. The generator is connected to a Liebig condenser by a heated in a coverd beaker containg 10 ml 0.01 N NaOH with the end of the condenser under the surface of the liquid. The condenser is then washed with distilled water. Since the amount of NaOH in the beaker is insufficient to neutralize the distilliation, until indicator changed colour. After adding a few more drops fo 0.1 N NaOH the distillate is evaporated to dryness in a fan blower drying chamber.

About half an hour before analysis, 0.5 ml of a mixture of 2 N Hcl and reference substance (ethyleneglycolmonoethylether, B.P. 135.1°C, 60 mmol/ lit) is injected through the membrane of the sealed bottle with a calibrated hypodermic syringe and the sample is carefully shaken up. A suitable amount of sample (0.2-0.6μl) is then transfered into the gas chromatograph by means of a 1μl Hamilton syringe equipped with a chaney adaptor.

The analysis is carried out in a dual column gas chromatograph with a differential flame ionisation detector, model Perkin-Elmer 800, connected to a Honeywall recorder, model 5401, scale 0-1 mv, and a Perkin-Elmer electronic integrator D2. The separation of the VFA is carried out in a 2 meter, 1/4" column of stainless steel filled with 20% polyoxyethyl ensorbit monooleate (Tween 80) and 2% orthophosphorus acid at a concentration of 85% on 60-80 mesh chromosorb W. Before use, the column material is heated to 170°C for 48 hours during which time the flow of nitrogen gas is slow. After packing, the columns are again heated to 170°C for 24 hours, the flow of nitrogen being 65 ml/min. The columns are placed in the chromatograph without connection to the detector. During analysis, the temperature of the column is 140°C and the flow of nitrogen is unchanged at 65 ml per minute. The injector temperature is 280°C only 50% of the total amount of gas which left the columns, is allowed to pass the detector. The flow of hydrogen gas to the detector chamber is 30ml/min. and the air flow 250 ml/min. A sensitivity setting of 50 is used for the analysis. The paper speed of the writer is 8.4 and 4.2 mm/min. respectively. The total time of analysis is about 15 min.

Procedure for Processing Rumen Liquor to Quantify the Concentration of Lower Volatile Fatty Acids

(Method of Cottyn & Boucque, 1968 Modified by Astrup and Associates, 1975 Agricultural University of Norway – Ås-NLH (NORWAY)

Deliver 10 ml rumen liquor in a 50 ml centrifuge tube and add 0.5 ml of 50 per cent formic acid. The addition stops further fermentation and solids are precipitated. After sedimentation the clear supernatant is sampled for analysis. In a similar way 0.5 ml 50 per cent formic acid is also added to 10 ml of standard VFA mixture prepared according to formula II. Five ml of supernatant is measured in stoppered glass test tube and stored in the freezer at -15°C. *The author followed this method during his Doctoral Research work at the Agricultural University of Norway,* Ås-NLH.

The Organic Acids in Silage as Determined by the Gas Chromatography

Lessard *et al.,* (1961) developed the original method for organic acids estimation and this method may be applied in the case of silage samples. He prepared acid esters and analysed by Gas chromatography fitted with a chromatographic column filled with 15 grams of 42-60 mesh crushed C-22 Johns-Manville firebrick, coated with 8 millilitres of DOW-Corning Silicone Fluid type 550. They obtained satisfactory resolution of the lower fatty acid esters with a column temperature of 100°C, a pressure of the helium carrier gas of 20 p.s.i. at the column inlet and a filament current at 250 milliamperes.

Amine Analysis in Biological Samples

It is very difficult to analyse amine by Gas chromatography because the peaks frequently tail badly. This tailing is caused by the absorption of the sample on the chromatographic support of adsorbent. The tailing problem becomes increasingly severe as the basicity of the amine increases., consequently, primary aliphatic amines and polyfunctional amines are the most difficult to analyse. Secondary aliphatic amines are less basic, and consequently, a lesser problem, while tertiary amines are the least difficult to analyse. Aromatic amines are weakly amines, but they do required a deactivated column. Deactivation in general is usually accomplished by adding a basic material to the packing.

Aliphatic Amines : 1. Methyl 2. Dimethyl 3. Ethyl 4. Trimethyl 5. Isopropyl 6. n-propyl 7. t. Butyl 8. Diethyl 9. see-Butyl 10. isobutyl 11. n-Butyl.

Heterocyclic amines : 1. Ethylenediamine 2. Piperidine 3. Pyridine 4. Morpholine 5. Piperazine 6. Cyclohexylamine.

Derivatization of Amines

Amines are frequently converted to a derivative to avoid the problems of tailing of the peaks. In general trifluoroacetic anhydride (TFA) has been used as a derivatizing agent for amines. TFA is very reactive, frequently being added directly to the sample with complete reaction after only a few minutes. In some cases pyridine is added and/or heat is used to promote the reaction. In the case of primary amines, TFA will react with only one hydrogen, it will react with a secondary amine, but not a tertiary amine. If an alcohol is present, it too will react with TFA to form an ester, water also reacts. In some instances a small amount of alcohol or water is added to the sample to react the excess TFA. The n-trifluoroacetyl derivative is stable in the presence of water (Clarke *et al.,* 1966).

Amino Acids

Amino acids are converted to a volatile derivative in order to be separated on a GC column. Gehrke *et al.* (1966) have developed method in detail for derivatization of amino acids.

Fatty Amines

Morrisette and Link (1965), Mc Curdy and Reiser (1966) and Clarke *et al.* (1966) have developed procedure for making derivatives.

Ehtanol Amines

Brydia and Persenger (1967) have developed a quantitative procedure for determination of the ethanolamines as the TFA derivative Both the amine and hydroxyl groups are reacted with TFA. A 5 foot x 1/4 inch column with 5% neopentyl glycol succinate on 60/80 chromosorb G is used for the separation. TC detector is found necessary to obtain good quantitative results.

Volatile Amines

Irvine and Saxby (1969) have studied the separation of a large number of volatile amines obtained from Latika tobbaco leaves. The amines are steam distilled and collected in an HCL solution which is subsequently dried. The amine hydrochlorides are treated with KOH and then extracted with ether. The amines are then added to an ion exchange column and the TFA derivatives are prepared by treating the column with TFA.

Aromatic Amines

Dove (1967) separated about twenty aromatic amines including aniline, toluidine, Xylidine, ethylaniline and n-methyl toluidine isomers as TFA derivatives. He used column packed with 9.5% Apiezon D,3.6% Carbowax 20 M on 80/100 Aeropak 30. The column is operated at 152°C with a flow rate of 100 ml/minute. The sample is dissolved in THF containing pyridine. TFA is added to the solution, which is held in an ice bath. After the addition of TFA the mixture is heated at 50°C for 10 minutes. The mixture is cooled and water added. It is then extracted with methylene chloride and dried. Brydia and Willeboordse (1968) have developed procedures for the separation of various isomers of diaminotoluenes as the TFA derivatives are prepared by adding TFA directly to the sample.

Polyamines

Tetraethylene pentanine (TEPA), triethylene tetramine (TETA) are examples of polyamines. Bergstedt and Widmark (1970) have developed procedure for the quantitative estimation of polyamines.

Column Materials for Separating Amines by Gas Chromatography

Following column materials are manufactured by Supelco, S.A. RTENDECELIGNY 3, 1299 CRANS, SWITZERLAND having a supplying agent M/s Universal Ferro and Allied Chemical Ltd., Liberty Building, Sir Vithaldas Thackersey Marg (New Marine Lines), Mumbai - 400 020.

Aliphatic Amines

Supelco Cat. Mo.	Description
1-1805	10% Carbowax 20 M 2 % KOH on 80/100 Chromosorb W AW Min./Max. Temp. 60/225°C
1-1806	10% UCON 50-HB-5100 2% KOH on 80/100 Chromosorb W AW Min./Max. Temp. 0/200°C
1-1893	10% Apiezon L/2% KOH on 80/100 chromosorb W AW Min./Max. Temp. 50/250°C
1-1887	GP Carbopack B/4% carbowax 20 M and 0.8% KOH

Aromatic Amines

Supleco Cat. No.	Description
1-1896	3% SP-2401-DB on 100/120 Supelcoport
1-1897	5% SP-2401-DB on 100/120 Supelcoport
1-1894	3% SP-2100-DB on 100/120 Supelcoport
1-1895	3% SP-2250-DB on 100/120 Supelcoport

Porous Polymer Packing

Chromosorb 103 is developed to separate both aliphatic and aromatic amines.

Chromosorb 103

Supleco Cat. No.	Description
2-0216	60/80 mesh
2-0217	80/100 mesh
2-0218	100/120 mesh

Note : Biogenic amines, e.g. *histamine, putrescine, Cadeverine and tyramine* may be estimated by gas chromatographic method using above column packing materials.

Derivative Formation in Gas Chromatography

Principle : Derivatives are used in G.C. separations for many reasons, such as increasing volatility, decreasing adsorption of the G.C. column, and improving separation. A number of derivatives are used, many of them being specific for certain functional groups. For example, a high molecular weight compound with polyfunctional groups is usually not amenable to direct gas chromatographic analysis as the "free" compound. The different functional groups make the compound very polar and generally reduce its volatility. Such polyfunctional compounds will exhibit long retention times, or will not be eluted from the column. By replacing some or all of the functional groups, a decrease in polarity is generally accomplished, volatility is increased, and the compound can be eluted from a G.C. column in a reasonable time compounds with low volatility and high polarity which do elute from a G.C. column in the free state usually shows signs of adsorption and/or breakdown. Quantitiative analysis is therefore very difficult, if not impossible, to achieve. When we analyse "free" cholesterol by gas chromatography then broad and tailing peaks are obtained, when "free" cholesterol is derivatised then sharp peaks are obtained.

Even at high concentrations of the free compound, the quantitative analysis can be impaired by adsorption, which is evidenced by tailing peaks. Since a tailing peak is a non-Gaussian peak, quantitative measurement is difficult to achieve by a manual integration method such as triangulation. This problem can be over-come by analysing a derivative of the compound. Hammarstand (1967) chromatographic system can also be due to improper choice of column, active sites, and/or excessive dead volume in the system. A derivative can improve the separation of two closely related compounds or make possible a separation that cannot be accomplished otherwise.

Derivaties of Different Functional Groups

Functional Group : OH

silyl ether, acetate, methyl ether, heptafluorobutyrate

Functional Group : COOH

methyl ester, butyl ester, silyl ester

Functional Group : NH_2

trifluoroacetyl, silyl ether, dipivalyl

Functional Group : NH

silyl ether

Functional group

Oxime, hydrazone

Formation of Methylester and Butylester Derivatives

The methyl ester is the most common derivative of the COOH group. This ester derivative has been widely used in the analysis of fatty acids (Hammarstrand, 1966 and Szymanski, 1964). The butyl esters and higher have been used mainly for short chain fatty acids (Sampugna *et al.*, 1966., Craig *et al.* 1963. Jones and Davison, 1965. Appleby and Mayne, 1967). The methyl ester derivatives has also been used for a wide variety of compounds. Some of these are urinary aromatic acids (Horning *et al.*, 1966) Krebs cycle acids (Simmonds *et al.*, 1967), Sugar phosphates (Wells *et al.*, 1964), fatty acids (Szymanski, 1964), amino acids (Szymanski., 1964) barbituric acids (Stevenson, 1966, Martin and Driscoll, 1966), and sulphonic acis (Kirkland, 1960).

Esterification Procedures

Methyl Esters

Method 1 : The boron trifluoride-methanol transesterification technique of Metcalfe, Schmitz and Pelka (1966) prepared in the apparatus described by Parodi (1967).

Method 2 : The Sealed tube methanolysis method of de Man (1964, 1967). Butyl esters.

Method 3 : The butanol-H_2SO_4 method of Gander, Jensen and Sampugna (1962).

Method 4 : The di-n-butyl carbonate method of sampugna, pitas and jensen (1966).

Method 5 : A boron-trifluoride-butanol method.

Method 5 is used for ester preparation for the gas chromatographic analysis of the fatty acids composition of butterfat. Parodi (1967) used the following method for preparing butyl esters.

Two hundred mg of fat is added to a stoppered 50 ml volumetric flask. Four ml of 0.5 N butanolic sodium hydroxide is added. The mixture is heated on a steam bath for five minutes. Five ml of boron trifluoride-butanol is added to the flask and the mixture is boiled for 5 minutes. The contents of the flask are cooled, and distilled water is added to the mark. The flask is shaken vigorously for one minute and the layers are allowed to separate. Due to the limited solubility of butanol in water a further floating-out step is required. Two ml of the butanol-ester layer is added to a modified Babcock bottle described by Parodi (1967) and enough distilled water is added to float the butyl esters into the neck of the bottle. After vigorous shaking for a few seconds the flask is centrifuged at 2000 rpm for 10 minute. This results in a sample of butyl esters ready for direct injection into the gas-chromatograph.

Quantitative Estimation of Fatty Acids by Using Gas-Liquid Chromatography (GLC)

Gas chromatograph fitted with dual column and equipped with dual flame-ionization detectors. The columns are freshly prepared 6′ x 1/8′ stainless steel packed with 15% diethylene glycol succinate (DEGS) on 8-100 mesh DMCS treated chromosorb W.

The samples are injected at an initial column temperature of 80°C, held isothermally for one minute and then temperature programmed at 8°/min. to 190°C. Carrier gas flow rates are selected to give similar retention times for methyl and butyl esters.

Sample size is selected so that the methyl or butyl myristate peak had on 80 to 100 percent full scale deflection on the recorder chart.

Fatty Acid Methyl esters

C_4, C_6, C_8, C_{10}, C_{12}, C_{13}, C_{14}, C_{15}, C_{16}, C_{17}, C_{18}, C_{18}^{-}, C_{18}^{2}, C_{18}^{3}, C_{19}, C_{20}, C_{21}, C_{22}.

Column Considerations in Fatty Acid Esters Analysis

The most commonly used liquid phase for this type of analysis is DEFS (Diethylene Glycol Succinate, LAC-3R-728) or EGS (Ethylene glycol Succinate, LAC-4R-886). These polyesters are very selective for fatty acid esters and will separate most of the esters including saturated and unsaturated ones. The only drawback of these liquid phases is their maximum operating temperature of 190°C to 220°C. Since the bleed rate is high at temperature programming when using highly sensitive ionization detectors.

Most analysis are performed on columns of 6 to 12 foot length packed with 10 to 20% Polyester on chromosorb W.

Gas Chromatographic Conditions

Instrument	:	Model 2100
Column	:	6′ x ¼″, 1% LAC-4R-886 on Aeropak 30, 80/100 mesh
Temperatures	:	Column : 170°C isothermal Inj/Det. : 250°C
		Carrier Gas : N_2, 35 ml-min
Detector	:	FID (H_2 = 30 ml/min., air = 300 ml/min.)
Sensitivity	:	32 x 10^{-11} afs
Sample size	:	0.4 µl
Chart speed	:	10″/h

Method for Determination of The Free Fatty Acids of Milk Fat

Bills *et al.* (1963) have published methodology for isolating free fatty acids from the fat by means of a basic anion exchange resin, converted to methyl esters and extracted with ethyl chloride. They also calculated appropriate factors for relating the quantity of added internal standards to that of the naturally occuring free fatty acids.

Jensen et al. (1967) have published an exhaustive review about the gas-liquid chromatographic analysis of milk fatty acids. They have also discussed some of the problems involved in GLC analysis of milk fatty acids.

Gas Chromatographic Analysis of Fatty Acids in Blood or Tissues

Lipid can be isolated from blood or tissue by the extraction method developed by Folch *et al.* (1957). This method gives a pure lipid extract, free from water soluble material such as amino acids, peptides and carbohydrates. If tissues is used, it first has to be homogenised. This can be done in a waring Blender for gram quantities of tissue. The Potter-Elvehjem homogenizer is better for amounts smaller than one gram. The homogenisation is carried out in a few millilitres of chloroform - methanol (2 : 1 v/v).

A. Extraction procedure

Choloform - methanol (2:1 v/v) is added to the blood, plasma or homogenate in a Erlenmeyer flask. Twenty ml of chloroform methanol per ml of blood should be used for 20 ml per gram of tissue. Swirl the contents around until thoroughly mixed. The protein fraction will precipitate and is removed by filteration.

The extract is filtered through a coarse fat free filter paper into a glass stopered graduate cylinder. Wash the flask and the filter paper three times with chloroform - methanol to achieve a quantitative transfer. To the extract in the cylnider, add an amount of 09% NaCl in water (saline) equivalent to 1/5 of the extract volume. Shake vigorously and allow to stand overnight or until the extract becomes clear.

Two phases will separate : one upper phase consisting of water-methanol-salt, and the lower phase consisting of chloroform. The water phase contains water soluble material which is discarded and the chloroform phase contains the lipids. Siphon off the upper water phase and discard. Wash the remaining surface with chloroform methanol-saline (3:47 : 48v/v) to remove traces of the water phase.

The remaining chloroform phase containing the lipids is then evaporated and processed further for analysis.

The total chloroform lipid extract can then be separated into its different lipid classes by the use of column chromatography on silicic acid, DEAE cellulose and so on (Barron and Hanahan, 1958, Birson and Ahrens, 1958., Fillerup and Mead, 1963, Rouser *et al.* 1963, Rouser *et al.* 1961). The different fractions can then be hydrolysed and the fatty acids are determined by gas chromatography.

B. Saponification of lipids and liberation of free fatty acids

In order to analyse for total fatty acids, the lipids from the original chloroform extract have to be saponified. The extract is treated with alkali. This hydrolyses the fatty acids from the cholesterol esters, triglycerides, and phsopholipids and converts them to water soluble soaps.

1. Saponification Procedure

The orignal chloroform extract from the extraction is taken to dryness in a 250 ml flat bottom flask equipped with a 20/40 standard joint. Add 50 ml of ethanol-ethyl ether (3:1 v/v + plus 0.5 ml of 10N KOH). Allow the flask to stand on a boiling water bath for two hours covered with a watch glass. If necessary, add ethanol to maintain constant volume. After saponification, add water to the soap solution. Ensure that the soap solution is diluted with the right amount of water to obtain a 50% ethanol-water solution of the soaps. To obtain a 100% recovery when extracting the sterols, the soap solution must be 50% + 50% ethanol in water.

Add about 75 ml of petroleum ether (30-60°C) and let stand overnight or shake the flask fitted with a 20/40 standard tapered stopper. Two phases will separate : The upper consisting of petroleum ether with the sterols (cholesterol), the lower consisting of water alcohol with the potassium salts of the fatty acids.

Siphon off the upper petroleum-ether phase containing sterols which, of course, can be separated and determined by gas chromatography or by colorimetric methods (Zlatkis *et al.,* 1953., Creech and Sewell, 1962, Wycoff and Parsons, 1957). Wash the surface layer three times with a few ml of petroleum ether and siplon off. A convenient way of siphoning off layers and transfering low boiling solvents like petroleum ether.

2. Free Fatty Acid Liberation Procedure

The fatty acids are then libreated by adding 10 ml of 1.5 N HCl to the water phase in the flask. Add 75 ml of petroleum ether, allow to stand overnight or shake the flask. The upper petroleum ether phase containing free fatty acids is then trasnferred to a 250 ml separatory funnel. Wash the flask three times with pertroleum ether for a quantitative transfer. Add a few ml of water to the lower water phase. After the two phases have separated, discard the lower water phase. This procedure will wash out traces of HCl in the extract. The remianing petroleum ether in the separatory funnel is first taken to dryness and then diluted with a few micro litres of a solvent. The fatty acids can then be analysed by gas chromatograph either as free acids or as methyl esters.

C. Methylation of free fatty acids

BF3 methanol method (Metcalf and Schmitz, 1961 and Metcalf *et al.,* 1966).

To the fatty acids, add the BF_3-methanol reagent. One hundred to two hundred mg of fatty acids can be methylated with 3 ml reagent. The reaction can be carried out in test tube. Boil the test tube mixture in a boiling water bath for two minutes. The reaction is then complete and the methy esters are extracted with a solvent such as heptane, hexane or petroleum ether. Transfer the mixture to a separatory funnel with 30 ml of petroleum ether (30-60°C), add 20 ml of water and shake vigorously. Discard the bottom water phase. The petroleum-ether phase is then filtered through a fine filter paper (to get rid of water droplets) into a flask. Evaporate the petroleum ether at a temperature below 40°C and discontinue when dry in order to prevent oxidation of the unsaturated methyl esters and evaporation of short chain methyl esters. The esters are then ready for analysis by gas chromatography.

☞ **Note**

BF_3 - methanol could be purchased from M/S Applied Science Laboratories, Inc., State College, Pa., 16801 or Lachat Chemicals, Inc., 10540, Wester Ave., Chicago, Ill., 60643 or Glaxo Laboratories (India) Ltd, Dr Annie Besant Road, Bombay 400 025).

D. Handling and storage of fatty acids and other liquids

Fatty acids and other lipids should be stored in a glass-stoppered test tube at -20°C (preferable-40°) dissolved in a solvent such as chloroform or petroleum ether (30-60°C). The atmosphere in the test tube should be inert. This can be done by flushing the tube with pure nitrogen. An antioxidant can be added to minimize oxidation (0.05-0.10%, w/w of a-tocopherol added to the lipids is useful). Other antioxidants are butylated hydroxy-toluene (BHT), butyl hydroquinone (BHQ) and butylated hydroxy anisole (BHA). A concentration of about 5-10 mg per cent is sufficient. Evaporation of solvents from a lipid mixture should be done in a stream of pure nitrogen or with a rotary evaporator. An antioxidant can be in the solution all the time during handling. Evaporations should be done at a temperature below 40°C. If the temperature is too high, the oxidation rate will increase and also cause a loss of short chain fatty acids. If oxidation of methyl esters occurs additional peaks due to oxidation products can be observed by a gas chromatograph. These peaks usually occur at a corresponding fatty acid carbon number of C_8-C_{12} and also around C_{17} on a DEGS column. Oxidized methyl linoleate gives different short chain aldehydes, esters, ketones and peroxy products.

Precautions

Solvents that are used in the extraction procedures should be reagent grade and eventually further purified. A test should be run to determine if they contain any lipids. This can be done by evaporating about one litre of solvent to dryness, saponify, and run the fatty acid methyl ester on gas chromatography. If any peaks appear, the solvents should be glass distilled. Petroleum ether (analytical reagent 30-60°C) has been known to contain triglycerides with C_{14}-C_{16}-C_{18} fatty acids. By distilling the pertroleum ether upto 55°C using a vigreaux column, a very pure solvent can be obtained. The filter papers used can easily be defatted in a soxhlet extractor. Grease and lubricants should be avoided for glass stopcocks and glass joints. To prevent them from freezing, graphite can be applied on the ground glass. An easy way to do this to apply the graphite with a soft pencil. Teflen stopcocks are preferred for separatory funnels.

Choice of Column

In preparation work for collecting acids and especially working with ^{14}C and/or ^{3}H labeled acids, it is desirable to use a long column that can take a large sample and at the same time give high resolution. Since it is possible to have a very high radioactivity in, for example, stearic acid and a very low radio-activity in oleic or cis-vaccenic acid, a complete separation of those acids is a must in order to get significant measurements of the distribution of the radioactivity.

For the analysis of the methyl esters, both polar and non-polar columns are being used. The most common polar columns are the polyesters like diethylglycolsuccinate (DEGS), diethyleneglycoladipate (DEGA) etc. These columns will give a complete separation of the fatty acids including those with double bonds. The two most common non-polar columns are silicone polymers like SE-30 and hydrocarbon greases like Apiezon - L. The SE-30 will only separate the saturated acids, while the Apiezon will separate the unsaturated except for those with two and three double bonds (linoeic and linolenic) which appear as one peak.

Free fatty acids up to the unsaturated C_{18} can be separated. James and Martin (1952) used silicone oil and stearic acid as a liquid phase. A significant advance in the analysis for free fatty acids was described by Metcalfe (1960, 1963) who used a polyester treated with phosphoric acid.

Most of the analysis of fatty acid methyl ester are performed with a 6-12 foot column packed with 10-20 % DEGS on chromosorb W or chromosorb P. Generally chromosorb P will give a better separation than the W. It has been experienced that Apiezon L is useful for long chain acids since it is quite heat stable - upper limit 300°C. Temperature programming can also be employed with this column.

Method for Determining Whether Acid is Saturated or Unsaturated

To the fatty acid methyl esters in a 250 ml flat bottom flask with a 20/40 joint, add 5 ml methanol. Add 10 mg of platinum Oxide as a catalyst. Flash the flask out with H_2 and let stand overnight on a magnetic stirrer with a glass stopper in place. The next day, the hydrogenated mixture is injected in the gas chromatograph. For identification purposes, the sample should be analysed before and after hydrogenation.

Quantitative Analysis

The best method to quantitate fatty acids is to use the internal standardization method. The standard used must not interfere with the other peaks in the chromatogram. Different compounds can be used, preferably a component similar to the ones in the unknown mixture (Napier, 1963). All odd chain fatty acid such as C_{17} can usually be used as an internal standard in biological samples after ensuring that the mixture does not contain any C_{17}.

Radioactivity Measurements

Fatty acids metabolism can be studied at the molecule level with the use of ^{14}C or ^{3}H. Different ^{14}C or ^{3}H labeled compounds can be used as precursors for *in vivo* or *in vitro* studies. For example, 1-^{14}C - sodium acetate can be metabolized by tissue or inject into an intact animal. After a certain time, the lipids in the tissue, blood or selected organs from the animal are extracted and the lipids separated by column or thin layer chromatography. The fatty acids from each lipid class can then be hydrolyzed, separated, and determined by gas chromatography.

Systems for measuring radioacitivity using some of the methods discussed are commercially available.

A method that is simple, efficient, and has been used by the scientist in investigating fatty acid metabolism in diabetes employs Collecting the acids in cigarette filters. The counting is then done by a liquid scintillation counter. Where both C and H can be determined. The filters used are Estron filtre rods (Estron filter rod, type FD-340) supplied by Eastman Chemical Products, Inc., Kingsport, Tennessee), which are cut to a length of 16 mm. After washing the filters in petroleum ether (30-60°C), they are siliconised by soaking in an 8 per cent solution of silicone oil (Dow Corning fluid 703) in petroleum ether and air dried.

The outlet of the gas chromatograph is fitted with an 8 mm long (15 gauge) hypodermic needle on which the filter is impaled. Collection efficiencies of at least 95 per cent are achieved. The filter is placed directly into a counting vial and a scintillation solution is added. A few minutes later, the vial is counted in a liquid scintillation counter. The quenching from the filter is only 3.7 per cent for C, using 4 g/litre of PPPO (2, 5-diphenyloxazole) and 100 mg/litre of POPOP (1, 4-bis - (5-phenyloxazol-2-yl) Benzene into toluene as a scintillation solution.

Supelco, S.A (Switzerland) supply the following column packing materials for analysis of long chain fatty acids.

1. G.P. 5 per cent DEGS-PS on 100/120 Suplecoport, 3 ft.X 2 mm ID glass, col. Temp. 200°C, Inlet and Detector : 210°C, Flow rate : 20 ml per minute, N_2, Sample : Quailmix FA, 1.0µl, Det. : FID, Sens. : 128 x 10^{-10} AFS.
2. G.P. 10% SP-216-PS on 100/120 Supelcoport, 3 ft. x 2 mm ID glass U, Col. Temp. : 130°C to 200°C, Prog. : 15°C. min. Flow rate : 20 ml/min., N_2.

Qualmix FA is fatty acid mixture containing 14:0, 16:0, 16:1, 18:0, 18:1, 18:2, 18:3, and 20:0 in $CHCl_3$ manufactured by Supelco. S.A. (Switzerland) under Catalogue No. 4-7057.

Analysis of Triglycerides by Gas Chromatography

Triglycerides are glycerol fatty acid esters of the general formula

H_2 C -COO - R

HC - COO - R′

H_2C - COO - R″

Where R, R′ and R″ are saturated and unsaturated fatty acids. Generally triglycerides are relatively high molecular weight compounds with high boiling points.

Column Requirements

1. *Short, low liquid loaded columns*
2. *Stable, high temperature liquid phases*
3. *Deactivated supports*
4. *Temperature programming*
5. *On column injection*
6. *Small samples*
7. *High flow rates*

Sample Preparation

One gram of butter is shaken vigorously with 10 ml of ether. After separation into a lower aqueous layer containing ether insoluble compounds and an upper organic layer, an aliquot of the ether solution is directly injected.

Gas Chromatographic Conditions

Column : 2′ x 2 mm internal diametre glass, 3% SE-30 on Aeropa K 30, 100/120 mesh

Temperatures

Column	:	210° - 340° programmed with 4°C/min.
Injection	:	360°C
Detector	:	350°C
Carrier gas	:	N_2. 40ml/min.

Detector	:	FID (H_2 = 30 ml/min., air = 300 ml/min.)
Sensitivity	:	128 x 10^{-11} afs
Sample size	:	0.5 µl
Chart Speed	:	10"/h

Procedure for Lipid Analysis

Fryer et al. (1960) conducted the first successful GLC analysis of triglycerides. Most of these compounds are of relatively high molecualr weight. For example, trimyristin has a molecular formula $C_{45}H_{51}O_6$. This compound has a boiling point of 313°C at the reduced pressure of 50 microns. As one might imagine this imposes strict requirements on the chromatographic system.

Lipid Analysis in Serum and Tissue

(Method of Entenmon *et al.*, 1961)

Lipids in serum or tissue must first be homogenized to allow solvent extraction. The chloroform/methanol (70/30) extract is evaporated to dryness and reextracted with ether-hexane (1:1) and washed with distilled water to remove water soluble compounds. The solvent is evaporated to dryness, this time under nitrogen to prevent oxidation. At this point the sample may be analysed for total fatty acids or the fatty acid pattern of the individual lipid classes via thin layer chromatography (TLC) and subsequent chromatography.

Choice of Column Material

The most successful liquid phases employed for triglyceride analysis have been the stable, high temperature silicones such as SE-30, OV-1, and J x R.

In order to obtain reasonable retention times, short (less than 2 feet) low liquid loaded columns (generally less than 3%) must be employed. This places strict requirements on the solid support material., any exposed, active sites on the surface of the support will result in tailing and distorted peaks. The support material may be deactivated using the method of Horning *et al.* (1959), Mc Nair and Bonelli (1967). In this method, the active sites, generally thought to be silanol (-Si-OH) groups are converted to the non-reactive trimethyl silyl (-Si-O-Si $(CH_3)_3$) derivatives. Deactivated materials recommended for lipid analysis are Aeropak 30, high performance chromosorb W and Gas chrom Q. A mesh size of 100/120 is usually employed. Triglyceride analyses demand temperature programmed operation to 350°C. Extremely high carrier gas flow rates (approximately 40-100 ml/min) are required. There is a need of a larger (>0.030") internal diametre flame tip.

Conditions for Coconut oil Triglycerides

2′ x 1/8′ S.S. 2% XJR on 100/120 chrom. W., Temperature program at 4°C/min. from 180°C to 340°C : Injector Temperature = 350°C : Detector Temperature = 350°C : 1.28 x 10^{-12} a.f.s. : Carrier Gas. N_2 at 125 ml/min. : Sample = 1μl (10% in ether).

Conditions for Triglycerides in Butter

2′ x 1/8″ S.S., 2% OV-1 on 100/120 chrom. W., High performance Temperature program at 8°C/min from 180°C to 340°C : Injector Temperature 375°C : Detector Temperature = 375°C : Carrier gas = Helium at 100ml/min. Sample 1.0 μl (10% in ether).

Conditions for Normal Serum Neutral Lipids

2′ x 1/8′ S.S. 3% EGSS-X on Aeropak 30, 80/100 mesh, Temperature program at 2°C/min. from 150°C to 205°C : Carrier Gas. N_2 at 30 ml/min.

(*Note* : The above packed column may be purchased from M/s varian aerograph 2700 mitchell drive/walnut Greek/California 94598, U.S.A.)

Vitamins Assay by Gas Chromatography

Recently several workers (Vecchi *et al.,* 1967., Richter *et al.,* 1967; Vecchi and Kaiser, 1967; Avioli & Lee, 1966) have established procedures for the estimation of vitamins as derivates by gas chromatography.

Sample Preparation

The successful gas chromatographic analysis of vitamins is only possible by converting the substances into volatile derivatives such as e.g. trimethyl silyl (TMS) derivatives.

Hexamethyldisilazane (HMDS) and trimethylchlorosilane (TMCS) in pyridine are used as reagents.

Procedure

To 1 mg dry vitamin 1 ml pyridine (dried over KOH), 0.1 ml HMDS and 0.05 ml TMCS are added and the mixture reacted at 50°C for about 30 minutes.

Gas Chromatography Conditions

1. For Vitamin B_1, B_6, and D_2 - TMS Derivatives

Column : 6′ x 2 mm id. glass, 3% SE-30 on Aeropak 30, 100/120 mesh

Vitamin Assay by Gas Chromatography

Conditions	**Vit. B_1**	**Vit. B_6**	**Vit. D_2**
Temp. Column	230°C	180°C	270°C
Temp. Inj/Det.	260°C	250°C	300°C
Carrier gas N_2ml/min	30	30	30
Detector FID ml/min	H_2 = 30 air = 300	H_2 = 30 air = 300	H_2 = 30 air = 300
Sensitivity, afs	8 x 10^{-11}	128 x 10^{-11}	32 x 10^{-11}
Sample size	0.2µl	0.5µl	0.5µl
Chart speed inch/h	10	10	10

2. For Vitamin C

Column	:	6′ x 2 mm id glass, 3% OV-17 on chrom W-100/ 120 mesh
Temperature	:	Column : 150°C isothermal Inj/Det. : 200°C
Carrier gas	:	N_2, 30 ml/min.
Detector	:	FID (H_2 = 30 min/min., air = 300 ml/min.)
Sensitivity	:	64 x 10^{11} afs
Sample size	:	0.1 µl
Chart speed	:	10^{11}/h

3. For Vitamin D_2

Column	:	6′ x 2 mm id glass, 3% SE-30, Aeropak 30, 100/ 120 mesh
Temperature	:	Column : 270°C isothermal programmed Inj/Det. : 300°C
Carrier gas	:	N_2, 30 ml/min.
Detector	:	FID (H_2 = 30 ml/min., air = 300 ml/min.)
Sensitivity	:	64 x 10^{11} afs
Sample size	:	0.5 µl
Chart speed	:	10^{11}/h

(*Note* : Above packed columns may be obtained from M/s varian Aerograph AG, Pelikan Weg 2, 4003 Basel/Switzerland).

Analysis of Carbohydrates by Gas Chromatography

Sample Preparation

The successful gas chromatographic analysis of sugars depends upon their conversion into stable, volatile derivates. The most widely used derivatization technique is the conversion of sugars into their trimethylsilyl (TMS) derivatives, utilizing as reagents nexamethyl - disilazane (HMDS) and trimethylcholorosilane (TMCS) in pyridine.

$$\text{-OH HMDS/TMCS/PYRIDINE-O-Si} \begin{cases} CH_3 \\ CH_3 \\ CH_3 \end{cases}$$

Procedure

To 10 mg dry carbohydrate 1 ml pyridine (dried over KOH). 0.2 ml HMDS and 0.1 ml TMCS are added and the mixture reacted at 50°C. The reaction is completed afterabout 10 minutes.

Sample (TMS - Derivatives) :

I:
1. L (+) Rhamnose
2. Xylose
3. D-Mannose
4. D (+) Gallactose
5. D (+) Glucose

II:
1. D (-) Arabinose
2. Xylose
3. D (-) Fructose
4. L-Sorbose
5. D (+) Glucose

Gas Chromatographic Conditions

A.	Column	:	6′ x 1/4″ glass, 3% SE-30, Aeropak 30, 100/120 mesh
	Temperature	:	Column : 170°C isothermal programmed Inj/Det. : 250°C
	Carrier gas	:	N_2, 30 ml/min.
	Detector	:	FID (H_2 = 30 ml/min., air = 300 ml/min.)
	Sensitivity	:	128 x 10^{-11} afs
	Sample size	:	0.2 µl
	Chart speed	:	10^{11}/h
B.	Column	:	6′ x 1/4″ glass, 3% OV-17 on chrom W-HP 100/120 mesh
	Temperatures	:	Column : 130°C isothermal programmed Inj/Det. : 250°C
	Carrier gas	:	N_2, 30 ml/min.
	Detector	:	FID (H_2 = 30 ml/min., air = 300 ml/min.)
	Sensitivity	:	64 x 10^{-11} afs
	Sample size	:	0.2 µl
	Chart speed	:	10^{11}/h

☞ Note

The above columns may be obtained from M/s Varian Aerograph AG, Pelikanweg 2, 4002 Basel/Switzerland.

Pesticides Residue Analysis in Biological Samples

The development of the ultrasensitive Electron Capture Detector and the selective phosphorus detector have made gas chromatography an important tool for the pesticide analyst. *Since most pesticides are "Sensitive" compounds which are easily decomposed on hot metal surfaces, therefore a total glass system is mandatory for their successful quantitative analysis.*

We may analyse the residues of the following pesticides

a.	*Lindane*	*b.*	*Aldrin*
c.	*Dieldrin*	*d.*	*Heptachlor*
e.	*P, P′ DDT*	*f.*	*Tedion*
g.	*Parathion*		

Gas Chromatographic Conditions

Column	:	6′ x 1/4″ glass, 5% DOW-11, on chrom W-AW / DMCS, 80/100 mesh
Temperature	:	Column : 180°C/195°C isothermal Inj/Det. : 210°C/ 215°C
Carrier gas	:	N_2, 30 ml/min.
Detector	:	EC
Sensitivity	:	64 x 10^{-10} x 10^{-10} afs
Sample size	:	1 µl/0.1 µl
Chart speed	:	10^{11}/h

☞ Note

The above packed column is available from M/s Varian Aerograph, AG Pelikanweg 2, 4002 Basel/Switzerland. We may further study the publication by Bonelli, E.J. 1966. Pesticides Residue analysis Handbook, Varian Arograph, Walnut Creek, Cal.

List of Indian Firms Engaged in the Manufacturing of Gas Chromatograph

1. M/s Netel chromatographs-manufacturer of Omega gas chromatograph supplier's address - M/s Universal Ferro and Allied Chemicals Ltd., Liberty Building Sir, Vithaladas Thackersey Marg (New Marine Lines) Mumbai (pin code 400 020) - India.
2. M/s Nucon Engineers, New Delhi (India).
3. M/s Toshniwal Brothers (P) Ltd., 3E/8, Jhandewalan Extension, New Delhi - 110 055 (India).

References

Appleby, A.J., Mayne, J.E.O. (1967). *J. Gas Chromatography.*, 5 : 266.

Astrup, H.N., Halvorsen, E.S. and Lindstad, P. (1973). Instt. Animal Nutrition, Agric. University of Norway, ÅS-NLH, Norway (*Personal Communication*).

Avioli, L.V and Lee, S.W. (1966). *Anal. Biochem.*, 16 : 193.

Barron, E.J. and Hanahan, D.J. (1958). *J.Biol.Chem.*, 231 : 493.

Baumgardt, B.R. (1964). Practical observation on the quantitative analysis of free volatile fatty acids (VFA) In Aqueous solution by Gas liquid chromatography, Bulletin Department of Dairy Sci., Univ., Wisconsin (USA).

Bills, D.D., Khatri, L.L and Day, E.A. (1963). *J.Dairy Sci.*, 12 : 1342.

Brydia, L.E. and Persenger, H.E. (1967). *Anal. Chem.*, 39 : 1318.

Brydia, L.E. and Willeboordse, F. (1968). *Anal. Chem.*, 40: 110.

Clarke, D.D., Wilk, S. and Gitlow, S.E. (1966). *J. Gas chromatography.*, 4 : 310.

Cliffe, A.J., Berridge, N.J. and Westgarth, D.R. (1973). *J.Chromatography.*, 78 : 333.

Coltyn, B.G. and Boucque, C.V. (1968). *J. Agr. Food Chem.*, 16 : 105

Craig, B.M., Tulloch, A.P., Murty, N.L. (1963). *J.Am.Oil Chemist's, Soc.*, 40 : 61

Creech, B.G., and Sewell, B.W. (1962). *Anal. Biochem.*, 3 : 119

Darbre, A. and Blau, K. (1963). *Biochem.* J., 88 : 8 p.

de Man, J.M. (1964). *J. Dairy Sci.* 47 : 546

de Man, J.M. (1967). *Lab. Practice.*, 16 : 150

Doelle, H.W. (1969). *J. Chromatography.*, 39 : 398.

Dove, R.A. (1967). *Analyt. Chem.*, 39 : 1188.

Entenmon *et al.* (1961). *J. American Oil Chemist's Soc.*, 38 : No. 10

Erwin, E.S., Marco, G.J., Emery, E.M. (1961). *J. Dairy Sci.*, 44 : 1768.

Fillerup, D.L., and Mead, J.F. (1963). *Proc.Soc. Exptl. Biol. Med.*, 83 : 574.

Folch, J., Lees, M., and Stanley, G.H.S. (1957). *J. Biol.Chem.*, 226 : 497.

Fryer, F.H., Ormand, W.L and Crump, G.B., (1960). *J. American Oil Chemist's Soc.*, 37 : 589.

Gander, G.W., Jensen, R.G. and Sampugna, J. (1962). *J. Dairy Sci.*, 45 : 323.

Gehrke, C.W. and Shahrokhi, F. (1966). *Anal. Biochem.*, 15 : 97.

Hogen, P. and Black, W. (1965). *Can. J. Biochem.*, 43 : 309

Hammarstrand, K. (1966). *Gas chromatographic analysis of steroids*, Varian Aerograph, Switzerland.

Hammarstand, K. (1967). *Gas chromatographic analysis of steroids*, Varian Aerograph, Swizerland.

Hirsoh, J., and Ahrens, E.H., Jr. (1958). *J. Biol. Chem.*, 233 : 311.

Horning, M.G., Knox, L.L., Dalgliesh, C.E., Horning, E.C. (1966). *Analyt. Biochem.*, 17 : 244.

Irvine, W.J. and Saxby, M.J. (1969). *Phytochemistry.*, 8 : 473.

James, A.T and Martin, A.J.P. (1951). *Biochem. J. Proc.*, 48 : VII.

James, A.T. and Martin, A.J.P. (1952). *Analyst*, 77 : 915.

Jensen, R.G., Quinn, J.G., Carpentre, D.L. and Sampugna, J. (1967). *J. Dairy Sci.*, 50 : 120.

Jones, E.P., Danson, V.L. (1965). *J. Ami.Oil Chemist's Soc.*, 42 : 121.

Kirkland, J.J. (1960). *Anal Chem.*, 32 : 1388.

Krishna, G. and Ekern, A. (1974a). *Z. Tierphysiol., Tierernährg. U. Futter mittelkde*, 33: 275.

Krishna, G. and Ekern, A. (1974b). *Z. Tierphysiol. Tierernährg U. Futtermittelkde*, 33: 281.

Krishna, G. and Ekern, A. (1974c). *Z. Tierphysiol. Tiernährg U. Futtermittelkde*, 33: 323.

Lamkin, W.M. and Gehrke, C.W. (1965). *Analyt. Chem.*, 37 : 383

Lessard, J.R., Briggs, R.A. and Scalelti, J.V. (1961). *Canadian J. Plant Sci.*, 41 : 507.

Mahadevan, V. and Zieve, L. (1969). *J. Lipid Res.*, 10 : 338.

Martin, A.J.B and Synge, R.L.M. (1941). *Biochem. J.*, 35 : 1358.

Martin, H.F. and Driscoll, J.L. (1966). *Anal Chem.*, 38 : 345.

Mc Curdy, W.H. and Reiser, R.W. (1966). *Anal Chem.*, 38 : 795.

Metcalfe, L.D. and Schmitz, A.A. (1961). *Anal Chem.*, 33 : 363.

Metcalfe, L.D. and Schwitz, A.A., Pelka, J.R. (1966). *Analyt. Chem.*, 38 : 514.

Morrisette, R.A. and Link, W.E. (1965). *J. Gas Chromatography.*, 5 : 67.

Napier, E.A., Jr. (1963). *Analyt. Chem.*, 35 : 1294.

Parodi, P.W. (1967). Austr. *J. Dairy Technology.*, Sept., Issue : 144.

Perry, T.L., Hansen, S., Diamond, S., Bulles, B., Mok, C. and Melancon, S.B. (1970). *Clin. Chem. Acta.*, 29 : 369.

Ramsey, W. (1905). *Proc. Roy. Soc.*, A76 : 111.

Ramsey, C. and Demigue, C. (1974). *Biochem. J.*, 141 : 85.

Richter, W., Vecchi, M., Vetter, W. and Walther, W. (1967). *Helve.*, 50 : 364.

Ross, J.P. and Kitts, W.D. (1971). *J. Dairy Sci.*, 54 : 1824.

Rouser, G., Kritchevsky, G., Heller, D. and Lieber, E.J. (1963). *J. Amer. Oil Chemist's Soc.*, 40: 425.

Rouser, G., Bauman, A.J., Kirtchevsky, G., Heller, D., O'Brien, J.S. (1961). *J. Amer. Oil Chemist's Soc.*, 38 : 544.

Sampugna, J., Pitas, R.E. and Jensen, R.G. (1966). *J. Dairy Sci.,* 49 : 1462.

Schmekel, J. (1966). Lantbrukshogskolane Annaler., 32 : 255.

Simmonds, P.G., Pettitt, B.C., Zlatkis, A. (1967). *Analyt. Chem.,* 39 : 163.

Simkins, K.L., Jr. (1965). Relationship of blood and rumen metabolites to food intake in ruminants. Ph.D. Thesis., University of Wisconsin (USA).

Stenvenson, G.W. (1996). *Anal. Chem.,* 38 : 1948.

Szymanski, H.A. (1964). *Biomedical applications of gas chromatography.* Plenum Press, New York.

Tswett, M. (1906). *Ber. dent. botan. Gas.,* 24 : 316.

Veechi, M. *et al.* (1967). *Helve.,* 50 : 1243

Veechi, M. and Kaiser, K. (1967). *J. Chromatography,* 26 : 22.

Wells, W.W., Katagi, T., Bentley, R., Sweely, C.C. (1964). *Biochim. et Biophys. Acta,* 82 : 408

Wiseman, H.G. and Irvin, H.M. (1957). *J. Agr. Food Chem.,* 5 : 213

Wycoff, H.D. and Parsons, J. (1957). *Science* 125 : 347.

Zlatkis, A., Zak, B., Boyle, A.J. (1953). *J. Lab Clin. Med.,* 41 : 486.

Text books and bulletins for further study

Ambrose, D. (1971). *Gas chromatography,* 2nd Edn., Butterworths.

Angele, H.P. (1970). *Four language technical dictionary of chromatography* Pergamon Press, USA.

Burchfield, H.P. and Storrs, E.E. (1962). *Biochemical applications of gas chromatography.* Academic Press.

Crippen, R.C. (1973). *Identification of organic compounds with the aid of gas chromatography,* Mc Graw Hill

Grab, R.L. (1977). *Modern Practice of gas chromatography,* John Wiley's Sons. U.S.A.

Jennings, W. (1978). *Gas chromatography with glass capillary columns.* Academic Press.

Jones, R.A. (1970). *An introduction to Gas-liquid chromatography.* Academic Press.

Laderer, E. and Laderer, M. (1957). *Chromatography.* Elsvier.

Mc Foden, W.H. (1973). *Techniques of combined gas chromatography/Mass spectrometry applications in organic analysis.* John Wiley & Sons.

Mc Nair, H.M. and Bonelli, E.J. (1969). *Basic gas chromatography.* 5th Edn., Consolidated Printers, Berkeley, California, Varian aerograph, Switzerland.

Morris, C.J.O.R. and Morris, P. (1964). *Separation methods in biochemistry.* Pitman.

Novak, J. (1975). *Quantitative analysis by Gas Chromatography,* Marcel Dekker.

Pethison, J.B. (1973). *A programmed introduction to gas - liquid chromatography,* Heyden and Sons, Ltd.

Sevcik, J. (1975). *Detectors in gas chromatography,* Elsevier, USA.

Smith, I. (1969). *Chromatographic and electrophoretic techniques (2 volumes).* Heinemaun.

Walber, J.Q. *et al.* (1975). *Chromatographic systems, maintenance and trouble shooting of gas chromatographs and liquid chromatographs,* 2nd Edn. Academic Press.

Chapter - 58

Atomic Absorption Spectrophotometry

Introduction

The first application of atomic absorption spectra to chemical analysis was made just over 100 years ago by Kirchoff (1860), who demonstrated the presence of various elements in the solar atmosphere. He and Bunsen, demonstrated shortly afterwards that atomic spectra, whether in emission or absorpiton, could be the basis of a powerful method of chemical analysis. Walsh (1955) recognized the potential advantages of the absorption method over emission method and devised simple and versatile apparatus applicable to the routine analysis of solutions of a wide range of elements. Alkemade and Milatz (1955) published papers describing the application of atomic absorption techniques to chemical analysis.

Principle

When a mist of droplets from a liquid sample is brought into a flame, the elements of the sample will affect the light emitted and light absorbed by the flame. Both effects may be used for the determination of the elements of the sample. The flame causes the molecules to dissociate into atoms. The emission comes about by heat exaltation of atoms, while absorption of light comes about by exalation of atoms by light. The remitted light from absorption (the resonance light) is emitted in all directions and thus escape detection by the photocell. *In emisssion photometry, light emitted is proportional to concentration, in absorption the "optical density" is proportional to concentration. The general advantage of absorption is that less heat is required, and less disturbance is included in the measurements, compared with emission spectrophotometry. However, the alkali metals are easily exaltated by flame and are determined by emission. Zinc and magnesium are particularly suited for absorption. Calcium may be determined both ways.*

Limits of Detection (in ppm)

Element	Absorption	Emission
Ca	0.1	0.05
K	-	0.02
Na	-	0.001
Mg	0.01	1
Zn	0.02	-
Cu	0.10	0.5
Fe	0.15	2

The instrumentation used for atomic absorption is similar to that used for flame emission, but the mechanism of atomic absorption is essentially the inverse of that for the emission technique. *In emission, the excited atoms emit radiation of characteristic wavelengths., in atomic absorption those same atoms in the non-excited, non ionized, ground states are capable of absorbing light at characteristic wavelengths.* Typically, the sample is converted to an atomic vapour by spraying the sample in solution into a flame. Since excitation of the component atoms of the sample is not required for atomic absorption, the flame temperatures needed are often lower than required for flame emission. In order to achieve proper dissociation, the design of the burner is very critical, and much research has been devoted to improve burner performance.

Parts of Atomic Absorption Spectrophotometer

1. *A light source emitting, under conditions which ensure the production of extremely sharp lines, the spectrum of the element to be determined.*
2. *A means of producing an atomic vapour of the sample to be analysed.*
3. *A wavelength selector to separate the resonance line required.*
4. *A detector, amplifier and readout system (metre or recorder).*

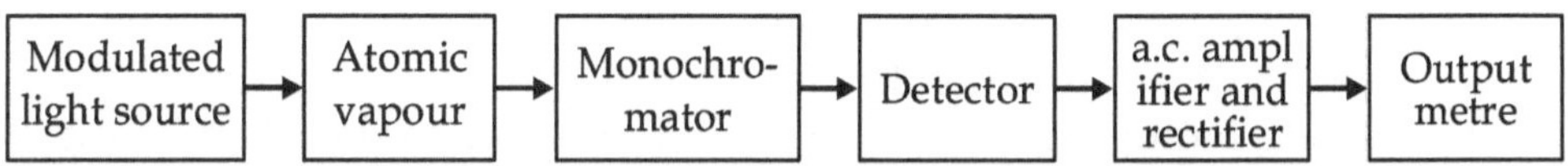

Schematic Diagram Illustrating Operation of an Atomic Absorption Spectrophotometer

A resonance line of some intensity is attenuated when passed through the flame containing atoms of the same element as the cathode of the generator lamp. A monchromator is used to isolate that line or wavelength from the remainder of the emitted radiation. The intensity of the radiation is measured with and without the sample to obtain a reading in either per cent absorption or absorbance, and the concentration of the element of interest is determined by comparing that reading to one obtained for a standard or series of standards. Many atomic absorption instruments can be calibrated to read directly in concentration through the use of absorbance readout and continuously variable scale expansion.

The typical design of an atomic absorption spectrophotometer utilising the single beam and double beam system is shown in Fig. 1.

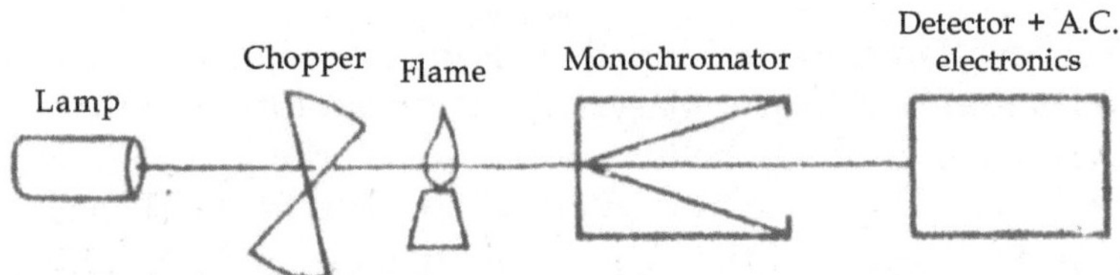

Fig. 1 : Single beam a.c. system. A chopper distinguished flame emission for lamp emission.

The single beam instrument is the more common design for atomic absorption spectrophotometers. A mechanical or electrical chopping of the lamp emission is used to distinguish between the emission generated by the flame and that emitted by the lamp. Chopping of the lamp is in phase with the tuned lock in, a.c. electronics.

Double beam instruments minimise the effect of lamp emission variations, detector sensitivity and electronic gain Fig. 2.

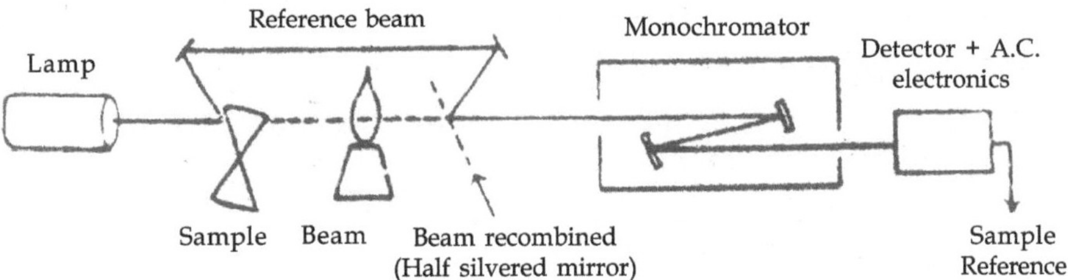

Fig. 2 : Double beam a.c. system. The effect of variations in lamp emission, detector sensitivity and electronic gain are cancelled out by this system.

The chopper shown here is a rotating sector mirror which alternately passes the hollow cathode lamp emission through the reference and sample channels. Both beams pass through the monochromater, which is used to isolate light of the wavelength of interest, and to the photomultiplier detector, which generated an electrical signal proportional to the intensity of the incident light. The electrical signals passes to the tube, lock in amplifier which will amplify only those signals with the same frequency as the chopped lamp emission.

Burners

Usually there are two types of burners (1) "Total consumption" of diffusion burner using for flame emission work, (2) the "premix" type in which sample, fuel and oxidant are mixed in a chamber before entering the flame in the total consumption burner, the fuel oxidant and sample are all passed through separate channels to a single opening from which the flame emerges.

The premix burner provides intimate mixing of sample and flame gases and a laminar flow flame. In addition, there is little dependence of absorption upon position of the sampling capillary in the sample solution, with the premix burner. It is possible to obtain better linearity of working curves and fewer interferences, and to determine more metals than with the total consumption burner. This is due to the fact that the premix flame is laminar and contains no large, unburnable sample dropletes, while the total consumption flame is turbulent and includes large droplets.

Name of Commercially Available Atomic Absorption Equipment

Manufacturers and Catalog No.	Types of instrument
Hilger and Watts. H909.	Single beam unmodulated
Perkin-Elmer 214	Double beam modulated
Jarrell Ash	Single beam unmodulated
Beckman	Double beam
Varian	Double beam
Techtron	Single beam, modulated

Addresses of Suppliers

Atomic absorption instrument are made under license to CSIRO, Australia, by several manufacturers.

1. Hilger and Watts Ltd., London, England
2. Perkin Elmer Corporation., Norwalk, Conn.

   Sole Selling Agents Blue Star N.Y. Blue Star Ltd. Bhandari Horse, 91 Nehru Place, New Delhi - 110024, India

3. Jarrell-Ash Company, Newtonvile, Mass.
4. Messrs. Jobin-Yvon, Areueil (Seine) France.
5. Techtron Pty Ltd., Melbourne, Australia.
6. Beckman Instruments Inc., Filerton California, USA, Sole Selling Agent in India is M/s. Systronics (P) Ltd., Baroda Industrial Estate. Ahmedabad, Gujarat (India).

Atomic Absorption Spectrophotometry vis-a-vis Flame Photometry

The atomic absorption method requires the use of resonance lines, and for the most elements there is little choice of line if high sensitivity is required. In flame photometry, particularly if a hot flame is used, there is sometimes a choice of lines, and some metals such as the alkaline earths form compounds in the flame which emit measurble band spectra. Since the non-metals mostly have their resonance lines in the vacuum ultravoilet (i.e., below 2000 A) special difficulties arise in both techniques. The limit of detection in flame photometry is set by the ability to distinguish the line emitted by the metal from the background emission of the flame. *In atomic absorption spectrophotometry, the limiting factor is the measurement of the small change in the intensity of the sharp line source caused by absorption by the metal atoms in the flame, which in practice is set by the noise level of the sharp line source.*

At present, flame photometry is slightly more sensitive than the atomic absorption method for strongly emtting metals such as lithium and sodium, at any rate in the absence of substance which would increase the background emission of the flame. The sensitivity of the atomic absorption technique, however, should improve considerably the development of double beam methods to overcome instability of the sharp line source and of multipass methods to increase the effective absorption path length in the flame.

Interferences

The three principal interferences can be grouped as chemical (or codensed phase), ionization and matrix bulb, viscocity interferences.

Chemical Interferences

The main reason for this type of interferences is the formation of stable compounds by the element of interest and some anion. This type of interference can be overcome by the addition of an excess of a "completing cation" or "releasing agent' to the sample solution. An alternate procedure is to use a higher temperature flame, one which has sufficient energy to break down the compound formed by the element of interest and the interfering anion.

Ionization Interferences

The generation of ions decreases the number of atoms and reduced atomic absorption and emission. This type of interference is most severe with high temperature flames such as nitrous oxide-acetylene. To overcome ionization interferences, a large excess of an easily ionized metal, usually potassium, is added to both standard and sample.

Matrix Interferences

Samples containing high dissolved solids concentrations or high acid concentrations will have different viscocities, etc., in comparision to simple aqueous standards. The problem can be solved by additional dilution of the sample, if possbile, or by matching the concentration of the major sample constituents in the standard.

Nebulizing Condition

Since the purpose of the nebulizer in both emission and absorption work is to inject into the flame a fine cloud of droplets of fairly uniform size, from which the metal to be determined can be efficiently converted to its atomic vapour. The spraying conditions are common to both techniques.

Preparation and Handling of Samples

Most determinations of metals in biological fluids such as blood serum and urine can be carried out on a diluted sample containing, if necessary a suitable material to suppress interferences, through sometimes it is desirable to remove proteins by precipitation with trichloroacetic acid (Willis, 1960). For other animal tissues and for plant materials, ashing is required. Wet ashing, using sulphuric nitric-perchloric acid mixtures, has been used by David (1958) and by Allam (1961) for plant materials, but for many metals dry ashing followed by solution of the ash in a few drops of hydrochloric acid is satisfactory. *Volatile elements such as antimony, arsenic, mercury and thallium, however require wet ashing under reflux.*

The alkaline earth metals seem to be quantitatively recoverable by dry ashing without critical control of the conditions, though it has recently been pointed out (Grove *et al.*, 1961) that prolonged heating above 550°C causes loss of sodium and potassium chlorides.

The process of wet chemical digestion of biological materials for mineral analysis is described elsewhere by author in volume I of this compendium.

Dry Ashing Procedure

This method is suitable for the determination of Ca, Cu, Fe, Li, Mg, Mn, K, Na, and Zn in plant tissue. We should try to avoid the contamination of sample by dust during drying and from grinding and sieving machinery. We should preserve the samples in tightly stoppered bottles and these should be stored in a dust free chamber.

We may follow the procedure of preparing mineral extract as already mentioned in the chapter entitiled, *"Calcium in biological material" and "Phosphorus in biological materials"* of this compendium. It will be advisable to use 5N HCl for preparing mineral extract, ash mixed with 5N HCl should be boiled on hot plate, but over heating should be avoided. Weigh about 1 g materials, ash at 550°C in muffle furnace for over night and make up the volume of mineral extract upto 100 ml in a volumetric flask, stopper the flask and seal with aluminium foil, keep it in a dust free place.

Use of Chelating Agents in Calcium and Magnesium Analysis

It has been observed that the presence of phosphate culminate some interferences in the calcium and magnesium assay. Therefore following chemicals may be used so as to avoid these interferences for getting accurate results of calcium and magnesium concentration in biological samples.

1. Lanthanum Chloride, 20 g/litre Solution

Weigh 25 g of lanthanum oxide in one litre volumetric flask and add 75 ml of hydrochloric acid. Allow to cool and make up the volume with distilled water upto the mark. Use 20 ml of this solution in 100 ml of calcium standard solution containing 10µg of calcium per millilitre. Some laboratories use Lanthanum at 1% (W/V) concentration, however we may check the recovery results using calcium standard solutions.

2. Oxine (8-hydroxyquinoline), 0.4% Solution

It is a buff colured crystalline compound almost insoluble in water, but readily dissolves in alcohol, acetone and acetic acid. It forms insoluble complexes with a number of metals. Dissolve 4 gram oxine in 25 ml acetic acid and make up the volume up to one litre in volumetric flask using distilled water. Stopper the flask and keep it in a dust free place. We should use 5 ml of this solution with 1 ml calcium standard solution containing 10 mg per cent calcium.

Measurement Conditions to Maintain Temperature of the Flame

It has been experienced that calcium and magnesium can be activated only at much higher temperatures and therefore require acetylene-oxygen or hydrogen-oxygen flames.

Pickett and Koirtyohann (1968, 1969) have described in detail the use of the nitrous oxide-acetylene flame for emission analysis.

Standard Solutions for Major and Minor Minerals

1. Calcium

2.497 grams calcium carbonate (dried at 105°C) is dissolved in 5 ml concentrated hydrochloric acid, and diluted to one litre. This will be 1000 ppm or 0.1 per cent solution. (Formula for one litre stock solution). 1 ml of this standard corresponds to 1 mg of calcium.

2. Cobalt

(a) Dissolve 1.0000 g cobalt in 1:8 HCl (Final concentration approx. 0.5 per cent). This represent 1000 ppm or 0.1 per cent solution.

(b) Formula for one litre stock solution

Dissolve 4.7694 grams cobalt sulphate ($COSO_4.7H_2O$) in distilled water, add 1 ml of concentrated sulphuric acid and make up the volume to one litre. Take one millilitre of this solution and make up volume to one litre with water in a graduated flask. This solution contains one microgram of cobalt per millilitre.

3. Copper

(a) Dissolve 1.0000 g copper in 1:2 HNO_3 (final HNO_3 concentration approx 1 per cent)

This represent 1000 ppm 0.1 per cent solution.

(b) *Formula for one litre stock solution*

Dissolve 0.393 grms cupric sulphate pentahydrate ($CuSO_4$, $5H_2O$) of analytical grade in distilled water, add a few drops of concentrated sulphuric acid and make up the volume to one litre in a graduated flask. Shake well. Pipette out 10 ml of this solution into a one litre graduated flask and make up the volume. This solution contains one microgram of copper per millilitre.

4. Iron

(a) Dissolve 1.0000 g Fe in 1:2 HCl.

(Final HCl concentration, approx 1 per cent)

This will give 1000 ppm or 0.1 per cent solution.

(b) Formula for one litre solution

Dissolve 0.7022 grams of ferrous ammonium sulphate ($FeSO_4$ $(NH_4)_2$ SO_4, $6H_2O$) in 100 ml of water, add 5 ml of concentrated sulphuric acid warm slightly and add potassium permanganate solution (approximately 0.1 N) drop by drop until the solution shows a slight pink colouration. Make up the volume to one litre in a graduated flask, Pipette 10 ml of this solution into a one litre graduated flask, add 100 ml hydrogen peroxide solution and make up the volume with water. This solution contains one microgram of iron per ml.

5. Magnesium

(a) Dissolve 1 mg in 1:100 hydrochloric acid (final HCl concentration approx. 0.5 per cent)

This will represent 1000 ppm or 0.1 percent solution

(b) *Formula For for one litre stock solution.*

Dissolve 40.4 grams of magnesium ammonium phosphate ($Mg\ NH_4$. PO_4. $6H_2O$) in 0.1 N hydrochloric acid and make up to one litre. Dilute 1 ml of the stock standard to 200 ml with distilled water. This solution contains 0.02 mg magnesium per millilitre.

6. Manganese

(a) Dissolve 1.5824 grams MnO_2 in concentrated hydrochloric acid, evaporate to dryness, dissolve residue in one litre water. This will represent 1000 ppm or 0.1 per cent solution.

(b) *Formula for one litre stock solution*

Dissolve 0.575 gram of dry potassium permanganate in about 50 ml of water in a beaker suitable size. Add 40 ml of concentrated sulphuric acid and reduce the permanganate by careful addition of sodium metabisulphite solution until the manganese solution just becomes colourless. Oxidise the excess sulphuric acid in the hot solution by the addition of a little nitric acid. Cool and transfer the solution quantitatively to a two litre graduated flask. Make up the volume and store the solution in a glass stoppered reagent bottle. This solution contains 0.1 mg of manganese per millilitre.

7. Potassium

Dissolve 1.9067 g potassium chloride in one litre water. This will represent 1000 ppm or 0.1 per cent solution.

8. Sodium

Dissolve 2.5421 grams sodium chloride in one litre water. This will represent 1000 ppm or 0.1 per cent solution.

9. Zinc

(a) Dissolve 4.5490 grams zinc nitrate hexahydrate Zn $(NO_3)_2.6H_2O$ in one litre water. This will represent 1000 ppm or 0.1 per cent solution.

(b) Dissolve 4.3987 grams $ZnSO_4.7H_2O$ in one litre water. This will represent 1000 ppm or 0.1 per cent solution.

Combined Standard for Ca, Mg, Na and K

Weigh 8.39 g Nacl, 0.286 g Kcl, 0.250 g $CaCO_3$ and 0.167 g $MgCl_2$. $6H_2O$ separately. Dissolve all the chemicals in one litre 0.1 N HCl. This combined standard mixture will represent 10 mg per cent Ca, 2 mg per cent Mg, 330 mg per cent Na and 15 mg percent K.

Role of "Emission and Absorption" Phenomenon in Mineral Assay

We should always remember that Ca, Na and K may be assayed directly without using any cathode lamp by emission spectroscopy while on the other hand minerals like Mg, Zn, Cu and Fe are always assayed by absorption spectroscopy where cathode lamp is needed.

Judging the accuracy of analytical procedures for mineral analysis by atomic absorption spetrophotometry.

Willis (1963) in the book entitled *"Methods of biochemical analysis"* suggested the following criteria for this purpose.

1. *The results obtained by atomic absorption spectrophotometry should agree, over the widest possible range of sample composition, with those of a reliable and well tested alternative method.*
2. *Different variations of the atomic absorption technique should give the same results.*
3. *Measurements on different quantities of the sample should yield the same final result in terms of concentration.*
4. *Known quantities of metal added to the sample should be quantitatively recoverable.*
5. *The standard deviation of the method should be statisfactory for the purpose for which the analysis is required.*

Assay of Individual Element by Atomic Absorption Spectrophotometry

Some 40 elements, all metals have their resonance lines in the spectral range 2000-10, 000 A, and most of these can be atomized in the flame. For the metalloid and non metallic elements the resonance lines lie below 2000 A and the use of the atomic absorption method is more difficult.

Magnesium, Calcium and Zinc in Biological Materials

If the mineral samples are soluble in HCl, 1 g of the solid is dissolved in 7 ml of 3N HCl and diluting to 50 ml. Some samples are first dissolved in 2ml of concentrated HNO_3 and 7 ml of concentrated HCl and evaporated to dryness, the residue is then redissolved in 7 ml of 3 N HCl and diluted to 50 ml. Many of the samples had to be further diluted to put the magnesium content within the analytical range.

Magnesium in Feed Samples

Two grams samples are ashed at 600°C until carbon free. They are then dissolved in 2 ml of concentrated HCl, evaporated to dryness, and redissolved in 2 ml of 3 N HCl and diluted to volume. Feed samples can also be prepared for analysis bydigestion with HNO_3 as described for tissue samples.

Magnesium in Tissue Samples

The tissue is weighed and digested in 2.3 ml of concentrated HNO_3 per g of tissue. This is done directly in 50 ml Kjeldahl flasks (calibrated at 50 ml) to avoid the need to transfer the solution. An aliquot of this solution is then diluted to the appropriate volume to put the magnesium in the range from 0.2 to 1.2 ppm. The diluent used supplied 0.1 per cent. $SrCl_2$ $6H_2O$ and sufficient HNO_3 to bring the concentration of HNO_3 to 0.1 N. The magnesium standards are prepared in the same solution.

Calcium in Feed and Tissue Samples

It is possible to prepare samples for calcium analysis by digestion with HNO_3, as described for magnesium, however, HNO_3 influences calcium absorption and it is advisable to adjust the HNO_3 concentration in both samples and standards to about 0.5 N where small changes in acid concentration do not measurably influence calcium absorption. Since HCl has very little influence on calcium absorption, dry ashing in a muffle furnace followed by dissolving the ash in HCl is a preferred method of sample preparation. The addition of 1 per cent strontium as $SrCl_2$. 6 H_2O to the final solution is found to reduce to less than 1 per cent the interference due to the phosphate present in most biological samples. A modification of the oxalate precipitation method described by willis (1961) is found to be suitable for the determination of small amounts of calcium in urine. A small amount of strontium is added to the urine samples prior to precipitation of the calcium by oxalate. The combined strontium and calcium oxalates gave sufficient precipitate to be conveniently separated by centrifugation. The same technique could be used to concentrate small levels of calcium in tissue samples. The use of trichloroacetic acid to precipitate proteins from blood plasma, as described by Willis (1967) gives precise results and good recoveries of calcium added to blood plasma.

It has been experienced that phosphate will reduce the apparent absorption of a solution of calcium and that the addition of strontium (David, 1958) or lanthanum (Willis 1960) will reduce or remove this inhibition. The additon of 10,000 ppm (1%) strontium will protect the calcium analysis up to phosphate levels of 100 ppm. All determinations are made against standards that contained an equal amount of strontium.

Example : Suppose a sample contained 5 ppm calcium and 500 ppm phosphorus, marked A. is the unknown. It is assumed that the sample B is **sample A** to which has been added 10 ppm calcium. The apparent calcium is 4.1 ppm using the standards. The addition of 10 ppm calcium produced an increase in absorbance of 0.216, while the 10 ppm calcium standard had an absorbance of 0.269 after correction for the blank. Sample A must, therefore, have been subjected to an inhibition of $\frac{0.216}{0.269}$ or 81 percent. If the apparent calcium content of **sample A** is corrected for this 81 per cent inhibition, the calcium exhibit the limits of experimental accuracy.

Zinc in Tissue Sample

A weighed amount of tissue (about 1 g), if available is dry ashed overnight in a muffle in a porcelain crucible at 600°C. The ash is dissolved in sufficient 3 N HCl to make the final HCl concentration in the diluted samples (0.36). The samples are diluted to the appropriate volume to give zinc concentrations ranging from 0.25 to 2.0 ppm and compared with zinc standards in 0.36 N HCl. Wet oxidation with sulphuric, nitric-percholoric acids is used to prepare some feed and blood plasma samples for zinc analysis. However, the reagent blank is relatively high for this method of sample preparation. It might be advantageous to use this technique after purification of the acids. The technique used by Allan (1961) and Willis (1962) for extracting Chelated metals into an organic solvent is found to work satisfactorly for copper and zinc. The method increases sensitivity and also makes it possible to concentrate samples to smaller volumes conveniently. In the the zinc extraction, where sodium acetate is used to adjust and buffer the pH to between 2.5 and 5.0, it is advantageous to extract a sodium acetate solution with the organic solvent in the presence of the chelating agent to remove the zinc contamination.

Solvent Extraction Techniques

Ammonium pyrolidine dithio carbonate (APDC) and methyl isobutyl ketone (MIBK), are the principal components of this system, useful to extract a large number of metals.

Principle

Solvent extraction is that process whereby two immiscible are brought into contact so as to effect a transfer of one or more elements from one liquid phase to the other. In the usual case, one phase is an aqueous solution of the sample, and the other is an immiscible organic solvent.

Because of their ionic nature, sample metal salts are usually much more soluble in aqueous media than in organic solvents. In order to extract a metal into an organic, it is first necessary to convert the metal ion to an uncharged species. Fortunately, this is frequently easy to accomplish. Most metals from stab, neutral, and extractable complexes with one or more members of a group of organic compounds known as chelating agents.

Table 1 : Examples of chelating agents.

Common term	Chemical designation
APDC	Ammonium pyrolidine dithiocarbamate
Cupferron	Ammonium salt of n-nitrosophenyl-hydroxylamine
Oxine	8-hydroxyquinoline
Dithiozone	Diphenylthiocarbazone
Acetylacetone	2, 4-pentanedione
TTA	Thenoyl trifluoroacetone
DEDC	Sodium diethyldithiocarbamate

The solvent used must completely dissolve the metal chelate and, of course, be immiscible with the sample solution. In additon, it should burn with a clear, steady flame, Esters and Ketones have been used extensively because of their good burning characteristics in both air-acetylene and nitrous oxide-acetylene flames.

In general, solvent extraction may be useful in atomic absorption analysis when the metals of interest are present in concentrations too low for direct analysis, when the sample matrix is such that it would interfere, or when the sample size is too small for direct analysis. Another important, when an organic solution is aspirated into the flame of a premix type burner. This increase in absorption is one the order of three to five times, depending upon the solvent being aspirated, and is primarily due to nothing more complicated than the fact that more sample actually reaches the flame. The apparent explanation for this is that the organic solvent forms more small sized droplete during aspiration, and these are more likely to pass through the burner mixing chamber without condensing. Two general tests on solvent extraction that have been useful are those of Morrison and Freiser (1957) and Stary (1964). Both of these references contain extraction procedures for nearly all metals.

The APDC/MIBK System

Malissa and Schoffman (1955) listed 30 metals which form chelates with APDC and most of those listed react over wide pH ranges. Allan (1961 a,b) found that the APDC chelate of copper could be extracted quantitatively into MIBK and use this system to determine low concentrations of copper in plant and soils. Copper obviously has received much more attention than the others. This is probably due to the ease with which it is extracted quantitatively over a very wide pH range. In fact, copper is frequently added and co-extracted as a kind of "internal standard" in studies of the extraction characteristics of other metals.

Procedure of Extraction

After adjustment of the pH to the desired range, the sample solution is transferred to an extraction vessel. APDC is added, usually as a 2 per cent or 5 per cent aqueous solution, followed by an accurately measured quantity of MIBK. The mixture is shaken thoroughly and the layers are allowed to separate. Centrifugation may be necessary in order to get a good, clean separation of phases. The upper MIBK, layer containing the metal is then aspirating directly into the flame. Ordinary glassware, such as separating funnels, centrifuge tubes, Babcock cream fat test bottles may be used for extractions. After shaking and separation of the two layers, the organic layer may be aspirated into the instrument directly.

This emphasis on the APDC/MIBK system is not meant to imply that it is the only suitable extraction system. In fact, it is only one of a number of excellent systems available to the atomic absorption analyst. *Oxine reacts with even more metals than does APDC, including aluminium, magnesium, calcium and other alkaline earths (Stary, 1964). Mansell and Emmel (1965) used oxine in chloroform to extract manganese, nickel and cobalt.*

Plasma Iron and Iron-binding Capacity Determination

The concentration of iron in blood plasma is useful in determining iron-deficiency states. The iron-binding capacity is low in septic and neoplastic states, with a saturation index exceeding 25 per cent.

Method

Heparinized blood samples are obtained and centrifuged as soon as possible, and the plasma is removed. The plasma is then diluted 1 : 1 with deionized distilled water. Small amounts of precipitated fibrinogen are removed with a wooden applicator before aspiration without affecting end results. When serum is used, plastic test tubes are not satisfactory because clots adhere to the sides. Acid cleaned glass test tubes should be used when using serum. All glass test tube should be used when using serum. All glassware is washed in 10 per cent nitric acid and rinsed in deionized water.

Standard solutions are prepared containing 3 per cent aqueous egg albumin with 50, 75, 100 and 150 µg/100 ml of iron, added as ferric chloride. These standards are aspirated into the flame and the absorption signals are recorded. An analytical curve is prepared for the standards, and the deflections of the 1 : 1 diluted plasma samples are compared to it.

To determine iron binding capacity, 2 ml of ferric chloride (500 µg per 100 ml) are mixed with 2 ml of plasma in a plastic tube, and allowed to stand for five minutes. About 0.4 g of magnesium carbonate is added and the sample is mixed at regular intervals for 40 minutes. After centrifugation for 10 minutes at 200 rpm, 0.5 ml of the supernatant liquid is removed and added to 0.5 ml of 6 per cent aqueous egg albumin. The mixture is then aspirated into the flame and the absorbance values obtained are compared to the analytical curve used above. *The iron concentration found from the curve, multiplied by four, represents the iron - binding capacity.*

Plasma iron is also determined colorimetrically by chelating the iron with the chromogen 2, 4, 6 tripyridyl-s triazine (TPTZ) in acid (0.1% chromogen dissolving in 2% acetic acid) after reducing the plasma iron to the ferrous state with ascorbic acid and precipitating the plasma proteins with a mixture of trichloroacetic acid and chloroform (Carraway, 1963 and Ramsay, 1958). The blue colour produced by the reaction is measured at 590mµ. Table 2 reveal the comparative study of results of atomic absorption and colorimetry for total iron binding capacity.

Table 2 : Comparative total iron binding capacity (µg/100 ml) of aliquot plasma samples.

Atomic absorption	TPTZ
240	248
280	288
240	246
380	378
200	200
180	200
280	272
256	256

Source : Zaino, E.C. 1967. Atomic Absorption News Letter, **6 :** 93.

Atomic absorption analysis does not distinguish between plasma iron and haemoglobin iron, so that care must be taken to obtain hemolysis free samples. With haemolyzed blood, the iron must either be chelated and determined by Zettner's method (Zettner *et al.*, 1966), or be determined colorimetrically. *Haemolysis, however, is not a problem when heparinized blood is used and the plasma is rapidly centrifuged.*

Direct Serum Analysis for Iron

If direct analysis is applied to iron in serum, three principal difficulties are encountered.

Sensitivity

Serum iron levels, especially those of clinical importance (less than 50 μg per 100 ml) range near the sensitivity limit of the AAS method. In as much as a minimal dilution 1 : 3 of serum is necessary to overcome severe matric effects, analysis have to be made on samples containing 15 μg/100 ml of iron or less after dilution. The signal of this iron concentration achieved under ideal instrumental conditions (slit width, lamp current, burner aligment etc.) is 2.4 absorption per cent (97.6 per cent transmittance). Thus, most clinically critical analysis would be based on absorbance values of 0.010 or less. Zettner *et al.*, (1966) have also investigated scale expansion techniques and have found that the advantages of sensitivity enhancement are partially lost in an analysis that is extremely noisy as a result of the complex matrix of serum.

Matrix Effects

Ferrichloride solution or hemoglobin is added to a serum pool until the undiluted serum, when aspirated into the flame, gave signal of approximately 60 per cent absorption. Dilutions are prepared in the ratios 1:2, 1:3, 1:4, 1:5, 1:10 and 1:20. The samples are directly aspirated and their absorbance values plotted against dilution. The non linear nature of the curve demonstrates the effect of serum constitutents on iron absorption, the non linearity worsens with increase in serum concentrations. The results are the same with serum treated with 0.2 N HCl and thioglycolic acid.

Haemolysis

In the direct determination, the AAS technique does not differentiate between serum or transferrin iron and haemoglobin iron. Serum collected routinely in tubes without grossly visible haemolysis contained from 5 to 20 mg per 100 ml of haemoglobin, raising the total iron level by 17 to 68 μg per 100 ml., thereby introducing serious analytical errors. Sufficiently accurate serum iron determinations by direct analysis in the low or normal range are precluded for the reasons stated above.

Iron Determination after Chelating and Solvent Extraction

Reagents

1. *Hydrochloric acid 1 N.*
2. *Thioglycolic acid*
3. *Trichloroacetic acid (TCA), 10 percent*
4. *Potassium acetate, 30 percent.*

5. Phenanthroline (4, 7-diphenyl-1, 10-phenanthroline), 25 mg per 100 ml solution in ethyl alcohol.
6. Methylisobutyl ketone (4-methyl-2-pentanone, isopropyl acetone).
7. Ferric ammonium citrate, 5 mg per 100 ml of Fe.
8. Buffer, pH 7.5 containing 0.11 M NaCl and 0.04 M barbital.
9. Amberlite IRA 410 resin.

Procedure

Place 2 ml of serum into a 15 ml test tube, add 1 ml of 1 N HCl and 1 drop of thioglycolic acid, mix by swirling, and let stand for 10 minutes. Add 8 ml of 10 per cent TCA, Cap with a small square of parafilm, shake vigorously for 10 seconds and let stand for 30 minutes.

After centrifugation, pipette 8 ml of the supernatant into a 15 ml test tube, add 1.5 ml 30 per cent potassium acetate and 2 ml of alcoholic solution of phenanthroline, mix, and let stand for 5 minutes.

Add 1.4 ml of methylisobutyl ketone, cap with a small square of wrap, and mix vigorously for 10 seconds. Let stand until the phases are separated. Then aspirate the organic layer into an acetylene air flame previously adjusted with MIBK. Read percentage of absorption at the resonance line of iron at 2483 A. Procedure can be carried out with half volumes of sample.

Procedure for Determination of Iron Binding Capacity in Serum by AAS

Place 1 ml of serum in a 10 ml test tube, add 0.1 ml of ferric ammonium citrate solution, and let stand for 10 minutes. Add 0.4 ml of dry amberlite IRA 410 resin, 4.9 ml of barbital buffer, and let stand for 10 minutes. Mix occasionally.

Centrifuge and pipette 4 ml of the supernatant into a 150 x 40 mm test tube, add 1 ml of 0.2 N HCl and 1 drop of thioglycolic acid, and let stand for 10 minutes.

Add 6 ml of 10 per cent TCA and proceed as described above for serum iron from this point on. *The iron value multiplied by 3 equals the iron binding capacity.*

Advantages of Using Chelating Chemical and Solvent Extractions in the Determination of Iron in Serum

1. Atomic absorption sensitivity of iron in MIBK is twice that of iron in water.

2. When iron is extracted into small volumes of organic solvents, iron concentrations greater than those originally present in the serum sample are obtained.
3. The interfering effects of serum constituents are eliminated as a result of the separation of iron from the serum matrix.
4. The occasional turbidity of the organic phase after extraction is inconsequential in the AAs analysis.
5. The standard deviation of the method is 0.7 µg per 100 ml of iron. Recovery experiments indicated excellent accuracy and precision of the method, even in the range of less than 10 µg per 100 ml of iron.

Copper in Milk

For many years it has been known that the off flavour of milk known as oxidized flavour results from abnormally high concentrations of copper in the milk. The copper content of feed and soils is conveniently determined by atomic absorption (Allan, 1961) and the copper content of blood is also no problem. However, the copper content of normal milk from cows except in the early stages of lactation varies from 0.02 to 0.04 ppm. Attempts have been made in past to analyse these low levels by dry ashing a 25 ml volume of milk and taking up the ash in HCl. Copper is extracted from the acid solution into a ketone using ammonium pyrolidine dithiocarbamate (APDC) using the method of Allan (1961). *The analytical range is from 0.01 to 1 ppm copper in the original milk sample.*

Reagents

Analytical grade HCl is used without further purification. A blank is carried through the full procedure and the small resulting signal is subtracted from the sample signals. Isopentyl methyl ketone (5-methyl-2-hexanone) is used although no advantage is found over the use of methyl isobutyl ketone recommended by Allan (1961). The ammonium pyrolidine dithiocarbamate (APDC) is prepared in the laboratory by the method of Malissa and Schoffman (1955).

Sample Preparation

A 25 ml sample of whole milk is acidified with 4 ml of 2.4 N HCl and evaporated to dryness. The dried sample is heated slowly in a muffle to 500°C, and left overnight at this temperature. This produces a grey ash. Two ml of concentrated HNO_3 is added and the sample is evaporated to dryness on a steam bath. The dried sample, still in the original beaker, is flamed for a few minutes. It is returned to a muffle at 500°C for one hour to produce a white ash.

The ash is taken up in 5 ml of 6 N HCl and dried on a steam bath. It is taken up again in 10 ml of 0.1 N HCl, brought to boiling and the solution transferred to a Babcock 50 per cent cream fat test bottle. The original beaker is rinsed again with 10 ml of acid solution, which is brought to a boil and transferred to the babcock bottle. Finally, the beaker is rinsed with 10 ml of deionized water, which is also added to the Babcock bottle. All of the copper has been converted to the chloride by this procedure. To the solution in the Babcock bottles are 1 ml of 1 percent APDC and 5 ml of isopentyl methyl ketone. The Babock bottles are shaken about 1 minute by hand. The bottles are centrifuged for 10 minutes and the separated organic phase is raised into the narrow neck of the bottle by addition of water. The bottles are respun for 10 minutes.

Atomic absorption analysis are run on the organic phase, directly from the Babcock bottles. The standards are prepared by extracting 1, 2, 3, 4, 5, 10, 20 and 30 μg of copper from 25 ml of 0.1 N HCl. The same procedure is being used routinely for the extraction of copper from water samples and diluted feed ashes.

About 200 samples have been analysed for copper with results that range from 0.03 to 0.8 ppm copper. Replicate samples indicate that the method is dependable to 0.01 ppm copper in the milk sample.

Sulphur in Biological Materials

The majority of existing methods for the determination of the organic sulphate are based on the formation of barium salts, usually barium sulphate, which may be estimated subsequently by standard gravimetric determination (Loeb and Benedict, 1927) or turbidimetric analysis (Berglund & Sorbo, 1960), by estimation of sulphate by precipitation with radioactive barium, or by flame photometric methods (Cullum & Thomas 1959). Atomic absorption spectrophotometry offers sensitive procedure for the estimation of barium, and thus of sulphate in the low concentrations that may be found in biological materials. In the procedure to be described, samples of urine, diet, faeces and biological tissues oxidised by one several techniques are added to a solution containing an excess of barium chloride. The resulting precipitate of barium sulphate is dissolved in disodium ethylenediaminetetracetic acid and barium concentration of the resulting solutions estimated by atomic absorption spectrophotometry.

Reagents and Methods

Oxidation Procedures

1. *Schoniger digestion, absorbant fluid for combustion flasks. Ammonium hydroxide, 6 per cent* NH_4 *OH : 100 ml concentrated* NH_4OH *+ 400 ml*

water, Hydrogen peroxide, 6 precent H_2O *: 100 ml* H_2O_2 *(30%) + 400 ml* H_2O.

2. *Benedict's digestion mixture : Copper nitrate, CU* $(NO_3)_2\ 3H_2O$ *: 200 g Potassium chlorate,* $KClO_3$ *: 50 g Distilled water to 1000 ml.*

Sulphate Determination

1. *Disodium ethylenediaminetetra acetic acid solution, 10 g EDTA, is dissolved in 500 ml distilled water, 100 g NaOH added, and the resultant solution made up to a total volume of 2000 ml with distilled water.*
2. *Barium chloride, 15 per cent W/V.*
3. *Lanthanum chloride solution, 5 per cent equivalent to 50,000 ppm of lanthanum.*

   Method 1. 58.64 g La_2O_3 *is dissolved in 100-200 ml distilled water, 250 ml hydrochloric acid (37.4%) is added carefully, and the mixture is allowed to cool, after which the total volume is brought up to 1000 ml with distilled water.*

   Method 2. Lanthanum chloride, 133.7 g dissolved in 1000 ml distilled water.
4. *HCl, 25% : concentrated HCl (37.4%) : water - 1:4 V/V.*

Barium Standards

1. *Stock solution, 1.5 gram barium chloride* $(BaCl_2.\ H_2O)$ *diluted to 1000 ml, this will represent 1000 ppm barium.*
2. *Working standards, containing 25-2000 ppm of barium are employed.*

   Note : All solutions are prepared with glass-distilled water and "Sulphate-free" reagents. Glassware is cleaned with a non ionic detergent, rinsed several times with tap water and three times with distilled water containing a trace of hydrochloric acid, and allowed to air dry.

Sulphate Standards

1. *Stock solution, sodium sulphate* Na_2SO_4 *: 1.479 grams dissolved in 500 ml distilled water, equivalent to 2000 ppm of sulphate.*
2. *Working standards, the concentration of solution used covered the range from 50-400 ppm of sulphate.*

Barium Estimations

The precision of barium determinations by atomic absorption spectrophotometry is evaluated by repeated estimation of barium in working standards, prepared from the stock solution of barium chloride.

Sulphate Estimation

Triplicate aliquots of the stock sulphate solution are pipetted into screw-capped tubes and the total volume of each tube is brought up to 5 ml with distilled water, 1 ml of the lanthanum chloride solution is added to each and 2 ml of 15 per cent barium chloride. The contents of each tube are mixed and then the tubes are centrifuged at 2600 rpm for 5 minutes. The supernatants are discarded and precipitates of barium sulphate washed with 5 ml of distilled water to remove the excess barium chloride. This step is repeated and then the precipitates are dissolved in 10 ml of the disodium EDTA solution. The samples are aspirated into the flame of the atomic absorption spectrophotometer.

Sample Analysis

Oxidation : The destruction of organic substances and the oxidation of the sulphur to the sulphate form is achieved in liquid samples, e.g. urine by Benedict's method (Benedict, 1909). Cumbustion and oxidation of solid samples, e.g. freeze dried diet, faeces, and biological tissues, is carried out in the Schöniger flask by a modification of the method employed by Lysyj and Zarembo (1959). Dry samples, 50-100 mg are weighed into methylcellulose capsules which are burnt in a500 ml Schöniger flask containing 10 ml each of 6 percent in ammonium hydroxide and 6 percent hydrogen peroxide. After completion of the oxidation process, the contents of the Schöniger flask are concentrated to 3-5 ml by boiling. Hydrolysis of conjugated sulphates in urine is performed by Folin's technique (1914).

Determination of inorganic sulphate concentrations in urine samples are made directly in an aliquots from which the sediment had been removed by centrifugation. *Lanthanum chloride solution is added to all prepared samples in order to eliminate phosphate interference in the atomic absorption spectrophotometric determinations of barium.*

Triplicate sulphate analyses are performed on all prepared samples as described for the standard sulphate solutions.

Calculations

Standard graph is prepared by plotting the values of absorbance and sulphate concentration. The total amount of sulphur in the samples is then calculated as follows.

Liquid samples (e.g. urine)

$$\frac{\text{ppm}\,SO_4^{-2}}{3 \times 1000} \times \frac{15\,\text{ml NaEDTA}}{5\,\text{ml urine}} \times \text{Total vol. urine} = \text{mg S}$$

Solid samples (e.g. faeces)

$$\frac{\text{ppm}\,SO_4^{-2}}{3\times1000}\times \text{ml NaEDTA}\times\frac{\text{Total dry wt.}}{\text{Wt. in capsules}}=\text{mg S}$$

One part per million of sulphate is equivalent to 1/3 x 1000 mg sulphur per ml of solution analysed.

Calculation in Atomic Absorption Spectrophotometry

We should take into consideration following factors so as to calculate the concentration of trace mineral in unkonwn or testing sample.

1. *The test analysis containing all reagents and the analytical sample.*
2. *The analysis blank containing only the analytical sample and serving as correction for intrinsic optical absorption.*
3. *The reagent blank containing the reagents without the analytical sample and giving the correction for the intrinsic absorption of the reagents.*
4. *The standard containing the standard solution and all reagents.*

Example

Estimate Concentration of Zinc in the given Sample A

$$\text{Zn (ppm) in sample} = \frac{a \times b \times 100}{c \times w}$$

where

a = Concentration of zinc in standard solution.

b = O.D. of unknown sample's extract

c = O.D. of standard solution.

w = Weight (g) of material on dry matter basis

100 = Volume (ml) of mineral extract

a = 0.4 ppm

b = 0.05

c = 0.1

w = 1 gram

$$\text{Zn (ppm) in sample} = \frac{0.4 \times 0.05 \times 100}{0.1 \times 1}$$

= 20 ppm

Result = The given sample A contained 20 ppm zinc

Note : we should deduct the O.D. of blank from the O.D. of unknown sample and only the net value after subtraction should be used.

Mineral Conversions

	Multiply by	Reciprocal multiply by
Calcium to calcium oxide	1.400	0.714
Calcium to calcium carbonate	2.500	0.400
Calcium Oxide to calcium carbonate	1.800	0.560
Chloride to sodium chloride	1.650	0.607
Manganese to mangansese sulphate	2.750	0.364
Phosphorus to phosphoric acid	2.290	0.436
Magnesium to magnesium Oxide	1.658	0.603
Copper to copper sulphate	2.510	0.398
Iron to iron sulphate	2.720	0.367

References

Alkemade, C.T.J and Milatz, M.W. (1955). *J. Opt. Soc. Am.*, 45 : 583.

Ailan, J.E. (1961). Spectrochem. *Acta.* 17 : 459

Anonymous, (1960). Analyst, 85 : 643.

Benedict, S.K. (1909). *J. Biol.Chem.*, 6 : 363.

Berglund, F. and Sorbo, B. (1960). *J. Clin. Lab. Invest.* 12 : 147.

Carraway, W.T. (1963). *Clin. Chem.*, 9 : 188.

Cullum, D.C and Thomas, D.B. (1959). *Analyst*, 84 : 113.

David, D.T. (1958). *Analyst*, 83 : 655.

Folin, O. (1914). *J. Bio Chem.*, 17 : 469.

Grove, E. L., Jones, R. A. and Mathew, W. (1961). *Anal. BIochem.*, 2 : 221.

Kirchoff, G. (1860). *Progg.Ann.*, 109 : 275.

Krishna, G., Paliwal, V.K., Yadav, K.R. and Khirwar, S.S. (1981). Note on alkaline earth metals in Agro-Industrial byproducts and Wastes of Haryana State. *Indian J. Anim. Sci.* 51: 1170-1172.

Krishna, G. and Mahadevan, V. (1969). Effect of copper supplementation on growth and utilization of nutrients in large white yorkshire growing pigs. *Indian Vety. J.* 46: 320-329.

Krishna, G. Paliwal, V.K.; Yadav, K.R. and Khirwar, S.S. (1981). Trace elements in Agro-Industrial byproducts and wastes of Haryana State. *Indian J. Dairy Sci.*, 34: 336-338.

Loeb, R.F. and Benedict, E.M. (1927). *J.Clin. Invest.*, 4 : 33.

Lysyj, I. and Zarembo, J.E. (1959). *Microchem., J.*, 3 : 173.

Mallissa, H.a dn Schoffman, E. (1955). *Mikrochem. Acta,* 1 : 187.

Mansell, R.E. and Enmel, H.W. (1965). *Atomic Absorption News letter*, 4 : 365.

Morgan, M.E. (1964). *Atomic absorption Newsletter*, Perkin Elmer corporation, Norwalk, Connecticut.

Morrison, G.H. and Freiser, H. (1957). *Solvent extraction in analytical chemistry.* John Wiley and Sons, New York.

Pickett, E.E. and Koirtyohann, S.R. (1968). *Spectrochimica Acta,* 23 B : 235.

Pickett, E.E. and Koirtyohann, S.R. (1969). *Analyt. Chem.*, 14 : 28A.

Ramsay, W.W.M. (1958). *Advances in Clinical Chemistry*, Vol. 1, Academic Press, New York.

Stary, J. (1964). *The solvent extraction in analytical Chemistry*, John Wiley and Sons, New York.

Walsh, A. (1955). *Spectrochem., Acta.*, 7 : 108.

Willis, J.B. (1960). *Spectrochem. Acta* 16 : 259.

Willis, J.B. (1961). *Analyt Chem.*, 34 : 556.

Willis, J.B. (1962). *Analyt. Chem.*, 34 : 614.

Willis, J.B. (1963). *Analysis of biological materials by Atomic absorption spectroscopy*, In methods of Biochemical analysis, *Vol XI*, Glick, D. (ed.), Inter Science, New York.

Zettner, A. sylva, L.C and Capacho Delgado, L. (1966). *Am. J. Clin. Path.*, 45 : 533.

References for further study

Allan, J.E. (1958). *Analyst*, 83 : 466.

Kolthoff, I.M., Elving, P.J. and Sandell, E.B. (1965). (eds.) : *Treatise on Analytical chemistry.* New York : John wiley & Sons. Part I (6), 3526.

Rusell, B.J., Shelton, J.P. and Walsh, A. (1957). *Spectrochim., Acta.*, 8 : 317.

Walsh, A. (1955). *Spectrochim. Acta,* 7 : 108.

Walsh, A. (1958). U.S. Patent, 2 : 847, 899.

Chapter - 59

Flame Photometry

Principles of Working

(Lundegårdh, 1929-1934 : Mac Intyre, 1961)

Flame photometry is the measurement of the concentration of an ionic material in a solution introduced in to a flame, where the intensity of light emitted by the flame under these conditions is measured. We should give credit to Kirchhoff and Bunsen (1860), who developed the idea of emission spectroscopy into quantitative inorganic analysis, later on Janssen (1970) made lot of developments in this direction. The main parts of flame photometer are: (1) burner, (2) atomizer which disperses the solution as a fine spray into the flame; a means of isolating from the spectrum (i.e., filtering system, diffraction gratting etc.) only that portion of the emitted light which is a specific characteristics of the substance being examined ; a photosensitive detector with or without amplifier; and a method of measuring the desired emission. In flame photometry the diluted biological fluid is atomized directly ino the flame without need of preliminary separation. The resulting emissions are those of all the inorganic ions present. For measurement the emitted light is passed through a monochromater where the wavelength most characteristics of the material analysis and which most closely follows Beer's law is selected. The background colour of the flame is important as it contributes to any reading produced. *Some instruments utilise a solvent containing a light-emitting substance such as lithium not usually found in clinical system. This gives a constant light emission which act as a standard base emission.* All other emissions can then be compared to this constant base. Such a system is known as the internal standard method of flame photometry. Instruments using no constant light emitter are said to be externally standardized systems. Generally, instruments utilising the internal standard system will show a curve, rather than a straight line, when the reading is plotted versus concentration. It has been experienced that the use of the internal standard system is most reliable.

In general, flame photometers are calibrated for particular metals by running a series of standards containing varying concentrations of the metal ion. No ashing other preliminary preparation of the sample is ordinarily required; sodium and potassium determinations on blood plasma or serum, for example, require merely appropriate dilution with water or we may estimate directly by mixing with oxine solution.

The sample in solution is introduced in the form of a fine continuous spray into a non-luminous gas flame using either natural, acetylene, propane or butane gas. Air or pure oxygen under pressure is used to maintain high burning temperatures and thereby keep the luminosity of the flame at a minimum. Sodium and potassium are easily activated and require, therefore, only a relatively low temperature flame such as the propane - air flame (1925°C). *For the estimation of calcium and magnesium, we require high temperature flame this can be obtained only by using acetylene - oxygen or hydrogen - oxygen flames.* By the use of a colour filter or diffraction gratting the emitted light, of wavelength characteristic for the ion being analysed, is isolated and focused on a phtoelectric cell. The electrical response of the photoelectric cell is measured on a suitable meter previously calibrated to convert the electrical impulse to ion concentration either by direct reading or by reference to a calibration curve. Lundegardh (1929-34) wrote two books describing results obtain with an ordinary spectrograph equipped with an acetylene - air flame source. It is possible, by using high-temperature flames (hydrogen-oxygen at 2900°C or cyanogen-oxygen at 4800°C), and separating the emission lines with a monochromator, to adapt the flame photometer to the determination of numerous other elements. For the estimation of plasma calcium an acetylene flame (high temperature flame photometry) at 622 nm is required. The choice of the hot acetylene flame almost completely eliminates interference from sodium, but when propane gas is used the strong effect of sodium must be taken into account. *Neutron activation may be used as a reference method for comparing the accuracy in the result of Na and K analyses.*

Sodium and Potassium : Flame Photometry

(Marti and Munoz, 1957; Henri, 1964)

Assuming that interfering substances such as salts of calcium, iron or aluminium are present, the ash is first boiled with ammonium oxalate solution. The potassium content is estimated from the measurement of the characteristic radiation at 766-770 nm, by using a suitable filter, from a flame into which a solution of the sample is sprayed.

Reagents

1. *Ammonia solution. Dilute 60 ml of ammonia solution of sp.gr. 0.800 with water to 200 ml.*

Potassium Stock Solution

Formula I

Dissolve 5.779 grams of potassium dihydrogen phosphate (dried at 105°C) in water and dilute the solution to one litre.

Dilute 50 ml of stock potassium solution to one litre with water (=100 ppm as K_2O). Prepare from the stock solution just before use.

Formula II

Prepare a stock standard by dissolving 2.229 grams of pure dry potassium sulphate in water in a one litre volumetric flask dilute with water to the mark, and mix, preserve with little toluene. This solution contains 1 mg of potassium per ml and is stable indefinitely. Prepare a working standard fresh daily by diluting 1 ml of stock standard to 100 ml water in a volumetric flask. This solution contains 0.03 mg of potassium in 3 ml.

Standard Sodium Solution

Exactly 1 gram of C.P. sodium chloride is dissolved in water and made up to a litre in a volumetric flask. Each ml of this solution contains 0.393 mg of sodium.

Potassium Standard for Use in Serum Analysis

Standard solution covering a range from 3 to 7 milli-equivalents of potassium per litre, at a dilution of 1:100 are usually adequate for calibration purposes. Prepare a stock standard containing 10 milli equivalents of potassium per litre by dissolving 0.746 grams of Kcl in water and diluting to one litre. Working standards equivalent to 3.0, 4.0, 5.0, 6.0 and 7.0 milli equivalents of potassium per litre, at a dilution of 1 : 100, are prepared by diluting respectively 3, 4, 5, 6, and 7 ml of stock solution to one litre with water. If the analytical procedure requires an internal standard such as lithium sulphate solution, add to these working standards 10 times the volume of such solution routinely added to the diluted plasma or serum before diluting to the one litre mark and mixing. Prepare a calibration curve from these standards as described for the determination of sodium.

Sodium Standard for Use in Serum Analysis

Standard solutions covering the range from 100 to 160 milli equivalents of sodium per litre, at a dilution of 1:100, are usually adequate for calibration purpose. Prepare a stock standard containing 100 milli equivalents of sodium per litre by dissolving 5.85 g of NaCl in water and diluting to one litre. Working standards are prepared from this stock standard by measuring out 10, 11, 12, 13, 14, 15 and 16 ml aliquots into one litre volumetric flask, and diluting to the mark with water. These standards represent respectively 100, 110, 120, 130, 140, 150 and 160 milli equivalents of sodium per litre at a 1:100 dilution. If the analytical procedure requires an internal standard such as lithium sulphate solution, add to each working standard 10 time the volume of lithium sulphate solution routinely added to the diluted plasma or serum, before diluting to the mark and mixing. To prepare a calibration curve, read each of these standards in the photometer, plot readings against equivalent sodium content in milli equivalents per litre, and draw a smooth curve to include the points.

Important Point

Standards should always be run both before and after analysing a series of unknown solutions, to be sure that the calibration is constant ; if there is considerble fluctuation, each unknown solution should be followed by a standard closely equivalent to it.

Table 1 : Sodium and potassium standards for use in serum/plasma analyses

Stock Standard	Sodium chloride (g/l)	Potassium chloride (g/l)	Sodium content (mEq/l)	Potassium content (m Eq/l)
I	6.43	0.149	110	2
II	7.01	0.224	120	3
III	7.60	0.298	130	4
IV	8.18	0.373	140	5
V	8.77	0.448	150	6
VI	9.35	0.522	160	7
VII	9.94	0.597	170	8

Common Standard for Sodium, Potassium and Magnesium for Use in Serum and Plasma Analyses

Formula I (For sodium and Potassium)

Generally a single standard is used in determining sodium and potassium. This is prepared diluting 10 ml of sodium stock solution and 3 ml of potassium stock solution to one litre. The final standard solution represents 100 milli equivalents of sodium and 3 milli equivalents of potassium at a dilution of 1:100. The remaining standards are prepared in a similar manner.

Formula II (For Sodium, Potassium, Calcium and Magnesium)

Dissove 8.39 grams NaCl, 0.286 gram Kcl, 0.50 gram $CaCO_3$ and 0.167 gram $MgCl_2.6H_2O$ in one litre 0.1 N HCl. This combined standard will represent 10 mg per cent calcium, 2 mg per cent magnesium 330 mg per cent (143.550 m Eq/l) sodium 15 mg per cent (3.855 mg/l) sodium and 15 mg per cent (3.855 m Eq/l) potassium.

Procedure in the Case of Feed and Fodder Sample

Method I (Pearson, D. 1973)

Incinerate a suitable amount of sample at not more than 500°C in a silica dish. Add 50 ml conc. HCl and evaporate to dryness on a water bath. Wash the residue into a 400 ml beaker with 125 ml water, add 50 ml saturated ammonium oxalate solution and boil for 30 minutes. Cool, add the ammonia solution slight excess, wash into a 500 ml volumetric flask with water, make up the solution to the mark, then mix and filter it. Dilute the mixture so that the final solution contains about 15 ppm of K_2O (Solution A).

Prepare a series of solutions from the standard diluted potassium solution containing 10, 12, 14, 16, 18 and 20 ppm of K_2O. Set the sensitivity of the flame photometer so that 100 scale divisions (full deflection) is equivalent to 20 ppm. Spray each standard solution at least against the 20 ppm solution. From the reading obtained, prepare a calibration graph.

Reset the instrument at 100 scale division with the 20 ppm solution and spray the diluted sample solution A. Estimate the potassium contents from the calibration graph after taking several readings.

Method II (Source : The Beckman Flame news, published quarterly by Beckman Instruments International S.A., Geneva, Switzerland, Issue 1.2.1972)

2 grams of corn starch sample is weighed on tissue paper and transfer the material in a 100 ml volumetric flask and dissolved in about 80 ml of distilled water. Before filling up to the mark the solution was treated with 10 ml of a 5 per cent La_2O_3 (Lanthanum Oxide) solution and 5 ml of 18 per cent

HCl. After filling up to the final volume this solution is ready for the determination of Na, K and Mg.

Method III (For Estimating Sodium and Potassium in Animal Feeds and Human Foods)

Prepare 0.5 per cent sodium standard by dissolving 6.3550 grams sodium chloride in 500 ml N/10 HCl and one per cent potassium standard by dissolving 9.5340 grams potassium chloride in 500 ml N/10 Hcl. Such concentration of sodium and potassium in the standard will cover up the range usually reported in animal feeds and fodders by Krishna *et al.* (1981). Weigh 1 g human food or animal feed sample in conical flask and follow up the process of wet chemical digestion as per method described in volume I of this compendium and made up the volume of digested material upto 100 ml. Run a blank without sample simultaneously. Spray first dimineralised distilled water and operate the zero control to return the galvanometer to zero, then spray blank solution and adjust zero again on the galvanometer, the spray sodium standard after putting the sodium filter in the socket, adjust galvanometer needle to 100 on the scale, again spray blank, the needle should come back to zero and then spray the unknown sample, record the reading from galvanometer. Repeat the process in a similar way with potassium standard and calculate the result using the following formula.

$$= \frac{\text{concentration of Na or K in standard x reading of unknown sample x volume (min.extract)}}{\text{100 (galvanometer reading with standard) x wt. of material on dry matter basis}}$$

= Concentration of sodium or potassium in per cent (g/100g) sample

Method I : Sodium, Potassium, Calcium and Magnesium in Serum

The procedure varies with different types of instrument. A serum dilution of 1:100 (1 ml serum diluted to 100 ml with water) is used for either sodium or potassium analysis unless otherwise specified by the instrument manufacturer. Standard solutions are used along with the unknown samples whenever analyses are carried out. If an internal standard, e.g. lithium salt, is required for the successful operations of the photometer, the required aliquot of a stock solution of such a substance is added to the volumetric flask before diluting to the mark. Ordinally, the same concentration of internal standard is used for both sodium and potassium analyses. In order to get the sodium content of the sample, the reading obtained is referred to a calibration curve previously obtained by the same procedure on a series of solutions of known sodium content.

Procedure

Standards and sample solutions should be read in the order : standards, samples, standards, samples and standards. Blank should be included each time that standards are read. Water may be aspirated after each standard or sample. Flush plenty of water after each series of readings. Sample concentration should not read directly on reading scales (recorder or meter) because of the curvature of the analytical working curves.

Method II: Estimation of Sodium, Potassium, Calcium and Magnesium in Serum Sample

Reagents

1. *Sodium, Potassium and calcium standard solution*

   Prepare common standard solution according to the formula II mentioned previously in this chapter.

2. *Oxine (8-hydroxyuinoline), 0.4 % solution. Prepare this solution according to procedure mentioned under chapter entitled, "Atomic absorption spectrophotometry" of this compendium.*

Procedure

Mix 1 ml standard solution, unknown solution, blank and distilled water with oxine solution as given below :

A.	1 ml distilled water + 5 ml oxine	Na, K and Ca, Nil	
B.	1 ml blank solution + 5 ml oxine	Na, K and Ca, Nil	
C.	1 ml standard solution + 5 ml oxine	Sodium 143.550 mEq/l Potassium 3.855 mEq/l Calcium 10 mg percent Magnesium : 2 mg per cent	
D.	1 ml unknown sample (serum) + 5 ml oxine	Sodium Potassium Calcium Magnesium	Result may be obtained by calculation

Run the above A, B, C and D in the following order

A	B	C	D
(Set Zero)	(Set Zero)	(Set 100)	Note the reading and calculate result

Galvanometer Scale

☞ Notes

1. *Plasma obtained by using anticoagulant (lithium or ammonium heparinate) may be used for estimating sodium or potassium. We should not use other anticoagulants in any way, otherwise accurate results will not be obtained.*

2. *In general red blood cell contain potassium at a concentration some 25 times that of plasma. In any case, haemolysed serum or plasma should accordingly not be used for potassium estimation.*
3. *The serum or plasma must be separated from the red blood cells within an hour as otherwise high values may be obtained.*
4. *High temperature (oxyacetylene or hydrogen oxygen) flame should be used for estimating calcium and magnesium.*

Normal Values

In the case of adult human subjects the concentrations of serum sodium and potassium is 142 and 5.0 m Eq/L, respectively. In the case of cattle, the normal concentration of serum calcium is 9-12 mg/100 ml, while normal serum sodium and potasium is 135 and 4.5 m Eq/l. The concentration of magnesium in the blood plasma of cattle, ranges from approximately 2 to 4 mg per 100 ml.

Unit of Expressions

In the case of sodium to convert mg per cent sodium into milli equivalents per litre, divide by 2.3.

In the case of potassium to convert mg per cent potassium into milli equivalents per litre, divide by 3.9.

Experssion of the concentration of electrolytes of plasma, serum and extracellular fluids has confusion. Ions are usually expressed in terms of their chemical equivalents by stating their concentration in milli equivalents per litre, rather than a milligrams or grams per 100 ml.

$$\text{Concentration (meq / L)} = \frac{\text{Concentration (mg / 100ml)} \times 10}{\text{Ma}} \times V$$

Where v is the valence and Ma is the atomic weight. The normal values for electrolytes in human serum and plasma, formulas for conversion to milliequivalents per litre are presented in the following Table.

Table 2 : Normal values of cations in human serum (Thomas, 1952).

Cations	Normal Values (mg/100ml)	Atomic Weight	Valency (V)	Conversion of conc. C in mg/100 ml to mEq/L Formula	Factor	Normal values (mEq/L)
Na^+	313-333	23	1	$\left(c x \frac{10}{23}\right) x1$	= 0.435	136-145
K^+	14-19	39	1	$\left(c x \frac{10}{39}\right) x1$	= 0.257	3.5-5.0

References

Henri, R.J. (1964). *Clinical chemistry. Principles and Techniques*, New York, N.Y. Hoeber.

Janssen, J. (1870). *C.R. Acad. Sci.*, 71 : 626.

Kirchhoff, C. and Bunsen, R. (1860). *Ann.Physik, Chem.*, 110 : 161.

Krishna, G., Paliwal, V.K., Yadav, K.R. and Khirwar, S.S. (1981). Note on alkaline earth metals in Agro-Industrial byproducts and Wastes of Haryana State. *Indian J. Anim. Sci.* 51: 1170-72.

Krishna, G. (1985b). Major mineral components and calorific value of Agro-Industrial byproducts and Tropical Wastes. *Agricultural Wastes*. 13: 149-154.

Lundegaardh, H. (1929-1934). *The quantitative spectral analysis of the elements*. Fischer, Jena, Vol 1 and Vol 2.

Mac Intyre, I. (1961). *Adv. Clin. chem.*, 4 : 1.

Marti and Ramirez - Munoz. (1957). *Manual of flame photometry*, American Elsevier Publishing co., Inc., New York.

Pearson, D. (1973). *Laboratory techniques in food analysis*, First edn., Butterworths, London, pp 111.

Thomas, H.H. (1952). *A syllabus of laboratory examinations in clinical diagnosis*. Cambridge, Massachusetts, Harvard Univ. Press.

Chapter - 60

Direct and Indirect Calorimetry

Quantitative heat production estimation is necessary to know the net energy of feeds and fodders. *In the case of ruminants approximately 8 per cent of the gross energy consumed is lost as methane, therefore it becomes necessary to know this important loss in terms of methane energy so as to assess the metabolisable energy of any particular feed.* In human subjects, heat production studies are conducted to know the effect of planes of nutrition on basal metabolism as affected by different environmental conditions.

In the important laboratories of world, *heat production and methane production studies were conducted by respiration chamber (open circuit and closed circuit), since in our country respiration chamber has been installed at IVRI, Izatnagar, Bareilly* (U.P.) India, therefore, this technique is mentioned in brief in this chapter. *Indirect calorimetry involving the use of face mask and Douglas bag is followed at present in our country at NDRI, Karnal (India) so as to study the basal metabolic rate (BMR), heat production in human subjects and animals,* Krishna *(1973)*. Some laboratories in the country are interested to study respiratory quotient at different levels of feeding in human subjects and animals. The methods of estimation of RQ (respiratory quotient) is expressed in detail in this chapter.

A. Direct Calorimetry

Lavoisier and Laplace (1780) confined a guinea pig in a chamber containing a given weight of ice, and estimated the heat production from the amount of ice melted. The carbon exhaled was also collected. They found that melting of a given weight of ice corresponds to the exhalation of a definite amount of carbon dioxide. *About one fourth of the body heat is dissipated by moisture vaporisation which can be measured by absorption in such reagent e.g.* H_2SO_4. *About three fourth of the heat is emitted by radiation, conduction and convection and can be measured by absorption in water.* The total heat produced is the sum of two. In brief, direct calorimetry measures the heat loss.

B. Indirect Calorimetry

It is based on the fact that normally, oxygen consumption and carbon dioxide production are closely correlated with heat production. In contrast to direct calorimetry in which physical methods of measuring heat emission (by radiation, conduction, convection and latent heat of water vaporisation) are used, indirect calorimetry methods are dependent upon measurements of chemical changes which occur when different nutrients are catabolised or stored in the body of the organism.

Table 5.1 summarises the average constants for protein, fat and carbohydrate when oxidised in the animal body. These values are recommended by a sub-committee (Brower, 1965) to be used calculations of energy metabolism and they are used as the basis preparing formulae for calculating heat production from oxygen consumption, carbon dioxide, methane production and urinary nitrogen excretion.

The subcommittee on constant and factors (Brower, 1965) recommended the use of a multiple regression equation for calculating the heat production of ruminants and a correction is included for methane production. The formula, which was adopted by general consent of the participants of the third symposium on energy metabolism is as follows :

Calculation of Heat Produced

$$HP = 3.866\ O_2 + 1.200CO_2 - 0.518\ CH_4 - 1.431\ N$$

where HP = Heat produced (kcal)

O_2 = Litres oxygen consumed

CO_2 = Litres CO_2 produced

CH_4 = Litres methane produced

N = Urinary nitrogen excreted

Table 1 : Constants for protein, fat and carbohydrate when oxidised in the animal body (Brower, 1965)

Compound	Carbon %	O_2 consumed on oxidation of 1 g		CO_2 produced on oxidation of 1 g		Heat produced kcal	Respiration quotient
		g	1	g	1		
Protein*	52.00	1.366	0.957	1.520	0.774	5.70	0.809
Fats	76.70	2.875	2.013	2.810	1.431	9.50	0.711
Starch	44.45	1.184	0.829	1.629	0.829	4.20	1.000
Saccharose	42.11	1.122	0.786	1.543	0.786	3.96	1.000
Glucose	40.00	1.066	0.746	1.746	0.746	3.74	1.000

* Assuming the composition is 16 per cent, N, 52 per cent C and 5.7 kcal/gram calorific value.

However, in the last it may be mentioned that indirect calorimetry measures the heat production of an animal.

Calculation of Heat Production based on Oxygen Consumption Data Only

Weir (1949) has proposed a method of computation of heat produces which require only a knowledge of oxygen consumption and the per cent protein in the diet. Weir's equation is

$$HP = \frac{(Oi - O_e) \times 0.0504}{1 + 0.082p} \times \text{litres expired air}$$

where Oi = oxygen in inspired air

O_e = oxygen in expired air

p = decimal fraction of protein in diet

Countries where Respiration Chambers are Working

The first measurements of energetic effects of feeds in animals were made by Gustav Kuhn. He conducted the first energy balance trials in farm animals with a respiration apparatus during the years before 1900 at the Agricultural experiment station of Mockern near Leipzig, Germany. His successor, Oscar Kellner, determined in comprehensive experiments the energy gain in animals produced by pure nutrients and feeds which led to the establishment of the starch equivalent value. In the USA, Henry Armsby investigated the energy utilisation of a great number of feeds with the respiration calorimeter. After world war second, a number of respiration calorimeter were built under the leadership of Blaxter (England), Breirem (Norway), Brower (Netherland), Colovos (USA), Denissov (USSR), Flatt (USA), Kleiber (USA), Lerby (France), Nehring and Coworkers (Germany), Thorbek (Denmark), Tomme (USSR) and Wohbler (Germany).

C. Characteristic of Closed Circuit (Regnault-Reiser) System

The distinguishing characteristics of a closed circuit system is that the same air is recirculated through the system. By analysis of a sample of air at the beginning and at the end of an experiment, it is possible to learn from the changed composition, the amount of oxygen absorbed and the amount of CO_2 given off. Regnault and Reiset (1849) build the first closed circuit apparatus which provided for the absorption of the CO_2 as rapidly as it was produced and its replacement by oxygen. A fall in pressure in the whole apparatus occurs as a result of the absorption of oxygen by the animal, and oxygen is admitted to the system in proportion to this fall in pressure. Gas analysis is limited to checks of air composition to ensure that the CO_2, O_2 content of the air in the system are the same at the begining and end of an experiment.

D. Characteristic of an Open Circuit (Pettenkofer) System

In the open circuit respiration apparatus, out-door air is passed through the chamber of the instrument, and the changes in its oxygen, methane and carbon dioxide content are measured. If the amount of air which passes through the apparatus and the incremental changes in gas concentrations are known, the total amounts of carbon dioxide and methane produced and of oxygen consumed can be computed.

E. Different Parts and Working of Open Circuit Respiration Chamber

Sundstϕl *et al.* (1973) of Agricultural University of Norway, have described parts and working of respiration chamber (open circuit).

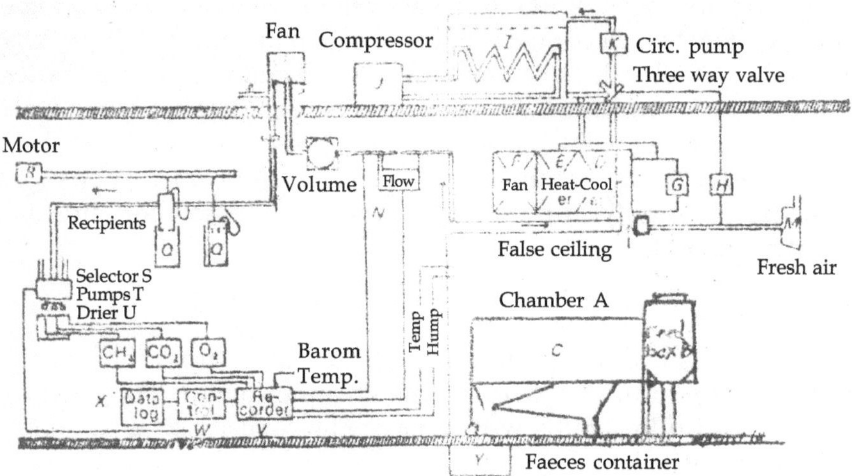

Fig. 1 : Open circuit respiration chamber installed at the department of Animal Nutrition, Agricultural University of Norway, ÅS - NLH (Norway). (*Source :* Sundstϕl et al. 1973).

Different Parts

Various parts of open circuit respiration chamber are illustrated in Fig. 5.1 The two chambers A are made of steel plated on a frame of angle iron with heavy insulation and the inside wall are covered with vinly felt. The inner measurements of the chambers are 190 x 120 x 200 cm high, and may be used for studies on calves, sheep, goats, pigs, and even flocks of poultry. The two chambers are placed sidewise 90 cm apart with a joint inspection airlock entrance in between. When animals are placed in the chambers, they can see each other through windows at the side wall. Each chamber is equiped with two more inspection windows, and even the top lid of the feeding box is made of glass, enabling inspection without opening. The feeeding box itself B measures 65 x 40 x 90 cm high, and the trough can be moved up and down by the compressed air. At feeding, when the trough is elevated to the upper position, it is locked air tight against a rubber gasket, securing a minimum loss of chamber air. If required, the trough may be fixed at any position between top and bottom. Water is supplied from a small reservoir at the top of the chamber through drinking cups operated by the animal itself.

The animal cage C is used inside and outside the chamber. The chambers are fully air-conditioned by a climatic control unit at the top of each. Each unit consist of a cooling radiator and electric heat exchanger E and Ventilation fan F. The temperature of the tank supply of cooling liquid is maintained constant by a compressor J operating on the basis of freon evaporation. The cooling liquid is circulated from tank I, through the cooling radiator and back again to the tank. The degree of cooling is regulated by the rate of flow of cooling liquid through the radiator which is again directed by a three way valve L. The overall control of this valve as well of the degree of heating of unit E is provided by two electronic proportional and integral regulators G, H according to the preset values of temperature and humidity from devices located at the conditioning unit. Each chamber can be operated Independently at constant temperature (+0.5°C) and humidity (+1-2%) within the range of +5 to 35°C and 30-100% relative humidity, respectively. Any emergency switch turns off the power supply to the heater if the chamber temperature rises above a maximum level.

Ventilation

The fan F maintained a constant internal flow of air from the chamber through the climatic unit and back to the chamber again. The chamber ventilation is provided by a fan F with a maximum capacity of 30 m^3/hours. The fan is placed on the left above the chamber and is sucking the air out of the chamber and thus create a small negative pressure inside the box. On the steel pipeline between the chamber and the ventilation fan two flow metres.

One thermocouple and one dry gas metre are located. After passing the ventilator, a small part of the chamber air is directed through the gas analysis apparatus and to provide chamber gas for the 24 hours composite sample collected in recipient Q with the bell placed in oil/water bath. In 24 hours the recipients are lifted by an electric motor at a constant speed collecting a 15 litre gas sample. Each chamber is provided with two receipients for gas sampling.

Analysis and Recording System

From the membrane pumps T the gas flows through a drier unit to the CO_2 and CH_4 analysers (infra-red, Hartmann and Braun). The concentration of CH_4 (0-0.15%), CO_2 (0.-1.5%) and O_2 (19-21%) in the gas is recorded together with barometric pressure, gas metre temperature, gas flow and chamber and humidity on the 24 points recorded V and the data logger (X, paper tape) for direct computation. The interval between each cycle (24 records) can be varied from 2.5 minutes to 24 hours. The number of records per cycle and per chamber can also be directed from the control W. *The gas analysis is done with the help of Haldane gas analysis apparatus as well as on the automatic Hartmen and Braun equipment.*

Heat production is calculated by using Brower's equation (1965) constant as mentioned in Table 1.

F. Actual Working of Indirect Calorimetry for Heat Production Studies (Method of Brody, 1945)

Indirect calorimetry is based on the fact that, normally, oxygen consumption and carbon dioxide production are closely related to heat production. Pfluger's *"Calorie coefficient of oxygen"* is the ratio of heat produced in calories to oxygen consumed in grams, which is about 3.5 for carbohydrates, 3.3 for fat and 3.2 for protein oxidation. Since the calorie equivalent of oxygen consumed and carbon dioxide produced varies with the nature of substance oxidised, it is theoretically necessary to know the compostion of the fuel mix (carbohydrate, fat and protein) oxidised.

Respiratory Quotient

The relative amounts of fat and carbohydrate oxidised are determined from the non-protein respiratory quotient (RQ). *The respiratory quotient is the ratio of mole or volume of CO_2 produced to moles of volumes O_2 consumed. For the oxidation of carbohydrates the RQ is unity, conversely, when the non-protein RQ is 1.00, it is assumed that carbohydrate is oxidised. The RQ for mixed fat is 0.71, although each fat has its distinctive RQ. The short chain fats have an RQ nearer 0.70.* The RQ for mixed protein is 0.81, although, as in the case of fat, each protein and amino acid has its distinctive RQ. *The oxidation of the amino acid alanine may yield an RQ of 0.83.*

Benefit of Indirect Calorimetry Over Direct Calorimetry

1. For most purposes, when the reaction are not endothermic or partly anaerobic and the caloric equivalent of O_2 is known indirect calorimetry is more reliable than direct, and the measurement of oxygen consumption alone gives as good, sometimes better results than measuring CO_2 production and the RQ.
2. Direct calorimetry involves a very costly and sophosticated equipments, it is difficult to instal such type of respiration chambers in the country. However, heat production studies could be conducted by simple apparatus using indirect calorimetry.
3. *The author of this compendium has conducted heat and methane production studies on zebu cows, using technique of indirect calorimetry at the National Dairy Research Institute, Karnal (Haryana), India, under the guidance and supervision of Late Dr. S.N. Ray, Ex-Director, NDRI, Karnal, Haryana (India), (Krishna, 1973).*

Method I : Closed circuit spirographic face mask method for farm animals and human subjects (Method of Brody, 1945)

Its use for measuring human basal or standards metabolism was made generally known by Benedict and Associates. It consists in connecting the pulmonary system of the subject to an oxygen spirometre, and measuring the rate of oxygen consumption by the rate of decline of the oxygen bell. This apparatus is illustrated below in Fig. 2.

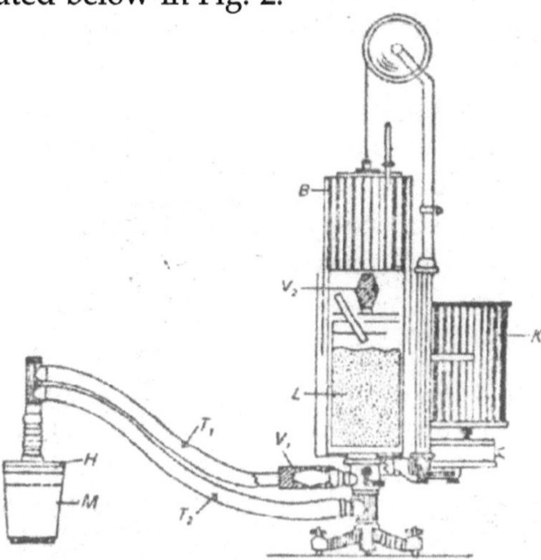

Fig. 2 : Benedict Roth Collins clinical metabolism apparatus (*Source :* Brody, S. 1945. Bioenergetics and Growth, Rein Hold Publication, New York, pp 314).

The air is circulated freely through the porous soda lime in one direction by the valves V. The oxygen bell, B which floats freely in the water seal, is counterbalanced by a weight, and so will not rise or fall except when acted upon by the circulating air. The decline of the bell is recorded graphically on the kymograph drum K. It should be noticed that animals are entirely at ease in natural positions, completely under the operator's control. The clock kymograph records the rate of oxygen consumption graphically.

The oxygen bell is of a size to produce an oxygen consumption line of reasonable slope. The oxygen bell used for human metabolism by the Benedict Roth method has a volume of 20.73 ml per 1mm height. This oxygen volume has a calorie equivalent of 0.1 cal (under) STP conditions, assuming an RQ of 0.8 with a calorie equivalent of 4.825 cal per litre. This bell size was adopted to facilitate computation. Benedict Roth measured the decline in slope for 6 minutes corresponds to a heat production 50 cal per hour. When using the Benedict Roth size spirometre, the slope of the spirograph in mm per 6 minutes multiplied by a factor to reduce it to standard temperature, pressure and humidity. The resulting value corresponds to the heat production in terms of cal per hour. If there is a temperature rise in the oxygen bell during the 5 minutes, 1/2 mm per degree centrigrade is added to the rise of the oxygen consumption line before the other computations are made.

As previously noted, the advantage of using this graphic spirometric method for measuring ruminant metabolism is that the digestive tract CO_2 exhaled by these animals is absorbed in soda lime and is thus eliminated as a complicating factor.

This method would indeed be ideal for ruminants except for the fact that they also exhale some methane (after its absorption into the blood stream from the rumen) which may accumulate in the oxygen bell, so that the decline in the oxygen bell due to the consumption of its oxygen will be less by the volume of methane accumulated. The oxygen consumption is measured regularly before the morning feeding. The graphic spirometre methods of course, involves only a part of the methane eliminated, not that eliminated by rectum or regurgitated by the oesophagus, because such more or less sudden gas elimination is graphically recorded, and the metabolism is measured by the smooth slope of the graphic record, not by the absolute change in height of the oxygen bell.

Method II: Open circuit mask method using Douglas bag & gas analysis (Method of Brody, 1945), followed by Krishna (1973) at NDRI, Karnal (Haryana), India

Apparatus

1. Face mask
2. Wet gas metre
3. Douglas bag
4. Haldane gas analysis apparatus

1. *Face Mask* : This Face Mask was originally developed by Author at NDRI, Karnal (Haryana), India. Fig. 5.3 gives an elevation (half in section) of the face mask in which the general dimensions are given. This figure shows at part No. 1 the exhaust pipe for connecting the rubber pipe to a Douglas bag at No 2 the rubber gasket for making the unit air tight. Part No. 3 comprises an outlet valve made of mild steel for enterance of outside air into the face mask.

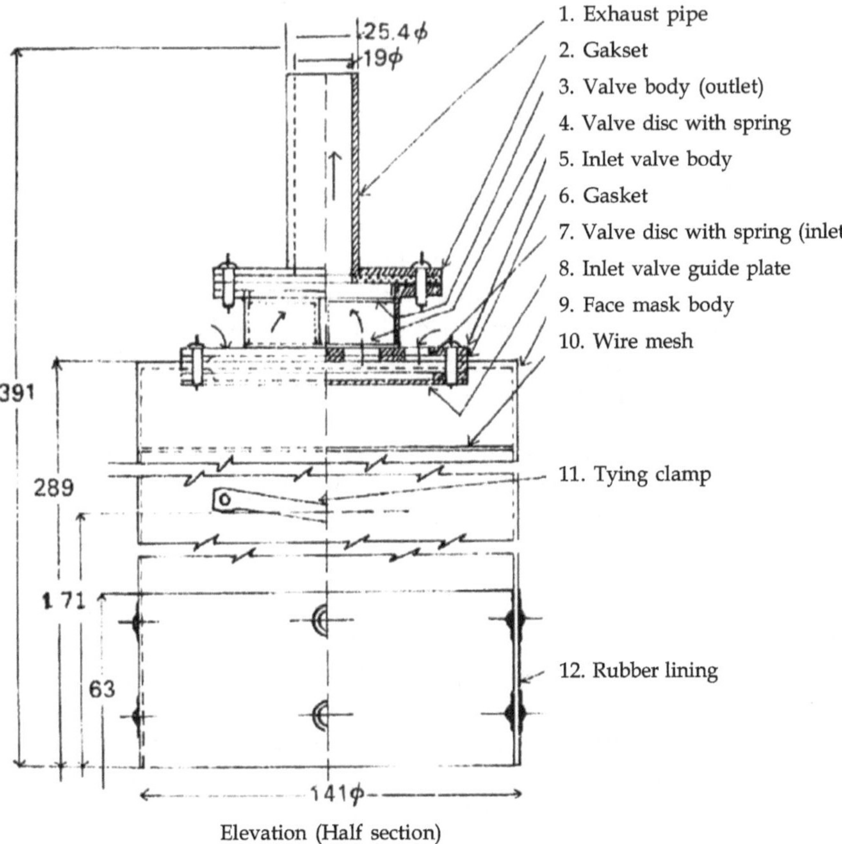

Fig. 3 : Elevation (Half section) of face mask. (*Source :* Krishna, G. 1973. Studies on energy and protein requirements for milk production in Indian dairy animals, Ph. D. Thesis, Agra University, Agra, India). Designed and prepared at NDRI, Karnal (Haryana) by the author with the assistance of Dairy Engineering Division.

There are eight circular holes in its body for inlet and four holes for outlet, part No. 6 shows the rubber gasket between inlet valve body for making the unit air tight at this joint. Part No. 7 is the aluminium valve disc with spring (steel for inlet valve No. 8 is the inlet valve guide plate made of mild steel and fitted with the inlet valve body No. 9), the face mask body made of ordinary tin having tin coating inside and outside. Circular wire mesh (Part No. 10) is provided for preventing the particles going inside the valves and choking the passage of air. Part No. 11 comprises the tying clamps made mild steel for tethering the mask by rope to the face of the animal and No. 12 is the rubber lining inside and outside of the apex of face mask body which has been provided for prevention of injury to the face of the animal. The mild steel parts which remain in the contact with expired air are nickle coated to prevent the parts from being rusted.

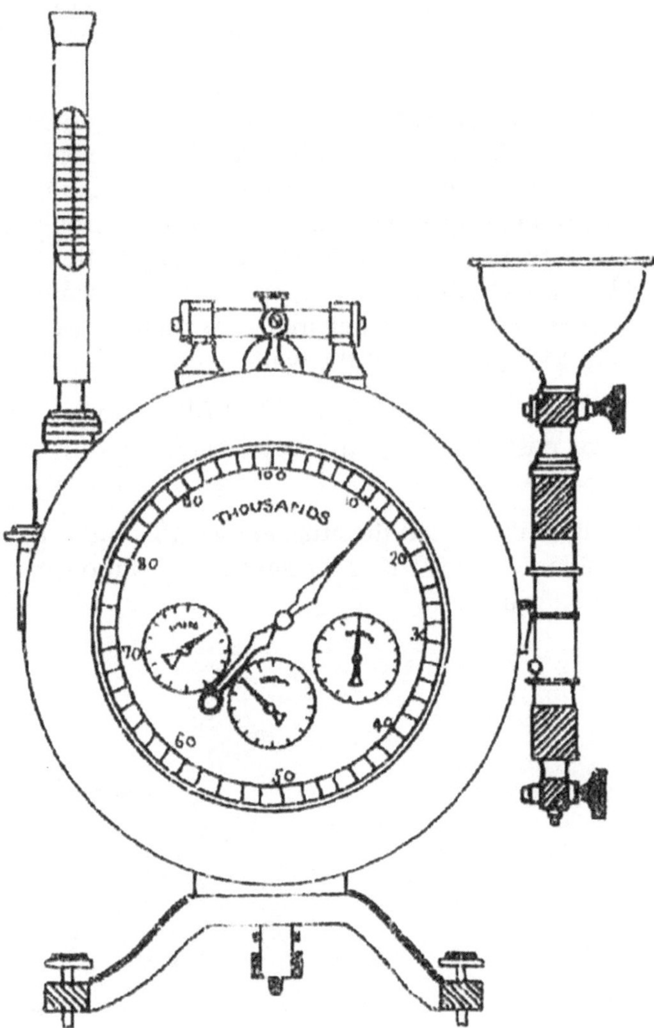

Fig. 4 : Wet gas metre for measuring gas volume filled in Douglas bag. (*Source:* Dennis, D.M. and Nicholoas, M.L. 1929. Gas analysis, The Mac Millan Co., New York, pp 22).

2. *Wet gas metre :* The gas metre is illustrate in Fig. 4. It consist of a cylinderical casing of either cast iron, steel or brass, protected by a coating of tin, nickel, enamel.

Enclosed in the casting is a rotating, horizontal drum made of some metal or allow like tinned brass, German silver or monel metal to withstand the corroding action of gases. The dials of the metres are so graduated that one complete revolution of the drum and the large pointer corresponds to one tenth or one twelth cubic foot or three litres, while the small pointers record the total volumes of gas that has passed through the metre. The metre is also equipped with a level indicator generally two spirit levels at right angles to each other, leveling screws at the base, a water level indicator and a thermometre.

A metre of this type is prepared for use in the following manner. It is first set at absolutely level by adjusting the leveling screws at the base, and is next filled with water until the water is slightly above the gauge mark. The metre is then connected with the gas supply, and gas is passed through it until the water is saturated with the gas. Both the inlet and outlet opening are disconnected and left open to the air, and the pointer is set at zero. The water level is then adjusted exactly to the gauge mark, the metre is run through one more revolution, and the ajustment of the water level is verified.

If the temperature, pressure and humidity of the gauge are unknown, the volume which has passed through the metre may be reduced to standard conditions.

3. *Douglas bag :* Fig. 5 illustrated the attachment of Douglas bag with face mask through adapter. This bag is air tight and expired gas collected, is not allowed to be leaked.

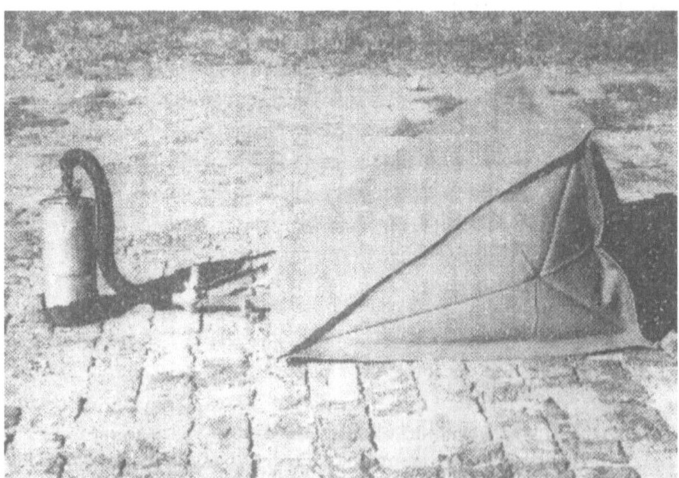

Fig. 5 : Author conducting indirect Calorimetry studies at NDRI, Karnal, India.
(*Source :* Krishna, G. 1973. Studies on energy and protein requirements for milk production in Indian dairy animals, Ph.D. Thesis, Agra University, Agra, India).

As shown in the Fig. 5, the experimental cow is confined in a pen in recumbent position. The newly designed face mask is attached to the face & is connected to a Douglas log through rubber tubing and a three way valve.

The three way valve is first opened to open the face mask to the outside air. Then the animal is permitted to respire for five minutes, after which the three way valve is closed from the outside contact and opened to the inside passage between face mask and Douglas bag. The desired volume of expired air sample is collected in the bag noting the exact time taken for the collection **Haldane gas analysis apparatus**. *The Haldane gas analysis apparatus is illustrated below in Fig. 6.*

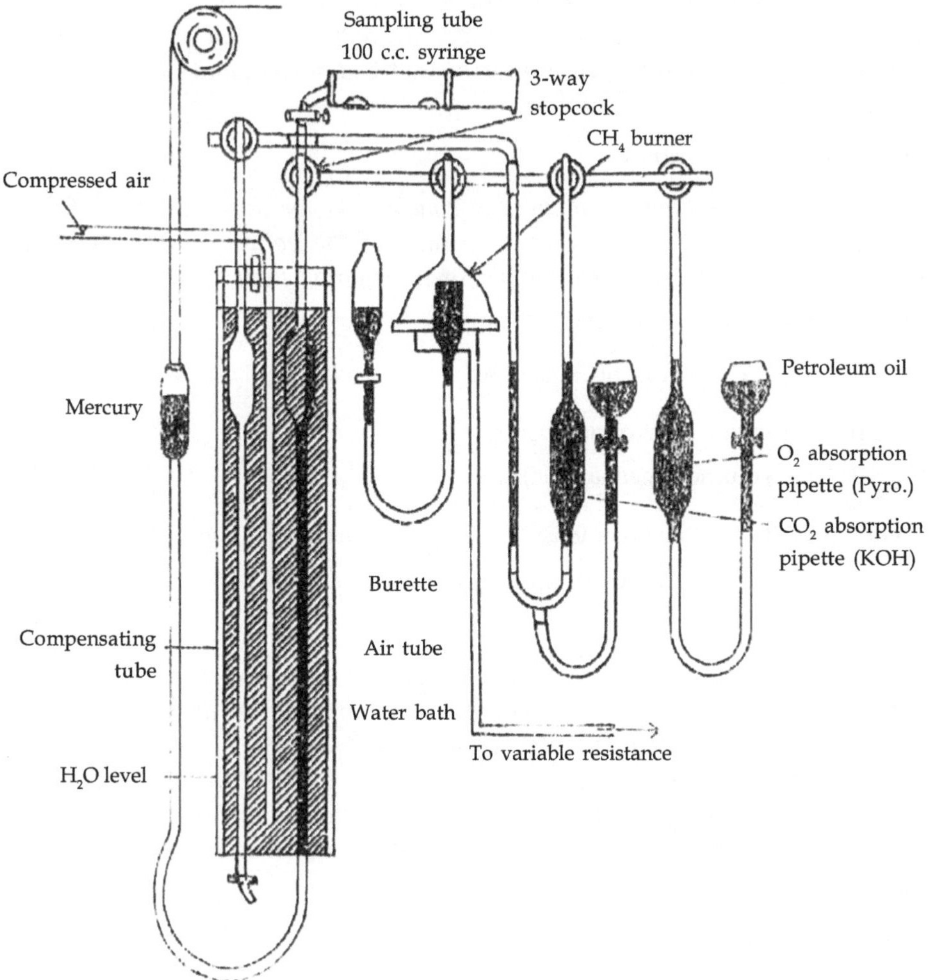

Fig. 6 : Haldane gas analysis apparatus. (*Source :* Brody, S. 1945. Bioenergetics and Growth, Reinhold Publ. Corp. New York, pp 338).

As shown above, the apparatus is composed of a 10 ml burette in which the gas sample is confined. This burette is connected to a levelling bulb where the gas sample can be drawn in or forced out, and attached to 30 ml absorbers, one for CO_2 (Carbon dioxide) and one for O_2 (Oxygen). The burette is also connected to a combustion pipette for oxidising the CH_4 to CO_2. *The CO_2 absorber contains a 20 per cent solution of KOH, the oxygen absorber contains a solution made by dissolving 10 grams pyrogallic acid in 100 ml saturated solution of KOH (sp. gr. 1.55).* Temperature, barometric pressure and water vapour changes are adjusted by a compensating tube of the same and shape as the gas burette. Both burettes are kept in a water bath. Some distilled water is kept in a water compensating burette. The potash absorption pipette connects the air between the control and same tubes. *The methane is burned by heating the platinum wire in the combustion chamber to white heat (from a 4 volt current). The resulting CO_2 is measured by absorption in the KOH burette, and CH_4 computed from the equation.*

$$CH_4 + 2O_2 = CO_2 + 2H_2O \qquad \text{......... (A)}$$

From the above equation, 1 volume (or 1 mole) CH_4 produces 1 volume CO_2, so that the CH_4 per cent is the percentage ratio of the volume CO_2 formed in combustion divided by the total gas sample, or in equation form.

$$CH_4\% = \frac{\text{Volume } CO_2 \text{ formed in combustion}}{\text{Total volume of gas sample}} \times 100 \qquad \text{......... (B)}$$

$$= \frac{\text{Volume shrinkage due to combustion}}{2\,(\text{Total volume of gas sample})} \times 100 \qquad \text{........... (C)}$$

$$= \frac{\text{Volume shrinkage due to combustion} + \text{Vol. } CO_2 \text{ formed in 2 combustion}}{(\text{Total volume of gas sample})} \times 100$$

$$\text{........ (D)}$$

Equation follows from the fact, shown in equation (A), that, discounting the water which condenses, volume CH_4 produces one volume carbon dioxide, equation (C) follows from the fact, shown by equation (A), that the volume of methane present is half the contraction on combustion, equation (D) follows from the fact, shown by equation (A) that when the CO_2 has been absorbed, there is a diminution of half of the volume. Equation (A) also shows that twice as much oxygen as methane disappers in the combustion of methane.

Composition of Outdoor Air

Under ordinary cases, it is assumed that the inspired air is pure outdoor air contains 0.031 per cent. CO_2, 20.93 per cent oxygen and 79.04 per cent N_2 and that no change occurs in the volume of nitrogen.

Example : **Analysis of barn yard air (Krishna, 1973)**

Volume of air taken into burette	*9.663 ml*
Volume after CO_2 absorbed	*9.659 ml*
CO_2 asborbed	*0.004 ml*
Carbon dioxide	*0.040 %*
Volume after oxygen absorbed	*7.663 ml*
Oxygen absorbed	*2.026 ml*
Oxygen	*20.97 %*
Nitrogen % = 100- (0.04 + 21.04)	*78.92*

It is very important to have appreciable amounts of acidulated water in the burette, or the burette becomes alkaline and stores CO_2 with resulting apparently low CO_2 values.

Actual Procedure of estimating heat production in dry cow using Face mask, Douglas bag and Haldane gas analysis apparatus (Method of Brody, 1945) as per experience of author during Ph.D. degree research work conducted at NDRI, Karnal (Haryana), India under late Prof. Dr. S.N. Ray Ex Director NDRI (Karnal), Haryana.

Experimental cow of a breed Tharparkar and Sahiwal is fasted for 46 hours and the value of respiratory quotient 0.71 is observed, which indicate post absorptive stage. Colvos *et al.* (1964) also observed RQ value of 0.71 after 48 hours of fasting, which they considered the post absorptive stage in their experiment. Mullick and Kehar (1952) observed RQ value of 0.71 after 72 hours of fasting in tropics.

After 46 hours of fasting, cow is fed on experimental ration, sample of expired gas is collected after four hours of feeding at the time of active fermentation in rumen.

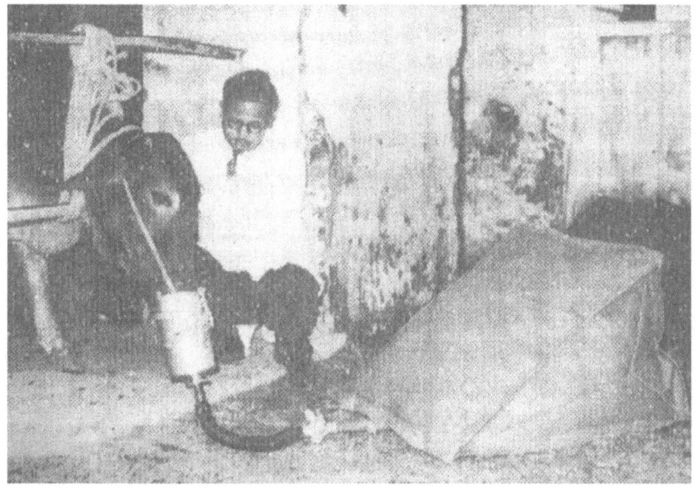

Fig. 7 : Author conducting indirect calorimetry studies at NDRI, Karnal, (Haryana) India. (*Source :* Krishna, G. 1973. Studies on energy and protein requirements for milk production in Indian diary animals, Ph.D. Thesis, Agra University, Agra, India).

Experimental cow is confined in a pen in a standing positon as shown in the above Fig. 7. The face mask is attached to the face and connected to Douglas bag through rubber tubing and a three way valve. The three way valve is first opened to connect the mask to the outside air. Then the animal is permitted to respire for five minutes after which the three way valve is closed from the outside contact and opened to the inside passage between face mask and Douglas bag. Expired gas is collected in Douglas bag for ten minutes. After collection of gas, contact between face mask and bag is disrupted by turning the three way valve. Care is taken to see that the animal did not feel any difficulty or obstruction in breathing while expired gas is collected. The animals are trained for this purpose before the acual experimentation.

The Douglas bag is filled with expired gas sample is brought to the laboratory and an aliquot of gas sample is taken in an gas sampler. The gas sampler is attached to the central tube of Haldane gas analysis apparatus. The volume of expired gas filled in the Douglas bag is measured by passing through wet gas metre. Average metre temperature and Barometric pressure is measured immediately. Expired gas sample is analysed by Haldane gas analysis apparatus, for knowing the per cent oxygen, per cent carbon dioxide and per cent methane.

Example : Calculation of heat production by indirect calorimetry in a zebu cow (Krishna, G. 1973).

Animal, Sahiwal cow 127 of NDRI (Karnal, India), diary herd.

1. *Volume air passed through gas metre in 30 minutes = 95.8 x 28.317 = 2712.768 litres*
2. *Average metre temperature = 18.3°C*
3. *Barometric pressure = 739.7 mm mercury pressure*
4. *Correction factor*

$$\frac{265}{273+\text{Met.Temp}} \times \frac{\text{Bar.Pressure}}{760} = 0.885$$

5. *Expired air at STP = 2712.77 x 0.885 (lit./30 mm) = 2400.799 litres*
6. *Volume expired air sample in the Haldane 10 ml analyser = 10 ml*
7. *Volume after CO_2 absorbed = 9.714 ml*
8. *CO_2 absorbed = 0.286 ml*
9. *CO_2 in exhaled air = 2.86 per cent*
10. *Volume after combustion of methane and absorption of resulting CO_2 = 9.629 ml*

11. *Methane produced = 1/3 (9.714-9.629) = 0.028 ml*

$$** \text{Per cent produced} = \frac{\text{Vol. shrinkage due to combustion} + \text{Vol. } CO_2 \text{ formed in combustion}}{3\,(\text{Total volume of gas sample})}$$

☞ **Note**

* *See table 8, pp 55, Carpenter's, Tables, factors and formulae for computing respiratory exchange and biological transformations of energy, Carnegie Instt. Washington Publ. 303 A.*

12. *Methane in expired air sample = 0.28 per cent*
13. *Volume after oxygen absorbed = 7.885 ml*
14. *Oxygen absorbed = 9.629-7.885 = 1.744 ml*
15. *Total oxygen absorbed, including that used for oxidation of* CH_4 *= Vlaue of column 14+2 x methane produced = 1.744 + 2 x 0.028 = 18.00 per cent*
16. *Oxygen in expired air = 18.00 per cent*
17. *Nitrogen in expired air = 100-(%* CO_2 *+ % methane + %* O_2*)*

    100 - (2.86 + 0.28 + 18.0) = 78.86 per cent

To compute the volume of oxygen retained by the animal, the volume of oxygen expired is deducted from the volume of oxygen inspired.

The total volume of expired air for the 30 minutes period, as measured by gas metre and corrected to standard conditions of temperature and pressure, is 2400.79 litres.

The percentage of nitrogen in this sample expired air is 78.86 per cent, as compared to 79.03 per cent, the known percentage in outdoor air. Since nitrogen is not retained by the animal, the same volume (STP) of nitrogen is expired as is inspired. The decrease in the percentage of nitrogen expired over that inspired means that the total volume of air expired is different (more in this case) from the total volume inspired. The reason for the change in volume in the air, on passage through the lungs is that the RQ is not equal to 1.

The air inspired during the 30 minutes period must have had such volume that the nitrogen percentage was 79.03 per cent instead of 78.86 per cent, the percentage found in expired air. The volume of inspired air may (having 79.03 per cent nitrogen) be computed by inverse proportion.

Volume inspired air : volume expired air : 78.86 : 79.03

Therefore, volume of inspired air =

$$\frac{\text{\% Nitrogen in expired air}}{\text{\% Nitrogen in inspired air}} \text{x volume of expired air at STP}$$

$$= \frac{78.86}{79.03} \text{x volume of expired air at STP}$$

= 0.997 x 2400.79 = 2393.596 litres

The content of oxygen in outdoor air is 20.94 per cent. Therefore vol. O_2 in outside air inspired (STP) = volume of inspired air x 0.2094

= 2393.596 x 0.2094 = 501.219 litres

= volume O_2 in expired air (STP)

= volume of expired air at STP x % O_2 in expired air

= 2400.790 x 0.18 = 432.143 litres

= volume O_2 consumed by the animal = 501.219-432.143= 69.076 litres

The oxygen consumed expressed as a percentage of expired air is then

$$= \frac{\text{Oxygen consumed}}{\text{Volume of expired air}} \text{x} 100$$

$$= \frac{69.076}{2400.799} \text{x} 100$$

= 2.87 per cent

The CO_2 in outdoor is approximately 0.03 per cent.

Volume CO_2 in expired air = expired air x % CO_2 in expired air = 2400.799 x 0.0286 = 68.60 litres

Volume CO_2 in inspired air = volume inspired air x 0.0003 = 0.7181

CO_2 increment = 88.660–0.718 = 87.942

CO_2 increment as a percentage of expired air =

$$= \frac{CO_2 \text{ increment}}{\text{expired air}} \text{x} 100$$

$$= \frac{67.942}{2400.799} \text{x} 100$$

= 2.82 per cent

$$\text{Respiratory quotient (RQ)} = \frac{CO_2 \text{ increment}}{O_2 \text{ retained}} x100$$

$$= \frac{2.82}{2.87}$$

= 0.982

Heat production = volume of expired air x % oxygen decrement times thermal equivalent of the oxygen at the given RQ

= 2400.799 x 0.0287 x 5.022

= 346.030 calories in 30 mts.

= 16, 609 calories/day

☞ Notes

1. *Thermal equivalent of the oxygen at the given RQ may be consulted from the following Table 2 (Lusk Table).*

Table 2 : Thermal equivalent of oxygen at the given RQ (Source : Lusk, G. 1928. The science of Nutrition, chapter 8). LUSK TABLE

RQ	Oxygen Cal/litre	RQ	Oxygen Cal/litre
0.70	4.686	0.89	4.912
0.71	4.690	0.90	4.924
0.72	4.702	0.91	4.936
0.73	4.714	0.92	4.948
0.74	4.727	0.93	4.960
0.75	4.720	0.94	4.973
0.76	4.752	0.95	4.985
0.80	4.801	0.96	4.997
0.85	4.863	0.97	5.010
0.86	4.875	0.98	5.022
0.87	4.887	0.99	5.034
0.88	4.900	1.00	5.047

2. *The basal metabolism in human subject is measured about 12 hours after the preceeding meal, when RQ is about 0.82.*

3. *The simplest and, under normal conditions, perhaps the most accurate, method for measuring energy metabolism is, then, by the rate of oxygen consumption as fed from a calibrated oxygen container, and computing the heat production by the calorie value of oxygen, e.g., 4.825 cal/litre corresponding to an RQ of 0.82.*

4. *For most purposes-when the reactions are not endothermic or partly anaerobic and the calorie equivalent of O_2 is known, indirect calorimetry is more reliable than direct, and the measurements of oxygen consumption alone gives as good, sometimes better, results than measuring CO_2 production and the RQ (Brody, 1945).*

References

Brody, S. (1945). *Bioenergetics and growth,* Rein hold Publ. Corp., New York.

Brower, E. (1965). *In energy metabolism,* pp 441. Ed. Blaxter, K.L. European Assoc. *Animal Prod. Publ.* 11. Academic Press. London.

Krishna, G. (1973). *Studies on energy and protein requirements for milk production in Indian dairy animals. Ph.D.* Thesis, Agra Univ., Agra (India), NDRI, Karnal (Haryana), India.

Krishna, G., Razdan, M.N. and Ray, S.N. (1976). Effect of different planes of nutrition on heat and methane production in dry cows. *Ind. J. Exptl., Biol.* 14:710-711.

Krishna, G., Razdan, M.N. and Ray, S.N. (1977). Studies on energy and protein requirements of zebu (Bos Indicus). *Z. Tierphysiologie und Tierernährung* und *Fultermittelkde.* 38: 281-284.

Krishna, G., Razdan, M.N. and Ray, S.N. (1978). Assessment of Calorific value of dairy cows ration in tropical / subtropical region of India (Short Communication). *Indian. J. Dairy Sci.* 31: 385-387.

Krishna, G., Razdan, M.N. and Ray, S.N. (1978). Effect of nutritional and seasonal variations on heat and methane production in *Bos Indicus. Indian J. Anim. Sci.,* 48: 366-370.

Lavoisier, A.L. and Laplace, (1780). Mem. del 1' Academic des Sciences. 1780, 355 (oeuvres, 2: 283. 1862).

Mullick, D.N. and Kehar, N.D. (1959). *Ind.J. Vet.Sci.,* 29:27.

Regnault, V. and Reiset, J. (1849). *Annal de chemie et de Physique,* 3 e Serie, 26 : 299.

Sundstϕl, F., Ekern, A. and Haugen, A.E. (1973). *Description of a respiration unit for sheep, goats, calves, and pigs.* Proc. Sixth Symposium on energy metabolism, West Germany.

Weir, J. B., De, V. (1949). *J. Physiol.,* 109:1.

Chapter - 61

Fat Soluble Vitamin and Ascorbic Acid Assay

Assay of Carotene, Tocopherol and Plant Pigments (Method of Astrup *et al.*, 1971). Agricultural University of NORWAY, ÅS-NLH, NORWAY

Introduction

A method which assays the carotene together with chlorophyll a and b and xanthophyll was given by worker (1957, 1958) and this was a successful approach towards a useful routine procedure. Worker's way of extraction is based on the use of aqueous acetone a technique which was studied by Davidson (1954). The separation is accomplished on an alumina column. Worker (1958) has used a double successive chromatography, once on magnesia and again on alumina, to obtain its separation from the other lipid components. *The method developed by Astrup et al. (1971) permits simultaneous assay of tocopherol, carotene and plant pigments using alumina column.*

Carotene and tocopherol are extracted into acetone and eluted through alumina column. Petroleum ether (for chromatography, B.P. 60-80°C) aids in eluting carotene, while 2 per cent acetone in petroleum ether and 1 per cent ethanol in petroleum ether help in eluting tocopherol. In the case of carotene O.D. is measured at 465 nm and in the case of tocopherol, light brown colour developed (by using dipyridyl and ferric chloride) is measured at 520 nm.

Apparatus : Column as shown in Fig. 1 having Rotafflo stopcock is used for carotene and tocopherol assay.

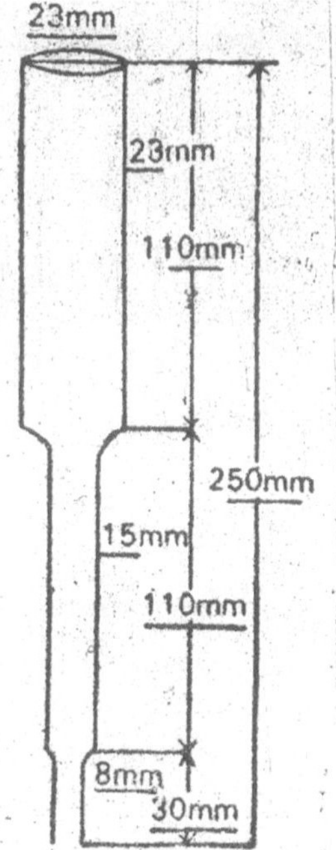

Fig. 1 : Carotene assay column fitted with Rotaflo stopcock

Reagents

1. Aluminium Oxide Activated

When cyrstalline aluminium oxide trihydrate is heated at 500°C, the anhydrous alumina is produced. By controlled heating at higher temperature, alumina of a suitable "activity" or retentiveness or adsorptive power, for various purposes may be produced. Activated alumina is procurable, ready made an obvious advantage-but with the disadvantage that most of the commercial preparations are hygroscopic. Freshly activated alumina may be too dry, thereby holding carotene too tenaciously or as purchased it may be suitable for use, but after the bottle has been opened a few times the powder becomes less adsorptive. If has been experienced that this moisture acts as a physical barrier between carotene and alumina, so that the adsorptive forces are active at a distance. This surface moisture is not water of crystallisation and is only driven off by moderate heat to restore the original activity. The surface moisture can be adjusted by exposing the powder to air for a few minutes or by washing it with aqueous alcohol (if too dry) or by heating (if too moist).

Preparation of "Activated Alumina"

Activated alumina is usually available in market, but it can be prepared in the laboratory as follows :

Pass crystalline alumina trihydrate through a 150 mesh sieve. Heat the 150 mesh crystals at 800°C (+20°C) for 7 hour. Allow the powder to cool completely.

Testing the Efficiency of Adsorbent

The alumina mix should allow quantitative recovery of carotene, while holding back carotenols, chlorophylls, lycopene and even carotenoid esters. The drier the mix the more firmly are pigments held. Since it is required that carotene be separated easily and other pigments retained on the column, a compromise is sought.

An extract of tomato provides an excellent solution for testing the satisfactoriness of this compromise. It is recommended that a quantity of tomato skin should be dried, and stored in the refrigerator, in order to be available for the tests at any season. Enough pigments for a quantitative test can be easily extracted from tomato skin directly into pertoleum ether (chromatography) without acetone. When the petroleum ether solution is drawn through the column, the pigments should form a pink band near the top. Enough solution should be used to produce a coloured band nearly 1 cm deep. when 2 per cent acetone in petroleum ether is passed through the column, it should easily elute the carotene as a faint orange band (about 2 mm deep) leaving most of the pigments, the lycopene, in a scarcely widened band at the top. A good absorbent should allow light petroleum to percolate through a column 5 cm high at a rate about 1 cm per second with suction.

2. Sodium Sulphate (Anhydrous)

The anhydrous sodium sulphate, AR grade as purchased may be suitable for use or it may be too moist. It is less likely to be too dry. If it is too moist, as judged by the test, it should be dried by heating in an oven at about 150°C for 12 hours or longer. The amount heated should be no more than enough to form a layer 2 cm. It should be finely grinded (about 200 mesh) otherwise there are chances of channeling. The word channeling means that the pigment runs down through the absorbent in little rivers, instead of in horizontal zones.

3. Distilled Acetone (AR)

It should be extra pure and of standard quality.

4. Ehanol, 96 per cent (AR)

5. Petroleum ether

60-80° C.B.P., specially for chromatography.

6. 2 per cent Acetone in Petroleum ether

(500 ml solution) 10 ml acetone and 490 ml petroleum ether.

7. 0.1 per cent ethanol in petroleum ether

(500 ml solution). 5 ml ethanol and 495 ml petroleum ether.

8. 0.8 per cent ethanol in petroleum ether

(500 ml solution). 40 ml ethanol and 460 ml petroleum ether.

9. 0.1 g $FeCl_3$ in 100 ml ethanol

10. 0.25 g 2.2' dipyridyl in 100 ml ethanol.

Procedure

Weigh 5 g sample in a 150 ml conical flask and add 80 ml acetone, keep it in a refrigerator for a overnight. Transfer the contents of flask in electric blendor and churned for ten minutes. Transfer the contents back in same conical flask. Filter the contenst of flask through sintered glass curcible by decantation and wash the residue with 80 ml acetone (AR grade).

Transfer the contents of filteration flask into 250 ml volumetric flask and make up the volume with acetone. Twenty ml of extract is taken in 50 ml beaker in duplicate, extract is evaporated at 60°C in the presence of nitrogen gas stream on water bath. Care is taken to avoid overheating Add 2 ml petroleum ether twice in the beaker. Fill the column at the bottom with glass wool and add 8 per cent ethanol in petroleum ether, allow it to run out, but retain 4-5 cm column, add 4-5 spoons alumina so as to make a height of 3.5-4.0 cm of column. Remove air from the column by tapping it with hand and allow the mass to settle down. Add one spoon of sodium sulphate (anhydrous) A.R. quality as cap material so as to absorb traces of water. Tap the column using tempering rod so as to resort through homogeneous packing of alumina as well as sodium sulphate. Add 2 ml alcohol and subsequently, add 4 ml petroleum ether, allow it to come upto glass wool by opening stop cock. Close the stop cock and then add 4 ml pigment mixture already present in 50 ml beaker on the top of the column. Now open, the stop cock, when the yellow colour has spread over three-fourth of the length of column, deliver 5-10 ml petroleum ether over the column and open the stop cock. When there is no yellow colour, in the narrow portion of the column (between stop-cock and packed below the column). Close the stop cock, place conical flask below the column, add 10 ml, 2 per cent acetone in petroleum ether and 10 ml, 1 per cent ethanol in petroleum ether till the green colour of cholorophyll appears on cotton wool and narrow neck above the stopper of column. Evaporate the content of conical flask at 60°C on water bath under nitrogen atomosphere to 0.5 ml and then add 5 ml 96 per cent ethanol and 0.2 ml each of dipyridyl and ferric chloride. Similarly prepare a blank in a conical flask by adding 5 ml ethanol, 0.2 ml dipyridyl and 0.2 ml ferric chloride. In the case of vit. E (Tocopherol), take the reading in Photoelectric colorimeter at 520 nm and take the reading at 465 nm in the case of carotene.

Calculation (Krishna, 1985a)

Calculate carotene and tocopherol contents in green sample of Doob grass (Cynodon dactylon). Analysis done by Author at CCS-HAU Hisar (Haryana), India

Net weight of green Doob grass taken for preparing acetone extract	=	5 grams
Dry matter in Doob grass	=	30.53g/100 g
O.D. x 142.5	=	carotene ppm on raw matter basis
O.D. in sample	=	0.469
0.469 x 142.5	=	66.832 ppm carotene on raw matter basis
Carotene on dry matter basis will be	=	$\frac{100 \times 66.832}{30.53}$
	=	218.807 ppm

Tocopherol

O.D. x 338	=	Tocopherol ppm on raw matter basis
O. D. in sample	=	0.108
0.108 x 338	=	36.504 ppm tocopherol on raw matter basis
Tocopherol on dry matter basis will be	=	$\frac{100 \times 36.504}{30.530}$
	=	119.51 ppm

Result : Doob grass (cynodon dactylon) contained 218.807 ppm carotene and 119.51 ppm tocopherol.

Assay of Vitamin A Using Carr-Price (1926) Reaction

(Method of Dann and Evelyn, 1938 Modified by AOAC, 1965)

Important Precaution

We require subdued light, high laboratory temperature should be avoided. All the steps of assay should be complete within a shortest possible time.

Principle

This method is based on the measurment of the unstable blue colour formed by the interaction of vitamin A and antimony trichloride. The absorbancy (optical density) of this solution at 620 mμ is a function of the concentration of vitamin A.

When antimony trichloride reacts with vitamin A in chloroform solution a blue colour develops. Carotene, which is also in the extract, is determine directly (without $SbCl_3$) and a correction is applied to the vitamin A value for the contribution of the carotene to the $SbCl_3$ colour.

The chief disadvantages of this procedure are given below :

The rapid fading of the blue colour resulting from the reaction, necessitating speed and expereince for the determination of its maximum intensity., the corrosive nature of the antimony trichloride necessitating careful handling., its extreme sensitivity to even minute amounts of moisture and the production of a typical colours or inhibition of colour development, due to the presence of various sterols, carotenoids and other interfering materials.

Reagents

1. *Potassium hydroxide solution : Dissolove 50 g pellets in 50 ml water.*
2. *Diethyl ether : USP. Hence forth, the term ether refer specifically to diethyl ether. This must be freshly redistilled, discarding the first and last 10 per cent.*
3. *Ethanol : USP, S.D. 3-A or S.D 30 are satisfactory.*
4. *Anhydrous sodium sulphate (granular). : This should be checked to determine that it retains no vitamin A as follows : Shake several g of sodium sulphate with 50 to 100 ml of ether containing 100 USP units of vitamin A. Decant the ether as completely as possible and wash the sodium sulphate several times with 10 to 15 ml portions of ether. If the washed sodium sulphate does not turn blue when treated with 2 or 3 ml of a 25 per cent solution of antimony trichloride in chloroform, it retains no vitamin A. Lots of sodium sulphate which give a blue colour should be rejected.*
5. *Pehnolphthalein : Dissove 1 g of phenolphthalein in sufficient ethanol to make 100 ml.*
6. *Choloroform : This should be free of moisture and phosgene gas. The latter forms especially in redistilled chloroform on standing and results in destruction of vitamin A. The chloroform may be dried by allowing it to stand over anhydrous Na_2SO_4 or $CaCl_2$.*
7. *Antimony Trichloride reagent : Care : Corrosive agent :*

   Weigh an unopened bottle 1/4 1b of antimony trichloride. Open the bottle and empty the contents into a wide-mouth, glass stoppered amber bottle containing approximately 100 ml of chloroform. By difference obtain the weight of antimony trichloride and then add sufficient chlorofrom to supply 100 ml for each 25 g. Dissolve by warming or shaking for several hours and filter through Na_2SO_4 into a clean, dry, amber bottle with ground glass stopper. This solution may be stored at room temperature but should be kept in the dark when not in use. The reagent is apparently stable for long periods for time, but it is convenient to make up sufficient amounts to last for one month. Rinse all *glassware coming in contact with this reagent with chloroform, a mixture of ethanol and ether, or dilute or concentrated HCl before washing.*

8. *USP Vitamin a Reference standard : A solution of purified vitamin A acetate crystals in cottonseed oil capsulated in gelatin tubes. Each g of this solution contains 3.44 mg of vitamin A acetate (3 mg of vitamin A).*

Equipments

1. Flasks (250 ml capacity) with ground glass joints fitted to air or water cooled condensers for saponification. In lieu of these, ordinary 250 ml Erlenmeyer flasks may be used in conjuction with cold finger condensers.
2. Separating funnels, Squib (pearshaped). 500 ml capacity. The lubricant used for the stop cocks should not be soluble in ether nor contain ether soluble substance which absorb ultraviolet light. Separatory funnels equiped with Teflon stop cocks can be used. The lubricant is not necessary with these funnels.
3. Flasks, 250 or 500 ml for solvent removal. The size to be used depends upon the volume of solvent to be removed.
4. Glass stoppered volumetric flasks.
5. Volumetric Transfer pipettes especially 1, 2, 5 and 10 ml.
6. Hot plate.
7. Vacuum pump or filter pump (aspirator) with vapour trap for solvent removal.
8. Cylinder of nitrogen.
9. Glass funnels, 6 cm or sintered glass plates.
10. Rapid delivery pipettes for addition of the antimony trichloride reagent. An all glass 10 ml automatic pipette with a short delivery time (1 to 2 seconds) is recommended.
11. Photoelectric colorimeter or spectrophotometer.

    Any instrument capable of making readings at 620 mμ and whose galvanometer registers maximum colour formation within 3 to 6 seconds after addition of the antimony trichloride reagent may be used.

Procedure

I. Saponification

(a) For food products, accurately weigh a sample estimated to contain at least 200 USP units of vitamin A. For products such as butter, cheese and fortified margarine, this usually will be 5 to 10g. As an alternative procedure for butter and margarine obtain a clear oil by liquefying the sample at 80-85°C and filter through whatman No. 1 filter paper. Determine the vitamin A content of the oil and calculate the potency of the original sample after a determination of its fat content. In the case of milk, use 50 to 100 ml. Extract the fat and carry out the vitamin assay on the saponified fat. Products containing starch or sugar should be dissolved in a minimum amount of hot water prior to saponification.

For vitamin A fortified feed concentrates, weigh a finely ground sample containing not less than 400 USP units of vitamin A into an extraction thimble and extract for 2 hours with ether in an extraction apparatus, evaporate the ether and saponify the residue. Should this be a premix of sufficiently high potency, it may be saponified directly. For this purpose, weigh a finely ground sample containing not less than 200 USP units into a saponification flask, using at least 1 g of sample.

(b) Add 30 ml of ethanol and 3 ml of KOH solution.

1. The above is advised for fish oils or concentrates. For margarine (5 to 10 grams sample) use 50 ml of ethanol and 5 ml KOH solution.
2. It is recommended that the volume of KOH solution be such as to contain an amount of KOH at least equal to one half of the weight of the assay sample.

(c) Heat under gentle reflux for at least 30 minutes, or until saponification is complete.

The time required for complete saponification varies with the nature of the product. In general, those materials containing long chain fatty acids will require a longer saponification time. For most samples, 15 minutes is adequate, but time exerts no detrimental effect on the content of vitamin A. Test for completeness of saponification by adding a small amount of water and shaking. If cloudiness appears, the reaction is incomplete and the same should be refluxed for an addition period of time. However, if usually high amounts of unsaponifiable material are present, cloudiness may occur even though saponification is complete. Occasionally, the soaps produced during saponification will solidify, but solution results upon the addition of water.

II. Extraction

(a) Wash the reflux condenser with about 10 ml of water, and transfer to a separating funnel.

(b) If the volume of ethanol used is more than 30 ml, the amount of water may be increased accordingly.

(c) Rinse the saponification flask with 50 ml of ether and add to the separatory funnel in (b) above.

1. Larger volumes of ether may be used when more than 30 ml of ethanol is used.

2. If the material remaining in the saponiification flask are of a sticky nature (candy etc.) the saponification flask should be rinsed with water prior to the first ether extraction and these rinsings included in the first separatory funnel.

(d) Shake the separatory funnel cautiously opening the stop cock at intervals to release pressure. Allow the phases to separate completely.

Emulsions may occur upon too vigorous shaking at any stage in this extraction and the subsequent extraction and washing procedures or if the proportions of ethanol, water and ether are incorrect. Should an emulsion form, the addition of a few millilitres of alcohol may break it. If this proves ineffective, the addition of water may be successful.

(e) Draw off the lower (aqueous) phase directly into a second separatory funnel and let the ether extract remain in the first.

It is also possible to carry out the ether extractions with the use of only one separatory funnel per sample. In this case, drain the aqueous phase into the flask used for saponifying the sample and then place the ether solution in a 500 ml flask. Repeat this procedure one to three times more, then discard the aqueous phase and place the combined ether extracts in the separatory funnel for the subsequent washing procedure.

(f) Again rinse the saponification flask with 35 to 50 ml of ether and add the rinsings to the second separatory funnel.

(g) Repeat (d) above.

(h) Draw off the lower (aqueous) phase into a flask and add the ether extract to that in the first separatory funnel.

(i) Return the contents of the flask from (h) above the second separatory funnel.

(j) Re-extract this material 3 more times with 35 to 50 ml portions of ether, adding with 35 ml to all ether extracts to the first separatory funnel. Discard the last aqueous layer removed.

Experience with some products has indicated that fewer than 5 ether extractions are necessary. If many assays are to be made, it may be time saving for the analyst to determine the minimum number of ether extractions necessary for removal of all the vitamin A.

(k) Add 50 to 100 ml of water to the combined ether extracts in the first separatory funnel, and swirl gently. Draw off and discard the lower (aqueous) phase.

An alkaline wash of 50 ml of 0.5 N NaOH or KOH solution is sometimes used to insure the removal of acid soaps which are ether soluble. It has been suggested that the use of tap water containing Ca or Mg accomplishes the same purpose.

(l) Continue the washing by shaking gently with 50 ml portions of water until the washings are free of alkali as determined by tested with phenolphthalein. This may require as many as 5 to 8 portions.

(m) After removal of the final water wash, allow the ether extract to stand for 10 minutes and carefully draw off any separated water.

III. Solvent Removal

(a) Filter the ether extract into 250-500 ml flask through several g of anhydrous sodium sulphate distributed evenly on a filter paper in a glass funnel or on a sintered glass plate.

Alternatively, the sodium sulphate may be added prior to or during the evaporation of the ether extract.

(b) Rinse the separatory funnel and sodium sulphate with two 25 ml portions of ether, adding the rinsings to the flaks in (a).

(c) Place a glass bead in the flask and evaporate the total ether extract, or a suitable aliquot, to dryness on a water bath in a hood, removing the flask from the source of heat during evaporation of the last few ml of solution. The ether removal may also be accomplished by heating the solution on a steam bath with the concurrent introduction of a stream of nitrogen until all of the ether is removed.

The evaporation may be carried out with the use of suction only. If nitrogen gas is used with heat for the solvent removal, or alongwith vacuum, the introduction of the gas may be delayed until a layer of ether about one-third inch deep remains in the flasks. The remaining ether can then be evaporated with the flask removed from any source of heat, thus insuring the maintenance of the residue in an inert atmosphere until the final solvent addition is made. Carbon dioxide gas may be used but often times its use results in turbid antimony trichloride reaction products.

(d) Immediately, take up the residue in chloroform, making dilutions if necessary, to a concentration between 7 and 15 USP units vitamin A per ml.

1. The final solvent addition must be made immediately after removal of the ether is complete to prevent possible oxidation of vitamin A. This is a very sensitive point.
2. The concentration indicated (7 to 15 USP units per ml) here applied to both colorimeter and spectrophotometer.
3. For the saponified USP vitamin A Reference standard, it is recommended that the final chloroform solution contains 8-10 USP units per ml.
4. For routine assays where only small amounts of unsaponifiable material remain, the dilution may be accomplished by adding a measured amount of chloroform directly to the evaporation flasks rather than by transferring to volumetric flasks and diluting to the mark. Thus, for a dilution to 10 ml, the addition of 10 ml of chloroform from a pipette will be sufficiently accurate for control purposes, although the chloroform plus the unsaponifiable matter may total 10.1 or 10.2 ml.

IV. Preparation of Calibration Curve

(a) Weigh accurately into a saponificaiton flask about 0.5 gram of USP vitamin A reference standard and proceed as described under D-1, 2 and 3. The final chloroform should contain at least 25 USP units of vitamin A per ml.

(b) Prepare a series of at least 5 chloroform dilutions containing from about 5 to 25 USP units of vitamin A per ml.

(c) Introduce 2 ml of chloroform into a colorimeter tube, place in the instrument and add 10 ml of $SbCl_3$ reagent from the rapid delivery pipette.

(d) With this solution in path of the light beam at 620 mμ, set the galvanometer at full deflection (100% transmittance).

(e) To a series of colorimeter tubes add 1 ml of each of the standards prepared in (b) and 1 ml of chloroform.

(f) Place each tube, in turn in the instrument in the path of light beam and add 10 ml of $SbCl_3$ reagent from the rapid delivery pipette.

Occasionally, a turbid solution occurs upon the additon of the $SbCl_3$ reagent, especially when the humidity is high. The addition of drop of acetic anhydride prior to the addition of the reagent will usually prevent cloudiness although it may decrease the absorbance as much as two percent

(g) Read the galvanometer at the pause point, obtaining the percent transmittance.

1. The pause point refers to the point of minimum light transmittance after the agitation of the mixture has ceased and should be reached in 3 to 6 seconds after addition of the reagent. The time required is influenced by the type of sample tested, concentration of the vitamin A, the intensity of the incident light beam and also by the degree of damping of the galvanometer used.
2. It must always be remembered that the blue colour formed as a result of this reaction is unstable. It usually appears to be more stable with materials of high potency or high degree of purity. The presence of certain impurities may render the determination invalid, in as much as the colours formed as a result of the reaction may not be blue, but rather violet, reddish, or even yellow or brown in colour. Observations of such off colours should be carefully noted.

(h) Convert all transmittance readings to absorbancy (2-10 g, G 620) where G 620 is galvanometer reading at 620 mμ.

For convenience, the term "absorbancy" is used throughout this procedure, although it must be realised that true absorbancy can be measured only with sources of monochromatic light.

(i) Plot the absorbance on rectangular coordinate paper and draw the best fitting smooth curve through the origin.

The calibration curve should be checked at frequent intervals, particularly when solutions are renewed.

Note : Carotene, or provitamin A, also gives a blue colour with $SbCl_3$ although it is of lesser intensity than that formed with an equal amount of vitamin A. In extracts where carotene occurs, correction of the blue colour for that contributed by carotene should be made. In order to accomplish this correction, treat 2 ml aliquots of a series of concentrations of carotene ranging from 0 to 50 mcg per ml of chlroform with $SbCl_3$ and plot the absorbancy against the concentration. Calculate the amount of carotene present in the 01 ml of chloroform extract taken for the $SbCl_3$ reaction of the unknown from the carotene assay of the sample as described previously. Employing the blue colour curve for carotene, determine the absorbancy due to the concentration of carotene present in the 1 ml of unknown. Subtract this absorbancy from the absorbancy found, thus getting the absorbancy as corrected for carotene. If other coloured materials are present as measured according to the directions for this step, corrections must be made for these also, as indicated.

Calculation

(a) Using the calibration curve, convert the absorbancy of the sample, measured into USP units of vitamin A per ml.

(b) Repeat above for absorbancy of the sample plus increment due to extraneous substances.

(c) Calculate the vitamin A content of the sample from the following formula:

USP units of vitamin A per

$$g = \frac{U \times R}{(I-U) \times W}$$

U = units of vitamin A per ml

I = Units of vitamin A in sample plus reference standard

R = units of vitamin A per ml in reference standard calculated.

W = g of sample represented in U.

Example Fish oil Concentrate

1. Original Weight of sample = 0.2355 g

   Saponified sample taken up in 100 ml chloroform, 2 ml aliquot diluted to 100 ml with chloroform. 1 ml of chloroform solution of sample

   (W) = 0.0000467 g

2. Original weight of Reference standard = 0.5200 g

   Saponified USP vitamin A reference standard taken up in 100 ml chloroform, 10 ml aliquot diluted to 50 ml with chloroform. 1 ml aliquot diluted to 50 ml with chloroform. 1 ml of chloroform solution of saponified reference standard (R) = 10.4 units.

Steps	Absorbancy	Units from curve
1	0.248	11.8 (U)
	0.444	22.3 (I)
	$\frac{11.8 \times 10.4}{(22.3-11.8) x 0.0000467}$	= 250,400 blue colour units vitamin A per gram.

Assay of Ascorbic Acid

(Titrimetric Method of Beesey, 1944 Modified by AOAC, 1965)

Principle

The visual titration method is based upon the reduction of the dye (2, 6-dichlorophenolindophenol) by an acid solution of ascorbic acid. In the absence of interfering substanecs, the capacity of an extract of the sample to reduce a standard solution of the dye, as determined by titration, is directly proportional to the ascorbic acid content. In this method, titration is conducted in the presence of acetic and metaphosphoric acids in order to inhibit aerobic oxidation catalyzed by certain metallicions, to inactivate enzymes, and to precipitate proteins and liberate protein bound ascorbic acid.

Reagents

The distilled water used in making acid solution for extraction of samples should be *"copper free"*. For this reason it may be desirable to redistil certain lots of distilled water from an all-glass still.

1. *6% Metaphosphoric acid solution (0.005 M EDTA). Without heating, dissolve 60 g of reagent grade HPO_3 sticks or pellets and 1.8 g disodium ehylenediamine tetraacetate in 900 ml water redistilled from glass. Dilute to one litre and store at 3°C when not in use. On standing in solution, HPO_3 is slowely hydrolysed to H_3PO_4., hence a fresh solution should be prepared weekly.*
2. *3 % Metaphosphoric acid solution (0.0025 M EDTA). Dilute 500 ml of the above 6 per cent HPO_3 solution to one litre with redistilled water.*
3. *Ascorbic acid standard : Dissolve 100 mg of ascorbic acid (preferably USP reference standard obtainable from United States Pharmacophial convention, Inc, 46 park Avenue, New York), in 3 per cent HPO_3 solution and dilute to 500 ml with the same solvent. As this solution is unstable, use immediately to standardise the dye.*
4. *0.025% 2,6-Dichlorophenol indophenol solution : Dissolve approximately 50 mg of the sodium salt of 2, 6 dichlorophenol indophenol (sodium 2, 6-dichlorobenzenone indophenol, distillation products Industries, Easter organic chemicals Department, Rochester 3, New York), in approximately 150 ml of hot water containing 42 mg $NaHCO_3$., Cool and dilute with water to 200 ml. Place in a brown bottle and store at 3°C, renewing once a week. Standardise daily as follows :*

   Dilute a 5 ml aliquot of the standard ascorbic acid solution (containing 1 mg ascorbic acid) with 5 ml of 3 percent HPO_3. Titrate with the dye solution to a pink colour which persists for 15 seconds. Since this volume of dye represents 1 mg of ascorbic acid, the ascorbic acid equivalent (T) of 1 ml of dye solution is equal to 1 divided by the volume in ml of the dye solution used in this titration.
5. *Source of Nitrogen : A cylinder of N_2 with facilities for saturating the gas with moisture. Water-pumped N_2 is preferable to oil-pumped N_2.*

Procedure

(a) Blend equal weights (200 to 300 g) of the sample and 6 per cent HPO_3 to yield a homogenous slurry.

1. The procedure described is applicable to food products, but it may be modified for use in the analysis of blood, etc.
2. A large sample is required to obtain representative sampling of a heterogenous mass of the material being analysed.
3. A solution of 3 per cent HPO_3 is not adequate for inactivating the enzymes in certain fresh vegetables. Therefore, 6 per cent HPO_3 is preferred.
4. An 8 per cent acetic acid solution has been recommended as an extracting medium for processed materials that may contain large amounts of Fe++. This condition may occur when canned foods have been stored for long periods of time prior to opening. When HPO_3 or oxalic acid is used as an extracting medium, Fe^{++} will reduce 2, 6 dichlorophenol indephenol, resulting in erroneously high values for ascorbic acid. If acetic acid is used, Fe^{++} will not react with the dye at a rate sufficiently rapid to affect the titration.
5. If the material is a liquid with a very low solids content, it is not necessary to perform this step.
6. When HPO_3 is rejected for economic reasons or because of difficulty in securing the reagent, 1 per cent oxalic acid may be used as an alternative stabilizing medium in analyses on substances other than animal tissue. Two per cent oxalic acid solution should be used as the initial extracting acid, thus resulting in a 1 per cent solution when equal parts of sample extractant are blended. If large amounts of protein material are present, undesirable turbid extracts may be result since this medium is not efficient as HPO_3 in precipitating proteins.
7. An inert atmosphere has been suggested for use during the blending of fresh biological material containing large amounts of oxidative catalysts. Such a step would minimise contact with atmospheric oxygen. A simple means of conducting this step is to introduce N_2 through a glass tube extending into the blendor bowl under the surface of the liquid extractant. If N_2 is bubbled into the bowl for 15-30 seconds before starting the blender, the possibility of oxidation by catalysis or enzymes which are liberated with the breaking of the sample tissues is somewhat lessened. This is particularly true if the extracting medium does not completely inactivate these catalysts.

(b) Weigh 10 to 30 g of this slurry (sufficient to yield 1 to 5 mg ascorbic acid) into a weighing pan, transfer to a 100 ml volumetric flask, and dilute to 100 ml with 3 per cent HPO_3.

1. At this point, it is advisable to make the required weighing and dilution of the sample as rapidly as possible to minimise oxidation due to failure of the stabilising any catalysts present.

2. On dilution of the blended samples the presence of foam may cause difficulty in ascertaining the proper liquid level in the flask. The addition of a drop of caprylic alcohol has been found to be quite satisfactory in breaking this foam.

3. A short stem, 3 inch funnel with a relatively large bore in the stem aids in transfering the slurry from the weighing pan to the 100 ml volumetric flask.

4. In the case of products that were sulphated during dehydration, the efffect of SO_2 can be eliminated readily by adding 20 ml of acetone before dilution to the mark.

(c) Filter the diluted sample, discarding the first few ml of filtrate.

Titration of reduced Ascorbic acid : Pipette a 10 ml aliquot of the filtrate from D-I (c) into a small Erlenmeyer flask.

In the case of products of low ascorbic acid potency (5 mg per 100 g or less), it is convenient to titrate a 25 ml aliquot. If it is desired to maintain the volume at 10 ml to facilitate detection of the end point, 0.01% 2, 6-dichlorophenol indophenol to a faint pink end point which persists for 15 seconds.

Titration of reduced ascorbic acid with 2, 6-dicholorophenol indophenol dye oxidises the reduced ascorbic acid to dehydroascorbic acid. The dye as made up in the dilute $NaHCO_3$ solution is blue, but in an acid medium such as the stabilizing solution used in this determination, it is pink. Therefore, the colour change in this method, at the end point, is from colourless to pink. In the titration of the extracts with the dye, it is desirable to add the dye quite rapidly until the pink colour does not immediately disappear. Then as rapidly as possibly, add the dye dropwise with constant mixing of the solution until the faint pink colour of the solution resulting from the unoxidized dye, presists for 15 seconds. A rapid titration and short-time end point are desirable because of possible interfering action of other constituents of the solution. In general, such materials react more slowly with the dye than does ascorbic acid, therefore, their effect should be kept at a minimum by rapid titration.

Calculation

Calculate the Ascorbic Acid according to the Following Formula

$\frac{V \times T}{W} \times 100$ = mg ascorbic acid per 100 g sample

V = ml dye used for titration of aliquot of diluted sample

T = ascorbic acid equivalent of dye solution expressed as mg per ml of dye.

W = g of sample in aliquot titrated.

Example

300 g Product

300 g extracting acid

30 g slurry diluted to 100 ml

10 ml filtrate used for analysis

3 ml dye required for titration

0.125 mg per ml of dye

$$W = \frac{300}{600} \times \frac{30}{100} \times 10 = 1.5 g$$

By substituting the values V, T and W the equation becomes

$$\frac{3 \times 0.125}{1.5} \times 100 = 25 \text{ mg ascorbic acid per 100 g}$$

The visual titration method, as described, measures reduced ascorbic acid, not total (reduced plus dehydroascorbic acid). Reduction with H_2S has been described as being satisfactory for reducing dehydroascorbic acid to ascorbic acid. If an acid extract of the sample is treated with H_2S, followed by removal of the H_2S by bubbling N_2 through the solution, the titration with the standard dye solution may be measure of ascorbic acid plus dehydroascorbic acid. The value of the H_2S procedure as a measure of dehydroascorbic acid is open to question. Photometric methods employing 1, 6-dichlorophenol indophenol may measure total ascorbic acid. Duplicate determinations on a single sample should yield values checking within 5 per cent. In many cases, especially with high-potency samples, better checks may be expected.

Assay of Ascorbic Acid

(Colorimetric Method of Roe and Kuether, 1943)

Principle

Ascorbic acid is oxidised to dehydroascorbic acid by shaking with activated charcoal in the presence of trichloroacetic acid, the dehydroascorbic acid is condensed with 2:4 dinitrophenyldrazine, and the resulting 2:4 dinitrophenylhydrazone is treated with sulphuric acid to produce a red solution. Dehydroascorbic acid and its inactive oxidation product, diketogulonic acid, couple with 2, 4-dinitrophenyl hydrazine to yield an oxazone which gives a red colour with strong sulphuric acid.

Method for Blood or Plasma

The following special reagents are required :

1. *2:4 Dinitrophenylhydrazine reagent :* Made by dissolving 2 g of 2:4 dintrophenylhydrazine in 100 ml of approximately 9 N sulphuric acid (3 parts of water and 1 part of concentrated acid) and filtering acid washed activated carbon. In a large flask 200 g of activated carbon is stirred with 1 litre of approximately 3 N hydrochloric acid, which is heated to boiling. The carbon is collected on a suction filter, then transferred to a large beaker and stirred thoroughly with 1 litre of water. The carbon is again separated by filtration and the washing repeatedly until the filtrate gives a negative or very faint positive, reaction for ferric ions and finally it is dried overnight in an oven at 110°C to 120°C.
2. *Sulphuric acid (95%) :* To 100 ml of water is carefully added 900 ml of concentrated sulphuric acid.
3. *Thiourea solution :* Thiourea (10g) is dissolved in 100 ml of 50% v/v aqueous ethyl alcohol. The reagents keeps for at least two months, but it is advisable to test it occassionally to ensure that it will readily reduce mercuric chloride or potassium permanganate.

Procedure

Five ml of whole blood (or plasma) is added, drop by drop, to 15 ml of 6 per cent aqueous solution of trichloroacetic acid contained in a centrifuge tube, and the mixture is stirred with a glass rod until a fine suspension is obtained. It is allowed to stand for at least five minutes and then centrifuged. To the separated supernatant fluid is added approximately 0.75g of acid washed charcoal, which is mixed in by vigorous shaking or stirring and then separated by filteration. Four ml of the filtrate is placed in each of two test tubes and a drop of thiourea solution is added to each. One of the tube is kept in reserve to serve as a blank, while to the other tube 1 ml of dinitrophenylhydrazine reagent is added. This tube is placed in a water bath maintained at 37°C and is kept there for exactly 3 hours being then transferred, together with the blank, to a beaker of ice water containing generous quantities of ice. To each of the tubes, while in the ice water bath, 5 ml of 95 per cent sulphuric acid is added very slowly . (The acid is added from a burette, a drop at a time, the whole addition taking about a minute, during which a tube is kept agitated so as to ensure rapid mixing). Finally 1 ml of dinitrophenylhydrazine reagent is added to the blank. Both tubes are shaken thoroughly, while in the ice bath, and are then transferred to a test tube rack. After 30 minutes the colour is measured in a photoelectric colorimeter, a filter having maximum transmission at 540 mμ being used. Appropriate standards are taken through the process together with the test and blank, or one may use a calibration curve previously constructed with standard solutions of ascorbic acid ranging from 0.25 to 15 μg per ml in 4 percent trichloroacetic acid. These are treated with acid washed charcoal, filtered, and taken through the rest of the procedure as described above.

Procedure in the case of Urine Sample

To 1 volume of urine are added 19 volumes of 4 per cent W/V TCA. This dilution will serve for a range of 1 to 300 mg of ascorbic acid per litre of urine. In such cases where urine contain larger amounts of ascorbic acid greater dilutions may be made, but dilutions of less than 1:20 should not be used. Forty ml of the diluted urine is shaken with approximately 1.5 grams of acid washed with carbon and filtered, 4 ml of the filtrate is taken through the rest of the procedure as described above.

Procedure in the case of Plant Tissues

An extracting fluid is prepared containing 5 per cent of metaphosphoric acid and 10 per cent of acetic acid in water. The plant tissues (10 g) is ground in sufficient of this extracting fluid to produce a concentration of 5 to 15 μg of ascorbic acid per ml and the extract is filtered. Fifteen ml of the filtrate is shaken vigorously with approximately 0.75 g of acid washed charcoal and filtered, and 4 ml of the filtrate is taken through the rest of the procedure as described for blood and urine.

Method mentioned above measures total ascorbic acid i.e., dehydro and reduced ascorbic acid, both of which are physiologically active. If it is desired to determine only the dehydroascorbic acid, the extraction is carried out in the presence of thiourea, to stabilise the reduced ascorbic acid, and the treatment with charcoal is omitted.

Dehydroascorbic acid (in plant tissues). The plant tissue is ground under, usually, 50 parts (never less than 20 parts) of a solution containing 5 per cent metaphosphoric acid and 1 per cent thiourea. After filteration, the extract is treated as described for blood and urine, omitting the treatment with charcoal.

Vitamin D_2 and D_3

(Colorimetric Method of Nield *et al.*, 1940 and 1943)

We may follow the method of Nield *et al.* (1940 and 1943) for estimating vitamin D_2 and D_3 in animal feeds, human foods etc. By proper control of the composition of an antimony trichloride reagent it can be shown that saturated sterols do not react there with as chromogens but unsaturated steriods do. Sterols with one double bond in ring B give a yellow colour with a low absorption maximum at 500 mμ sloping from the violet towards the red. Sterols with two double bonds in ring B show a maximum at 510 to 515 mμ. While vitamin D_2 and D_3 have the very sharp and high absorption at 500 mμ.

General Note : All the above mentioned methods related to the analysis of carotene, vitamin A, tocopherol, ascorbic acid and vitamin D have been adapted by the Association of vitamin chemists, New York and published by the chairman Dr. Myer Freed (1960) of this Association.

References

AOAC. (1965). *Official methods of analysis of the Association of official Agricultural Chemists.* 10th Edn., AOAC. Benjamin Franklin Station, Washington, D.C. pp 755.

Astrup, H.N., Halvorsen, E.S., Lindstad, P., Enturistle, Y. and Mathers, J.C. (1971). *A quick method for the simultaneous assay of tocopherol, carotene and plant pigments in pasture.* Instt. Animal Nutr., Agricultural University of Norway, Bulletin 373.

Bessey, (1944). *J. Assoc. Offic. Agr. Chemists,* 27: 537

Corr, F.H. and Price, E.A. (1926). *Biochem. J.,* 20:498.

Dann, W.J. and Evelyn K.A. (1938). *Biochem, J.* 32: 1008.

Freed, M. (1966). *Methods of vitamin assay,* editor Freed, M. Chairman, The Association of vitamin chemists. Inter-Science Publishers, New York.

Krishna, G. (1985a). Carotene and Tocopherol in Agro-Industrial byproducts and wastes of the tropics. *Agricultural Wastes.* 12: 235-239.

Nield, C.H., Russell, W.C. and Zimmerb, A. (1940). *J. Biol.Chem.,* 136: 73.

Nield, C.H., Russel, W.C. and Zimmerb. A. (1943). *J. Biol.Chem.,* 148: 245.

Roe and Kuether. (1943). *J. Biol. Chem.,* 147: 399.

Chapter - 62

Water Soluble Vitamin Assay

Riboflavin or Vitamin B_2

Introduction

Riboflavin (synonymous with lactoflavin, vitamin G and vitamin B_2) is a yellow green, fluorescent, water soluble pigment widely distributed in plant and animal cells. The organic formula of riboflavin is (6, 7-dimethyl)-9-(D,1-ribtyl)-iso-alloxazine. The empirical formula is $C_{17}H_{20}N_4O_6$. Riboflavin is very sensitive to both visible and ultraviolet light. All manipulations with riboflavin or riboflavin containing materials should be carried out in subdued light or in low actinic glassware. Even subdued daylight may be destructive but artificial light of an intensity of 6 candles per squarefeet or less is permissible. Irradiation of alkaline solutions yields lumiflavin (6, 7, 9-trimethylis-alloxazine) and in acid solutions lumich rome (6.7 dimethyl alloxazine) is formed, which is characterised by a blue fluorescence. *One of the distinguishing properties of riboflavin is its yellow-green fluorescence in neutral solutions which reaches a maximum at pH 6.7 to 6.8.*

In lining cells riboflavin generally occurs combined either with phosphoric acid or with phosphoric and adenylic acid, both of which may be combined with specific proteins to form oxidative enzymes.

In most of analytical procedure for riboflavin, it is necessary to treat natural products with acid or enzymes to get maximum values. This insures the liberation of riboflavin from its protein combination and makes it more readily extractable.

There are three general methods mentioned below may be used for the assay of riboflavin content.

1. Microbiological method
2. Fluorometric method
3. Animal assay

Microbiological Method Using *"Lactobacillus Casei"*

(Method of Snell and Strong, 1939, Modified by Strong, 1947)

Principle

Microbiological methods are based on the observation that certain micro-organism require specific vitamins for growth. Using a basal incomplete in all respect for the vitamin under test, growth responses of the organism are compared quantitative in standard and unknown solutions.

Equipments

1. *Incubator or water bath*
2. *Autoclave*
3. *Uniform, Lipless Pyrex tubes*
4. *Culture tube racks*
5. *Cotton culture tube plugs or metal caps*
6. *Inoculating needle and loop*
7. *Hypodermic syringe*
8. *Refrigerator*
9. *Centrifuge*
10. *Sterilising can for pipettes*
11. *pH metre*
12. *Filter rack and support*
13. *Filter paper*
14. *Burette 25 ml, 50 ml*
15. *Automatic pipette 5 ml*
16. *Glass stoppered graduated cylinder*

17. *Beaker*
18. *Pipettes volumetric transfer-assorted sizes including 1, 2, 3, 4, 5, 6, 10, 15 and 20 ml*
19. *Densitometre, Nephelometre or colorimeter*
20. *Erlenmeyer flasks, 125 ml*
21. *Volumetric flask, 100 ml*
22. *Volumetric flask, 1 litre*
23. *Filter funnels, 3 inch*
24. *Pipette graduated 5 ml and 10 ml*

Reagents

1. *Salt solution A : Dissolve 25 grams of K_2HPO_4 and 25 grams of KH_2PO_4 and dilute to 500 ml with water. Store under toluene.*
2. *Salt Soltion B : Dissolve the following amounts of salts and dilute to 500 ml with water.*

Magnesium sulphate ($MgSO_4$-$7H_2O$)	*10 grams*
Sodium chloride	*0.5 grams*
Ferrous sulphate	*0.5 grams*
Manganese sulphate	*0.5 grams*

Add 5 drops of concentrate HCl and store under toluene. Sodium chloride may be omitted when HCl hydrolysed casein is used.

3. *Enriches Agar medium for stock cultures*

Reagent	***Quantity***
Anhydrous glucose	*2 grams*
Peptone	*1 gram*
Cystine	*100 mg*
Salt solution A	*1 ml*
Salt solution B	*1 ml*
Agar	*3.5 grams*

Dissolve all ingredients but agar in approximately 15 ml of water. Adjust the pH to 6.8 and make to 200 ml volume. Add agar and steam to the mixture until agar is dissolved. Dispense into 20 test tubes, stopper tubes with cotton plugs and sterilise at 15 pound pressure for 15 minutes.

4. *Enriched culture medium*

Quantity	***Reagent***
Difco Peptone	*5 grams*
Difco yeast extract	*1 grams*
Anhydrous glucose	*10 grams*

Reagent	*Quantity*
Anhydrous sodium acetate	*10 grams*
Salt solution A	*5 ml*
Salt soluton B	*5 ml*

Dissolve above ingredients in 200 ml water in beaker. Adjust the pH to 6.8 with 1 N NaOH and dilute to 500 ml. Pipette 10 ml quantities into test tubes, plug with cotton, and sterilise at 15 pound pressure for 15 minutes.

5. *Isotonic salt solution : Weigh 0.9 gram sodium chloride and transfer to a 100 ml volumetric flask. Dilute to volume with water and shake until salt has dissolved. Transfer 10 ml quantities of this solution to culture tubes, plug with cotton, and sterilise in autoclave at 15 pound pressure for 20 minutes.*
6. *1 N sodium hydroxide : Since NaOH pellets often contain cosiderable water, amounts in excess of the calculated NaOH may be used. To prepare 18 litres of 1 N NaOH, 720 grams NaOH are needed. From 1 to 15 per cent in excess of this amount can be used, depending upon the water content of the NaOH pellets. Although this is not a standard solution, it is time saving to determine the volume which will just neutralise the acid used in the extraction of the samples.*
7. *0.1 N sodium hydroxide : Determine the normality of solution (1 N sodium hydroxide) by titration against a standard acid and dilute to a concentration of 0.1 N alkali proportions indicated by the following equation :*

$$\text{Vol. of 1 N NaOH} = \frac{0.1 \times \text{Vol. of 0.1 N alkali needed}}{\text{Normality of solution (6)}}$$

The alkali solution may also be standardised against potassium acid phthalate, H_2SO_4 or other acid of constant and known concentration. This reagent is used in titrating the acid produced by the test organism. It need not be exactly 0.1 N but it is well to have a standardised solution so that results between laboratories can be completed.

8. *Bromothymol blue indicator solution : Weigh 0.1 gram bromothymol blue indicator into a small beaker. Add 1.6 ml of 0.1 N NaOH and triturate with a stirring rod until the powder has dissolved. Dilute with water to 250 ml. The solution may also be made up by dissolving in a few ml of 95 per cent ethanol, adding 1.6 ml of 0.1 N NaOH, and diluting to 250 ml with water.*
9. *0.1 N hydrochloric acid (approx.) : Dilute 8.5 ml concentrate HCl to one litre with water.*

10. *Stock riboflavin solution A (25 μg riboflavin per ml in 0.02 N acetic acid).*

    Weigh accurately 50 mg USP reference standard riboflavin which has been dried in a vacuum desiccator or oven over concentrated sulphuric acid for 24 hours, and transfer quantitatively to a two litre volumetric flask. Add about 1500 ml water, 2.4 ml glacial acetic acid and warm to aid solution. After cooling to room temperature, make to volume with water. Preserve, under toluene, protected from light. in a refrigerator, when the more concentrated stock solution of 100 μg per ml heretofore recommended by most authors, is cooled in a refrigerator, riboflavin crystallises from solution.

11. *Stock riboflavin solution B (10 μg riboflavin per ml in 0.002 N acetic acid). Dilute 40 ml of stock riboflavin solution A to 100 ml with water. Preserve under toluene, protected from light, in a refrigerator.*

12. *Riboflavin working standard (0.1 μg per ml).*

    Dilute 1 ml of stock riboflavin B to 100 ml with water. Prepare immediately before use.

13. *Alkali treated peptone solution : Dissolve 40 grams of peptone (Difco, Bacto or Wilson's is suitable) in 250 ml of water, Mix the two solutions. Allow to stand for 18-24 hours, then neutralise with glacial acetic acid (approximately 25 ml). Add 14 grams of anhydrous sodium acetate (or 23.2 grams $NaC_2H_3O_2 \cdot 3H_2O$) and sufficient water to make to 800 ml. Preserve under toluene in a refrigerator.*

14. *0.1% Cystine solution : Suspend one grams of L-cystine in 20 ml of water and add concentrate HCl until the crystals are dissolved. No more than 10 ml should be required. Add sufficient water to make a volume of one litre. Keep under toluene at room temperature.*

15. *Yeast supplement solution : Dissolve 100 grams of yeast extract or autolysed yeast (Difco is suitable) in 500 ml of water, and 150 grams of basic lead acetate in 500 ml of water. Mix the two solutions, adjust the pH to red to phenolphthalein with concentrate NH_4OH, and filter through a Buchner funnel. Adjust the filtrate to pH 6.5 with glacial acetic acid, precipitate the excess lead with H_2S, and filter. Remove about 200 ml of water under vacuum to get rid of the dissolved H_2S. Preserve with toluene and chloroform in the refrigerator. An alternate method preparing riboflavin free yeast solution involves the use of Florisil which quantitatively adsorbs riboflavin at a pH of 4.5. Dissolve 20 grams of yeast extract in a beaker with 150 ml of water. Adjust the pH to 4.5 with acetic acid and add 10 grams of florisil. Stir for 30 minutes filter, adjust the pH to 4.5 and repeat the treatment with 10 additional*

grams of florisil. Filter and adjust the pH to 6.8 with 1 N NaOH and make to 200 ml with water.

16. *Basal medium stock solution (for 100 tubes).*

Reagent	***Quantity***
Alkali treated peptone sol.	*100 ml*
Cystine solution (0.1%)	*100 ml*
Yeast supplement solution	*20 ml*
Salt solution A	*10 ml*
Salt solution B	*10 ml*
Glucose (Anhydrous)	*10 grams*

Dissolve the glucose in the mixture of the solutions, adjust the pH to 6.8 with N NaOH, and add sufficient water to make 500 ml.

An advantage of this medium is that it may be used for folic acid as well as for riboflavin, and there are indications that it may be suitable for niacin, folic acid, pantothenic acid, and biotin as well.

17. *Culture medium for growing inoculum : To 250 ml of basal medium stock solution, add 5 ml stock riboflavin solution B and water to 500 ml. Mix well, add approximately 10 ml to test tubes, plug with non absorbent cotton, autoclave at 15 pound pressure for 15 minutes and store in a refrigerator. This medium contains 1 mcg riboflavin in 10 ml. Reagent 4 may be substituted for this reagent.*

Procedure

1. Preparation of stock culture, L. Casei ATCC 7469

   (a) Prepare stab cultures in two or more agar stock culture tubes (Reagent No. 3) using a pure culture.

   Pure cultures can be obtained from the American Type culture collection, 12301 Parklawn Drive, Rockville, Maryland (USA)

   (b) Incubate for 16-24 hours at 37°C + 0.5°C

   (c) Store in the refrigerator under aspetic conditions not longer than one week before transferring to new stab.

   1. One stab culture should be reserved unopened for use in the preparation of subsequent stock culture stab. The others may be used as many times as necessary in the preparation of inoculum provided they are not more than one week old and sterile techniques are observed.

2. Whenever the stock culture has not been used for several weeks or months, get new cultures or revive the old one by making daily successive stab transfers for at least 3 days before preparing the inoculum. Poor growth results from old cultures.

Preparation of Inoculum

(a) Transfer cells from the stock culture to be sterile tube of inoculum culture medium (Reagent 4 or 17).

Do not use an old inoculum for preparing a new inoculum. This practice may alter the nutritive requirements of the test organism making it unsuitable for the assay.

(b) Incubate this culture for 6-18 hrs at 37°C.

Inoculum incubated longer than 24 hours should not be used as the organism tends to become attenuated and poor growth refrigerated for 24 hours before use.

(c) Secure cotton plug with a rubber band, adhesive tape, or a pin and centrifuge.

An angle head centrifuge layers cells so that decantation is easy, but the conventional centrifuge is satisfactory.

(d) Dacant the supernatant liquid and resuspend the cells in 20 ml of sterile isotonic salt solution. This must be done aseptically.

20 ml of inoculum will inoculate 200 to 400 tubes.

(e) Fill the sterille syringe with the resuspended cells and use atonce.

1. Sterilise the needle and syringe (plunger removed) by wrapping in paper and autoclaving for 15 minutes at 15 pounds pressure. By pouring the resuspended cells into the open end of the syringe before inserting the plungers, the disadvantages of withdrawing the inoculum from a deep culture tube with a short needle can be overcome.
2. A tube drawn out to a capillary or a pipette can be used in place of a syringe.
3. Preparation of Sample : Extraction and hydrolysis.

   (a) Into a 125 ml Erlenmeyer flask, weigh a homogenous sample containing 10 or more μg riboflavin, add 50 ml 0.1 N HCl, and autoclave at 15 pounds for 15 minutes.

   When the concentrations of the various members of the B-complex (thiamine, riboflavin, niacin, biotin and inositol) are wanted on the sample or samples are following general enzymatic digestion procedure has been used for their simultanoeus release from plant and animal tissues. Dilute approximately 1 gram of finely minced tissue with 8 ml of 0.2 N sodium acetate buffer having a pH of 4.5 to 4.7. Add 1 ml of a freshly prepared enzyme suspension containing 20 mg of papain and 20 mg of takadiastase per ml. To prepare the enzyme suspension, mix 20 mg of papain with one drop of glycerine, add 20 mg of takadiastase, and make to 1 ml with water. In practice, when several samples are assayed simultaneously, a suitable multiple of these quantities is used. After mixing the enzymes with the sample, add a few drops of benzene or toluene, cover loosely, and inoculate for 24 hours at 37-45°C.

Since papain and takadiastase contain varying amounts of riboflavin (1 to 8µg/g) it is important especially with low potency samples, that the vitamin content of each lot of enzyme be determined and proper correction made in the calculation.

Heat the samples in flowing steam of autoclave for 10 minutes. Add a level teaspoonful (about 1 g) of filter cell or equivalent filter aid (must not absorb riboflavin), shake and filter through a conical paper. Collect the filtrate in a volumetric flask of suitable size. Wash the residue with small amounts of water and collect the washings with the filtrate.

Finally, dilute the extracts so that the riboflavin concentration is between 0.05 and 0.5 µg per ml. If the samples are to be stored, transfer to brown bottles and a few drops of toluene and refrigerator.

(b) Cool to room temperature adjust the pH 4.5 transfer to a 100 ml volumetric flask, make to volume and filter.

1. For most samples filtration at pH 4.56 is effective in removing growth stimulants and inhibitors, such as starch, fatty acids and phospholipids. Some workers find that the stimulating effect of starch may be avoided, and lower and more uniform values can be obtained with cereal products if, after autoclaving in 0.1 N HCl, the samples are digested at 50°C for one and half an hour with 5 ml of 6 per cent takadiastase in 2.5 N sodium acetate prior to pH adjustment and filtration. Also, some find that fat has a stimulating effect. In the case of high fat materials such as cheese, liver meal and fish meal by ether extraction. The difficulty is overcome after autoclaving with 0.1 N HCl, adjust to pH 4.5, make to volume, and filter. Extract a 50 ml aliquot of the filtrate three times with 30 ml portions of ether. Then adjust to pH 6.8 and dilute to 100 ml.

2. When urine is assayed without dilution as is sometimes necessary, when the riboflavin concentration is extremely low, case should be taken that the urea concentrated does not exceed 20 mg per tube. If more than this amount is present the growth of organism is inhibited. If it is impossible to keep the urea concentration below this level, a formula to correct the result has been devised (Isbell *et al.*, 1941).

(c) Measure 50 ml (or an aliquot containing about 5 mcg riboflavin) of the filtrate into a 100 ml volumetric flask, adjust the pH to 6.8, and dilute to 100 ml.

4. Preparation of standard tubes

   a. To duplicate tubes add 0.0, 0.5, 1.0, 1.5, 2.0, 2.5 and 3.0 ml quantities of the riboflavin working standard.

   b. Add sufficient water to bring the volume in each tube 5 ml.

   c. To each of these tubes add 5 ml of the basal medium stock solution.

   1. Adding the basal medium to the extract and water gives better mixing of the two solutions than adding the extract and water to the basal medium. Better mixing can be attained in this step by allowing part of the basal medium to run down the side of the tube and part to fall directly on the liquid surface.

   2. An automatic 5 ml pipette or pipetting machine is a valuable time saver in this step.

5. Preparation of assay tubes.

   a. To duplicate tubes add five levels of the sample extract ranging from 0.05 to 0.25 μg riboflavin. Volumes of unknown should vary by not less than 0.5 ml. Volume greater than 5 ml cannot be used.

   1. The test solution is used at several levels so that several tests will fall on the standard curve. The best index of the validity of the assay is agreement of the calculated results at different test levels.

   2. Some workers do not run duplicate at each level of sample, since each of the levels used already constitutes an independent observations of the same thing. They believe that for most practical purposes, use of single assay tube for each level will give satisfactory accuracy. The standard tubes, however are always run in duplicate. Add sufficient water to bring the volume to 5 ml. To each of these tubes add 5 ml of basal medium stock solution.

6. Sterilisation

   a. Mix the contents of each tube thoroughly by rotating the tube vigorously in the palm of the hand. Mixing without spilling is difficult and time consuming, but by adding the ingredients as indicated in procedure 4 sufficient mixing may be attained.

b. Plug with cotton or cover with caps.

c. Autoclave at 15 pound perssure for 15 minutes.

The minimum time in which sterilisation without undue caramelisation, can be accomplished is desired. Pressure above 15 pounds and periods longer than 15 minutes increase caramelisation of the sample. In some autoclaves sterilisation is accomplished in considerably less than 15 minutes at 15 pounds pressure.

7. Inoculation and Incubation

a. Cool all the tubes to the incubation temperature or below.

1. All tubes must be the same temperature all the way through the rack. Allow the culture tube to stand in water bath or at room temperature until there is no question that the temperature is uniform. This precaution is especially necassary when turbidimetric measurements are made. Since in that procedure the rate of growth, rather than the extent of growth, is being measured. Small differences in temperature, especially at the start of the assay, influence the rate of growth much more than the extent of growth over a long period of time.

b. Aseptically inoculate each tube with one drop of inoculum.

1. It is convenient to use 5 or 10 ml pipette with 5 mm tip bent at a 60° angle, so that the pipette may be held.

2. A 10 ml syringe fitted with a 20 gauge needle is satisfactory for delivery of drips of inoculum into the culture tubes. If the plunger is removed from the barrell of the syringe after starting the inoculum through the needle. Uniform drops will continue to fall from the needle. By mounting the syringe directly above a wire or block "stop", both hands are freed to remove the plugs and rapidly place the culture tubes into position against the "stop" so that the incoulation falls directly on to the surface of the basal medium.

3. The bacteriological technique of flaming tubes in inoculation has been omitted from the recommended procedure, since this has been found to be necessary and time consuming. In areas where the danger of contamination is high, however, it may be adivisable to introduce the flaming technique.

c. Incubate at 37°C for approximately 72 hours.

1. All tubes must be maintained at exactly the same temperature. The time of incubation can be extended by as much as 18 hours and shortened by as much as 12 hours, without appreciably affecting-the results of the assay. After incubation the tubes may be kept in a refrigerator overnight and titrate the following day.

2. The incubation period is 18-24 hours if turbidimetry is to be used.

8. Titration

a. Tranfer the contents of each tube to a 125 ml Erlenmer flask, and rinse the tube once with about 10 ml water, adding the rinsing to the flask. Add about 02 ml of 0.1% bromothymol blue about (most conveniently from a dropper) and titrate with 0.1 N NaOH to a green colour (about 6.8 pH) Hold a flask for a reference colour for about 10-20 titrations and then substitute a new flask. The colour in the reference flask changes on standing.

1. Two or three drops of indicator should be used. The end point may be taken where the yellow colour changes to green or the green changes to blue providing that all tubes are titrated to the same end point.

2. Instead of 0.1 per cent bromothymol blue, of which about 0.2 ml is used in each tube for the titration, some workers perfer to use a larger volume (about 40 ml) of a more dilute indicator solution (0.001% bromothymol blue), and to use this very dilute indicator solution for rinsing the test tubes. In this later procedure, after the incubation, fill all tubes at once with the 0.001 per cent indicator solution, and pour the contents of each tube into a 125 ml Erlenmeyer flask. Then fill each test tube once again with the dilute indicator, pour into the same flask, and titrate with 0.1 N NaOH. In this way the addition of indicator and the rinsing of the tubes is accomplished at once, and the total volume and amount of indicator are kept satisfactorily constant.

3. In order to compare results between laboratories, it is advisable to plot curve using ml of 0.1 N NaOH although assay results can be obtained with other strengths of alkali. However, the whole series of tubes be titrated with the same lot of NaOH.

4. Coloured extracts may be encountered in the assay of certain foods. This colour may interface by obscuring the end point and necessitate the use of another indicator or an electrometric titration.

5. Titration values in excess of 2 ml for the tubes containing 0.0 ml of the standard vitamin solution indicate an excessive amount of vitamin being tested in the basal medium and invalidate the assay.

6. Instead of titration, turbidity may be used of as a measure of microbial growth. For greatest convenience, matched colorimeter tubes are used for setting up the assay. Great care must be excercised to add exactly the same amount of inoculum to each tube. The time of incubation is 18-24 hours. The turbidity is measured in a turbidimeter or a photoelectric colorimeter with a filter in the region of 640 mμ. Shake well to suspend the organisms uniformly and if air bubles are present in the solution, allow to stand for approximately 30 minutes. After this time the contents must again be suspended uniformly.

From the turbidimetric values of the standard vitamin tubes, a standard curve is plotted - density against μg of vitamin. The density of the inoculated blank need not be subtracted from the readings. The turbidimetric method has the advantage of being more rapid but where coloured or turbid solutions are encountered, before the addtion of the organisms, the titration procedure is indicated.

7. A glass electrode assembly has been described for titrating. The pH metre may be set for constant indication of pH or the key pressed intermittantly. When approximately pH 6.5 is reached, add alkali, more slowly to pH 7. The assembly is simple and rapid and eliminates the colour end point.

8. The high blank and drift are two types of errors which occasionally appear in microbiological work. Which the investigator should understand when the titration value of the standard tube containing no vitamin under test (usally 0.5 ml) exceed 2 ml, the blank is too high. The cause is excessive amounts of the vitamin under test in the basal medium stock solution. The remedy is to examin carefully each constituent of the basal medium and to replace those constituents which contain the excessive vitamin.

9. Calculation

a. From the titration values of the standard riboflavin tubes perpare a standard curve plotting ml 0.1 N NaOH against μg of riboflavin.

b. Using standard curve, determine the riboflavin content corresponding to the titration value each tube or to the average value of duplicate tubes. Divide the riboflavin in content per tube by the volume of the sample aliquot added to it getting the concentration of riboflavin in terms of μg per ml sample extract. Riboflavin values of less than 0.05 or more than 0.30 μg per tube cannot be used since they are beyond the useful range of the standard curve.

1. Except for the most precise work, if the titrations for duplicate tubes check within 0.2 ml the values may be averaged before calculating the content per millilitre. Titrations above 10 ml may be averaged if they do not differ by more than 0.4 ml.

c. Determine the average concentration of riboflavin per ml of sample extract, using only those values which do not differ from the average by more than 10 percent.

The term upward drift is applied to data in which the calculated values for μg riboflavin per ml of test solution consistently increase as the size of the sample is increased. Downward drift relate to a corresponding progressive decrease.

The cause of upward drift is the presence in the sample of some growth factor which is inadequately supplied in the basal medium. The remedy is to enrich the basal medium. For this purpose, the use of 14 grams of anhydrous sodium acetate in the preparation of the alkali treated peptone and 10 grams of glucose per 250 ml of basal medium has been recommeded. The above procedure specifies such a medium. Some workers find that this is all that is necessary. Others prefer to further enrich their medium with 6 ml of 1 per cent asparagine, 25 mcg of pantothenic acid per 250 ml of medium and to double the amount of cystine. Still others use 1 mg of niacin per 250 ml of medium as the only enrichment source. Some workers use as much as 15 grams of glucose in the preparation of the medium, but this is not desirable since caramelization during autoclaving makes subsquent titration difficult. As little as 5 grams of glucose may be used.

Downward drift may be due to some toxic or inhibiting factor in the sample. In these cases the remedy is to remove these factors, downward dirft may also be due to some factor which stimulates at low but not at high concentration of sample.

The nature of some of these growth promoters and inhibitors and method for removing them are discussed under extraction and hydrolysis. This whole problem of stimulation and inhibition, and enrichment of medium, has been ably discussed by strong (1947).

d. Calculate the riboflavin content of the sample from the following formula

$$\mu g/g = \frac{\text{Avg.}\mu g\text{ per ml extract x volume}}{\text{wt.of sample}} \text{x dilution factor}$$

For samples of potencies such that the procedure can be followed exactly, the volume is 100 ml, and the dilution factor is 100/50. Effectively, this is equivalent ot setting the equal to 200 ml.

Fluorometric Method of the U.S. Pharmacopeia

(Freed, M. 1966)

Principle

Riboflavin flourescence in light of wavelength 440 to 550 mμ. The intensity of fluorescence in proportional to the concentration of riboflavin in dilute solutions. The riboflavin is measured in terms of the difference between the fluorescence before and after chemical reduction.

Equipment

1. *Autoclave*
2. *Erelenmeyer flask*
3. *Funnels*
4. *Filter paper (Whatman No. 12)*
5. *Beakers or flasks 100 ml capacity*
6. *Pipettes assorted sizes 0.5, 1.4, 10 and 50 ml*
7. *Graduated cylinder, 100 ml*
8. *Graduated cylinder, 1000 ml*
9. *Volumetric flask, 1000 ml, 2000 ml, 100 ml, 50 ml*
10. *Matched cuvettes to fit fluorophotometer of choice*
11. *Test tubes, 15 to 18 x 150 mm*
12. *Racks for test tubes*
13. *Flurophotometer - Coleman Model 12-A with filters B-2 an dPC - 2 and voltage stabilizer, Pflatz and Bauer Model B with voltage stabilizer or model C. Lumetron, Klett, Coleman Model 14. All of these require appropriate filters, cuvettes.*
14. *pH meter*

Reagents

1. *10 N hydrochloric acid : Dilute 850 ml of concentrate HCl to 1 litre with water*
2. *1 N hydrochloric acid : Dilute 100 ml of 10 N HCL to 10 litre with water*
3. *0.1 N hydrochloric acid : Dilute 100 ml hydrochloric acid 1 N HCl to 1 litre with water*

4. *10 N sodium hydroxide* : Dissolve 400 grams NaOH pellets in sufficient water to make 1 lite
5. *1 N sodium hydroxide* : Dilute 100 ml of 10 N NaOH to one litre with water
6. *0.1 N sodium hydroxide* : Dilute 100 ml of 1 N NaOH to 1 litre with water.
7. Glacial Acetic acid.
8. *3% potassium permanganate* : Dissolve 3 grams in sufficient water to make 100 ml. Prepare fresh solution every week.
9. *3% hydrogen peroxide* : Prepare this solution at the time of use by diluting 30 per cent H_2O (Merck superoxol) 1:10 with water.
10. Stock riboflavin solution (25 μg riboflavin/ml). See back under microbiological method.
11. Riboflavin working standard (0.5 μg riboflavin per ml) : Dilute 1 ml of stock solution to 50 ml with water. Prepare immediately before use. It may be necessary to test different concentration of the working standard with the particular instrument to be used as the various instruments differ in sensitivity. This particular concentration is suitable for a Coleman Mode 12-A.
12. Stock solution of sodium fluorescein : Dissolve 50 mg of sodium in fluorescein sufficient water to make 1 litre.
13. Dilute solution of sodium fluorescein : Dilute 1 ml of stock sodium fluorescein to 1 litre with water
14. Sodium hydrosulphite (Dithionite).

The fluorometric method is not applicable to samples which contain high concentrations of iron unless it is removed or to those, which have been heated so that interfering colours like caramel may be present. *Since riboflavin is light sensititive and is most readily destroyed by light in the blue and violet regions, it is necessary to perform all operations in the absence of strong light. The use of red or amber glassware or a darkened room is advantageous.* The higher the pH of the solution, the greater will be the destruction of riboflavin in the presence of light.

Extraction

a. Weight a sample estimated to contain 5-10 μg of riboflavin and transfer to a 125 ml of Erylenmeyer flask. After adding 50 ml of 0.1 N HCl to the flask, autoclave for 30 minutes at 15 pound pressure.

1. When a sample solution contains a high concentration of inorganic iron, this iron may be removed by the addition, immediately after autoclaving of an excess of phosphoric acid, sodium phosphate or potassium phosphate and precipitating and filtering at pH 4.5 to 6.6.
2. Some materials, such as dry mineral vitamin feed supplements may contain enough basic substances to neutralise or more than neutralise 50 ml of 0.1 N HCl. Where an appreciable amount of basic substances is present, an excess of dilute HCl should be added. For many types of samples, even after adjustment to proper acidity, it has been found necessary that the volume of 0.1 N HCl be equal in ml to not less than ten times the dry weight of the sample in grams.
3. If an autoclave, pressure retort or pressure cooker is not available, extraction may be accomplished in a boiling water bath agitating every 5 minutes for one hour.
4. An acid acetone extraction has been used by some workres to eliminate troublesome cloudiness which occurs with some samples. The acetone flocculates colloidal suspensions and prevents the adsorption of riboflavin from solution by proteins.

Precipitation of Interfering Impurities

a. After autoclaving, cool the sample and adjust to pH 6.0 with NaOH, Since riboflavin is unstable in alkaline solution the extract should swirled constantly during the addtion of alkali. To prevent local areas of high pH. Immediately add 1 N HCl to bring the pH to 4.5.

1. Some workers prefer to add sufficient 2.5 M sodium acetate to bring the pH to 4.5 without any pre-adjustment to pH 6.0. However, this procedure may not be as effect to precipitation in the pH range of 4.5 to 6.0.
2. It is necessary to remove interfering substances by precipitation through a pH range of 4.5 to 7.0 followed by oxidation at an aid pH. In some products it may be necessary to include further purification steps, it is better to use the microbiological procedure for the analysis of samples which are highly coloured or difficult to purify. Absorption and elution techniques have been used for this purpose.

Dilute the solution to 100 ml with water and filter. To a 50 ml aliquot of the filtrate, add 1 N HCl dropwise until no more precipitate form. Follow by an approximately equal number of drops of 1 N NaOH with constant shaking. Dilute the aliquot to 100 ml with water and filter if necessary.

Care must be taken not to add an excess of NaOH so that the pH is raised above 6.6. If an equal number of drops of HCI and then NaOH are added, no such difficulty should be encountered.

Acidification of Extract

(a) Add 10 ml or sample solution and 1 ml of water to each of 2 test tubes and mix.

The addition of 1 ml of water compensates for the extra dilution of the sample by the standard in the following step and thus simplifies the calculation by eliminating the volume correction.

Add 10 ml of sample solution and 1 ml of riboflavin working standard (0.5 μg per ml) to each of 2 other test tubes and mix.

This and the preceding step may be carried out directly in the cuvettes. If test tubes are used, transfer the contents to cuvettes prior to the measurement of fluorescence. The oxidation and fluorometry are carried out in duplicate for each sample.

Add 1 ml of glacial acetic acid to all 4 tubes and mix.

Oxidation

Add 0.5 ml of 3 percent $KMnO_4$ to each tube, mix. and allow to stand for exactly 2 minutes.

Removal of the interfering fluorescent substances and pigment which occur in extracts may also be accomplished by treatment with $SnCl_2$ and Na_2SO_4. These reagents reduce the interfering fluorescent substances and the riboflavin to the non-fluorescent form. Shaking in the presence of air oxidises the riboflavin and fluorescence may then be measured.

After 2 minutes add 0.5 ml of 3 percent H_2O_2 and mix thorough. The red colour should disappear within 10 seconds.

Sufficient H_2O_2 should be added to just decolourise the tubes. Avoid an exesss of hydrogen peroxide because bubbles will form and interfers with the reading of the fluorescence and the use of sodium sulphate for reading the blank.

A fine precipitate of MnO_2 may be formed at this point. Centrifugation will settle this precipitate and result in a clear solution. Usually, however, solutions are clear.

Fluorometry

The following instructions apply to the coleman Model 12-A photofluorometer.

Using the dilute sodium fluorescein (50 μg per litre) adjust the instrument to give a deflection of 80 on the galvano-meter scale. Check the adjustment immediately before reading each series.

Before attempting to measure the fluorescence of solutions containing riboflavin. It should be determined that the instrument use gives a linear response to different concentrations of standard fluorescent substances.

Measure fluorescence of the extracts containing added water (reading A). Add with mixing approximately 20 mg of sodium sulphate and fluorescence with 10 seconds (reading C).

Sufficient mixing may be accomplished by tapping the cuvettes against the finger. Care should be taken not be scratch the cuvette if a stirring rod is used.

Excessive quantities of sodium sulphate should be avoided since high salt concentrations may change the fluorescent properties of the blank. Since the blank my change on stand, it should be read immediately after addition of the sodium sulphate.

Instead fo sodium sulphate, 0.5 ml of 5 percent solution prepared by dissolving 5 grams of sodium sulphate in 100 ml of an ice cold sodium bicarbonate solution (2 grams or sodium bicarbonate per 100 ml) may be used. The addition of the solutions instead of the solid prevents use of an excess of sodium sulphate. With care, howeve an excess can be avoided. Even with the solid, the use of the solution has two disadvantage it is stable for only 2 to 4 hours even in an ice bath and corrections for a change in volume are necessary.

(4) During the fluorescence measurements, care should be taken to avoid excess exposure of the solution to the ultraviolet light, which causes rapid destruction of riboflavin.

Measure fluorescence of the extracts containing added riboflavin (reading B).

Calculations

Calculate the riboflavin content of the sample from the following formula:

$$\frac{A-C}{B-A} \text{x} \frac{\text{riboflavin increment}}{\text{100 ml aliquot}} \text{x dilution factor x} \frac{1}{\text{sample wt.}} = \mu g / g$$

The factor $\frac{A-C}{B-A}$ x riboflavin increment equals μg/10 ml aliquot. This is divided by 10 equals concentration per ml. If the dilution recommended above can be used, the formula will reduce to:

$$\mu g/g = \frac{A-C}{B-A} \times \frac{0.5}{10} \times \frac{100}{50} \times 100 \times \frac{1}{Weight}$$

$$= \frac{A-C}{B-A} \times \frac{10}{Weight}$$

☞ **Notes**

1. *This method is applicable only to those extracts having low blanks and little, if any, interfering fluorescent substances. Whenever it is employed for a new product, the results should be checked by the increment technique.*
2. *These calculations do not take into accounts the possibility of loss of riboflavin during the procedure.*

   If such corrections are desired, treat 6 ml of stock riboflavin solution exactly as the sample including extraction, precipitation oxidation and fluorometry. Calculate the percent recovery, and, to correct values for the loss of riboflavin during the procedure, divide each by this percentage.
3. *All there readings may be made on one aliquot by first taking reading A, adding 1 ml of standard, mixing and taking reading B, followed by addition of sodium sulphate and taking reading C in this case the calculations is identical except that reading B and C must be multiplied by 11/10 to correct for changes in volume.*

Colorimetric Method for the Estimation of Niacin (B_3)

(Method of Melnick, 1942)

Principles

The chemical method is based upon the reaction of niacin with cyanogen bromide to give a pyridinium compound. The latter undergoes rearrangement yielding derivatives that couple with aromatic amines to produce coloured compounds. Under proper contitions the density of the colour produced is proportional to the niacin present and may be measured with a photoelectric colorimeter.

Equipments

The following equipment provides for the simultaneous analysis of eight samples.

1. *Centrifuge tubes*
2. *Packs to hold centrifuge tubes*
3. *Glass stirring rods*
4. *Burette (50 ml)*

5. *Wash bottle*
6. *Boiling water bath*
7. *Funnel, 3 inch diametre*
8. *Filter paper, Whatman No. 1, 15 cm*
9. *Beakers, 50 ml capacity*
10. *Volumetric transfer pipettes 1, 3, 4, 10 and 15 ml*
11. *Graduated pipette*
12. *pH Meter*
13. *Centrifuge*
14. *Photoelectric colorimeter*
15. *Volumetric flask, 200 ml capacity*
16. *Glass stoppered flask, 250 ml capacity*
17. *Constant temperature bath*
18. *Photoelectric colorimeter*

Reagents

1. *Concentrated hydrochloric acid*
2. *10 N sulphuric acid*
3. *2 N sulphuric acid*
4. *0.2 N sulphuric acid*
5. *10 N sodium hydroxide*
6. *Lloyd's reagent. hydrated aluminium silicate*
7. *0.5 N sodium hydroxide*
8. *Lead nitrate, pulverised*
9. *1% phenolphthalein in 70% ethyl alcohol*
10. *Potassium phosphate crystals, Tribasic*
11. *20% phosphoric acid*
12. *Indicator paper pH 4.5 . Nitrazine of p-hydrion paper is satisfactory*
13. *Standard Niacin stock solution : Place 500 mg USP reference standard Niacin (dried over P_2O_5) in a 500 ml volumetric flask. Add 5 ml of 10 N H_2SO_4 and when crystals have been dissolved, dilute to the mark with water. This stock solution is stable for at least one year if stored in the refrigerator and protected from sunlight. Each ml contain 100 μg of niacin.*

14. *Working Standard : Dilute 5 ml of the standard niacin stock solution to 200 ml with water. This solution contains 25* µg *of niacin per ml. Prepare fresh each day.*

15. *10% Potassium phosphate monobasic : Dissolve 25 grams* KH_2PO_4 *in water in a 250 ml volumetric flask and dilute to the mark. This solution should be prepared at frequent intervals, since molds may grow in the solution.*

16. *0.5 M Cyanogen bromide solution.*

    This is most easily prepared from CNBr crystals (Eastmen)

    Caution : Cyanogen bromide is extremely poisonous.

    All operations involing this reagent should be carried out in an efficient hood. Do not breath any vapours, and if solution come in contact with the skin, wash immediately with water.

    Weigh by difference 53 grams of CNBr Crystals into an Erlemeyer flask calibrated at 1000 ml. Dissolve the crystals in water and dilute to the mark. This preparation should be carried out under a hood. The solution is stable and can be stored in a glass stoppered, brown bottle for several months. If crystals are not available, the reagent may be prepared under a hood from bromine and NaCN as follows:

    Weigh quickly on a triple beam balance 80 grams cold bromine by pouring approximately 27 ml into a tared cold 25 ml graduated cylinder. Immediately transfer the bromine to a glass stoppered 1000 ml volumetric flask which contains 500 ml cold water. Cool in a bath of ice water. Prepare a 10 percent solution of NaCN by dissolving 50 grams in water in a 500 ml volumetric flask and diluting to the mark. Place part of this solution in a burette and slowly add in small portions to the bromine water, which should be constantly shaken. Until the reaction mixture become colourless. Add an excess of 10 drops of NaCN. Dilute to the mark with water and store in a glass stoppered brown bottle.

    Weigh by difference 53 grams of CNBr crystals into an Erlenmeyer flask calibrated at 1000 ml. Dissolve the crystals in water and dilute to the mark. This preparation should be carried out under a hood. The solution is stable and can be stored in a glass stoppered, brown bottle several months. If crystals are not available, the reagent may be prepared under a hood from bromine and NaCN as follow: Weigh quickly on a triple beam balance, 80 grams cold bromine by pouring approximately 27 ml into stared cold 25 ml graduated cylinder. Immediately transfer the bromine to a glass stoppered 1000 ml volumetric flask which contains 500 ml volumetric flask and dilution to the mark. Place part of this solution in a burette and slowly add in small portions to the bromine water, which should be constantly shaken, until the reaction mixture becomes colourless. Add an excess of 10 drops of NaCN. Dilute to the mark with water and store in a glass stoppered brown bottle.

17. *5 percent buffered cyanogen bromide (optional).* It may be convenient to add the CHBr solution and potassium phosphate buffer in one operation. Dissolve 12.5 grams KH_2PO_4 in 250 ml of stock CNBr solution. This solution should be stored in the refrigerator in a glass stoppered brown bottle and should be freshly prepared every 2 months.
18. 8 N hydrochloric acid. Prepare stock solution by diluting 670 ml conc. HCI to 1000 ml with water.
19. 0.5 N HCI
20. 5% metol (photol or pictol). This solution is light sensitive and should be prepared immediately prior to use each day. Place 10 gram metol in an amber or a red 250 ml glass stoppered bottle and dissolve it in 200 ml 0.5 N HCI. Metol which has darkened or which has a purplish tinge in solution should be replaced with fresh reagent or may be purified.

Hydrolysis Extraction

Weigh a sample to contain 100 μg niacin (usually 2-3 grams) and transfer to a centrifuge tube. Dilute to 15 ml with water. Insert stirring rod in each tube.

(1) Add from a burette 5 ml concentrated HCI. The function of the acid is to convert niacin derivatives such as co-enzymes and niacinamide into free niacin which is estimated by this procedure.

(2) 2 N H_2SO_4 is also highly satisfactory. It produces a lighter extract and liberates less interferig substances. However, with unfortified yeasts it was found to yield low results unless the hydrolysis time is increased. Alkaline hydrolysis may also be used. NaoH, however, yields dark extracts. A procedure using $Ca(OH)_2$ is described below:

(3) With yeasts and other samples of very high niacin contents. It is usualy convenient to conduct the hydrolysis in a 100 ml volumetric flask to facilitate higher dilution.

(4) Place centrifuge tube in rack in boiling water bath and allow to remain for 1 hour, stirring occasionally.

Utilise this period to weigh the Lloyd's reagent and lead nitrate to be used later.

(5) Remove rack containing centrifuge tubes from hot water bath and cool tubes to room temperature by placing in cold water bath. Rinse stirring rods with small amount of distilled water.

(6) Dilute to 25 ml with water and shake well.

Extract samples which contain a large amount of fat with chloroform . Add 5 ml chloroform, stopper, and shake well. The fat contains interfering substances and should be removed.

Whenever it is necessary to prepare a large number of sample that can be handled in one day, the analysis may be interrupted at this point. Extracts may be stored in the refrigerator for a period up to one week.

Filter into small beaker or centrifuge 20 minutes at 2000 rpm. Usually centrifugation is the better method since niacin may be absorbed on some filter paper. However, with many samples, filtration is more satisfactory since the extracts may remain clot following centrifugation.

For the sample treated with chloroform, the bottom layer which contains the fat is discarded. An aliquot is pipetted from the top layer and is used in the next step.

Adsorption and Elution-partial Decolourisation

Transfer a 10 ml aliquot with volumetric pipette to a 50 ml beaker. Add approximately 2 ml 10 N NaOH, cool, and adjust by dropwise addition of 10 N NaOH, cool, and adjust by dropwise addition of 10 N NaOH or concentrate HCI to pH 0.5-1.0. using a pH meter.

At this pH the Lloyd's reagent used in subsequent operations adsorbs niacin quantitatively from solution. Transfer the aliquot from the beaker quantitatively to a centrifuge tube containing 2 grams Lloyd's reagent using a small amount of 0.2 N H_2SO_4 in a wash bottle for this purpose.

Stir for one minute. Wash rod and sides of tube with 0.2 N H_2SO_4. Centrifuge about 5 minutes at 2000 rpm. Discard the supernatant liquid.

Wash the precipitate with 10 ml of 0.2 N H_2SO_4. stirring sufficiently to break up clumps of Lloyd's reagent. Wash rod, side of tube, and centrifugate, as before. Discard supernatant liquid, draining completely.

Add 15 ml of 0.5 N NaoH. Stir for one minute after breaking up lumps. Wash rod with distiled water. Dilute to 21.2 ml with distilled water. Stir to mix thoroughly, centrifuge as above but do not discard the supernatant liquid.

At this alkaline pH the niacin is eluted from the Lloyd's reagent and it is contained in the supernatant liquid. The volume occupied by the solid Lloyds's reagent is 1.2 ml. therefore the volume for the solution at this point is 20 ml.

Drain the supernatant liquid completely into a centrifuge tube containing 1 gram of pulverised lead nitrate and one drop of phenolphthalein solution. Stir until the pink colour disappears, centrifuge as above. The lead nitrate is converted to the hydroxide which adsorbs much of the dark colour in the extract.

Decant the solution into a centrifuge tube containing one drop phenlophthalein solution. Add just sufficient crystals of K_3PO_4 to obtain a pink colour. Cautiously add enough 20 percent H_3PO_4 solution to bring the pH back to 4.5, using indicator test paper. A very small drop is usually sufficient.

It is important to use a minimum of both reagents in order not to disturb volume relationships. pH 4.5 has been found to be optimal for the subsequent colour reaction.

Colour Development

All method of hydrolysis may cause decomposition of substances other than niacin in the sample. These decomposition products yield colour and also interfere with the reaction of niacin and the reagents. Much of this interfering material is eliminated in the preceding treatment with Lloyd's reagent and lead nitrate. However, in some cases interfering materials remain in the extract. These are of three types: (1) substances which react with aromatic amines to yield a yellow colour (2) substances which on reaction with CNBr yield colour and (3) inert coloured material. Each of these blanks are required to correct for the three errors introduced by the above steps. To illustrate the efficacy of this blank correction system, purified sugar produces an intense yellow colour when reacted with CNBr and amine reagents, but if all blank corrections are applied a zero value for niacin is obtained upon calculation.

The actual determination of each sample then requires 4 tubes, 3 for the blank corrections and other for the total colour to which these corrections are applied according to the following formula:

Corrected colour = total density - (1) + (2)-(3)

It is best to set up a definite physical arrangement of tubes to facilitate handling additon of reagents with minimum confusion and reading of tubes on a time basis. The following arrangement suggested in the diagram below shows the actual content of each tube. The actual order of addition and procedural treatments follow the diagram. The tubes are arranged in arrow of 4 for each sample being assayed. The standard requires only 1 tube, however, since USP Niacin standard is pure and does not requires correction. An additional row of 4 tubes for instrument blanks precedes the arrangement, and these are used to adjust the instrument before reading the corresponding series of tubes.

Set up in a rack a series of 4 tubes for each sample. 4 for the instrument blank and 1 for the standard niacin as shown in diagram below. All tubes have a final volume of 20 ml.

Total colour series	Amine Corr. series	CNBr. series	Colour Corr. series
Instrument blanks	1	2	3
7 ml water	9 ml water	7 ml water	9 ml water
1 ml KH_2PO_4	1 ml KH_2PO_4	1 ml KH_2PO_4	1 ml KH_2PO_4
2 ml CNBR	—	2 ml CNBr	—
10 ml Metol	10 ml Metol	—	—
–	—	10 ml 0.5 NHCl	10 ml 0.5 N HCl

Standard

1 ml niacin working standard
6 ml H_2O
1 ml KH_2PO_4
2 ml CNBr
10 ml Metol

No corrections are needed for The standard (USP)

Sample of A tubes

4 ml extract A	4 ml extract A	4 ml extract A	4 ml extract
3 ml water	5 ml water	3 ml water	5 ml water
1 ml KH_2PO_4	1 ml KH_2PO_4	1 ml KH_2PO_4	1 ml KH_2PO_4
2 ml CNBr	Nil	2 ml CNBr	Nil
10 ml Metol	10 ml Metol	Nil	—
		10 ml 0.5 N HCl	10 ml 0.5 N HCl

Sample B tubes, etc., same as for sample A tubes. Usually it is found possible to simplify the procedure so that only one blank need be run. After assaying a certain types of sample a number of times, it will generally be found that the amine correction (1) and colour correction (3) or that the CNBr correction (2) and the colour correction are nearly equal. In the case of meat, for example, (1) and (3) are nearly equal. Therefore, the significant correction to be considered is that of the CNBr, (2). In subsequent assays corrections (1) and (3) may be omitted. With cereal product the pronounced effect is that of the amine reactive materials. Corrrections (2) and (3) are usually very close, so that they may be omitted.

(a) After having set up the tubes as shown in D-3 (a) transfer 4 ml aliquot of sample extracts to the proper tubes. To the standard tube add 1 ml of working standard containing 25 μg of of niacin.

1. The increment technique may be preferred over the external standard. Because this involves additional work and has not been found to improve the accuracy of the method, the increment technique may find

application only in checking recoveries and is not necessarily recommended for routine use.

(b) To all tubes and 1 ml 10% KH_2PO_4. If a buffered CNBr solution is used, omit the KH_2PO_4 and add 1 ml water.

(c) Add water to tubes in amounts shown above.

(d) Place all tubes for 5 minutes in water bath adjusted to 70°C. This is a convenient time to prepare Metol reagent. This reagent should be made sufficiently prior to use to insure complete solution of the Metol. It should be kept in the dark. Do not heat to hasten solution.

(e) From a burette add 2 ml CNBr to tubes indicated in D-3 (a) at intervals of 15 seconds. Mix by swirling. This operation should be carried out under a hood in diffused light.

(f) Five minute after the addition of CNBr to the first tube, transfer this tube to a water bath held at 25° C. Transfer the next tube containing CNBr to water bath 15 seconds later, etc. Removal of blank tubes need not be strictly timed.

(g) Add 10 ml of freshly prepared acid Metol solution to those tubes indicated above and mix.

1. HCI in the amine reagent prevents darkening of the reagent, stabilises the colour, and permits maximum reaction with the aromatic amine.

2. Other amines, aniline, P-aminoacetophenone, m- phenylene diamine may be used.

(h) Add 10 ml 0.5 N HCI to those tubes indicated as above and mix. Place the tubes in a dark place for one hour. Before reading the colour wipe off the tubes with a soft lint free cloth.

(i) Read the colour intensities of all solutions in a photoelectric colorimeter using the 500 filter or wavelength band. Before reading a series, set the instrument to read 100 with the instrument blank of that series, e.g., for the total colour reading, adjust the instrument with the blank for the total colour series.

If the extract contains much colour, the 420 mμ filter is to be preferred, This yields somewhat lower readings but reduces the effect of amine reactive substances, thereby increasing the specificity of the procedure.

4. Calculation

(a) Convert all galvanometer reading to colour density. This is done by subtracting the log (base 10) of the galvanometer reading from 2.

(b) Correct the colour density of the sample by subtracting the colour density of the appropriate corrections or corrections.

1. If all three corrections are used:
   Corrected density = Total density -(1) +(2)-(3)
2. If the amine correction only is used:
   Corrected density = Total density - (1)
3. If the CNBr correction only is used:
   Corrected density = Total density - (2)
   Calculate according to the formula:

$$\mu g \text{ of niacin per gram testing material} = \frac{25}{\text{colour density of standard}}$$

$$\text{multiplied by} = \frac{\text{corrected colour density of sample}}{\text{SampleWeight}} \text{x dilution factor}$$

☞ General Note

All the above mentioned methods related to the analysis of riboflavin and niacin have been adapted by the Association of vitamin chemists. New York and published by the Chairman Dr. Myer Freed (1966) of this Association. I have referred this publication as well as original articles while preparing the text of this chapter.

References

Freed. M. (1966). *Methods of Vitamin Assay*. 3rd edn, Interscience publishers, a division of John Wiley & Sons, New York.

Isbell, H., wolley. J.G. and Fraser, H.F. (1941). *The inhibiting effect of urea on the microbiological assay of riboflavin*. U.S. Public Health Rep. 56:282.

Melnick, (1942). *Cereal Chem.* 19: 553.

Snell and strong, (1939). *Ind. Eng. Chem., Anal Ed.,* 11: 346

Strong.F.M.I. (1947). *The microbiological determination of Riboflavin, Biological symposia* XII. Jacques Cattel. Lancaster. Pa. pp 143-165.

Chapter - 63

Protein Quality Evaluation Techniques

Introduction

All the amino acids have in common an amino group and a carboxyl group attached to the α -carbon atom; however, they differ in having distinctive side chains, usually called R groups, as is shown in the following generalised structural formula

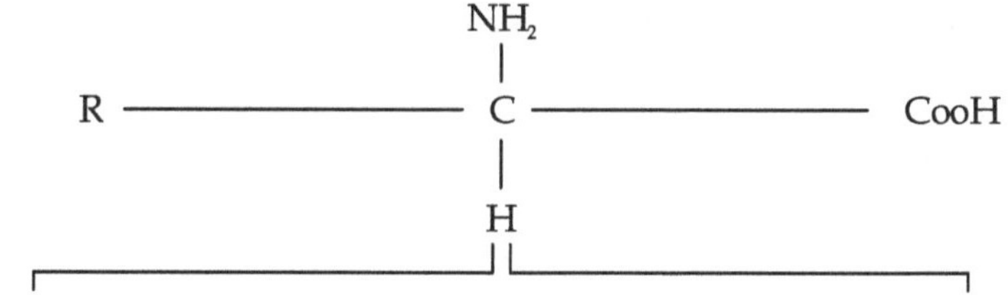

R groups of the various amino acids differ in sizes, shape and polarity. Some are highly polar and carry an electrical charge at the pH of the cell, such as the R group of glutamic acid and lysine; such R groups are water soluble or hydrophilic (water liking). However, the R groups of other amino acids such as isoleucine and phenylalanine, are non polar and thus are only in nature or hydrophobic (water-hating). Two amino acids may be covalently linked by the peptide bond, which joins the α -amino group of one and the α -carboxyl group of the other. When two amino acids are so joined, the product is a dipeptide.

Following methods are commonly used for analysing amino acids in biological materials.

1. Separation of ethyl esters by fractional distillation.
2. Van slyke's nitrogen distribution method.
3. Methods based on specific reactions of the various R groups of the individual amino acids, which yield either substances suceptible to gravimetric determination of colorimetric estimation.
4. The isotope dilution method.
5. The isotope carrier method.
6. Microbiological procedures, involving frequently but not exclusively the use of acid-producing micro-organisms which requires certain amino acids for normal growth, and give essentially linear curves relating acid production to concentration of a required amino acid in synthetic media.
7. Chromatographic ion-exchange method.

Protein-hydrolysis for Analysing by Automatic Amino Acid Analyser (Method of Weidner and Eggum, 1966)

The following is the description of method usually practised at the department of Animal Physiology, Copenhagen (Denmark).

The hydrolysis of protein materials still presents a great problem, as inevitably some amino acid decomposition is associated with the fragmentation process. The degree of destruction depends on the species of protein and conditions of the hydrolysis. A determination of the greatest possible precision with which an amino acid analysis can be performed will require a series of hydrolysis. An evaluation procedure of this nature deserve the attention ordinarily devoted to an experiment of singular dimensions.

The folloiwng method is a modification of standard procedure worked out by the different scientists (Krampitz, 1957; Moore *et al.*, Krampitz, 1960).

For every protein material to be analysed, two separate hydrolyses are required. In the oxidised (o) hydrolysis, methionine is determined as methionine sulphone, and cysteine, cystine are jointly detected in the form of cysteic acid. In addition, the determination of the oxidative resistant amino acid, aspartic acid, serve as a control for comparison of the two separate hydrolyses. Some of the amino-acids, other than methionine sulphon, cysteic acid and aspartic acid, are decomposed to varying degrees by the process of oxidation. They are therefore determined in a hydrolysate of the non- oxidised material (hydrolysate U). Tryptophan, which is acid labile, is unobtainable in both hydrolyses.

Preparation of Hydrolysate (the non-oxidised hydrolysate)

Reagents

1. *Stannous Chloride Sncl$_2$, 2H2O.*
2. *Hydrochloric acid (6 N). Measure 491 ml conc, hydrochloric acid (37%) in a one litre measuring cylinder, transfer to a litre volumetic flask, make up the volume with distilled water.*
3. *Buffer (pH 2.22)*

   Weigh 105g citric acid and 42 g sodium hydroxide in a beaker containing 70 ml concentrated hydrochloric acid, later on dilute this mixture upto five litre.
4. *Sodium hydroxide (percent)*

   Weigh 30 g sodium hydroxide and add to a beaker containing 100 ml distilled water.
5. *Methionine sulphone solution*

   Weigh 0.3624 g DL methionine sulphone in a beaker containing 200 ml distilled water.
6. *Phenol*

Method of Hydrolysis

An amount of sample containing 9-10 mg nitrogen is weighed into a 2 litre flask, and 60 mg stannous chloride is added as both catalyst and antioxidant, hydrochloric acid is added to give a total volume of 500 ml 6 N HCI. The mixture is then boiled under reflux for 24 hours on a sand bath, the time being taken from the moment that boiling begins.

After 24 hours, the hydrolysate is immediately cooled on a water bath and filtered on a Büchner funnel through a 7 cm open filter, two filter papers being used to obtain a clear solution. The filter papers are then washed with water and kept for analysis.

The hydrolysate and washings are immediately evaporated under vacuum using a Büchi evaporators, and the final volume must not fall below 30 ml. The temperature of the water bath must not exceed 50°C.

The concentrated hydrolysate is quantitatively transferred to a beaker and washed over with 30-40 ml of pH. 2.22 buffer solution. The beaker is then placed in a cooling mixture (ice, water, Nacl), and the hydrolysate adjusted to pH 2.5-3.0 with a 30% sodium hydroxide solution, dripped in slowly from burette so that the temperature does not exceed 50°C. The hydrolysate is then permitted to reach room temperature before being adjusted to pH. 2.22 with hydrochloric acid.

This hydrolysate is filtered through a 11 cm open filter into a 150 ml standard flask. The filter paper is washed with pH 2.22 buffer and kept for analysis. 100-150 mg phenol is now added to prevent microbial growth, and exactly 3 ml of the methionine sulphone solution is added for control. The solution is diluted to the 150 ml mark with pH 2.22 buffer and thoroughly mixed (2 ml hydrolysate contain 0.3 µmol methionine sulphone).

The hydrolysate is stored in a refrigerator at about 4°C, but is warmed to room temperature before use. For the determination of the amino acids, 2 ml of this hydrolysate is applied to the column.

Preparation of Hydrolysate II (the oxidised hydrolysate)

Reagents

1. *Hydrogen peroxide (30 percent)*
2. *Formic acid (98-100 percent)*
3. *Sodium pyrosulphite*
4. *Hydrochloric acid (6 N)*
5. *Buffer (pH 2.22)*
6. *Sodium hydroxide (30 percent)*
7. *Phenol*

Procedure for Oxidation

A portion of sample containing 9-10 mg nitrogen is weighed into a small beaker. Liquid samples, such as urine are freeze dried prior to oxidation.

In another beaker 0.5 ml 30 percent hydrogen peroxide is added to 4.5 ml concentrated formic acid, previously heated to 50°C. This mixture is allowed to stand for 3 minutes on a water bath at 50°C.

The performic acid solution is then poured on to the sample. This mixture is heated on water bath at 50°C for 15 minutes, under constant stirring.

At the end of the oxidation period, excess peroxide is removed by the addition of sodium pyrosulphite. The mixture is then quantitatively transferred to a 2 litre round bottomed flask using 500 ml 6 N hydrochloric acids, reagent grade.

The remaining steps are identical to those described under "method of hydrolysis" of hydrolysate I, except that neither stannous chloride nor methionine sulphate are added.

Precautions

1. To affect the least amount of amino acid loss during the evaporation stage, this operation is performed under high vacuum, thereby facilitating rapid completion. The volume of the hydrolysate must not fall below 30 ml during evaporation. Moreover, during neutralization, the NaOH should be added very slowly as the temperature of the hydrolysate must not exceed 50°C.
2. With many of the automatic amino acid analysers in the market, the recommended concentration of amino acids in the hydrolysate is lower than that employed here. In such case. It would be advantageous to neutralise with a NaOH solution weaker than 30 percent.
3. Reagent grade HCI could be replaced in the place of analytical grade in the oxidative process.
4. The amount of humin material in the hydrolysate may be used as a criterian for judging the quality of the hydrolysis, since humin is a direct result of amino acid decomposition. The filter papers from the two filtrations, mentioned above, are put into the same Kjeldahl flask and analysed for nitrogen. Normally the nitrogen content of the precipitate is less than 0.1 mg. However, if the nitrogen content is above 0.3 mg. hydrolysate is discarded and a new one is made.
5. For control purposes, it is not necessary to determine two hydrolysates for each of the oxidised and non-oxidised samples. Since aspartic acid is not destroyed in the oxidative processes, it may be determined from both the I and II hydrolysates. In this way, the double determination serves as a control between the two hydrolysates.

Practical Applicability

Hydrolysis, as determined according to the method described in this paper, has demontrated a high degree of reliability and when the amino acids are separated on an Ion-exchange column, there are no difficulties in the calculation (Mason, 1963).

Comparison of Amino Acid Analyses Carried out in Different Laboratories.

The values for the sulphur containing amino acids, cysteine and methionine, examplify rather well the extent of agreement between the various laboratories. This seems to indicate that the oxidation technique of Krampitz (1960)works satisfactorily. Between the remaining amino acids, there is a lesser degree of agreement, However, in most case the differences were small and do not reduce confidence in the figures found by the various laboratories.

Estimation of Lysine in Human Foods and Animal Feeds

(Colorimetric Method of Rao *et al.*, 1963) Modified by Indian Standards Institution, IS: 1374-1979

Principle

Lysine is estimated by the ion exchange chromatographic technique.

Reagents

1. Sodium Citrate Buffer (pH 5.28 ± 0.02)

Dissolve 98.2 g of citric acid (AR), 57.6 g of sodium hydroxide in 27.2 ml of conc. hydrochloric acid and dilute to 4 litres. Adjust the pH of the solution to 2.20 ± 0.03 and then preserved by adding 0.1 ml of caprylic alcohol (0.01 percent).

2. Sodium Citrate Buffer (pH 2.20 ± 0.03)

Dissolve 105 g citric acid and 42 g of sodium hydroxide in 80 ml of concentrated hydrochloric acid. Mix and dilute to five litres. Adjust the pH to 2.20 ± 0.03 and then add the preservative = 0.1 ml of caprylic alcohol (0.01 percent).

3. Hydrindantin

Dissolve 20 g of ninhydrin in 500 ml of distilled water maintained at 90°C. To this add by constant stirring a solution of ascorbic acid (20 percent) maintained at 40°C, Crystalline hydrindantin (reduced form of ninhydrin) is precipitated and the crystalization is allowed to proceed for 30 minutes at room temperature . Filter and wash the hydrindantin free of ascorbic acid by repeated washing and dry under vacuum by keeping overnight, over phosphorus pentaoxide. Store hydrindantin in dark bottle for further use.

4. Sodium Acetate Buffer (pH 5.5)

Dissolve 544 grams of sodium acetate in 700 ml of distilled water. To this solution add 100 ml of glacial acetic acid and make the volume to one litre. Adjust the pH to 5.5 with the addition of an alkali or acetic acid.

5. Methyl Cellosolve (Ethylene glycol-Monoethyl ether)

Peroxide free. To make methyl cellosolve free of peroxide, distil at 180°C before use.

6. Ninhydrin-hydrindantin Reagent

Dissolve 2 grams of ninhydrin and 300 mg of hydrindantin in 75 ml of methyl cellosolve. Then add 25 ml of sodium acetate buffer solution and thoroughly mix. This reagent should be prepared fresh for use. Reagent when discoloured should not be used.

Procedure

a. Preparation and Hydrolysis of Sample

Take 100 mg of finely ground fat-free material and hydrolyse with 5 ml of standdard hydrochloric acid in a sealed pyrex tubes at 110°C for 18 to 24 hours. On hydrolysis, make the volume to 10 ml with distilled water. Take an aliquot of 2 ml and evaporate to near dryness to remove the excess acid. Using sodium citrate buffer (pH 2.2), make the volume to 10 ml. In case the sample is not used immediately, the hydrolysates are kept under refrigerated condition.

b Preparation and Operation of The Column

The chromatographic column is poured with a slurry of the treated resin, Amberlite - IR 120 (300 to 400 mesh), in standard sodium hydroxide solution. A total length of 16 cm is poured in 3 to 4 sections. The first few centimetres of the column are allowed to settle by gravity and the rest is packed with a pressure of 1 to 1.5 kg/cm^2 from an air compressor connected to the column. When the required length of the resin column is poured and packed, the supernatant alkali is removed and the resin equilibrated with sodium citrate buffer (pH 5.28 ± 0.02).

The resin column is brought to a constant temperature (50° ± 1°C) by circulating warm water from a thermostatic water bath. 2 ml of the protein hydrolysate is added on top of the column without disturbing the top layer and a pressure of 1 to 1.5 kg/cm^2 is applied. As the hydrolysate enters the top layers of the column, two to three washings with 0.5 ml portions of citrate buffer of pH 5.28 are given. A separating funnel filled with the buffer is fitted to the column and pressure applied to maintain an affluent flow rate of 24 ml per hour. The collection of the affluent is started leaving the first few tubes, and subsequent 2 ml fractions are collected by means of a 2 ml syphon. A total of 24 tube is collected. The first 9 or 10 tubes which consist of neutral and acidic amino acids are discarded. To each of the later 12 tubes exactly 1 ml of the ninhydrin hydrindantin reagent is added. A reagent blank is similarly treated. The tubes are heated in a vigorously boiling water-bath at 100°C for exactly 15 minutes removed from the bath the immediately chilled in an ice bath. After making the solution to volume, the colour is read in a spectrophoto meter at 590 nm against a reagent blank.

c. Standard Curve

Lysine standard solutions of 0.05 to 0.25 kg/ml concentration are prepared and the colour developed as in the unknown solutions. A standard graph is plotted against which the concentration of the unknown may be read.

☞ Notes

Neutral amino acids - Contain one amino and one carboxyl group.

a. *Aliphatic aminoacids - Glycine, alanine, serine, threonine, valine, leucine, Isoleucine*

b. *Aromatic amino acids - Phenylalanine, tyrosine.*

c. *Sulphur containing amino acids - Cysteine, cystine and methionine*

d. *Heterocyclic amino acids - Tryptophan, proline hydroxy proline 3-hydroxyproline.*

e. *Acidic amino acids - contain an excess of carboxyl groups example - aspartic acid, glutamic acid.*

f. *Basic amino acids - contain in excess of basic nitrogen-histidine, lysine, arginine, hydroxylysine.*

Estimation of Methionine in Human Foods and Animal Feeds

(Colorimetric Method of Horn *et al.*, 1946 Modified by Indian Standards Institution, IS: 1374-1979)

Principle

Methionine forms a coloured complex with sodium nitroprusside. This reaction is taken advantage of in the determination of this amino acid in food proteins.

Reagents

1. *Standard sodium hydroxide solution - 5 N*
2. *Sodium Nitroprusside - 10 percent in water The solution is prepared a fresh every time before use.*
3. *Glycine - 3 percent solution in water.*
4. *Phosphoric acid - 85 percent*
5. *Hydrochloric acid - 6 N*
6. *Phosphotungstic acid*

Procedure

Take 100 mg of finely ground fat-free material and hydrolyse with 5 ml of standard hydrochloric acid in sealed pyrex tubes at 110°C for 18 to 24 hours. At the completion of hydrolysis, open the tubes and transfer the contents to a 10 ml volumetric flask with repeated washings. Add 50 mg of activated charcoal (previoulsy treated with standard hydrochloric acid) and 50 mg of phosphotungstic acid to the flask. Mix well and make the volume to 10 ml with distilled water and filter. Take 2 ml of acid hydrolysate and add 2 ml of water, 1 ml of standard sodium hydroxide solution, 1 ml of standard methionine solution and 0.1 ml of sodium nitroprusside solution. Shake the mixture thoroughly for 10 minutes in a mechanical shaker. Subsequently add 2 ml of glycine solution and again shake for ten minutes and read the colour at 540 nm in a spectrophotometer.

Prepare standard solution containing 200 to 1000 μg/ml of methionine. Treat this solution similarly mentioned at in above paragraph and prepare a standard graph. Run an identical reagent blank. The amount of methionine is expressed as grams per 16 grams of nitrogen.

Determination of Amino Acids in Protein Hydrolysates by Paper Chromatography

(Method of Consden *et al.*, 1944; Synge, 1944 Modified by Smith, 1960)

A paper chromatograph is prepared as follows. A drop of the solution containing the compounds to be separated is placed near the end of strip of paper and allowed to dry. The strip is then placed so that a few millimeters of it dips into a solvent, but it is essential that the dried spot is not immersed in this, otherwise it will dissolve into the solvent. The solvent then commences to flow along the paper, over the spot and towards the far end of the paper, When the strip is withdrawn and rapidly dried. To prevent evaporation from the surface of the paper, the operation is conducted in an air tight container. The fundamental measurement in chromatography is that of Rf which is defined as follow:

$$Rf = \frac{\text{Distance a substance travels from the origin}}{\text{Distance a solvent travels from the origin}}$$

With amino acids practically all run with the solvent front when water of acetic acid is the solvent, and nearly all remain at the origin when butanol or proppanol is the solvent. Adding water to butanol increases the Rf of most of the amino acids, but even in butanol saturated with water the Rf's are not sufficiently large to render the solvent mixture useful. Extra water can, however, be introduced into the butanol if acetic acid is also added and an excellent butanol-acetic acid-water mixture can be prepared. The protein hydrolysate is spoted on a strip of paper using a borax lead platinum 1000. About 10 ml of the solvent to be examined is placed in a cylinder and the strip is suspended from a paper clip, so that it just dips into the solvent. Runs of 7 to 10 cm, which take very little time on a whatman No.4 paper, are sufficient to indicate the desired information. The location of amino compounds by means of ninhydrin is carried out using 0.2 percent ninhydrin in acetone (w/v). Immediately before use some 2 percent pyridine is routinely incroporated into the reagent, directly in the dip tray, as an effective colour stabiliser and the paper is dipped through the reagent. The paper is then hung up in the cold or after the acetone has evaporated and heated for 2 to 3 minutes in an oven at 105°C. All the alpha amino acids react with this reagent in the cold, usually within 3 hours and certainly overnight giving the main purple colour.

If a compound yields a colour on heating but not when kept overnight in the cold, It is almost certainly not an alpha amino acid (smith 1960). Quantitative determination of amino acids can be carried out on the spots on filter paper by elution or direct colorimetry, after developing the colour with ninhydrin (Consden *et al.*, 1944; Synge, 1944).

Available Lysine in Foods

(Method of Carpenter, 1960; Carpenter and Ellinger, 1955)

Available lysine content is considered as the most important chemical (non-biological) indicator of nutritional quality fo protein because low values reflect loss due to heat processing. Since lysine is a limiting amino acid, its fortification should be viewed in the light of the concept of suitable and reliable method of analysis which gives repeatable and reproducible results. *There are mainly two methods, namely, chemical and microbiological, for analysis of lysine, of these, chemical method is more precise and accurate.* This compendium therefore, prescribes chemical method for analysis of available lysine. It is expected that this method will help in achieving uniformity in the analysis of lysine thereby facilitating uniform interpretation and comparison of results.

For the purpose of this standard, the following definition shall apply.

Available Lysine. *That fraction of lysine which reacts with fluorodini-trobenzene (FDNB) associated with biologically active fraction of lysine.*

Principle

The method is based on the conversion of lysine residues with the reactive epsilon amino groups in food proteins into yellow epsilon dinitrophenyl (DNP) lysine by treatment of the material with FDNB and colorimetric estimation of the DNP lysine obtained by a subsequent acid hydrolysis.

Ether soluble interfering compounds are removed by extraction and the extinction of the residual aqueous layer is measured. A blank value is obtained by treatment with methoxy carbonyl chloride and extraction of the ether soluble lysine compound, which results. The reaction of fluoro 2:4 dinitrobenzene (FDNB) with the free -NH groups of lysine in purified proteins, so that a stable, coloured DNP-lysine compound is formed on acid hydrolysis, has been used in studies of molecular structure (sanger, 1945) and of the reaction of casein with carbohydrates (Lee and Hannan, 1950) where a reduction in the number of free amino groups was paralleled by a fall in nutritional value (Henry and kon, 1950).

Apparatus

1. *Autopipette of suitably graduated pipettes.*
2. *Burette 25 ml capacity, graduated to 0.05 ml. Conical flasks.*

☞ Notes

It is not advisable to clean the flasks with chromic acid; but, if this is done, they should be soaked in dilute sodium hydroxide and rinsed with distilled water thoroughly.

3. *Photoelectric colorimeter Absorbance at 435 nm.*
4. *Round bottom flasks 100 of 150 ml capacity with 8 cm long necks and standard joints 24- 29 for fitting to condensers.*
5. *Stoppered test tubes Graduated at 10 ml.*
6. *Water Bath for temperature of 100°C.*

Reagents

Unless specified otherwise, pure chemicals and distilled water shall be employed in tests.

☞ Note

Pure chemicals, shall mean chemicals that do not contain impurities which affect the test results.

1. Mono F-N-Dintrophyenyl lysine Hydrochloride Monohydrate (DNPL)

Dissolve 314 mg of lysine in 250 ml of 8.1 N hydrochloric acid. Dilute 10 ml standard DNPL solution wtih water to 100 ml. Use this diluted solution as a standard for the routine tests. A 2 ml. aliquot contains the equivalent of 0.1 mg of lysine when diluted to 10 ml has a net absorbance of about 0.4 at 435 nm in a 1 cm cuvette.

The sample used as a reference standard of dinitrophenyl (DNP)-lysine hydrochloride is prepared according to the procedure of Porter and Sanger (1948). The lysine unit in this molecule represents 39.9 percent of its weight.

☞ Note

This compound dissolves slowly. It is, therefore, desirable to allow a day for the process.

2. Flouro-2-4-dinitrobenzene (FDNB)

If the FDNB is solid, place the bottle in warm water for a few minutes before dispensing it with a autopipette. Prepare FDNB solution in ethanol every day. Each sample will require 12 ml of ethanol solution containing 0.3 ml of FDNB. Actual measurement of FDNB may not be essential.

☞ Notes

It is a vesicant and, therefore disposable gloves of polyethylene, not rubber, should be worn during its use. All operation involving the use of the vesicant including its addition to the sample may be performed on sheet of paper which may be disposed of later.

3. *Methoxycarbonyl Chloride (MCC) : 8 percent (W/V).*
4. *Sodium Bicarbonate Solution : 80 grams in one liter of distilled water.*
5. *Buffer Solution : 19 parts of 8 percent sodium bicarbonate and 1 part of 8 percent sodium carbonate adjusted suitably to pH 8.5.*
6. *Hydrochloric acid Concentrated, : 1 N and 8.1 N.*
7. *Diethyl Ether : Peroxide free.*
8. *Phenolphthalein Indicator solution 0.1 g in 100 ml of 50 to 60 percent ethanol.*

Procedure

Carry out the procedure in duplicate and away from direct or strongly reflected sunlight.

Take 50 grams of the material finally ground to pass through 425-micron sieve. Take samples for the determination of nitrogen also in duplicate at this time. Then take two portions each containing an estimated 30 to 50 mg of nitrogen into round bottom flasks and to each add 8 ml of 8 percent sodium bicarbonate. Shake gently to disperse the material and leave for 10 minutes. The sample should not be widely scattered. Add 0.3 ml FDNB, previoulsy dissolved in 12 ml of ethanol to each flasks, stopper the flask and shake gently on a mechanical shaker for two hours. Remove the stoppers and allow the flask to stand in boiling water to remove the ethanol. Add immediately 24 ml of 8.1 N hydrochloric acid to one flask. To the other flask add only 12 ml of 8.1 N hydrochloric acid, a quantity that contain the equivalent of 8 mg lysine which serves as an internal standard. Add DNPL after the FDNB reaction has been stopped by the acid; otherwise it will be converted to bis-DNPL which will be eliminated by extraction with ether. Reflux the contents of the flask gently for 16 hours. Disconnect the flasks after the condensers have been washed with water. Cool the flasks in ice for two hours to keep for easy filtration. Filter the contents through a whatman filter paper No. 41 or equivalent, with water washings into a 250-ml volumetric flask. Make the filtrate to the volume and mix. Dilute an aliquot or the filtrate so that 2 ml of the dilute material contains an estimate of approximatley 50 μg of the available lysine.

Estimation of "Available Lysine" in Protein Concentrate

(Method of Carpenter and Elinger, 1955)

Ground material containing 0.05 g N is dispersed in 8 ml 10 percent (w/v) $NaHCO_3$ in a 50 ml round botton flask, Add 0.3 ml FDNB in 12 ml ethanol. After 2 hours shaking ethanol is evaporated off, 24 ml 5.5 N-HCI is added and the whole refluxed for 24 hours. The cooled contents are filtered with washings, and made to 50ml. 5 ml are extracted 4 times with 50 ml ether, adjusted to pH 5 with 1 ml glacial acetic acid and NaOH, diluted to 50 ml, centrifuged (if necessary) and read in the spekker absorptiometer (filter 601).

Replication without FDNB gives the blank DNP-lysine solutions provide a standard. To claim that the method in its present form measure "nutritionally available lysine" would involve the assumption that, with all the crude materials used, DNP lysine is the only compound formed, that remains to give an extinction, also that the lysine molecules reacting with FDNB, and only those, are available to the chick.

☞ Notes

A precipitate of dinitrophenol may form. The precipitate should be allowed to settle and avoided during the pipetting. It should not be transferred during the next stage, but should be removed by ether.

Pipette 2 ml from each diluted filtrate into each of the two glass stoppered test tubes marked 'A' and 'B' and a small conical flask marked 'C', Extract the contents of the tube thrice with 5.0 ml of ether. Discard as much of the ether as safely as could be by taking it off with a dropping pipette or autopipette. Hold the tube in hot water (about 80°C) untill effervescence from the residual ether had ceased and cooled off. Make up tube 'A' to 10 ml with 1 N hydrochloric acid and keep for the final readings.

Dilute the contents of flask 'C' with water and titrate with 2 N sodium hydroxide, using a drop of phenolphthalein indicator, Note the quantity of sodium hydroxide needed and then add the same volume to tube 'B'. followed by 2 ml of buffer solution. Further additions should be continued without pause as DNP-compounds are less stable at this pH. Add methoxy carbonyl chloride (0.045 to 0.055 ml permissible) and shake the tube vigorously to disperse and dissolve the compound. After 5 to 10 minutes, and carefuly 0.75 ml of concentrated hydrochloric acid. Extract again the contents 4 times with 5 ml ether. Discard the ether washings. Evaporate the residual ether in the aqueous layer by standing the tube in hot water bath, Cool the tube and make up the contents to 10 ml with water.

Read the absorbance of the contents of tubes A and B at 435 nm against water. Reading A minus reading B (the blank)is the net absorbance attributable to DNP-lysine.

Calculations

Available lysine in g per 100 grams of material.

$$= \frac{(A - C)}{(B - D) - (A - C)} \times \frac{x}{w} \times 100 \frac{40}{100}$$

where

A = Sample reading,

B = Sample and extra DNP-lysine

C = Blank for sample

D = Blank for sample and extra DNP-lysine,

W = Sample mass equivalent in g of 2-ml aliquot

A-C = Correct sample reading and

B-D = reading for extra DNP-lysine (X gram) in 2-ml aliquot.

☞ Note

The method is not suitable for measuring added lysine or free lysine in hydrolysed product. This yields di-DN-P-lysine which is lost in the first ether wash.

Microbiological Assay of Amino Acids in Human Foods and Animal Feeds (Method Published by Barton Wright, 1952 Later Adapted by Indian Standards Institution Vide IS: 7815-1975)

Principle

The method is based on the observation that certain micro-organisms require specific nutrients for growth. Using a basal medium complete in all respects except for the amino acid under test, growth responses of the organisms are compared quantitatively in standard and in unknown solutions. Either the acid or the turbidity produced by the organisms is measured to determine the extent of growth and thereby the amount of nutrient in the test solution.

Test Organisms

Leuconostoc Mesenteroides (ATCC No. 8042) For use in assay of all amino acids except threonine.

Streptococus faecalis (ATCC Nol 9790). For use in assay of threonine.

☞ **Note**

Lactobacillus plantarum (ATCC No. 8014) may also be used in assay of isoleucine, leucine, methionine, phenylalanine, tryptophan and Valine.

Preparation and Maintenance of Stock Culture

Prepare stock culture of agar tubes and inoculate with the pure culture (appropriate organism to be used for the different assays). Incubate the tubes for 16 to 24 hours at 37°C and store at 4°C. Transfer the cultures into new agar tubes every fortnight.

Preparation of Stock Culture Tubes

Salt solution A : Dissolve 20 grams each of dibasic potassium phosphate (K_2HPO_4) and monobasic potassium phosphate (KH_2PO_4) in water and make up to 250 ml with water.

Salt solutions B : Dissolve the following salts in 250 ml of water to which are added a few drops of concentrated hydrochloric acid to obtain a clear solution. Store under toluene.

Magnesium sulphate ($MgSO_4 . 7H_2O$)	*10.0g*
Sodium chloride (NaCI)	*0.5g*
Ferric sulphate ($FeSO_4 . 7H_2O$)	*0.5g*
Manganese sulphate ($MnSO_4 . H_2O$)	*0.5g*

Dissolve the following ingredients in 200 ml of distilled water, adjust the pH to 6.8 and make the volume up to 250 ml. Separately dissolve 7.5 grams of agar in 250 ml distilled water by heating. Mix well both the solution together. While the solution is still hot, take 10ml of the solution into test tubes. Plug with cotton, and autoclave for 15 minutes at 82 KN/m2 (0.84 kgf/cm^2) pressure. After cooling to room temperature store the tubes at 2 to 4°C and use for maintaining stock cultures.

Peptone	*5.0 g*
Yeast extract	*1.0 g*
Glucose, anhydrous	*10.0 g*
Sodium acetate 3 H_2O	*17.0 g*
or	
Sodium acetate, anhydrous	*10.0 g*
Salt solution A	*2.5 ml*
Salt solution B	*2.5 ml*

Preparation of Inoculum Broth

Prepare the inoculum broth in the same way as the culture medium excepting that instead of the agar solution, use more of distilled water (after adjusting the pH to 6.8) to make up the volume to 500 ml. Take 10 ml of the solution into test tubes, then plug with cotton, autoclave for 15 minutes at 82 KN/m^2 (0.84 Kgf/cm^2) Pressure, cool to room temperature and store at 2 to 4°C.

Preparation of Inoculum

A day prior to use, inoculate inoculum broth tube with a loopful of culture from the stock culture and incubate at 37°C for 16 to 18 hours. Use a centrifuge tube pluged with cotton, an all glass syringe, a 0.8 mm needle, and some saline (0.9 percent) in a conical flask. Sterilise saline by autoclaving for 15 minutes at 103 KN/m2 (1.05 Kgf /cm2) pressure and syringe, needle and centrifuge tube by hot-air oven at 160°C for one hour. Transfer the cells from the inoculum tube to the centrifuge tube and centrifuge, decant off the supernatant and resuspend the cells in sterile saline and centrifuge. Report the process two or three times. Again make up the washed cells to a suspension using the saline. Take resuspended cells in the sterile syringe and inoculate the assay tubes with one drop each of the inoculum. The optical density of the inoculum should be about 0.1.

Preparation of Solutions for Assay Tubes

Salt Solution A : Dissolve 12 grams each of dibasic potassium phosphate (K_2HPO_4) and monobasic potassium phosphate (KH_2PO_4) in water and make up to 100 ml with water.

Salt Solution B : Mix and dissolve the following in water to make 100 ml.

Magnesium sulphate ($MgSO_4$ $7H_2O$)	*4.0 g*
Manganese sulphate ($MnSO_4 . 4H_2O$)	*0.4 g*
Ferric sulphate ($FeSO_4 . 7H_2O$)	*0.2 g*
Sodium chloride (NaCI)	*0.2 g*

Adenine-Guanine : Uracil (AGU) solution. Dissolve 0.2 gram of each of adenine sulphate, guanine hydrochloric acid and uracil in 100 ml of water using concentrated hydrochloric acid dropwise for dissolving.

Xanthine Solution : Dissolve 0.2 gram of Xanthine in water using liquor ammonia dropwise for dissolving and make up to 100 ml with water.

Vitamin Solution

Para-aminobenzoic acid (PABA)	*2.00 g*
Biotin	*0.02 mg*
Ca-Panthothenate	*10.00 mg*
Folic acid	*0.20 mg*
Niacin	*20.00 mg*
Pyridoxal HCI	*6.00 mg*
Pyridoxamine 2 HCI	*20.00 mg*
Pyridoxine HCI	*10.00 mg*
Riboflavin (see note)	*10.00 mg*
Thiamine	*10.00 mg*

Dissolve in water and make up to 100 ml.

☞ Note

Riboflavin is weighed separately dissolved in a few millilitres of acetic acid and mixed with the other solution.

Non-essential Amino Acid Solution

dI-alanine	*4.0g*
1-asparagine	*8.0g*
1-aspartic acid	*2.0g*
1-cystine	*1.0g*
1-glutamic acid	*6.0g*
Glycine	*2.0g*
1-proline	*2.0g*
dI-serine	*1.0g*
1-tyrosine	*2.0g*

Dissolve each of these amino acids in water and make up to 100 ml using concentrated hydrochloric acid dropwise for dissolving.

Essential Amino acids	*g/100ml*
1-arginine HCI	*4.85*
1-histidine HCI	*1.24*
dI-isoleucine	*5.00*
1-leucine	*2.50*
1-lysine HCI	*5.00*
dI-phenylalanine	*2.00*
dI-threonine	*4.00*
dI-tryptophan	*0.80*
dI-valine	*5.00*
dI-methionine	*2.00*

Disslove each of these amino acids in water and make up to 100 ml using concentrated hydrochloric acid dropwise for dissolving, and keep each amino acid solution in separate bottles.

Composition of Basal Medium

For Leuconostoc Mesenteroides

Glucose	*5.0g*
Sodium acetate	*4.0g*
Ammonium chloride	*0.6g*
Salt solution A	*1.0 ml*
Salt solution B	*1.0 ml*
AGU solution	*1.0 ml*
Xanthine solution	*1.0 ml*
Vitamin solution	*1.0 ml*
Non-essential amino acid solution	*1.0 ml*
1-arginine HCI	*1.0 ml*
1-histidine HCI	*1.0 ml*
dl-isoleucine	*1.0 ml*
1-lysine HCI	*1.0 ml*
dl-phenylalanine	*1.0 ml*
dl-threonine	*1.0 ml*
dl-tryptophan	*1.0 ml*
dl-valine	*1.0 ml*
dl-methionine	*1.0 ml*
1-leucine	*1.0 ml*

Mix well the solution, adjust the pH to 6.8 and make the volume up to 100 ml with water.

For Streptococcus Faecalis

Hydrogen peroxide (H_2O_2) treated peptone	*75 ml*
1-methionine	*100 mg*
1-cystine	*100 mg*
1-tyrosine	*100 mg*
dl-tryptophan	*200 mg*
glycine	*100 mg*
Glucose (anhydrous)	*20 g*
Sodium acetate (hydrated)	*33 g*
Ammonium chloride	*6 g*
AGU solution	*12 ml*
Xanthine solution	*12 ml*
Salt solution A	*5 ml*
Salt solution B	*5 ml*

Vitamin Additions

Aneurine	*1000 μg*
Calcium pantothenate	*1000 μg*
Nicotinic acid	*2000 μg*
Riboflavin	*2000 μg*
Pyridoxine HCI	*1600 μg*
P-amino benzoic acid (PABA)	*50μg*
Water to make	*500 ml*

Mix the solution well, adjust the pH to 6.8

☞ **Note**

In the preparation of the basal medium, the amino acid to be assayed is omittted.

Preparation of Stock Standard Solution

Use for the preparation of standard solutions 1 form of the amino acids. Dissolve 50 mg of the amino acid in 100 ml of water to make 500 μg / ml. A few drops of concentrated hydrochloric acid may be needed to dissolve some of the amino acids. The standard stock solution should be prepared fresh every three months.

Working Standard Range

	***Range* (μg)**	***Dilution (ml)***
Arginine	*0 to 40*	*4 to 50*
Histidine	*0 to 10*	*2 to 100*
Isoleucine	*0 to 25*	*2.5 to 50*
Leucine	*0 to 25*	*5 to 100*
Valine	*0 to 25*	*1 to 50*
Methionine	*0 to 10*	*1 to 50*
Phenylalanine	*0 to 10*	*1 to 50*
Threonine	*0 to 20*	*1 to 100*
Tryptophan	*0 to 10*	*1 to 50*
Lysine	*0 to 30*	*3 to 50*
Cystine	*0 to 5*	*1 to 100*
Tyrosine	*0 to 10*	*2 to 100*

☞ **Note**

Make the dilutions from a stock standard solution containing 500 μg amino acid per ml.

Standard Levels

Take 0, 0. 1, 0. 2, 0. 3, 0. 4, 0. 5, 0. 6, 0. 7, 0. 8, and 1 ml in triplicate, add enough water to make 1 ml and follow by 1 ml or basal medium. Cover the tubes with cotton wool plugs and wrap with brown (Kraft) paper to protect the cotton wool plugs from getting wet during autoclaving. Altermatively use aluminium caps.

Preparation of Sample

Acid hydrolysis : Add 1 gram of the sample to 25 ml of 2.5 N hydrochloric acid. Autoclave the mixture for 6 hours at 103 KN/m^2 (1.05 Kgf/cm^2) pressure. Cool and add 2 ml of 2.5 percent sodium acetate. Adjust the pH to 4.5 and make the solution up to a known volume and filter. Take an aliquot and adjust the pH to 6.8 with sodium hydroxide, and dilute to the required concentration.

Alkali Hydrolysis for Estimatin of Tryoptophan and Tyrosine only

Add 1 gram of the sample to 25 ml of 2 N sodium hydroxide and autoclave the mixture for 6 hours or add 5 gram of barium oxide to 25 ml of water and autoclave for 8 hours at 103 KN/M^2 (1.05 kgf/cm^2) pressure. Then cool to room temperature, adjust pH to 4.0 with either hydrochloric acid or acetic acid and make up to a known volume and filter. Adjust pH of the aliquot at 6.8 and dilute to get the required concentration. *Recemiation takes place during this treatment and the amino acids will all be in dl form.*

Sample should be preserved and stored under toluene at 4°C and used for analysis preferably within a month's time.

Sample Levels

Take 0.2, 0.4, 0.6, 0.8 and 1.0 ml in duplicate, add enough water to make to 1 ml and follow by 1 ml of the basal medium. Cover the tubes with cotton wool plugs and wrap with brown (kraft) paper to protect the cotton wool plug from getting wet during autoclaving. Alternatively use aluminium caps.

Procedure

Standard tubes : Sterilize the tubes of basal medium containing standard levels of amino acid as mentioned above by autoclaving at 120° C for 10 minutes. Cool to room temperature and inoculate 3 tubes of each standard with the inoculum as mentioned above (under heading preparation of inoculum). For acidimetric titration method, incubate the inoculated tubes at 37°C for 16 to 20 hours.

Sample tubes : Sterilize the tubes of sample as mentioned above.

Acidimetric Method

Standard solution : 0.02 N sodium hydroxide and 0.1 percent bromothymol blue indicator solution.

Transfer the contents quantitatively to a 150 ml conical flask, rinsing the tubes with distilled water twice. Add about 0.2 ml of 0.1 percent bromothymol blue indicator and titrate the solution against 0.02 N sodium hydroxide to an end point of greenish blue colour around pH 6.8. A pH meter may be used in place of the indicator solution.

Calculation

Draw a standard curve for the assay by plotting the volume of 0.02 N sodium hydroxide on the Y-axis against concentration of the amino acid per tube in the standard series on the x-axis. It is preferable to plot these on logarithmic scale in order to obtain a straight line or a type of curve where the straight line of the curve can be utilised to determine amino acid content in the sample tubes. Determine amino acid content of the tubes in the x unknown series by interpolation of the title values on the standard curve. Calculate the average for 1 ml of test solution from values obtained from not less than three tubes which do not vary by more than 10 percent of the average. Calculate the amino acid content of the test solution using the following relationship.

μg of test amino acid/g sample

$$= \frac{\text{Average } \mu g \text{ per ml x volume x diluting factor}}{\text{Mass of the sample}}$$

Turbidimetric Method

Apparatus

Nephalometer (Turbidimeter)

Method : Take nephalometric reading of the growth using the tube supplied with the nephalometer. Transfer the same known volume of growths in the standard tubes. commencing with the lowest amount of amino acid, that is, the highest dilution made. Draw a standard curve for the assay by plotting the turbidimetric readings on the Y-axis against concentration of the amino acid per tube in the standard series on the x-axis, It is preferable to plot these on a logarithmic scale in order to obtain a straight line or a type of curve where the straight line of the curve can be utilised to determine the amino acid content in the sample tubes. Determine the amino acid content of the sample tubes by interpolation of the turbidimetric values on the standard curve. Calculate the average for 1 ml of test solution from values obtained for not less than three tubes which do not vary by more than 10 percent of the average. Calculate the amino acid content of the test solutions.

☞ Note

It is essential that the standard curves should be constructed each time that an assay is undertaken since conditions of autoclaving, temperature of incubation, etc.

Which influence the standard curve readings, cannot be duplicated exactly from time to time.

Repeatability

The method should be repeatable within the range of 10 percent.

Practical Implication of Amino Acids Picture in Human and Non-ruminant Nutrition

The importance of amino acid was recognised long back by Rose *et al.*, 1948 at the University of Illinois. *Rose defined an essential amino acid as one which cannot be synthesised in the body at a rate required for normal growth. He found that, for maintenance, rate needed the same ones as for growth, with the exception of arginine.* Early studies with poultry indicated that while glycine was synthesised in the body, this synthesis was not adequate to meet, the metabolic needs for rapid growth, and thus this amino acid was classed as a dietary essential for the growth of this species.

Table 1 : Classification of amino acids with respect to their growth effects in the rat

Essential	Non-essential
Lysine	Glycine
Tryptophan	Alanine
Histidine	Serine
Phenylalanine	Cystine *
Leucine	Tyrosine +++
Isoleucine	Aspartic acid
Threonine	Glutamic acid**
Methionine	Proline ***
Valine	Hydroxyproline
Arginine +	Citrulline

Cystine	Cystine can repalce about one-sixth of the methionine requirement but has no growth effect in the absence of methionine.
Tyrosine +++	Can replace about one-half of the phenylalanine requirement but has no growth effect in the absence of phenylalanine.
Glutamic acid ** and Proline ***	Can serve individually as rather ineffective substitutes for arginine in the diet. This property is not shared by hydroxyproline.

Arginine + Arginine can be synthesized by the rat, but not at sufficiently rapid rate to meet the demand of maximum growth. Its classification, therefore, as essential or non-essential is purely a matter of definition.

Pigs require the same 10 amino acids for growth as do rats. For maintenance they do not require arginine, histidine or leucine. Requirement fo each essential amino acid when all other amino acids of nutritive importance are provided, in the case of growing animals are presented in Table 2.

Table 2 : Essential amino acid requirements for optimum growth of chickens, pigs and rats (Percent of diet).

Amino acid	Starting	Starting Poults	Pigs (20-35 kg)	Rats
Dietary protein	20.0	28.0	16.0	20.0
Arginine	1.2	1.6	0.20	0.20
Glycine	1.0	1.0	None	None
Histidine	0.4	?	0.18	0.30
Isoleucine	0.75	0.84	0.50	0.50
Leucine	1.4	?	0.60	0.80
Lysine	1.1	1.5	0.70	0.90
Methionine*	0.75	0.87	0.50	0.60
Phenylalanine+	1.3	?	0.50	0.90
Threonine	0.7	?	0.45	0.50
Tryptophan	0.2	0.26	0.13	0.15
Valine	0.85	?	0.50	0.70

Cystine* Can replace 45 percent of the needs for methionine by starting chicks: 40 percent by starting poults, 40 percent by pigs, and 33 to 50 percent by rats.

Tyrosine+ Can replace 50 percent of the needs for phenylalanine by starting chick; 30 percent by pigs and 33 percent by rats.

Source Maynard, L.A. and Loosli, J.K. 1965. *Animal Nutrition* 6th edn., Mc Graw-Hill Book Co, New York, pp 457.

Some of the workers have divided amino acids into three categories: Indispensable. dispensable and semidispensable. In the case of the rats the semidispensable list includes arginine, which is not required for slow growth and cystine and tyrosine because of their interactions with methionine and phenylalanine, respectively, as previously discussed, The indispensable ones include those listed as essential in the table, except arginine, and the dispensable ones are those listed as non-essential, except cystine and tyrosine.

Estimated amino acid requirements for adult human subjects, infants and children is given in Table 3.

Table 3 : Estimated amino acid requirement of adults

Amino acid	Some reported amino acids requirement (mg/day)			Combined adult value (mg/kg/day)[d]	Suggested pattern (mg/g)
	Men[a]	Women[b]	Recalculated[c]	d	Protein
Histidine	0	0	0	0	0
Isoleucine	700	450	550	10	18
Leucine	1100	710	730	14	25
Lysine	800	700	545	12	22
Methionine + cystine	1100	550	700	13	24
Phenylalanine +tyrosine	1100	700	–	14	25
Threonine	500	310	375	7	13
Tryptophan	250	160	168	3.5	6.5
Valine	800	650	622	10	18

Source: World Health Organisation Technical Report Series. 1973. No. 522.
(a) Rose, 1957. (b) Irwin & Hegsted, 1971. (c) Hegsted, 1963 (d) Derived estimate emphasizing the upper range of individual requirements (e) Assuming a safe level of protein intake (0.55 kg/ day), (averaged value for men and women).

Table 4 : Estimated amino acid requirements of infants

Amino	Estimated requirements mg/kg/ day[a]	mg/kg/ day[b]	Composite of lower values (mg/kg/day) d	Suggested pattern (mg/g of protein) c
Histidine	34	28	28	14
Isoleucine	119	70	70	35
Leucine	229	161	161	80
Lysine	103	161	103	52
Methionine + cystine	45+cys	58	58[d]	29
Phenylalanine + tyrosine	90+Tyr	125	125d	63
Threonine	87	116	87	44
Tryptophan	22	17	17	8.5
Valine	105	93	93	47

Source : World Health Organisation Technical Report Series. 1973. No. 522.
(a) Holt and Synderman. 1967. (b) Fomon and Filer, 1967. (c) Based on a safe level of intake of 2 gram protein per kg per day, the average of suggested levels for the period 0-6 months. (d) The values for cystine and tyrosine were estimated on the basis of methionine: cystine and phenylalanine: tyrosine ratio in human milk.

Table 5 : Estimated amino acid requirement children.

Amino acid	School Children 10 to 12 years	
	Observed requirement mg/kg/day[a]	Suggested pattern (mg/g of protein)[b]
Histidine	0	0
Isoleucine	30	37
Leucine	45	56
Lysine	60	75
Methionine +cystine	27	34
Phenylalanine+tyrosine	27	34
Threonine	35	44
Tryptophan	4	4.6
Valine	33	41

Source : World Health Organisation Technical Report series. 1973. No. 522.
(a) Nakagawa *et al.*, 1961, a, b., 1962, 1963. (b) Based on a safe level of protein intake ot 0.8 g per kg per day, the average of safe levels of protein for boys and girls in that age group.

If we have amino acid picture of any food, then the requirement of amino acid being supplied by a particular diet could be checked after consulting above tables. If any amino acid is limiting in the diet then it could be supplied from synthetic source so as to meet the requirement or individual subject. Almost all foods are limited by lysine or methionine and both of these are manufactured on the factory scale, and so are available as supplements. The most obvious approach to amino acid supplementation is to fortify cereals with lysine, as this is the limiting amino acid. However, all complete diets that have been examined are limited by methionine so that even if the cereal staple has an enhanced BV through lysine addition, this will not improve the diet as a whole. In developing countries where protein is in short supply and where amino acid fortification could be an advantage, supplies and facilities for adding it to a staple food are not available. Methionine is added to some of the protein-rich food that have been developed for infant feeding and both methionine and lysine are added to animal feeds in certain cases. *However, it is often cheaper to obtain extra protein for animal feed than to add synthetic amino acids.*

Amino Acid Pictures of Food and Chemical Score

Block and Mitchell (1946) suggested that since all amino acids must be presented at the site of protein synthesis in adequate amounts for protein synthesis to proceed, an equal percentage deficit of any essential amino acid would limit protein synthesis to a comparable degree. Thus, if the composition of an Ideal protein", i.e. one containing all the essential amino acids in sufficient amounts to meet requirements without any excess, were known then it should be possible to compute the nutritive quality of a protein by calculating the deficit of each essential amino acid from the amount in the "ideal protein". The most limiting amino acid is that which is in greatest deficit, would presumably determine the nutritive value. *In practice they suggested the protein of whole egg as the "ideal", since this was known to have a biological value closely approaching 100. Block and Mitchell compared biological values with "amino acid deficits" calculated using egg protein as a standard. A high correlated between two suggested that the procedure was valid.*

The amino acid score of a protein or mixture of protein is calculated as follow:

$$\text{Amino acid score} = \frac{\text{mg of amino acid in 1g of test protein}}{\text{mg of amino acid in reference pattern}} \times 100$$

The data presented in Table 6 clearly demonstrate the idea of Block and Mitchell (1946) for calculating chemical score for wheat.

Table 6 : Calculation of Block and Mitchell's chemical score for wheat.

Name		Amino acids	
	% in egg protein	% in wheat protein	% deficiency in wheat
Arginine	6.4	4.2	- 34
Histidine	2.1	2.1	0
Lysine	7.2	2.7	- 63
Tyrosine	4. 5	4.4	- 2
Tryptophan	1.5	1.2	- 20
Phenylalanine	6.3	5.7	- 10
Cystine	2.4	1.8	- 25
Methionine	4.1	2.5	- 39
Cystine + methionine	6.5	4.3	- 34
Threonine	4.9	3.3	- 33
Leucine	9.2	6.8	- 26
Isoleucine	8.0	3.6	- 55
Valine	7.3	4.5	- 38

Source : Block and Mitchell, 1946, Nutr. Abstr. Rev., **16:** 249.
Note : Chemical score for wheat, based on amino acid in greatest deficit, is 100-53 =37.

Oser's EAA Index Method of Chemical Evaluation

In general to take into account all the essential amino acids, Oser has proposed an essential amino acid (EAA) index, which is the geometric mean of the ten egg ratios found by comparing the content of the ten essential amino acids in a feed protein with that found in whole egg protein. Algeberically the index is expressed as:

$$\text{EAA Index} = 10\ \frac{100^{a}}{a_e} \times \frac{100^{b}}{b_e} \ldots\ldots \frac{100\,j}{j_e}$$

in which a, b................j are the percent of essential amino acids in the food protein and ae, be ....je are the percent of the respective amino acids in whole egg protein.

References

Barton-Wright, R.C. (1952). *The microbiological assay of the vitamin B complex and amino acids, Pitman publishing corporation*, London.

Block, R.J. and Mitchell, H.H. (1946). *Nutr. Abstr. Rev.,* 16: 249.

Carpenter, R.J. and Ellinger, G.M. (1955). *Biochem. J.*, 61: XI (Abstr.)

Carpenter, K.J. (1960). *Biochem. J.* 77: 604.

Consden, R., Gordon, A.H. and Martin, A.J. P. (1944). *Biochem. J.* 38: 224.

Hegsted, D.M. (1963). *Fed. Proc.*, 22: 1424.

Henry, K.M. end kon, S.K. (1950). *Biochem. Biophys. Acta,* 5: 455.

Horn, M.J., Jones, D.B. and Blum, A.E. (1946). *J. Bio. Chem.*, 166: 313.

Indian standards Institution (1975). *Method for estimaton of amino acids in food*. IS: 7815. (BIS), Manak Bhavan, New Delhi (India).

Indian standards Institution (1976). *Method for determination of available lysine in foods.* IS : 8168. (BIS), Manak Bhavan, New Delhi (India).

Indian Standard Institution (1979). *Specification for poultry feeds* (Third Revision), IS: 1374. (BIS), Manak Bhavan, New Delhi (India).

Irwin, M.I. and Hegsted, D.M. (1971). *J.Nutr.* 101: 539.

Krampitz, G. (1957). *Experientia*, 13: 239.

Krampitz, G. (1960). *Zfür Tierphysiologie, Tierernährung und Futter mittelkunde*, 15: 76.

Krishna, G. & Günther, K.D. (1987). Nutrient Composition and amino acid content of some Agro-Industrial byproducts and wastes used as livestock feeds. Z. *Landwirtschaftliche Forschung*. 40: 277-280.

Lea, C.H. and Hannan, R.S. (1950). *Biochem. Biophys.* Acta, 4: 518.

Mason, V.C. (1963). Amino acids in Nutrition. (Licentiate Thesis Copenhagen, Denmark)

Moore, S., Spachman, D.H. and Stein, W. (1958). *Anal. Chem.*, 30: 1185.

Nakagawa, I., Takahasi, T. and Suzuki, T. (1961a). *J. Nutr.*, 73: 186.

Nakagawa, I., Takahasi, T. and Suzuki T. (1961b). *J. Nutr.* 74: 401.

Nakagawa, T., Takahasi,T., Suzuki, T. and Robayashi, K. (1962). *J. Nutr.*, 77: 61

Nakagawa, I., Takahasi, T., Suzuki, T. and Kobayashi, K. (1963). *J. Nutr.*, 80: 305

Porter, R.R. and Sanger, F. (1948). *Biochem. J.*, 42: 287

Rao, S. R., Carter, F.L. and Frampton, N.L. (1963). *Analyt. chem.*, 35 : 1927.

Rose. W.C. and Co-workrs, (1948). *J. Biol. Chem.*, 176: 753.

Rose, W.C. (1957). *Nutr. Abstr. Rev.*, 27 : 631

Sanger, F. (1945). *Biochem. J.*, 39 : 507

Smith, I. (1960), *Chromatographic and Electrophoretic techniques.* Vol. I. Chromatography. William. Heinemann. Medical Book Ltd. London.

Synge, R.L.M. (1944). *Bio chem. J.*, 38 : 285

Weidner, K. and Eggum, B.O. (1966). *Acta Agriculture Scandinavica*, 16: 115.

Chapter - 64

In Vitro, Nylon Bag and Cellulase Digestibility Techniques

A. *In vitro* Rumen Fermentation Technique for Forage Quality Evaluation

The term *in vitro* means "in a glass" in contrast to *in vivo* which is defined as "within the living body". *In vitro* implies a close relationship to an *in vivo* measurement an *in vitro* reaction is used as a substitute for a reaction which normally occurs and is observed within a living body. the terms "artificial rumen" and "*in vitro* rumen fermentation" are often used interchangeably.

The main advantage of the *in vitro* techniques rests in the ability to use them to study activity of micro-organisms away form the control and influence imposed by the host animal.

I. Continuous Flow System

In these technique provision in the apparatus invariably has to be made for regular additions of nutrients in somewhat the same way as might be achieved in the actual rumen of the animal as well as for constant removal of the end products when properly designed, conducted and interpreted, the continuous flow or chemostat techniques offer the possibility of studying rumen microbial processes as they occur in the intact rumen. Therein the processes of synthesis and absorption can be stimulated and studies made of the effects of various environmental or nutrient treatment on anabolic or catabolic proceses within the microbial culture. To accomplish this very exacting control must be maintained on nutrient input, endproduct removal, pH, nutrient concentration, oxidation-reduction potential rate of agitation etc. Example is RUISTEC system developed at Hannah Research Institute Ayr., Scotland (U.K.) Author has working experience with this system, as he has worked at Hannah Research Institute, Ayr. Scotland (U.K.), [Krishna *et al.*, 1986; Agricultural Wastes. 17: 99-117]

II. Closed Systems

(Johnson, 1963)

As reviewed by Johnson (1963), however, a series of papers from OHIO (USA) (Dehority *et al.*, 1960., el-Shazly *et al.*, 1961a,b) have demonstrated quite well that bacteria propagated *in vitro* can be truly representative of those in the intact rumen itself. Thus, the assumption can be made that the activities being measured are similar to those occurring in the intact animal. In such a system the possibility of enriching the culture for a particular species of micro organisms is always present and undoubtedly occurs to some extent in practically all closed system. This, however, does not make the system invalid for studying certain metabolic processes, since this in fact may enhance quatitative measuremens without necessarily changing them qualitatively. The possibility of culturing species with aberrant metabolic pathways should be kept in mind when using closed systems and should be checked by microbial techniques when possible. Another major criticism of closed system, as far as studying mixed rumen microbial cultures is concerned, it the almost invariably elimination of protozoa from the population.

Variables Affecting *in vitro* Rumen Fermentation Studies with Forages

Van Dyne and Hong (1968) have listed the following four major variables.

1. *Variations in microbial populations:*
   - *(a) Diet of host animal,*
   - *(b) Animal to animal differences,*
   - *(c) Inoculum processing differences,*
2. *Variations due to different storage, grinding and processing techniques in sample preparation.*
3. *Difference attributable to medium:*
   - *(a) Sample : inoculum ratio,*
   - *(b) Buffer used,*
   - *(c) Nutrient medium*
4. *Procedural variations such as length of fermentation, criteria of digestibility and laboratory errors.*

The largest single source of error or variability in the *in vitro* system is the inoculum. Among the known factors which can contribute to variability are:

1. *Diet of the animal,*
2. *Feeding system (time, etc.),*
3. *Time of removal of rumen contents,*
4. *Method of processing rumen contents,*
5. *Handling of rumen liquor between animal and in vitro vessel.*
6. *Treatment in the laboratory prior to inoculation. Mostly the workers are of the opinion that rumen liquor should be taken after a 12-18 hours fast because shortly after feeding the rumen is tightly packed and difficult to sample. Further more, sampling of liquor during this time involves removing a considerable portion of "diet solubles" Which may contribute more nutrients than desired to the medium.*

III. A Two Stage Technique for Screening Forage Sample (Tilley & Terry, 1963)

Principle

The two stage *in vitro* digestion technique used at the Grassland Research Institute, Hurley, England differs from earlier published methods in that the digestion with rumen micro organisms is followed by a digestion with acid pepsin solution.

The first stage of the procedure, digestion of structural carbohydrate by micro organisms for 48 hours, does not go to completion, it is known that greater amounts of digestion can be obtained if the first stage is continued for a longer period. The choice fo incubation time was made because the *in vitro* dry matter digestibilities thus obtained seemed to give the best agreement with *in vivo* data. Since the first stage does not got to completion, it must be operated under completely standard conditions. The second stage, digestion with acid pepsin solution, was introduced to remove bacterial protein and unchanged feed protein. The conditions for this stage are not as critical as the first stage.

Using 146 sample of grass, clover and lucerne of known *in vivo* dry matter digestibility coefficient (Y)) the regression equation Y = 0.99 y = 0.99 + -1.01 x (S.E. ± 2.31) has been calculated where x = *in vitro* dry matter digestibility coefficient.

Brief Summary of Method

Herbage sample are oven dried at 100°C and ground in a mill fitted with a 0.8 mm screen. 0.5 gram of sample is weighed and transferred to centrifuge tube of 100 ml capacity fitted with Bunsen gas release valve. A mixture of 40 ml of buffer solution and 10 ml of strained rumen liquor is added to each tube, incubated at 38°C for 48 hours. The tubes are gently shaken twice a day. Rumen micro organism fermentation is stopped by cooling cold water or by use of 5 percent $HgCI_2$ the tubes are centrifuged at 2500 rpm and supernatant decanted. The residue is stirred with 50 ml of 0.2 percent pepsin in 0.1 N HCI and incubated for a further 48 hours at 38°C. The undigested residue is then collected in an Alumina crucible, washed, dried and weighed and ashed if organic matter digestibility is required.

Equipments

1. *100 ml centrifuge tubes, plastic or glass, and racks to hold tubes.*
2. *Rubber stoppers (Fig. 1) fitted with bunsen valve for gas release and shown in Fig. 1.*
3. *Expendable laboratory supplies:*

   Beakers, Erlenmeyer flasks, thermometers, desiccator, graduate cylinders, cheese cloth, Buchner funnel, rubber tubing, insulated jug, side arm suction flask, sintered glass crucible, tongs and glass tubing.
4. *Permanent laboratory, equipments:*

   Analytical balance, pH meter with electrodes usuable in 100 ml centrifuge tubes. drying oven, centrifuge, incubation bath , Co_2 cylinder with regulator.

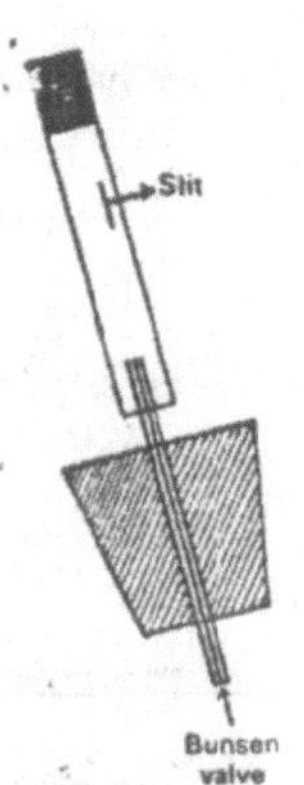

Fig. 1 : Bunsen valve showing outlet slit for escape of gases.

Reagents

1. *Buffer-nutrient solution (Mc Dougall, 1949). The following quantities are for one litre solution.*

$NaHCO_3$	-	*9.80 g*
$Na_2HPO_4 . 7H_2O$	-	*7 g or 3.71 g (anhydrous form)*
KCl	-	*0.57 g*
NaCl	-	*0.47 g*
$MgSO_4 . 7H_2O$	-	*0.12 g*
$CaCl_2$	-	*0.04 g*

Mix the first 5 chemicals in ± 500 ml water in onelitre volumetric flask and stir until dissolved. Adjust to volume and store. Just before use, add the $CaCl_2$, keep at 39°C, and bubble CO_2 into solution until pH is 6.8 to 7.0.

2. *5% W/V mercuric chloride: 5g $HgCl_2$ per 100 ml.*
3. *1 N Na_2CO_3 : 143 g $Na_2Co_3.10H_2O$/litre*
4. *1 N HCl: 86 ml conc. HCl/litre distilled water*

5. *Pepsin soluiton : Two grams of 1:10,000 pepsin is dissolved in 100 ml of 1 N HCl.*
6. *Rumen filuid: Donor animal is a rumen fistulated cow or steer regularly fed twice daily medium quality alflafa hay (12% grass) plus minerals and salt.*

Homogeneous rumen liquor sample is drawn from different parts of rumen by suction, using plastic tube about 30 mm in diameter, with several 9 mm holes in the lower two inch portion Precautions are taken to minimise contact with the rumen wall. The bottle containing rumen liquor is placed in a bucket containing water at ± 40ºC. Rumen fluid is filtered through 8 layers of cheese cloth in the buchner funnel. Filtering is done and fluid obtained by applying gentle suction to side arm of flask. Rumen fluid is collected mid-morning, two hours after feeding. The animal should not have any access to feed and water between one and two hours post feeding. Fluid is transported to the laboratory with temperature maintained at 37 to 39º C in an insulated jug or other apparatus. In the laboratory, Co_2 is bubbled into the rumen fluid for 60 seconds and the rumen fluid is used immediately.

It has been usual to feed *ad libitum* the sheep from which rumen inoculum is taken. The rumen liquor is then rich in food particles and the weight of "blank" residue after incubation is about 0.06 gram. Since the weight of dry residue from 0.5 gram of forage with an *in vitro* digestibility of 80 percent is only 0.10 gram, a large proportion of the undigested residue is derived not from the forage under test but from the rumen liquor inoculum. It has to be assumed, moreover, that the weight of the final residue from the inoculum is same, whether or not herbage is present during the incubation.

Procedure

Forage samples of about 0.5 gram are weighed on weighing paper or similar material by using an analytical balance. Weighed samples are quantitatively transferred to numbered centrifuge tubes. Exact sample weights and tube numbers are recorded. Separate duplicate samples are weighed into dry tared containers for dry mattter determinations. Sample are weighed out prior to the day of incubation and samples for all three runs are weighed at the same time.

Forty ml of prepared buffer is added to the centrifuge tube containing the forage sample. The tubes are allowed to stand at 39ºC for 15 minutes and then 10 ml of rumen fluid is added as inoculum. The surface of the tube contents is flushed with CO_2 gas for 15 seconds before stoppering tightly with a rubber stopper containing a bunsen value. Tubes are then placed in a water bath or incubator and incubated at 39ºC for 48 hours. Tubes are gently swirled to dispense particles at 2, 4, 20 and 28 hours after initiation of incubation. Immediately after inoculation, the pH of rumen fluid and unicubated reagent blanks is measured.

After 48 hours incubation, the pH is measured on the contents of all tubes, an 1 ml $HgCl_2$ and 2 ml $Na_2 CO_3$ are added to all tubes. The tubes are centrifuged at 2,000 grams for 15 minutes and the supernatant decanted.

Fifty ml of HCl-pepsin solution are added to each tube and the precipitate resuspended. Tubes are incubated without stoppers for 48 hours at 39° C. Tubes are again gently swirled at 2, 4, 20 and 28 hours after initiation of incubation.

After 48 hours. material in tubes is filtered through a tared sintered glass crucible. The crucibles with residue are dried at 100° C for about 24 hours to attain constant weight. Crucibles are weighed within 5 to 15 minutes after removing them from the oven into a desiccator or they are weighed directly from the oven on a single pan analytical balance. Material remaining in the crucible is the residual or undigested dry matter.

Two types of blanks are used for the study and are designated as unicubated and incubated reagent blank are outlined below:

1. Unincubated reagent blank or inoculum or zero hour blanks incubated buffer and rumen fluid with pH measured, $HgCl_2$. and Na_2CO_3 added immediately., and filtered as soon as possible without incubation.
2. Incubated reagent blanks, or simply reagent blanks, incubated buffer and rumen fluid processed through both the anaerobic fermentation and pepsin incubation stages. Four blanks of each type are interspersed throughout the forage samples during each *in vitro* run.

Routine Use of Method

It has been found convenient to analyse 20 to 40 forage of unknown digestibility, together with two standard herbages, in a single experiment. Each standard should be analysed in triplicate or quarduplicate. The two "standard" samples are selected of "high" and "low" digestibility relative to the unknown materials analysed. The "mean" digestibility of each of these samples is calculated from its performance in at least 10 different *in vitro* experiments (these mean value are closely similar to the *in vivo* digestibilities of the standard). Comparison of the mean digestibilities of the standard with the values found in a given experiment enabled and assessment to be made of the digestive efficiency of the particular rumen liquor preparation and pepsin solution used. Appropriate corrections are made if the values for the standard forages are higher or lower than their mean digestibilities.

A graph is constructed for each experiment on which the "mean" digestibilities of standard samples are plotted along the Y axis, and "found" digestibilities along the x-axis. The points for the "high" and "low" standard are joined with a straight lines and the correct digestibilities for the unknown samples are estimated as the Y values corresponding to the digestibilities found (X values).

Calculation

Estimate *in vitro* dry matter and organic matter digestibility using two stage Tilley and Terry technique.

Sample - W

The digestibility of dry matter (%) is : -

$$\left[1-\left\{\frac{(d_s-c_s)-(d_i-c_i)}{a_s}\right\}\right]\times 100$$

The digestibility of organic matter (%) is : -

$$\left[1-\left\{\frac{(d_s-e_s)-(d_i-e_i)}{a_s \times b_s}\right\}\right]\times 100$$

where,

a = dry sample, g

b = organic matter-g, per sample, g

c = dry crucible + filterdisc, g

d = dry crucible + filter disc + undigested dry matter, g

e = dry crucible + filter disc + undigested ash, g

Subscript "s" pertains to sample

Subscript "i" pertains to inoculum

☞ Note

A difference up to one unit between duplicate assays is within permissible limit.

We can estimate *in vitro* dry matter digestibility using polyethylene bags as per method developed at Swift Current Research Station, Saskatchewan (Canada) by Troelsen (1970, 1971).

In vitro Cellulose Digestibility in Forage Sample

(Method of Bentley *et al.*, 1954 and 1955)

Since the discovery of the requirements for certain short chain fatty acids and biotin as growth factors for cellulolytic rumen micro organisms by Bentley *et al.* (1954 a, b, 1955) and Bryant and Doetsch (1955), *valeric acid and biotin have become standard ingredient of the in vitro fermentation media used in labotratory when cellulose digestion is the variable being measured. Both nutrients are especially critical when separated cells or washed inocula are being used. A number of other laboratoris have adopted this procedure.*

In cellulose digestibility studies, use of artificial saliva (Mc Dougall, 1949), should be replaced by "OHIO" *in vitro* fermentation media.

The detailed constituenst of "OHIO" *in vitro* fermentation media are given below:

Ingredient	**ml/100ml**
Na_2CO_3 200 mg/ml	1.0
Mineral mixture*	2.0 (mg/100 ml)
$Fecl_3$, 4.4 mg/ml	1.0
$Cacl_2$, 5.29 mg/ml	1.0
Urea, 126 mg/ml	1.0
Biotin, 10 µg /ml	2.0
Valeric acid, 5 mg/ml	5.0

* Composition of mineral mixture used in the above media.

Na_2HPO_4	-	56.5 g
NaH_2PO_4	-	54.5 g
KCl	-	21.5 g
NaCl	-	21.5 g
$MgSO_4 . 7H_2O$	-	5.82 g
K_2SO_4	-	7.50 g

V. *In vitro* Dry Matter Digestibility in Forage Samples (Barnes and Accociates, 1971) Modification of Two Stage Technique

Main Modification

If centrifuge is not available in the laboratory then Barnes & Coworkers (1971) method may be adopted. The modified Tilley and Terry technique as suggested by Barnes and Coworkers is mentioned below:

Principle

The *in vitro* rumen fermentation technique attempts to stimulate the breakdown of structural carbohydrate components into soluble components by enzymes produced by rumen microorganisms under anaerobic conditions of controlled temperature and pH. The second stage of the two-stage *in vitro* rumen fermentation technique attempts to stimulate the breakdown of proteinaceous material by the enzyme, pepsin, in the lower gastrointestinal tract of the ruminant.

Procedure

The *in vitro* system consisted of 250 mg samples of substrate in 50 ml centrifuge tubes fitted with gas release valve. The buffer nutrient solution added to each tube is 20 ml of CO_2 saturated phosphate carbonate buffer. Five ml of strained rumen fluid per tube served as inoculum blank tubes, designated reagent blanks, are included to which only buffer nutrient solution and rumen fluid are added. The gas CO_2 is passed over the surface of the tube contents for 10 seconds, and tubes are immediately stoppered and incubated at 39°C. Tubes are swirled gently during incubation to resuspend the substrate. After 48 hours, 2 ml of 6 N HCl and 0.1 gram pepsin powder are added to each tube and mixed thoroughly. The tubes are incubated for an additional 24 hours and filtered through tared whatman No. 54 filter paper. About 25 ml or distilled water is used in rinsing the tube and washing the residue. The residue on the filter paper is dried at 100° C overnight and weighed for determining the dry matter content of the residue and *in vitro* dry matter disappearance (IVDMD) is calculated by using following formula:

In vitro dry matter digestion (IVDMD)

$$\text{IVDMD} = 100 \times \frac{\text{Sample dry matter - Residual dry matter - Residual dry matter of reagent blank}}{\text{Sample dry matter}}$$

VI. *In vitro* Dry Matter Digestibility of Forage Samples
(Method of Goering and Van Soest, 1970)

The acid-pepsin digestion stage stimulates the *in vivo* breakdown of feed and microbial protein by the digestive enzymes of the abomasum in the ruminant. A greater amount of dry matter is solubilized by the Neutral detergent solution compared to acid-pepsin. This has been attributed to the solubilization of the bacterial cell wall and other-endogenous products by the neutral detergent solution. Thus, the two-stage *in vitro* procedure with neutral detergent has been proposed for the estimation of the true digestibility of herbages rather than the apparent digestibility. Second stage neutral detergent (IVDMD) analysis proposed by Goering and Van Soest (1970) have given satisfactory correlations with *in vivo* digestibility.

Apparatus

1. *Rumen-content source from an animal on a high cell-wall roughage (preferably a fistulated animal).*
2. *Erlenmeyer flasks, 125 ml (Pyrex, requiring No. 6 stoppers).*
3. *Shaking water bath at 40° C with holder for 18 flasks.*
4. *Manifold for 18 flasks constructed over water bath (See Fig. 2).*

5. *Waring Blendor.*
6. *CO_2 source.*
7. *Cheese cloth.*
8. *Glass wool and enclosed funnel assembly.*
9. *10 ml syringe.*
10. *Glassware refluxing apparatus used for detergent preparations.*

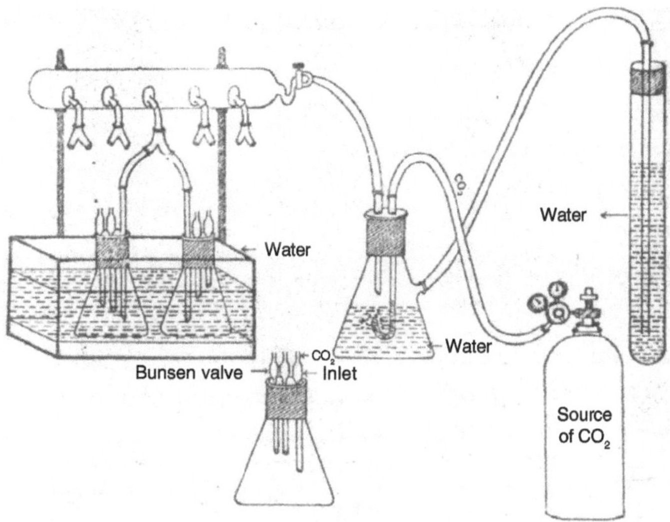

Fig. 2 : *In vitro* rumen fermentation system suggested by Goering & Van Soest (1970).

Description

Fermentations are conducted in 125 ml pyrex Erlenmeyer flasks (wide mouth), 0.5 gram substrate, 40 ml medium and 10 ml inoculum are used. Fermentation flasks are placed in a shaking water bath (Capacity, 02 liter) and closed with No.6 rubber stoppers. Stoppers are fitted with three opening: (1) an inlet tube, (2) a bunsen valve-both flush with the botton of the stopper and (3) a gassing tube connected to a common manifold. The inlet tube is closed on the outside a rubber sleeve and a glassrod. The gassing tube should stop about 1 cm above the surface of the liquid. The manifold is connected to a supply of carbon dioxide and in parallel with a water manometer with a capacity of 60 cm water pressure.

Reagents

1. *Trypticase : a pancreatic digest of casein, USP.*
2. *Sodium sulfide nonhydrate (Reagent grade).*

3. *1 N Sodium hydroxide : Dissolve 4 gram in water and dilute to a litre.*
4. *Cystein HCI.*
5. *Resazurin 0.1 percent W/V solution.*
6. *6 N HCI Dilute concentrated HCI (about 12 N) with an equal amount of water. Need be standardised.*
7. *Toluene Commercial grade.*
8. *In vitro rumen buffer solution.*

   Distilled water = *one litre*

   Ammonium bicarbonate = *4.0 g*

   Sodium bicarbonate = *35.0 g*
9. *In vitro rumen macromineral solution.*

   Distilled water = *one litre*

   Na_2HP_4 *anhydrous* = *5.7 g*

   KH_2PO_4 *anhydrous* = *6.2 g*

   $Mg_2\ SO_4.\ 7H_2O$ = *0.6 g*
10. *In vitro micromineral solution.*

    $CaCl_2.\ 2H_2O$ = *13.2g*

    $MnCl_2.\ 4H_2O$ = *10.0 g*

    $CoCl_2.\ 6H_2O$ = *1.0 g*

    $FeCl_3.\ 6H_2O$ = *8.0 g*

    Add to volumetric and bring volume to 100 ml with distilled water.

Procedure

The *in vitro* rumen procedure is designed so that a true digestibility value can be obtained. The predicted true digestibility value is based on undigested cell-wall constituents. The *in vitro* procedure yielding true digestibility values is a faster method and requires little extra equipment in a laboratory containing a detergent apparatus.

1. Weigh sample weigh 0.5 gram sample (20 mesh or 1 mm into a 125 ml Erlenmeyer flask).
2. Prepare medium, Add in order 2 gams of trypticase, 400 ml water, add 0.1 ml micromineral solution and agitate to dissolve. Then add 200 ml buffer solution. 200 ml macromineral solution, and 1 ml resazurin. Mix and add 40 ml per 125 ml flask.
3. Equilibration. Assemble and put stoppers and flasks in bath, admit carbon dioxide presssure (about 30 to 40 cm water), and check bunsen valves.

Open the inlet tubes and swirl flask while open and then close. Next prepare the reduction solution. Add 625 mg cysteine hydrochloric acid, 95 ml water, 4 ml 1 N sodium hydroxide and dissolve, then add 625 mg sodium sulphide nonayhdrate and dissovle. Reduce carbon dioxide pressure to 3 to 4 cm, and inject 2 ml reducing solution through the inlet tube with a syringe., open and close each tube in turn. Swirl all flask. Watch for reduction of medium, which is a change from a red colour (oxidized) to colourless (reduced).

4. *Inoculum Preparation :* Collect ingesta from a fistulated animal in a litre beaker, fill, cover with a watch glass to eliminate airspace. Discard the top layer of the ingesta, and blend 400 ml of the remainder in a waring blendor for 2 minutes under carbon dioxide. Squeeze the blended mass through cheese cloth and filter through glass wool into a warm flask, there after keep the filtrate under carbon dioxide. Inoculate 10 ml of the filtrate with a syrings through inlet tubes of each fermentaion flask.
5. *Fermentation :* Seal tubes and incubate 48 hours with shaking at a rate not to produce splashing. Adjust carbon dioxide pressure to 2 cm water. Flasks may be stored before proceeding with 6.1 ml toluene as a preservative and refrigerate. Stopper with cork.
6. Neutral - detergent procedure for estimation of true digestibility. Remove flasks from water bath after digestion or from refrigerator if stored. Wash with 100 ml neutral detergent solution into a 600 ml Berzelius beaker to make a total volume of 150 ml. Add 2 ml decahydronaphthalene. Reflux for one hour, and filter on previously tared 50 ml, 40 mm plate, coarse-porosity fritted glass crucibles. Wash twice with hot water and twice with acetone, and suck dry. Dry in oven at 100°C and weigh , Blanks are not necessary.
7. *Calculations :* Calculate true dry matter digestibility: 100 - Percent ND residue = true digestibility.

VII. *In vitro* Abomasum Protein Digestion Technique (Gutcho, 1973)

Reagent

Gastric Fluid

Dissolve two grams sodium chloride (NaCI) in 950 ml distilled water. Add 3.2 grams pepsin in this solution and deliver 7 ml conc hydrochloric acid to this solution, adjust the pH to 2 with aqueous sodium hydroxide.

Procedure

Add 60 mg testing material to a glass flask (*in vitro* vessel), containing 20 ml gastric fluid. Incubate this material in the *in vitro* vessel for 2 hrs at 39°C.

Digestion of protein is then determinecd by ammonia analysis, the greater amount of ammonia produced the greater the amount of protein digested.

VIII. *In vitro* Intestinal Protein Digestion Technique (Gutcho, 1973)

Reagent

Intestinal Fluid

Dissolve two grams sodium chlorice (Nacl) in 950 ml distilled water. Add 3.2 grams pepsin in this solution and deliver 7 ml conc. hydrochloric acid to this solution, adjust the pH of this solution to 7.0 with 0.1 N sodium hydroxide. Add pancreatin enzyme (10 mg/ml of solution).

Procedure

Add 60 mg testing material to a glass flask (*in vitro* vessel) containing 20 ml intestinal fluid. Incubate the material in the *in vitro* vessel for 2 hrs at 39°C. Digestion of protein is then determined by ammonia analysis, the greater the amount of ammonia produced the greater the amount of protein digested.

B. Nylon Bag Technique for Screening Forage and Feed Sample (Method of Lowrey. 1970)

Digestion trials have been the primary *in vivo* procedure used to measure forage quality. Such trial are expensive, time consuming, require large amount of forage, and thus, cannot be used in an extensive evaluation program. If plant breeders are to satisfy the needs of animal scientists by developing high yielding, high quality forage crops, it is essential that a technique be developed which requires only small amount of material to evaluate a forage and provides measurements which highly correlate with animal performance, thereby, allowing them to economically and effectively evaluate hundreds of new genetic creations.

In this technique, bags made of an indigestible material such as dacron or nylon are filled with the substrate in question, usually forages, and tightly tied. These bags are then placed in the rumen of a fistulated animal by a variety of techniques and removed after various periods of time to determine digestion of the contents. Precautions must be taken to insure a mesh sufficiently fine that particles of the test substrate cannot pass through the material and in addition to insure that there are no holes in the bag. Most workers made provisions for suspending the bags in the rumen in such a way that they would not lodge in the bottom or in any particular pocket of the rumen.

Hopson *et al.* (1963) compared this technique with determination of digestibility by *in vitro* procedure. *Generally, the coefficients of variation for the dacron bag technique were very high for digestibility values at early time periods from 6 to 24 hours. The digestion curves obtained from using these techniques, however, were similar to digestion curves obtained using in vitro fermentation.*

Luck *et al.* (1962) conducted two trials comparing cellulose digestion by both the nylon bag technique and total collection technique. They reported correlation value of 0.66 ($P<0.05$) and 0.83 ($P<0.05$) for the two trials, respectively. These workers used a 3 gram sample with the bags weighted in the ventral part of the rumen. Recently, Neathery (1969) used this technique to study dry matter digestibility of high fiber, poorly digested roughage.

Actual Procedure

Procure simple nylon bacterial filter cloth of 100 mesh from Garware Nylon Ltd. Bombay (India). The bags of 5 x 15 cm size stitched with double seams (nylon thread) that enclosed the raw edges of the cloth and made a smooth interior, should be prepared. Bags of this size are easy to fill, tie and clean, Before filling, the bags are dried at 110°C in a forced draft oven for at least 5 hours and weighed and kept in desiccator .The forage sample is ground through the 1 mm wiley mill screen and about 10 grams sample is filled in the nylon bag and again the net weight of bag and material is noted upto fourth place after decimal. It is not necessary that material should be exactly 10 grams but exact weight of material inside the bag should be known. Two blank bags without material should also be weighed so as to know the weight of any infiltered material. All the bags and blank bags should be kept in the desiccator. At the same time a sample for moisture determination is weighed. Filled bags are closely secured by tying with nylon line (minimum of 9.1 kg test) which is turn is tied having a knot at one end on the cap of a 250 ml polyethlene bottle. Eight bags are attached to the cap which is attached on to the bottle filled with water. The bottles with the bags attached are embeded in the rumen ingesta. The water filled bottle had a specific gravity similar to rumen fluid so that it moved around with the rumen contents and did not float. The bottle also prevented the bags from being regurgitated and assisted in locating the bags. As many as six bottles containing six bags each are placed in the rumen without any noticeable harmful effects. The bags filled with material should be embeded inside rumen for 72 hours. After completing this period, remove the bags along with bottle and adhering ingesta is rinsed off with a small amount of water using camel hair brush. Bag attachements are cut and the bags are dried overnight at 80°C in a large forced draft oven. Afterwards they are transferred to a small laboratory oven, dried at 110° C for a minimum of 5 hours and weighed.

The weight of infiltered material if any is find out by weighing blank bags it before and after embeding in the rumen. Now weigh the bags after embeding and find out the weight of digested material by difference deduct the weight of any infiltered material from the weight of digested material.

☞ **Note**

It is very important that fistulated cattel/buffalo for nylon bag technique should be maintained on good quality Iucerne hay (medicago sativa). Three bags of forage of known dry matter digestibility should be used per run per animal. Simultaneously three bags (blank) containing no material should also be tied with every set. Recently orskov et al. (1980) have published the use of nylon bag technique for the evaluation of the feedstuffs.

C. Cellulase Digestibility Method for Screening Forage Samples

(Method of Jarrige *et al.* 1970 modified by Jones and Hayward, 1973, 1975)

Jarriage *et al.* (1971) found this technique to be more reproducible than the two stage Tilley and Terry method for *in vitro* digestibility. Jones and Hayward (1973) also found is to be reproducible both within and between different analytical batches, different operators etc. and over several months of use. A good correlation has been established between the solubility of herbage in cellulase solution and *in vivo* digestibility (Jones and Hayward, 1973).

The two-stage enzyme technique is considered to be a simpler and more precise alternative to the conventional *in vitro* method using rumen inoculum and has obvious advantages for laboratories without access to fistulated animals. The technique is currently being applied in plant breeding programme aimed at improving the nutritive value of herbage.

Reagents

1. *Buffer solution (pH 4.6). 106.5 ml of 0.1 M citric acid (19.2 g of anhydrous citric acid /litre) is mixed with 93.5 ml of 0.2 M-disodium hydrogen orthophosphate (28.4 g) of anhydrous salt/litre.*
2. *Acid pepsin solution (0.2% 1:10000 units in 0.1 M HCI).*
3. *Enzyme solution Dissolve 6.25 g of Trichoderma Koningi cellulase in one litre of buffer solution immediately prior to use.*

Procedure

1. Weigh 200 mg of ground (1 mm sieve) forage in a 125 ml capacity Erlenmeyer flask.
2. Add 20 ml of acid-pepsin solution and incubate the flask at 39°C for 24 hours.
3. Remove the supernatant using stick filter and incubate the residue with 20 ml enzyme (cellulase) solution at 39°C for 48 hours.

4. Keep circle of whatman filter paper No. 54 in oven and weigh.
5. Filter the content of flask through filter paper 54.
6. Dry the digested sample & forage and filter paper in forced draft oven at 100°C for overnight.
7. Weigh the filter paper and digested material.
8. Calculate the cellulase digestibility of the material by deducting the weight of filter paper dried material from the weight of filter paper.

☞ **Note**

Always use fresh enzyme (cellulase) solution and enzyme should be procured fresh. Stored enzyme (cellulase) preparation usually lost their activity during storage period.

References

Barnes, R.F. Muller, L.D. Bauman, L.F. and Colenbrandor, V.F. (1971). *J. Anim. Sci.*, 33: 881.

Bentley. O.G. Johnson. R.R., Hershberger, T.V., Cline, J.H. and Moxon. A.L. (1955). *J.Nutr.*, 57: 389.

Bentley. O.G. Johnson, R.R., Venecko, S. and Hunt, C. H. (1954a). *J. Anim. Sci.* 13: 581.

Bentley, O.G., Lehm Kuhl, A., Johnson, R.R., Hershberger, T.V. and Moxon, A.L. (1954b). *J. American Chem, Soc.*, 76: 500.

Bryant, M.P. and Doetsch, R.N. (1955). *J. Dairy Sci.*, 38: 340.

Dehority, B.A., El-Shazly, K. and Johnson, R.R. (1960). *J. Anim. Sci.*, 19: 1098.

El-Shazly, K., Dehority, B.A. and Johnson, R.R. (1961a). *J. Anim. Sci.*, 20: 268.

El-Shazly K,- Johnson, R.R., Dehority,B.A. and Moxon, A.L. (1961b). *J. Anim. Sci.* 20: 839

Goering, H.K. and Van Soest, P.J. (1970). Forage fiber analysis, Agricultural Research Service, *USDA, Agriculture Handbook* No. 379.

Gutcho, M.H. (1973). Feeds for livestock, poultry and pets (NDC) Noyes data corporation, *Food Technology Review* No. 6, Park Ridge, New Jersey, London.

Hopson, J.D. Johnson, R.R. and Dehority, B.A. (1963). *J. Anim. Sci.*, 22: 448.

Jarrigge, R., Thivend, P. and Demarquilly, C. (1970). *Proc. 11th Inst.Grassld. Congr.* (Queensland, Australia) pp 762-766.

Johnson, R.R. (1963). *J. Anim Sci.*, 22: 792

Jones. D.I.H. and Hayward, M.V. (1973). *J. Sci. Fd. Agric.*, 24: 1419.

Jones, D.I.H. and Hayward, M.V. (1975). *J.Sci. Fd. Agric.*, 26: 711

Krishna, G. and Günther, K.D. (1987). The usability of Hohenheim gas test for evaluating *in vitro* organic matter digestibility and protein degradability at rumen level of some agro-industrial byproducts and wastes used as livestock feeds. Z. *Landwirtschaftliche Forschung*. 40: 281-287.

Krishna, G. and Günther, K.D. (1987). Comparative performance of existing *in vitro* methods for testing the nutritional value of agro-industrial byproducts and wastes. Z. *Tierphysiologie U. Tierernährung*. 58: 108-115.

Krishna, G. Czerkawski, J.W. and Breckenridge, Grace, (1986). Fermentation of various preparations of spent hops (*Humuus lupulus* L.) using the Rumen simulation Technique (RUSITEC). *Agricultural Wastes*. 17: 99-117.

Krishna, G. (1985c). Nylon log dry matter digestibility in Agro-Industrials byproducts and wastes of the Tropics. *Agricultural Wastes*. 13: 155-158.

Lowrey, R.S. (1970). *Proceeding of the National Conference on forage quality evaluation and utilization, edited by Barnes and Associates, published by Nebarska centre for continuing education*, Lincoln, Nebraska pp 0-1 to 0-12.

Lusk, J.W., Browning, C.B. and Miles, J.T. (1962). *J.Dairy Sci.*, 45: 69.

Mc Dougall, E.I. (1949). *Biochem. J.*, 43: 99.

Neathery, M.W. (1969). *J. Dairy Sci.*, 52: 74.

ϕrskov, E.R. Hovell, D.D. and Mould, F. (1980). *Tropical Animal Production*, 5: 195.

Tilley. J.M.A. and Terry. R.A. (1963). *J. British Grassl. Soc.*, 18: 104.

Van Dyne, G.M and Haug, P.T. (1968). *Variables affecting in vitro rumen fermentation studies in forage evaluation: An annotated bibliography*. Oak Ridge National Laboratory TN-1973.

Chapter - 65

Techniques for Studying *in vivo* Utilization of Nutrients under Stall and Range Conditions in Tropics

Techniques to Conduct Digestion Trial Under Stall Conditions

Digestibilty definition. The digestibility of a food is most accurately defined as that proportion which is not excreted in the faeces and which is , therefore, assumed to be absorbed by the animal. It is commonly expressed in terms of dry matter and as a percentage, the digestibility coefficient. For example, if a cow ate 11 kg of hay containing 10 kg of dry matter and excreted 4 kg dry matter in its faeces, the digestibility of the hay dry matter would be

$$\frac{10-4}{10} \times 100 = 60 \text{ percent}$$

For poultry, the determination of digestibility is complicated by the fact that faeces and urine are voided from a single orifice, the cloaca. The compounds present in urine are mainly nitrogenous, and faeces and urine can be separated chemically if the nitrogenous compounds of urine can be separated from those of faeces. The separation is based either on the fact that most urine nitrogen is in the form of uric acid or that most faecal nitrogen is present as true protein.

The chemical comoposition of feeds and fodders does not give us any idea about their feeding value to the various classes of livestock. It is, therefore, very essential to know the amounts actually digested from the different types of foods eaten by the animal. By conducting digestion trial we evaluate animal utilisation of a particular or nutrient, feedstuff or ration.

The method of digestibility determination commonly used was originally proposed by Henneberg and Stohmann in Germany. Normally, apparent digestibility of nutrients is estimated since faeces contain bile juices and debris of intestinal tissue etc, in this metabolic faecal losses are not taken into consideration.

There are following three periods which are necessary for the assessment of nutritive value of feeds and fodders :

1. *Adaptation period - (10 to 12 days)*
2. *Preliminary period - (10 days)*
3. *Collection period - (10-12 days in the case of ruminants and 6-8 days in non ruminants and human subjects)*

With simple- stomached animals or human subjects the faeces resulting from a particular input of food can be identified by adding an indigestible coloured substance such as ferric oxide or carmine to the first and last meals of the experimental period the beginning and the end of collection are then delayed until the dye appears in and disappears from the excreta. With ruminants this method is not successful because the dyed meal mixes with others in the rumen, and instead an arbitral time lag of 24 to 48 hours is normally allowed for the passage of food residues, i.e., the measurement of faecal output begins 1 to 2 days after that of food intake.

In all digestibility trials, and particularly those with ruminants, it is highly desirable that meals should be given at the same time each day and that the amounts of food eaten should not vary from day-to-day. When intake is irregular there is the possibility, for example that if the last meal of the experimental period is unusually large the subsequent increase the faecal output may be delayed untill after the end of faecal collection. In this situation the output of faeces resulting from the measured intake of food will be underestimated and digestibility overestimated.

Digestibility and Nutritive Value of Unknown Feed in Ruminants

Concentrate such as oil cakes and gram cannot be fed in large quantitites so as to keep an animal in normal conditions, hence it is necessary to feed roughage along with concentrate. The digestibility co-efficient of roughage to be fed during the digestion trial in such cases should be determined separately. The basic roughage used under such circumstances should be a maintenance ration containing at least 8 percent digestible protein. It should preferably be hay from leafy fodders. A roughage with a high content of protein may greatly exceeds the share of nutrients fed from the concentate and thus there is the possibility of an associated effect. Insuch cases, however, it is highly probable that the crude fiber digestibility of the cake will be effected but the total intake of fiber from the share of concentrate is so small that no significant error will be introduced due to this factors.

As it is well-known that the straws in general and the inferior quality fodders are poor in protein, they can not therefore, support an animal even if any quantity fed to them. In such cases concentrate like oil cakes is added in quantities just sufficient to make up the protein part of the ration. The concentrate is fed separately and not by mixing with the roughage. When such addition of concentrate become obligatory, care should be taken to see that the nutrients added from the concentrates do not exceed those consumed from the roughage under examination. The results are wrong if the nutrients so added greatly exceed those from the roughage due to the associated effect of other feed nutriens. In this way a combined digestibility data is obtained from which by simple calculations the digestible portions of the different constituents are deducted on the basis of known digestible coefficient of the concentrate used in experiment. Hence in such experiments it become very necessary that the digestible coefficients of the concentrates to be used during trial should be known previously, otherwise it has to be determined by conducting a separate digestion experiment prior to the actual trial.

Crampton and Harris (1969) have recommended that in cattle rations one must usually employ hay as the basal ration, in which case the coefficients for the hay (B) in the first trial, and for the hay plus meal (T) in the second trial might be as

$T = 60$

$B = 50$

Let us asume that the proportion of meal was 40 percent of the total dry ration. Then the digestibility of the meal mixture would be according to the formula suggested by Crampton and Harris (1969).

$$S = \frac{100\,(T - B)}{s} + B$$

where

S = Digestibility of supplement

T = Digestibility of total ration (Hay + meal)

B = Digestibility of basal ration (Hay)

s = Proportion of supplement (meal) in total ration taking the above data into consideration:

$$S = \frac{100\ (60 - 50)}{40} + 50 = 75\%$$

Example

Estimation of nutritive value of groundnut cake by difference method in ruminant (Adult cattle)

We could not estimate nutritive value of groundnut cake by feeding it alone, therefore it is fed with maintenance oat hay having determined nutritive value by conducting digestion trial separately. Oat hay was found to contain 2.3 percent DCP and 6.36 percent TDN. For determining nutritive value of groundnut cake, feed about 1 kg on dry matter basis alongwith maintenane oat hay to an adult cattle, the intake of hay remains at 10 kg per day per head. The composition of groundnut cake is : crude protein, 50 percent; ether extract 4 percent; crude fiber 4 percent and NDF 35 percent. The faeces excreted during the 10 day is 62 kg with 52 percent moisture giving a total dry matter faecal excretion of 33 kg. The composition of the dung on dry matter basis is crude protein 10 percent; ether extract 1 percent; crude fiber 37 percent; and NFE 46 percent.

The calculation steps are given below:

Parameters	CP	E. Ext	CF	NFE
Intake from hay	5	1	30	55
Intake from G.N. cake	5	0.4	0.4	3.5
Total intake	10	1.4	30.4	58.5
Total excreted in dung	3.3	0.33	12.2	15.2
Total digested	6.7	1.07	18.2	43.3
Digested from hay as found in a separate experiment	2.3	0.76	18.0	41.5
Digested from G.N. cake	4.4	0.31	0.2	1.8
Digest Coef. G.N. cake	88	77.5	50.0	51.0

Summary : The groundnut cake contained DCP 44 and TDN 71 percent respectively.
Source : Late Prof. Dr. S.N. Ray (Ex Director NDRI, Karnal (India) Personal Communication as student (Dr. G. Krishna, Ph.D. Thesis, Agra University, Agra)

Calculation of Nutritive Value Index (NVI) and Relative Intake (RI)

The proposal to use the voluntary intake of a forage as a quantitative measure of its nutritive value was made by Crampton in 1957 and later elaborated as the Nutritive value index (NVI) scheme (Crampton *et al.*, 1960) which took into consideration in its calculation both voluntary (Relative) intake and gross energy digestibility measurement. The NVI calculation was designed to obtain a single value which might best describe the contribution of a forage in meeting the animal's digestible energy requirements, and was based on the axiom as stated by Reid *et al.* (1959) that forage intake is equal to intake of forage dry matter times the concentration of energy in the forage. Whereas NVI represents a relative measure useful in the comparison of different forage, the same criteria involved in its calculation can also be used to express the absolute digestible energy intake potential of a forage in terms of DE per unit metabolic body size ($W^{0.75}$ kg).

Crampton *et al.* (1962) recommended the formula to calculate NVI (Nutritive value Index).

Sheep

$$NVI = \frac{100 \times (\text{g daily forage intake})}{80\,(W^{0.75}\,\text{kg})} \times \%\,\text{digestibility of energy}$$

Cattle

$$NVI = \frac{100 \times (\text{g daily forage intake})}{100\,(W^{0.75}\,\text{kg})} \times \%\,\text{digestibility of energy}$$

NVI could be expressed as:

NVI = Relative intake X digestibility of energy.

Relative intake : According to Crampton and Harris (1969), in the equation for computing the NVI of a forage, the relative intake (RI)is merely the observed intake of the forage under test, divided by the expected intake of the standard forage, and the quotient multiplied by 100. It is the amount of forage voluntarily eaten by a sheep or steer relative to each 100 units it would be expected to eat of the standard forage.

Crampton and Harris (1969) have demonstrated relative intake and NVI by the following example.

Example

A sheep weighing 50 kg, ate 1,100 gram of a forage in 24 hours. The expected intake of the standard forage would be (50 kg 0.75) X 80 =18.8 X 80 = 1,504 grams.

The relative intake of this forage is then (as a whole number)

$$RI = \frac{1{,}100 \times 100}{1{,}504} = 73$$

Suppose energy digestibility in the case of standard forage is 70 percent and testing forage is 60 percent then NVI of testing forage will be

NVI = RI X % digest
= 73 X 60% = 43.8

For the standard forage, NVI is by definition.

NVI = 100 X 70% = 70

Effective feeding value of testing forage will be 43.8/0.70 = 62.5 percent.

Intake Measurement and Faecal Collections

1. On the first day of the experiment the sheep are weighed and placed in individual metabolism cages, in these cages there is no need of using faecal bags since urine and faeces are separated automatically.
2. Voluntary intake measurement is recorded by adjusting the quantity offered to each sheep daily to provide between 100 and 200 grams of refused hay each day. The sheep are fed once daily and refusal re-weighed just before feeding. We should watch carefully if sheep leaves less than 100 grams on any given day, the amount offered is increased by 100 grams, but if no refusal are left, the amount offered is increased, 200 grams over the amount offered the day before.
3. The first 14 days of the experiment are considered as a preliminary period during which the amount of forage offered is adjusted to achieve voluntary intake, as defined above.

Experimental calender

Day	Job
1	Weigh sheep. place in metabolism cages, attach faeces bags, start experimental diets.
2 to 14	Adjust feeding to *adlibitun* intake, remove residue each day.
15	Collect forage sample.
16	a. Collect forage sample
	b. Collect refusal.
17	a. Collect forage sample
	b. Collect residue
	c. Collect faeces.
	Continue all these activities from 17th to 22nd day.
23rd	a. Collect faeces.
	b. Weigh sheep.

Procedure of Sampling of Forage Offered

During the peiod of 7 days (faecal collection duration) proceed as below:

(a) Weigh about 100 grams of chaffed fresh forage sample offered daily to sheep, in a tray for dry matter determination. Collect daily dried sample of forage in a plastic bag. Mix thoroughly dried cumulative sample of forage offered and ground through a Wiley mill using 4 mm and 1 mm screen.

(b) Weigh about 50 grams fresh sample of forage daily in kjeldahl flask and digest for nitrogen estimation. Daily sample of forage offered should be analysed for nitrogen since there may be variation from place to place in the field.

(c) Similarly, the residue sample of forage should be processed for dry matter and nitrogen estimation.

(d) The weight of daily faeces voided is recorded and one-tenth aliquot is weighed in the tray for dry matter estimation, one-twenteeth aliquot of fresh faeces voided is weighed separately and mixed with 10 ml 30 percent H_2SO_4 and kept in wide mouth bottle daily. The cumulative sample of dried faeces of seven days period mixed thoroughly and ground through 4 mm and 1 mm screen. Fresh sample of faeces kept in wide mouth bottle is weighed and exact amount collected in the bottle is calculated by deducting the weight of bottle. Amount of added sulphuric acid in faeces should also be calculated by deducting the weight of faeces and sulphuric acid added from the actual amount of faeces taken in the bottle for nitrogen estimation. Mix thoroughly the contents of bottle containing fresh faeces, in a separate polyethylene trough, the sample should be mixed thoroughly. Weigh 20 grams faeces on the filter paper and transfer as such in the kjeldahl for digesting so as to estimate nitrogen.

Example

1. Wt. of bottle (empty) without lid = 302 gram
2. -do- + faeces = 836.5 grams
3. Actual weight of faeces + acid = 534.5 grams
4. Actual wt. of faeces + acid = 21.1485 grams
5. Actual wt. of faeces in bottle without acid = 458 grams
6. Net wt. of acid free faeces taken for nitrogen estimation = 18.121 grams

(e) The ground sample of forage offered, forage residue and dried faeces is analysed for other proximate principles (ash, ether extract, crude fiber, moisture and nitrogen free extract).

(f) All the results of analysis of proximate principles in forage offered, forage residue and dried faeces are converted on wet basis from 100 percent dry matter basis.

(g) Digestibilities of nutrients is expressed on as fed basis.

Calculations

A = average daily dry matter offered

$$A = \frac{\%\text{ dry matter of forage X average daily forage offered}}{100}$$

B = average daily dry matter refused

$$B = \frac{\%\text{ dry matter of residue X average weight of residue}}{100}$$

C = average daily dry matter voided in faeces

$$C = \frac{(\%\text{ dry matter in faeces voided) X (wt. of fresh faeces voided)}}{100}$$

D = % digestibility of forage organic matter (O.M.)

$$D = \frac{\text{Weight O.M. eaten - Wt. O.M. in faeces}}{100} \text{ X 100}$$

Similarly digestibility of other nutrients may be calculated by adopting the following formula

$$\frac{\text{Nutrient in feed - nutrient in faeces}}{\text{Nutrientin feed}} \text{X100}$$

Digestion and Balance Trial for Sheep

Weighed amount of experimental feed is fed to sheep for a definite period of time and the excreta resulting therefrom are collected quantitatively for chemical analysis. By knowing the proximate principle in feed and faeces, digestion coefficients and digestible nutrients can be calculated. If we analyse the urine end products such as milk or wool the amount of source of the nutrients absorbed and retained in the body or stored as a product may be calculated by difference.

Aparatus

1. Metabolism cages with an arrangement at the floor for separation of urine and faeces.
2. Urine collection containers simple glass bottles or plastic containers.
3. Faeces containers plastic bags or plastic buckets.
4. Meat grinder.
5. Weighing balance- To weigh animals, feed, faeces and urine.
6. Wide mouth glass bottles.
7. Sample tray for moisture determination.
8. Plastic bottles.

Feeding and Watering

(a) Experimental sheep should be fed at the same time each day early in the morning at about 9 a.m. The amount of experimental ration should be exactly weighed.

(b) Experimental sheep should be allowed to drunk clean and wholesome water at least three tims a day in winter season and six times in summer season. If trace mineral balance or Ca & P balance studies are to be conducted then these contents should be analysed in water consumed. About one liter of water (representative sample) should be evaporated in a clean double distilled water washed pyrex glass beaker. The volume of water drunk by sheep should be recorded during the period of metabolism trial (5-7 days).

Preliminary period

(a) The main purpose of the preliminary period is to acquaint the animal with the metabolism cages or stall, to make the necessary adjustment in order that the faeces and urine are collected properly, and to adjust the animal to its intake of feed in relation to the excretion of faeces and urine.

(b) Always deworm the experimental sheep before starting preliminary period. Experimental sheep should be healthy in all the respect so as to study the normal nutrient metabolism.

(c) Preliminary period and adaptation period is usually of three weeks duraton.

Collection Period

(a) Bring the animal to the collection cage 7 days before the collection period starts.

(b) Weigh the experimental sheep at 7 a.m. before offering water and experimental ration, on three consecutive days. Take the average weight of three days recording for consideration in the calculation of digestion trial data. Similarly take the weight of experimental sheep after the completion of collection period.

(c) Usually collection period in sheep is of 5-7 days duration, If the animal is on *ad libitum* feeding, the collection period should be at least 14 days long. The collection period should begin on the morning after the animal has been eating a constant amount of feed.

Sampling

Samples of feed (offered and residue) and faeces should be processed as per procedure mentioned earlier. Measure the volume of daily voided urine and take aliquot one-thenth in a glass bottle and add 1 ml of 30 percent H_2SO_4 so the fungus may not grow. If gross energy of urine sample is to be determind then take aliquot 1/100th in a screw capped polyethylene bottle and keep sample in refrigerator at 1°C. At the end of collection period mix thoroughly the sample of urine and transfer 20 ml measured volume in the Kjeldahl flask so as to estimate total nitrogen.

Calcuim, phosphorus and nitrogen balance

Balance = mineral in feed minus mineral in faeces and urine.

Example

Adult sheep of Nali breed - 35.8 kg, Metabolic body size, $W^{0.75}$ kg - 14.94

Feed offered

1.	Lucerne hay (*Medicago sativa*)	=	738 grams
2.	Malt sprout	=	90.95 grams
3.	Crushed maize (*Zea mays*)	=	68.95 grams
4.	Molasses	=	112 grams
	Total intake	=	1009.90 grams
5.	Total residue	=	Nil
6.	Net intake	=	1009.90 grams
7.	Fresh faeces voided	=	808 grams

Fig. 1 : Calculation of Digestibility of nutrient in adult sheep (Expressed on as fed basis) based on research carried by Author at CCS-HAU, Hisar (Haryana), India

Parameters	Lucerne hay	Malt sprout	Crushed maize	Molasses	Total intake	Total residue	Net intake	Faeces voided(g)	Digested	Digest coeff
Amount offered (g)	738	90.95	68.95	112	1009.90	-	-	808	-	-
DM%	93.52	94.27	92.31	76.33	-	-	-	44.84	-	-
DM consumed (g)	690.17	85.73	63.64	85.48	925.05	-	925.05	362.3	562.75	60.82
OM%	87.16	87.08	89.49	62.85	-	-	-	37.13	-	-
OM consumed (g)	643.24	79.19	62.19	70.39	855.02	-	855.02	300.02	568.00	64.91
CP%	16.92	19.04	8.97	2.37	-	-	-	6.18	-	-
CP consumed (g)	124.86	17.31	6.18	2.65	151.01	-	151.01	49.93	101.06	66.93
E.Ext %	2.7	0.695	3.34	-	-	-	-	0.874	-	-
E.Ext consumed (g)	19.92	0.632	2.32	-	22.87	-	22.87	7.06	15.81	60.90
NFE%	37.89	44.20	72.46	60.48	-	-	-	15.06	-	-
NFE consumed (g)	279.62	40.19	50.35	67.73	437.91	-	437.91	121.71	316.20	72.20
CF%	29.66	23.15	4.71	-	-	-	-	14.92	-	-
CF consumed (g)	218.89	21.05	3.27	-	243.22	-	243.22	120.55	122.66	50.43
Gross energy-kcal/g	3.47	3.85	4.17	1.62	-	-	-	1.308	-	-
GE consumed kcal	2560.86	350.16	287.52	181.44	3379.98	-	3379-98	1057.21	2322.80	68.72

Table 2 : Calculation of DCP and TDN

Proximate Principle	% on raw matter basis	Digestible coefficient	Digestible nutrient	Total digestible nutrient	% contri bution to TDN
Crude Protein	14.95	66.93	10.00	10.00	17.79
Ether extract	2.26	54.85	1.24x2.25	2.76	4.91
NFE	43.36	72.20	31.30	31.30	55.69
CF	24.08	50.43	12.14	12.14	21.60
			Total digestible nutrients	56.20	

The experimental ration fed to sheep contained 10 percent DCP and 56.20 percent TDN.

Further Calculations

I. Actual DE (digestible energy) of experimental ration fed to sheep.

Please examine the data of Table 1&2 Experimental feed consumed contained 2.48 Mcal DE/kg.

II. According to NRC (1971), TDN figures may be converted to DE and ME by using the following factors

1 kg TDN = 4.409 Mcal DE
1 kg TDN = 3.616 Mcal ME

DE may be converted to ME by multiplying with 0.82, According to NRC (1971)

(a) 1000 g TDN is equivalent to 4.409 Mcal DE, 562 g TDN will be equivalent to

$$= \frac{4.409 \times 562}{1000} = 2.48 \text{ Mcal DE}$$

(b) 1000 grams TDN is equivalent to 3.616 Mcal ME, 562 gram TDN will be equivalent to

$$= \frac{3.616 \times 562}{1000} = 2.03 \text{ Mcal ME}$$

Therefore it is clear that 1 kg experimental ration fed to sheep contained 2.48 Mcal DE and 2.03 Mcal ME, while actual figure based on digestion trial and bomb calorimetry was 2.32 Mcal DE/kg.

(c) SE (kg) = 0.995 TDN (kg) - 0.051 digestible CP (kg/kg feed)

Source : Gohl, Bo, 1981. Tropical feeds, feed information summaries and nutritive values. FAO Animal production and Health Series No. 12, FAO, Rome

III. Calculation of DE and ME using Rostock equations

Rostock equations published by Schiemann *et al.* (1971) may be used to calculate DE and ME of experimental ration. The following example will clear the concept of using these equation.

DE=5.72x Dig CP + 9.05x Dig. E. Ext + 4.48xDig. CF+4. 06xDig.NFE

DE=5.72x10+9.05x1.24+4. 38x12.14+4.06x31.30 = 2:42 Mcal/kg

ME=4.49xDig. CP+9.05xDig.E. Ext.+3.61xDig CF+3.66xDig NFE

ME=2.14 Mcal/kg

Result

According to Rostock equation (1971) 1kg experimental ration contained 2.42 Mcal /kg DE and 2.14 Mcal/kg ME.

Conclusion

The nutritive value of experimental ration was assessed by using conventional method of conducting digestion trial and figures obtained are mentioned below:

DCP = 10%

TDN = 56.20%

	By Dig. Trial	NRC (1971)	Rostock equations (1971)
Digestible energy (Mcal /kg)	2.32	2.48	2.42
Metabolizable energy (Mcal/kg)	-	2.03	2.14

IV Digestion and balance trial in cows. buffaloes and bullocks

Procedure for conducting metabolism trial is same as mentioned in the case of sheep except the following mentioned points:

1. In the case of male animals (bullocks), use of urine bags are advised, while faeces is collected manually and kept in the plastic buckets. In the case of female animals (cows and buffaloes), polyethylene tube fitted in the urethral orifice and supported by the adhesive tap fixed on the labia majora, is used for collection of urine. *At National Dairy Research Institute, Karnal (India) and Indian Veterinary Research Institute, Izatnager (U.P.), especially designed conduct system made from galvanised sheet, is used for collecting urine in the case of female animals. Faeces is collected manually in the plastic buckets. Author has used especially designed conduct system made from galvanised sheet for collecting urine from experimental cows at NDRI, Karnal (Haryana), India (Krishna, 1973) during his Ph.D. research work under Late Prof. Dr. S.N. Ray Ex-Director of Research.*

2. Aliquoting of biological samples. Aliquot of urine (1/1000) is taken directly into the kjeldahl flask for nitrogen estimation; another aliquot of urine (1/1000) is taken in clean polyethylene bottle and kept in the refrigerator at 1°C for the estimation of calorific value. Aliquot of faeces (1/400) is taken and preserved with dilute sulphuric acid (30%) for nitrogen estimation. Another aliquot of faeces (1/200) is taken for dry matter estimation. Aliquot of milk (100 ml per litre of milk produced) is taken at each milking; samples of three times milking of every day are pooled up and kept in polyethylene bottles at 4°C in a refrigerator. Another aliquot (1/1000) out of this three times pooled samples is taken in duplicate, one is used for nitrogen estimation and another is kept at 1°C in refrigerator for the estimation of gross energy. Seven days samples of urine specified for gross energy estimation is also kept in refrigerator at 4°C.

Digestion and balance trial in pigs. Preliminary and adaptation period may be reduced from 21 days to 10 days and collection period may be reduced from 7 days to 5 days. Pigs should be weighed on two consecutive days and average weight should be taken into consideration in the computation of ration and growth data. Faeces is collected manually in the case of male and female pigs, while urine collection bags should be used in the case of male and female pigs. Method of feeding experimental ration and recording the residue is same as mentioned in the case of sheep. Clean and wholesome water should be offered *ad libitum.*

Aliquoting of faeces and urine sample. Daily amount of faeces voided is recorded and 1/50th of total weight is taken for dry matter estimation and preserved daily in paper bags. Another aliquot of faeces 1/100 is carefully weighed in a watch glass, transferred to a glass mortar and mixed with 5 ml 30 percent sulphuric acid for fixing the nitrogen, the mixed sample is taken in wide mouth glass bottle. Amount of faeces collected in the bottle during a period of five days is weighed and weight of sulphuric acid added is deducted from the total weight so as to know the actual weight of faeces in the bottle. Weigh 20 grams faeces on the filter paper and transfer to kjeldahl flask for digestion and estimating total nitrogen by macro-kjeldahl method. The sample of urine is carefully aliquoted using standard graduated pipette. An aliquot 1/100 is taken in the kjeldahl flask for nitrogen estimation and duplicate aliquot 1/100 is taken in a clean screw capped bottle, mixed with 1 ml sulphuric acid. The cumulative sample of five days period is collected in the kjeldahl flask and then digested as such. If copper or other trace element in the urine is to be determined then another aliquot 1/100 is taken in the glass bottle rinsed with glass distilled water, and 1 ml of distilled sulphuric acid is added to each bottle so as to prevent fermentation.

For estimation of mineral contents in the urine a suitable aliquot 1/100 is taken in duplicate in tared vitreosil basins and kept over hot water bath to dry.

Calculation of digestibility of nutrients is done in the same way as demonstrated in the case of sheep.

Determination of Metabolizable Energy of Poultry Feeds

(Method of Hill and Andersen, 1958)

Reagent

Acetic acid *(2 percent)*
Sulphuric acid *(5 percent)*

Apparatus

Brooder
Glass bottles

Procedure

Select 25 three week old healthy chicks (white leghorn or any breed) and place them in a brooder and rear them on the experimental feed for an 8 day acclimatization period. Then on the 2nd day of the fifth week, give the chicks the requisite amount of accurately weighed experimental feed at a fixed hour in the morning. Simultaneously, spread the polyethylene sheets on the faeces trays for the collection of excreta. Collect a representative sample of feed for dry matter percentage and proximate analysis. Next day at the same hour collect the remaining feed and faeces excreted and weigh them. A representative sample of the remaining feed is again collected for dry matter percentage. The difference in dry mass of feed offered and the remaining feed gives the amount of dry matter consumed during 24 hours. Collect the aliquots from excreta, after mixing it well, for dry matter and nitrogen estimation separately (one twentieth and one hundredth parts respectively) in wide mouth and glass-stoppered bottles, and keep them in a refrigerator. For nitrogen estimation, samples in duplicate should be preserved in 5 percent sulphuric acid. Repeat the same procedure on the next two alternate days and pool together the three-day samples of excreta for the analysis. For dry matter estimation add about 10 ml of 2 percent acetic acid for every 50 g of the excreta and dry it in an oven at about 80°C till constant mass is obtained. We may calculate the dry matter voided in three days.

Estimate actual gross energy of feed and the excreta by using Bomb calorimetry according to standard procedure compiled by author in volume I of this compendium.

Calculation

ME, Mcal/kg feed	=	Ediet – E excreta – N x 8.22
Ediet	=	Gross energy, Mcal/kg feed
Excreta	=	Gross energy, Mcal/kg excreta
N	=	Nitrogen (g) balance per kg of the feed

☞ **Note**

Recently Farrell (1980) has developed the "Rapid method" of measuring the metabolizable energy of feedstuffs in poultry. We may adopt this method if a large number of poultry feeds are to be screened for feed formulation purpose.

Digestion trial under range conditions

(Method of Harris, 1968)

Professor Reid of Cornell University and Professor Harris of Utah State University have been pioneer workers in this field. Several reviews related to this field have been published by Schneider *et al.* (1955), Vallentine (1956), Reid and Kennedy (1956), Raymond *et al.* (1956), and Bohman *et al.* (1967). *Long back, at the Animal Nutrition Division, Indian Veterinary Research Institute, Izatnagar, systematic studies were carried out by a team of scientists headed by Kehar so as to evolve regression equations for use under Indian Conditions (Gupta et al. 1962; Gupta 1966; Chaudhury and Majumder, 1962). At UP Veterinary College, Mathura (India) student of Talapatra used acid insoluble residue as an internal indicator (Shrivastava and Talapatra, 1962a, 1962b).*

The use of well established range research techniques for evaluating the nutritive value of pasture is demonstrated below, however, interested scientists should consult the publication (Harris, 1968) for knowing the details of techniques.

Following two techniques are in practical use for studying the nutritive value of pasture.

1. Ratio techniques

By determining the ratio of the concentration of the reference substance to that of a given nutrient in the feed and the same ratio in the faeces resulting from the feed, the digestibility of the nutrient can be obtained without measuring either the food intake or faeces output. If the digestibility of a component of a diet and its faecal output are known, then the intake can be calculated. Feacal output can be measured by fitting a grazing animal with a faeces bag to collect the total output or by feeding the animal an external indicator. *The external indicator permits estimation of the faecal output without using a faeces bag.*

If the herbage ingested is properly sampled, and the internal indicator is completely indigestible, **dry matter intake can be calculated as follows:**

$$\frac{\text{Weight of internal indicator in total faecal output}}{\text{level (\%) of indicator in forage}} \quad \text{(Formula I)}$$

The following data Will demonstrate the practical utility of this technique. (Harris, 1968)

(i) A grazing sheep fed on a mature pasture grass

1. Fed — 10g chromic oxide per day.
2. Mature pasture grass — 13.0% lignin (dry basis)
7.7% protein (dry basis)
3. Faeces — 1.15% chromic oxide (dry basis)
22.6% lignin (dry basis)
6.0% protein (dry basis)
4. Faeces output 870 g (dry basis-collected with bag or calculated by formula V).

$$\frac{870\,\text{(dry wt. of faeces)} \times 22.6\,\text{(\% lignin in faeces)}}{13\,\text{(\% lignin in mature pasture grass)}} \quad \text{(Formula I)}$$

= 1512 grams dry matter consumed

The apparent digestion coefficient for each nutrient is calculated as follow:

(ii) Apparent digestion coefficient (%) (Formula II)

$$= 100 - \left(100 \times \frac{\text{\% Int. indicator in forages}}{\text{\% Int. indicator in faeces,}} \times \frac{\text{\% nutrient in faeces}}{\text{\% nutrient in forage}}\right)$$

$$= 100 - \left(100 \times \frac{\text{13\% lignin in pasture grass}}{\text{22.6 (\%lignin in faeces)}} \times \frac{\text{6.0 (\% protein in faeces}}{\text{7.7 (\% protein in pasture grass}}\right)$$

100- (100 x 0.575 (DMindigest.xo.779)) = 55.2% apparent digest of protein and

$$100 - \left(100 \times \frac{\text{13.0(\% lignin in pasture grass}}{\text{22.5(\%lignin in faeces)}} \times \frac{\text{100(\% dry matter in faeces)}}{\text{100(\% dry matter in forage)}}\right)$$

100- (100x0.575 X1) = 42.5% apparent digestibility of dry matter.

Indigestible internal indicators which have been used in the ratio technique included lignin, silica and methoxyl group. *The ratio technique works well if (1) a method is used to obtain an accurate sample of the forage consumed by the animal (2) if the indicator is completely indigestible.*

Methods which have been used to sample the forage to estimate the diet of a grazing animal include (1) the before and after method, (2) the *esophageal fistula* method, and (3) the rumen-evacuation method. Is has been observed that the internal indicator is not always indigestible and also it is sometimes difficult to obtain an accurate sample of the animal's diet. To overcome these difficulties, the faecal index technique has been developed.

2. Faecal Index technique

In this technique, it is necessary to clip forage and feed it in a conventional digestion trial in which the forage intake and faeces are quantitatively measured. The feed and faeces are then analysed for an internal indicator such as chromogen, lignin, nitrogen, methoxyl group or silica and for gross energy, organic matter, nitrogen, silica free dry matter or dry matter. The internal indicator does not need to be indigestible, although that would be ideal. Correction is made for digestibility by using a regression equation.

While the conventional trial is being conducted, animals equipped with faecal bags or animals fed an external indicator or grazed on the pasture, and the concentration of the internal indicator in their faeces is determined. Regression equations for the data on the animals fed in the conventional digestion trial are then calculated as indicated above and are used to calculate the digestibility of the forage.

Once a regression equation has been established for a particular set of pasture conditions, it is not necessary to have animals fed clipped forage for subsequent trials. Digestibility can be calculated from the concentration of the internal indicator in the faeces. According to the experience of Harris (1968), *"A Regression equation under one set of conditions does not work under all sets of condition. Therefore, each research worker should determine his own regression equation or should make sure that someone else's equation applies to his own experimental conditions". The regression formula for the line will not be linears, however, the steeeper the slope, the more reliable the estimate will be.*

Given the data in the previous sample the dry matter intake can be calculated as follow:

(iii) % Indigestibility of dry matter (Formula III)

= 100 – digestibility of dry matter

= 100-42.5

= 57.5% indigestibility of dry matter

Note : In actual practice the digestibility of dry matter, 42.5 percent, would be predicted from the regression equation.

(iv) Dry matter consumption (Formula IV)

$$= \frac{\text{Total amount of dry matter in faeces} \times 100}{\text{\% indigestibility of dry matter}}$$

$$= \frac{870 \text{ (g dry matter in faeces)} \times 100}{57.5 \text{ (\% indigestibility of dry matter)}}$$

= 1513 g dry matter consumed.

Estimation of total faeces by grab samples

Grab sampling is a process of removing part of faecal sample from rectum manually. Total faeces output for a grazing animal can be determined (1) by using a collection bag (2) by feeding a quantitative amount of an external indicator to an animal and collecting grab sample of faeces. Total faecal dry matter can be calculated from grab samples.

(v) Faecal dry matter output

$$= \frac{\text{amount external indicator fed} \times 100}{\text{\% external indicator in faeces grab samples (dry basis)}}$$

$$= \frac{10 \text{ (g chromic oxide)} \times 100}{1.15 \text{ (\% chromic oxide in faeces) grab samples}}$$

= 870 g faecal dry matter output

Using formula I and II under the ratio method or the regression equation and formula III and IV under the faecal index method, the dry matter consumption and digestibility can be calculated by collecting grab samples of faeces without a faecal bag. *Chromic oxide appears to be the best external indicator for this purpose.* Blank samples containing faeces without chromic oxide should be run to correct for naturally occurring materials.

Harris (1968) has suggested the following method of chromic oxide administration.

1. Administer paper or cellulose impregnated with chromic oxide and enclosed in a gelation capsule or mix chromic oxide in the feed. If it is

administered in the feed, make up a paste of flour, or a portion of one of the ingredients in the diet and chromic oxide. Make the paste and grind through a mill, then mix it with the feed. The dose of chromic oxide ranged 1.0 to 2.5g/100 pound of body weight per day.

2. The preliminary period should be at least 10 days in length.
3. The collection period should be at least 7 days in length. Collect at least 50 grab samples from each animal.
4. To overcome diurnal variation, collect random samples of faeces in the pasture or pen. Each dropping can be marked with lime. If more than one animal is in a pasture, coloured polyethylene particles may be administered to the animals so the faeces from one animal may be distinguished from another.

Obtaining samples of actual forage ingested

1. The "Before and After" method. The dry weight and chemical composition of the available forage of each species on a pasture are determined before and after grazing (Cook *et al.*, 1948). The difference represent the animal's diet.
2. *Esophageal Fistula method.* The esophageal fistula provides accurate samples of a sheep's diet under most conditions. However, if used for chemical analysis certain corrections need to be made for contamination by the saliva (Bath et al., 1956; Van Dyne and Torell, 1964). There seems to be little contamination of protein, but considerable contamination of minerals has been reported.
3. Rumen evacuation method. To sample the grazing animal's diet by the rumen evacuation technique, a cannula is inserted into the rumen. For diet sample collection the contents of the rumen and reticulum are removed thoroughly (Lesperance *et al.*, 1960). It is usually advisable to quickly rinse the rumen and remove the water with a small pump before sampling. The animals are then allowed to graze for 0.5 to 2 hours depending on the availability of the forage. The forage sample is removed from the rumen and reticulum and the origninal contents are put back in.

Chromic Oxide Content of Faeces and Feeds

1. (Method of christian and Coup, 1954)

Reagents

1. *Potassium bromate. 4.5% W/V solution.*
2. *Phosphoric acid/manganese sulphate* = *Add 30 ml 10%* $MnSO_4.4H_2O$ *in 1 litre Analar orthophosphoric acid*

3. *Sulphuric acid/manganese sulphate : Dissolve 5 ml 10% $MnSO_4$. $4H_2O$ in 1 litre. 50% sulphuric acid.*

4. *Clearing mixture : Dissolve 125 g ammonium sulphate and 70 ml Analar hydrochloric acid in 1 litre of water.*

5. *N/20 ferrous ammonium sulphate : Dissolve 100 g ferrous ammonium sulphate made up to 5 litre with 5% sulphuric acid.*

6. *Standardisation of ferrous ammonium sulphate : To 25 ml N/20 potassium dichromate, add 100 ml water, 6 ml Analar orthophosphoric acid, 5 ml analar sulphuric acid and 2 drops ferroin. Titrate with ferrous ammonium sulphate. 1 ml N/20 ferrous ammonium sulphate = 1.266 mg Cr_2O_3.*

Procedure

Four to five gram of dried milled faeces or feed sample are ashed overnight at 600°C in a nickel crucible. The ash is brushed into a 250 ml conical flask, and the crucible washed with 4 ml of water. Five ml of phosphoric acid/ manganese sulphate solution and 3 ml potassium bromate solution are added and the mixture immediately digested on a hot plate until effervescence ceases and a purple colour appears (7-15 minutes). After cooling for 15-30 seconds, 10 ml sulphuric acid/manganese sulphate solution and a further 4 ml potassium bromate solution are added. Any solid material adhering to the flask is dispersed with a glass rod and the solution boiled for 5 minutes until it turns orange red from free bromine (plenty of silica chips are added to avoid "bumping"). Hundred millilitre water and 5 ml clearing solution are added and the mixture boiled until starch-iodide paper show it to be free from bromine (about 10 minutes). It is then titrated with ferrous ammonium sulphate, using ferroin as an indicator.

II. (Method of Gehrke *et al.*, 1950)

Procedure

1. Ash 5 grams of faeces or 10 grams of feed in a 145 ml porcelain crucible overnight in a furnace at dull red heat. The ash must be free of all organic matter at the end of the heating period.

2. Add 20 grams Na_2O_2 mix thoroughly, then fuse carefully over a Fisher burner until molten. Increase the heat gradually to prevent spattering. When the sample-peroxide mixture is completely molten it is removed from the flame. The crucible must be covered during the fusion. The fusion temperature is between 1000-1200°C.

3. Cool the molten material, then place the crucible containing the melt in a covered 600 ml beaker. Transfer the fused material quantitatively with water (using about 200 ml) to the beaker.
4. Add 30 grams of C.P. ammonium carbonate and heat to the boiling point. If no insoluble residue is present, this step may be omitted (Scott's standard methods of chemical analysis, 5th ed., Vol I, p.284).
5. Cool, add 1:1 H_2SO_4 until neutral, then 40 ml in excess. This step must be done carefully. When the evolution of Co_2 ceases, the neutral point has been reached.
6. Add 10 ml of 1:1 syrupy 85 percent H_3PO_4 to improve the sharpness of the end point. Add an excess of standard ferrous ammonium sulphate (0.1 N for feed and 0.2 N for faecal sample), about 40 ml for the sample weights of feed or faeces given in step 1.
7. Back titrate the excess ferrous ammonium sulphate, using standard $KMno_4$ (0.1 N for feeds and 0.2 N for faecal sample) to a faint pink colour resulting from a slight excess of the $KMnO_4$ solution.
8. Make blank determinations of feed and faecal samples containing no chromic oxide.
9. Calculate the percentage of chromium oxide from : (ml of ferrous ammonium solution) X normality $= \frac{151.992}{6000} =$ g Cr_2O_3 in sample.
10. $\frac{g Cr_2O_3 \text{ in sample}}{\text{sample weight}} \times 100 =$ % chromium oxide in sample

Validity of method

The accuracy and precision of the analytical method for chromic oxide and the high recovery of added Cr_2O_3 from feeds and faeces demonstrate the applicability of this method to digestibility studies with farm animals in which the chromic oxide ratio technique is employed.

Chromogen in Feeds, Fodders and Faeces

(Method of Reid and associaes, 1950 and 1952)

Introduction

The amount of light absorbed by a solution containing 1 mg percent Na_2CrO_4 is termed equivalent to one unit of "chromogen" per 100 ml of extract. For the particular instrument used in this study, the relationship of the concentration of chromogen in extracts to the quantity of light absorbed is expressed by the equation.

$$Y = 49.2379 - 23.8010\ x$$

Where Y = unis of chromogen per 100 ml of extract and x = log of the percent of transmitted light.

For all forages examined in these studies, the analyses for chromogen (s) are conducted on faeces as voided (undried) and on forage material in the same state as that fed to the animals. All moisture measurements are made by the toluene distillation method. Care is taken to protect all samples and their extracts from light as this is possible. All samples not in immediate process of analysis are kept in a refrigerator at 1-5°C.

Procedure

Samples are weighed on a filter paper of a diameter commensurate with the bulkiness of the sample and tansferred with the paper to a 500 ml boro-silicate waring blendor cup equipped with a large rubber stopper covered with aluminium foil. A glass tube extending from the base of an trough, the stopper approximately 6-8 inch above the cup is found to prevent leakage from around the stopper caused by pressure due to increased temperature accompanying blending. Two hundred fifty to 400 ml of 85% (by volume) acetone (depending upon the final volume of extract desired) is added to the weighed sample and the blending is started. The blender is allowed to run approximately 3-7 min, during which the cup is removed at intervals from the motor units and placed in an ice water bath. The number of times cooled during an extraction is determined by the degree of heating. The contents of the cup are transferred quantitatively to a Buchner funnel containing whatman No.42 paper, filtered by suction and the macerate is washed with 85% acetone. The residue is then returned to the blendor cup and extracted in the same manner two or more times, depending on the degree of pigmentation of the successive extract.

The extract is made to a known volume and a portion of this sufficiently large to prepare a final dilution is filtered by gravity through whatman No. 40 or 42 filter paper.

An absorption measurement then is made on the properly diluted extract at 406 mμ using a Beckman spectrophotometer. The units of chromogen (s) per gram of matter is calculated according to the equation shown above.

Calculation of Apparent Digestibility of Proximate Nutrient

Substitution of the chromogen (s) values in the following equation allows the derivation of the apparent digestion coefficient for any nutrient or the dry matter without a knowledge of the total quantity of faeces produced or of the forage consumed.

Apparent digestibility =

$$100 - \left(100 \frac{a \times \text{in faeces}}{b \times \text{in forage}}\right) \times C$$

a = units of chromogen per g faeces

b = units of chromogen per g forage

c = percent of specific nutrient

Calculation of daily dry matter intake

When the total yield of faeces is known, daily dry matter intake may be determined according to the following equation.

Dry matter consumption (g/day) =

$$\frac{\text{(Unit of chromogen (s)/g dry faeces) x (g of dry matter in faeces/day)}}{\text{unit of chromogen (s) / g dry matter in forage}}$$

☞ Notes

1. *Chromogen is light labile*
2. *Faeces should be kept in refrigerator at 1-5°C*
3. *Extract of the material should be kept in dark at room temperature.*
4. *Dry matter intake estimate are somewhat higher than those determined by the simultaneous dry matter consumption- excretion ratio method.*
5. *The digestibility of dry matter of grazed grass is seen higher than that of the barn fed clipped grass, indicating that grazing animals tend to select the more nutritive portion of the grass.*

Approximation of Calorific Value of Animal Feed and Fodder by using Rostock-equations

(Method of Schiemann *et al.* 1971)

In Germany, a team of scientists headed by Schiemann *et al.* (1971) developed a set of regression equations to calculate gross energy (GE), digestible enegy (DE), metabolisable energy (ME), net energy for fattening (NEF) using digestible nutrients of any feed. These equations are mentioned below for use in cattle, sheep, swine and Hens.

Gross energy (Common for all species)

Y = 5.72 X CP% + 9.50 X E. Ext. % + 4.79 X CF% + 4.17 X NFE%

Cattle

$$DE = 5.79 \times X_1 + 8.15 \times X_2 + 4.42 \times X_3 + 4.06 \times X_4$$
$$ME = 4.32 \times X_1 + 7.73 \times X_2 + 3.59 \times X_3 + 3.63 \times X_4$$
$$NEF = 1.71 \times X_1 + 7.52 \times X_2 + 2.01 \times X_3 + 2.01 \times X_4$$

Sheep

$$DE = 5.79 \times X_1 + 9.05 \times X_2 + 4.38 \times X_3 + 4.06 \times X_4$$
$$ME = 4.32 \times X_1 + 9.05 \times X_2 + 3.61 \times X_3 + 3.66 \times X_4$$
$$NEF = 1.82 \times X_1 + 8.39 \times X_2 + 1.90 \times X_3 + 1.90 \times X_4$$

Swine

$$DE = 5.78 \times X_1 + 9.42 \times X_2 + 4.40 \times X_3 + 4.07 \times X_4$$
$$ME = 5.01 \times X_1 + 8.93 \times X_2 + 3.44 \times X_3 + 4.08 \times X_4$$
$$NEF = 2.56 \times X_1 + 8.54 \times X_2 + 2.96 \times X_3 + 2.96 \times X_4$$

Hen

$$ME = 4.26 \times X_1 + 9.50 \times X_2 + 4.23 \times X_3 + 4.23 \times X_4$$
$$NEF = 2.58 \times X_1 + 7.99 \times X_2 + 3.19 \times X_3 + 3.19 \times X_4$$

where

X_1 = Digestible crude protein (g)
X_2 = Digestible crude fat (g)
X_3 = Digestible crude fiber (g)
X_4 = Digestible NFE (g)
X = Multiplication sign

Correction factors for swine and hens

Deduct 0.15 kcal per g disaccharide.
Deduct 0.30 kcal per g monosaccharide.
Add 1.0 kcal per g milk protein.
Deduct 1.0 kcal per g milk fat.

Krishna and Ranjhan (1977 a, b) tried the use of Rostock equations for calculating DE, ME and NEF of Indian feeds and fodder in the case of sheep and cattle. On the basis of these studies, they concluded that Rostock equation could be used under Indian conditions. They also compared values of DE and ME obtained from Rostock equations with figures calculated on the basis of already established factors by Crampton and Harris (1969), Moore et al. (1952), NRC (1971).

If bomb calorimeter is not available in the laboratory then values of DE and ME could be calculated using the figures of digestible nutrients of any

Indian feeds and fodders. If any research worker is interested to countercheck the values of gross energy estimated by bomb calorimeter then Rostock equations are of great help for this purpose.

References

Bath, D.L. Weir, W.C. and Torell, D.T. (1956). *J.Anim. Sci.,* 15 : 1166.

Bohman, V.R., Harris, L.E., Lofgreen, G.P., Kereber, C.J. and Raleigh, R.J. (1967). Techniques for range livestock nutrition Res. *Ut. Agr. Expt. Sta. Bul.* 471.

Chaudhary, H.P.S. and Majumdar, B.N. (1962). *Ann. Biochem. Exptl. Med.* 22: 292.

Christian, K.R., and Coup, M.R. (1954). *N.Z.J. Sci. Tech.,* 36(A), 328-30.

Cook, C.W., Harris, L.E. and Stoddard, L.A. (1948). *J.Anim. Sci.,* 7:170.

Crampton, E.W., Donefer, E. and Lloyd, L.E. (1960). *J. Anim. Sci.,* 19:538.

Crampton, E.W. Donefer, E. and Lloyd, L.E. (1962). J. Anim. Sci., 21:628.

Crampton, R.W. and Harris, L.E. (1969). *Applied Animal Nutrition,* 2nd Edn., W.H. Freeman & Co. San Francisco.

Farrell, D.J. (1980). Feedstuffs, No. 3, pp 24.

Gehrke, C.W. Mayer, D.T., Pickelt, E.E. and Hunyon, C.V. (1950). *The quantitative determination of chromic oxide in feed and faeces.* Miss.Agr. Expt. Station Bulletin

Gupta, B.N., Majumdar, B.N. and Kehar, N.D. (1962). *Ann. Biochem. Exptl. Med.,* 22 :105.

Gupta, B.N. (1966). *Ind . J. Dairy Sci.,* 19: 66.

Harris, L.E. (1968). *Range nutrition in an arid region.* Honour Lecture series, Utah State University, Logan, Utah.

Hill, F.W. and Andersen, D.L. (1958). *J. Nutr.,* 64 : 587.

Krishna, G. and Ranjhan, S.K. (1977a). *Indian J. Anim. Sci.,* 47: 299-303.

Krishna, G. and Ranjhan, S.K. (1977b). *Indian J.Anim. Sci.,* 47: 283-285.

Krishna, G. (1973). Studies on energy and protein requirements for milk production in Indian Dairy Animals. NDRI, Karnal (Haryana) India, Agra University, Agra (U.P.) India.

Krishna, G. (1982). Nutritional evaluation of a new maintenance ration fodder for feeding adult buffaloes. *World Review of Animal Production.* 18: 29-37.

Krishna, G. (1984). Possibilities of ensiled paddy straw and Agro Industrial byproducts for rearing cross bred calves in tropics. World Review of Animal Production. 20: 39-43.

Krishna, G. (1983). Note on nutritive value of paddy straw ensiled with some Agro-Industrial byproducts and its effect on the growth of calves. *Tropical and Animal Science Research.* 1: 194.

Krishna, G., Mandal, A.B., Paliwal, V.K. and Yadav, K.R. (1991). Fermenter Yeast as a feed for adult sheep. *Indian Vety. J.* 68: 1126.1129.

Lesperance, A.L. Bohman, V.R. and Marble, D.W. (1960). *J.Dairy Sci.* 43: 682.

Moore, J.E. (1960). *Procedure for determining voluntary intake and nutrient digestiblity of hay with sheep.* univ. of Florida, Deptt. of Anim.Sci., unpublished. cited Harris, L.E. 1970. Nutr. Res. *Techniques for domestic and wild animals, Vol. 1, an international record system and procedure for analysing a sample. Highland drive, Logan Utah.* 84321.

Moore, L.A., Iroin, H.M. and Shaw J.C. (1952). *Relationship between TDN and energy values of feeds,* U.S. Deptt. Agric. Bur. Dairy, Ind. Inf. 139.

National Research Council, (1971). *Nutrient requirements of domestic animals No.3 Nutrient requirements of dairy cattle,* 4th revised edition, National Academy of Sciences, Washington, D.C.

Raymond, W.F. Minson, D.J. and Harris, C.E. (1956). *The effect of management on herbage consumption and selective grazing.* Proc. 7th International grassland congress. Massey Agr. College. New Zealand.

Reid, J.T. Woolfolk, P.G. Richards, C.R. Kaufmann, R.W. Loosli, J.K. Turk, K.L., Miller, J.I. and Blaser, R.E. (1950). *J. Dairy Sci.,* 33: 60.

Reid, J.T. and associates, (1952). *J. Nutr.* 46: 225.

Reid, J.T. and Kennedy, W.K. (1956). *Measurement of forage intake by grazing animals.* Proc. 7th International Grassland Congress.

Reid, J.T. kennedy, W.K., Turk, K.L., Slack S.T., Trimberger, G.W. and Murphy, R.P. (1959). *J. Dairy Sci.,* 42 : 567.

Schiemann, R., Nehring, K., Hoffmann. L., Jentsch, W. and Chudy, A. (1971). *Energetische fütter bewer tung und Energinormen. Berlin.* VEB. Deutch Lantwirtschaftsverlag, Berlin.

Schneider, B.H. Soni, B.K. and Ham, W.E. (1955). Methods for determining consumption and digestiblity of pasture forages by sheep. *Wash Agri. Expt. Sta. Bul.* 16.

Shrivastava,V.S. and Talapatra, S.K. (1962a). *Ind. J. Dairy Sci.,* 14: 137.

Shrivastava V.S. and Talapatra, S.K. (1962b). *Ind J.Dariy Sci.,* 14: 154.

Vallentine, J.F. (1956). *J.Range Mgnt.,* 9 : 235.

Van Dyne, G.M. and Torell, D.T. (1964). *J. Range Mgnt.,* 17 : 7.

References for further study

Schneider, B.H. and Flatt, W.P. (1975). *The evaluation of feeds through digestibility experiments.* Univ. of Georgia Press, Athens, Ga.

Chapter - 66

Enzyme Assay in Biological Samples

The main groups of some diagnostically important enzymes are as below:

1. Oxido Reductases

Glucose 6-phosphate dehydrogenase, Isocitrate Dehydrogenase, Lactate dehydrogenase, Malate dehydrogenase, Sorbitol dehydrogenase.

2. Transferases

Alanine transaminase (GPT)
Aspartate transaminase (GOT)
Creatin binase
Hexose-1 phosphate uridyltransferase

3. Hydrolases

Acetylcholinesterase
phosphatases
Amylases
Pepsin
Trypsin
Lipase

Glucose-6-phosphatase
β-Glucuromidase
5-Nucleotidase

4. Lyases

Enzymes which remove groups from their substrate without group transfer and add group to double bonds-*Aldolase*.

Alkaline Phosphatase in Blood

(Adaptation of the method of King and Armstrong, 1934)

Principle

Serum or plasma is incubated with disodium phenyl phosphate for 15 minutes at pH10. The enzyme phosphatase liberates phenol, which is estimated by measurement of the colour produced with Folin-Ciocalteu reagent and sodium carbonate. The unit of phosphatase is defined as the quantity of phenol expressed in miligrams liberated under the standard conditions.

1. *0.1 Disodium phenyl phosphate : Dissolve 2.18 grams disodium phenyl phosphate in one litre of water. Heat quickly to boiling, then cool immediately. Store at 4°C with a few drops of chloroform as preservative.*
2. *Bicarbonate buffer, pH10 : Dissolve 6.36 grams anhydrous sodium carbonate and 3.36 grams sodium hydrogen carbonate in distilled water and make to one litre. Check the pH and store in the refrigerator.*
3. *Folin-Ciocalteu reagent : This can be purchased or prepared according to the instructions mentioned below:*

   Dissolve 100 grams AR sodium tungstate and 20 grams AR sodium molybdate in about 700 ml of water in a two litre flat bottomed flask with a B_{34} neck. Add 50 ml phosphoric acid (sp. gr. 1.75), followed by 100 ml of concentrated hydrochloric acid.

   Add a few glass beads to prevent "bumping", fit with a condenser and reflux the mixture for 10 hours. Allow to cool and then add 150 grams lithium sulphate, about 50 ml water and a few drops of bromine. The solution must be cold before the bromine in added. Boil the contents of the flask without the condenser for about 15 minutes to remove excess bromine. The solution should be a golden yellow colour with no trace of green.

   Make to one litre with water, filter and store in a brown bottle in the refrigerator. The reagent keeps indefinitely, but it must be discarded if any green colour forms.

   Before use, dilute it 1 in 3 with distilled water.

4. *15 percent W/V sodium carbonate.*

5. *Stock standard phenol : Dissolve 0.1 gram pure phenol in 0.1 N hydrochloric acid and make to 100 ml. The solution must be standardised. Pipette 25 ml of the phenol standard into a 250 ml conical flask and add 50 ml 0.1 N sodium hydroxide. Heat over a bunsen burner to 65°C and then add 25 ml of 0.1 N iodine. Mix well, stopper and allow to stand to room temperature for 35 minutes.*

   Add 5 ml concentrated hydrochloric acid, mix well and titrate the free iodine with 0.1 N sodium thiosulphate until the solution is a pale yellow colour, then add a few drops of soluble starch and continue the titration to the point where the blue colour is just discharged. One ml of 0.1 N sodium thiosulphate is equivalent to 1.57 mg phenol.

   One ml of stock standard phenol is equivalent to 1 mg phenol.

6. *Working standard : Prepare before use by pipetting 5 ml of the above stock solution into a 500 ml volumetric flask. Add 100 ml of Folin Ciocalteu reagent previously diluted a fresh 1 in 3 and then make to 500 ml with distilled water. One ml of this is equivalent to 0.01 mg phenol.*

   Label two 15 ml centrifuge tubes "Test" and "Control" and add to each 2 ml of the substrate and 2 ml of the buffer. Mix well, stopper the tubes and incubate in a water bath at 37°C for 5 minutes.

   Add 0.2 ml of serum to the test, mix well and incubate with the control at 37°C for 15 minutes. Add 1.8 ml of dilute Folin-Ciocalteu reagent to each, followed by 0.2 ml of serum to the control. Stopper both tubes and mix by inversion; allow to stand for about 3 minutes, then centrifuge.

Set up the following in glass stoppered test tubes:

1. *Test = 4 ml of supernatant*
2. *Control = 4 ml of supernatant*
3. *Standard = 4 ml of the combined phenol*

Standard and Folin Ciocalteu reagent

Blank = 3.2 ml of water and 0.8 ml of dilute Folin Ciocalteu reagent

Add 2 ml 15 percent sodium carbonate to each. Stopper, mix by inversion and incubate at 37°C for 10 minutes. Measure the optical density of each at 680 mμ or with a filter transmitting maximally at that wavelength zeroing the instrument with water in the reference cell.

Calculation

The original king-Armstrong unit was modified by king and wooton, who defined it as that amount of the enzyme in 100 ml of serum which releases 1 mg phenol from phenyl phosphate under the conditions of the method. King Armstrong units per 100 ml of serum are given by:

$$\frac{\text{OD of (Test - control)}}{\text{OD of (Standard - Blank)}} \text{X}\, 30$$

This is derived as follow:

$$\frac{\text{OD of Test}}{\text{OD of Standard}} \text{ X Conc. of Standard X Dilution}$$

$$\text{X 100/ Amount of serum}$$

Which equals:

$$\frac{\text{OD Test}}{\text{OD Standard}} \text{X } 0.04 \text{ X } \frac{6}{4} \text{X} \frac{100}{0.2}$$

$$\frac{\text{OD Test}}{\text{OD Standard}} \text{X}\, 30$$

☞ Note

The Folin-Ciocalteu reagent is very sensitive to traces of organic material with which it reacts to give blue coloured products. For this reason, all glassware should be free from trace of soap and detergents. A common source of contamination is the stoppers of test tubes and volumetric flask which are not always cleaned as carefully as the flasks and tubes themselves.

Acid Phosphatase in Blood

(Adaptation of the method of Fishman and Lerner, 1953)

Principle

Serum is incubated with phenyl phosphate with or without tartrate. Protein is precipitated and the phenol liberated is measuring using the Folin and Ciocalteu reagents. In this method citrate buffer (pH) is used.

The procedure for the determination described in this work depends upon the reaction.

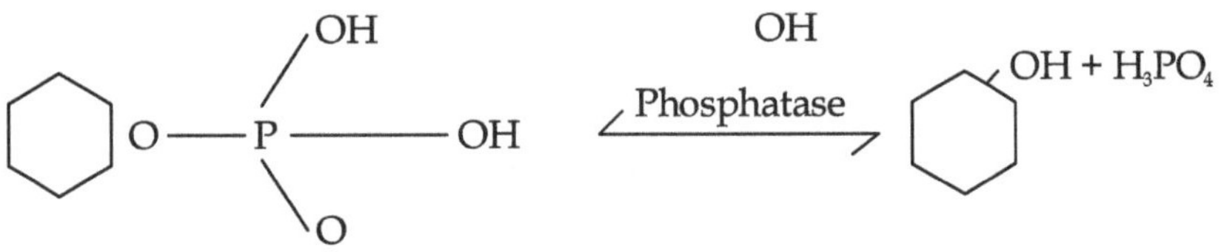

OH

O—P—OH

O

Phosphatase

OH

OH + H_3PO_4

The free phenol produced in the reaction from the phenyl phosphate being determined colorimetrically by its reaction with Folin-Ciocalteu's reagent.

In serum, alkaline phosphatase is stable. King (1965) reports a slight increase on storage at 4°C. At 0°C serum acid phosphatase is stable for about two week. At room temperature the acid phosphatase is labile and may reduce 50 percent of its activity in summer heat (Woodward 1957). Serum for the assay must be free from haemolysis.

Reagents

1. *Citrate buffer, pH 4.9 : Dissolve 42 grams citric acid in about 300 ml of water and add 376 ml N sodium hydroxide. Mix well and make to one litre with water. Check the pH and adjust it if necessary.*
2. *Formaldehyde Solution : Add 2 drops of phenolphthalein indicator to 50 ml of 40 percent formaldehyde and then add 0.1 N sodium hydroxide drop until the solution just turns pink.*
3. *Tartrate solution : Dissolve 15 grams L (+) tartrate in about 70 ml of water and then add 18.5 ml 10 N sodium hydroxide from a safety pipette. Mix well, check the pH and adjust it to 4.9. Make to 100 ml with water, and store in the refrigerator when not in use with a few drops of chloroform as preservative.*
4. *Other reagents as previously mentioned in the case of alkaline phosphatase.*

Set up the following in glass stoppered test tubes

Reagent	Total	Control 1	Formal Stable	Control 2	Tartrate Labile
Buffer	2	2	2	2	2
Substrate	2	2	2	2	2
Formaldehyde Solution	–	–	0.05	0.05	–
Tartrate Solution	–	–	–	–	0.05

Stopper all tubes and place them in a water bath at 37°C for 5 minutes. Add 0.2 ml of serum to all tubes except the controls. Stopper, mix the contents by tapping the tubes and place them in the water bath for exactly one hour. Add.1.8 ml of freshly diluted (1 in 3) Folin-Ciocalteu reagent to each, followed by 0.2 ml serum to the controls. Mix well by inversion, allow to stand for about 3 minutes and then centrifuge. Transfer 4 ml of each supernatant, which must be clear, to another series of glass stoppered test tubes. Next set up a standard and Blank as described previously under "Alkaline phosphatase".

To each then add 2 ml of 15 percent sodium carbonate. Stopper all the tubes, mix by inversion and measure the optical density of each as described previously with water in the reference cell.

Calculations

The activity of the serum is then calculated as already described for "Alkaline phosphatase". that is:

$$\frac{\text{OD (Test control)}}{\text{OD (S tan dard blank)}} \times 30 = \text{King-Armstrong units per 100 ml serum}$$

For total acid phosphatase substitute total control 1 in the above formula, and for Formal stable use control 2. The Tartrate labile is derived from total – Tartrate labile.

Glutamic- Oxalacetic Transaminase and Glutamic pyruvic transaminase

(Adapted method of Karmen *et al.*, 1955 modified by Wroblewski and LaDue, 1956)

Principle

The transaminases are concerned with the synthesis and degradation of amino acid, and play a key role in intermediary metabolism. As shown below, the enzymes reversibly transfer amino groups from glutamic acid to either pyruvic or oxaloacetic acid. This results in the formation of an oxo-acid corresponding to the original amino acid. At the same time an amino acid corresponding to the original keto-acid is formed. In these transfers, pyridoxal phosphate, which is the prosthetic group in both enzymes, plays an important part.

Go-Transaminase (GOT)

Aspartic acid + Ketoglutaric acid GO-T oxalacetic acid + Glutamic acid

As there is no readily measurable change in OD in the above reaction, we couple it with the following:

Oxalacetic acid + B – DPNH $\xrightarrow{\text{MDH}}$ Malic acid + B – DPN as B-DPNE has a high OD at 320 mμ, and B-DPN has no OD at this wavelength, we can readily follow the overall reaction by measuring the rate of decrease in OD at 340 mμ.

For GP - Transaminase

1. Alanine + Ketoglutaric acid GP-T Pyruvic acid + Glutamic acid
2. Pyruvic acid + B DPNH $\xrightarrow{\text{LD}}$ Lactic acid + B – DPN. Measure decrease in OD as in SGO-T reactions above.

In both assays, alanine or aspartate is added, depending upon the transaminase, together with the addition of reduced coenzyme 1 to each. Prior to the addition of oxoglutaric acid, some time is required for the reduction of oxo-acids already present in the serum to take place due to added dehydrogenase and the dehydrogenases present as normal constituents. Addition of oxoglutaric acid triggers off the reaction in accordance with the above equation. The rate of production of the new oxo-acid is then measured, the latter acting as the substrate for the appropriate dehydrogenase in the presence of $NaDH_2$.

Karmen *et al.* (1955) developed a spectrophotometric (kinetic) method, by which in the GOT determination the oxalacetic acid formed, is converted into malic acid by malate dehydrogenase (MDH) in the presence of suitable H_2 donor and by which in the GPT determination, the pyruvic acid formed is converted into lactic acid by lactic dehydrogenase (LDH) in an analogus way.

Reduced β-nicotinamide adenine dinucleotide ($NaDH_2$) is used as the H_2 donor. The decrease of $NADH_2$ as expressed as a decrease of the light absorption at 340 nm, is determinative for the GOT and GPT content respectively, if these enzymes are present in the reaction as a limiting factor.

$$\text{Oxalacetic acid} + NADH_2 \xrightleftharpoons{\text{MDH}} \text{malic acid} + NAD$$

$$\text{pyruvic acid} + NADH_2 \xrightleftharpoons{\text{LDH}} \text{lactic acid} + NAD$$

In the case of colorimetric methods in alkaline solution 2:4-dinitrophenylhydrazine reacts with oxo-acids to give red coloured dinitrophenylhydrazones, and this froms the basis of the colorimetric method employed. In the procedure mentioned below, oxaloacetate formed by aspartate transaminase is converted to pyruvic acid by treatment with aniline citrate, and the above colour reaction then applied.

Reagents

1. *Sorensen's phosphate buffer, pH 7.4 Dissolve 13.97 dipotassium hydrogen phosphate (anhydrous) and 2.69 grams potassium dihydrogen phosphate in water and make to one litre. Store in a refrigerator.*

2. *0.2 M Aspartate. Dissolve 2.66 grams L- aspartate in about 70 ml of the above buffer. Add 20 ml N sodium hydroxide. mix well and check the pH. Adjust to pH 7.4 if necesary and make to 100 ml with the buffer. Store in the refrigerator.*

3. *0.1 M- Oxoglutaric acid. Dissolve 1.47 gram of the acid in 20 ml N sodium hydroxide. Make to 100 ml with phosphate buffer. Check the pH and store in the refrigerator.*

4. *Malate dehydrogenase. Preparations are available with an assay of the activity in terms of optical density units. Dilute afresh with phosphate buffer to give 1, 000 units/ml. The diluted solution does not keeps.*
5. *Reduced coenzyme. This contains 1 mg/ml of buffer. The solution must be kept frozen.*
6. *Potassium dichromate. 0.0001 N*
7. *0.4 M Alanine. Dissolve 3.56 grams alanine in buffer and make to 100 ml.*
8. *Lactate dehydrogenase. This contains 500 μg/ml of buffer.*

The solution is unstable and only enough for the alanine transaminase assay should be prepared. If kept, it must be frozen.

Aspartrate Transaminase (GOT)

Erythrocytes contain transaminases, therefore haemolysis should be avoided. King (1965) reports no significant changes in serum left at room temperature for 48 hours, or after three weeks in a refrigerator at 4°C. The enzymes are inactivated by prolonged freezing. Anticoagulants such as oxalate, citrate, EDTA and heparin have no effect.

Procedure

First, allow all reagents to come to room temperature before the assay. Switch on the spectrophotometer and give it ample time to stabilize. Set up the following in two cuvettes:

	Test	**Control**
0.1 M phosphate buffer	1.3 ml	2.3 ml
Serum	0.2 ml	0.2 ml
0.2 M Aspartate	1.0 ml	–
Coenzyme solution	0.2 ml	0.2 ml
Malate dehydrogenase	0.1 ml	0.1 ml

Mix the contents of each with a fine glass rod. Use a different rod for test and control.

Fill a cuvette with the dichromate solution and use this to zero the instrument. Measure the optical densities at 340 mμ until the solution stabilises, that is by two consecutive readings duplicating one another. This preliminary stage may take about 10 minutes.

At this stage, King (1965) suggests that if low optical densities result, a further 0.1 ml of coenzyme should be added and the optical density changes again followed until the system stabilizes. If additional coenzyme is not required, then 0.1 ml buffer is added to the test and the control.

Add 0.2 ml oxoglutarate to each and mix rapidly with a fine glass rod but avoid forming air bubbles. Start a stopwatch on the addition of the oxoglutarate, and measure the optical density at 340 mμ at 2 minute intervals for a period of 16 minutes.

The readings are then examined to establish the period where the reduction in the reading show a linear fall with time. Check the temperature of the cell compartment at the end of the assay.

Calculation

Using 0.2 ml serum

OD/min X 2, 500 X Temperature

Correction factor = mμ/ml.

Note : A number of laboratories still report result of the assay in Karmen units, that is, one unit is the amount which produces a fall in the optical density at 340 mμ of 0.001 per minute per millilitre under the conditions of the method. The Karmen unit can be converted to mμ/ml by multiplying by 0.48.

Definition of unit of SGO-T or SGP-T

One unit of transaminase activity is defined as that amount of enzyme which will cause a decrease in OD of 0.001 per minute at 25°C, and per Cm light path. This is equivalent to the formation of 4.82 x 10^{-4} μm of oxalacetic acid (or pyruvic acid) per minute.

One international unit (I.U.) of any enzyme is defined as that amount which will convert 1 μm of substrate per minute per litre of serum. The conventional units of Transaminase as used may be converted to International units by multiplying by 0.48.

Table 1 : Temperature correction factors for transaminases (After Wilkinson, 1962, Courtesy of Edward Arnold)

Temperature measured	Factor for GOT	Factor for GPT
20	1.51	1.75
21	1.39	1.51
22	1.20	1.35
23	1.16	1.22
24	1.09	1.10
26	0.94	0.92

As noted previously, fluctuations in the temperature of the assay mixture can cause serious errors. The presence of glutamic oxaloacetate apoenzyme in samples of malate dehydrogenase causes erroneously high results. The apoenzyme is aspartic transaminase without pyridoxal phosphate. When such samples are used the apoenzyme is activated by the pyridoxal phosphate present in the serum. Reliable sources of supply of malate dehydrogenase are therefore essential. The slight increase in optical density which occurs when the oxoglutaric acid is added to initiate the transamination is due to the absorption of this compound at 340 mμ. It disappears once the reaction commences.

Alanine Transaminase (GPT)

Reagents

The reagents required are as above.

Procedure

The procedure for alanine transaminase is the same as that described previously, except that alanine replaces aspartic acid and lactate dehydrogenase is used in place of malate dehydrogenase.

Set up the following in cuvettes.

	Test	Control
0.1 M phosphate buffer	1.3	2.3
0.4 M Alanine	1.0	–
Serum (free from haemolysis)	0.2	0.2
Coenzyme solution	0.2	0.2
Lactate dehydrogenase	0.1	0.1

Mix well and proceed as described previously.

Precautions

1. Haemolysed serum should not be used for assay of GO-T and GP-T
2. Richterich (1969) has reported that a blank serum is unnecessary since the pre run always reaches a fixed absorbance if it is long enough.
3. Richterich (1969) has experienced that if the determination cannot be carried out within 4 hours of blood collection, the serum should be frozen. Serum and plasma give results of same range.

Ceruloplasmin assay in serum

(Enzymatic with p-phenylenediamine)

(Method of Ravin, 1961 modified by colombo and Richterich, 1964)

Introduction

In normal human blood plasma about 90-95 percent of copper exists in the form of cuproprotein termed "ceruloplasmin". The remainder of the plasma copper is loosely bound to the other proteins, chiefly albumin. *Ceruloplasmin a blue alpha globulin of plasma with a molecular weight of 151000 and containing about 0.34 percent copper which corresponds to 8 atoms of copper per molecule. Ceruloplasmin contains hexosamine, hexose, neuraminic acid.* Its physiological function is unknown, its *in vitro* enzymatic activity as an oxidase towards certain polyphenols and polyamines particularly p-phenylenediamine (PPD) is well known. *Ceruloplasmin, like haemoglobin, albumin, haptoglobin, transferrin is heterogenous.*

Principle

Many quantitative method for ceruloplasmin in plasma (or serum) have been proposed which are based on four principles.

1. *By measurement of the absorption of light of 605 mμ by ceruloplasmin before and after destruction its blue colour.*
2. *By measurement of total copper after removal of free or loosely bound copper.*
3. *By measurement of the rate of oxidation of phenylenediamine.*
4. *By immunochemical precipitation of ceruloplasmin and quantitative estimation of the specific precipitate.*

Long back, Houchion (1958) developed enzymatic procedure for the estimation of ceruloplasmin. He confirmed that a strong positive linear correlation exists between the total copper content of human serum and the PPD oxidase activity. According to procedure of Houchin (1958), colour intensity is produced when the serum sample is incubated with a buffered solution (pH 5.2) of PPD. Rice (1961) modified the acetate buffer by adding a small quantity of EDTA to suppress nonenzymatic oxidation of the substrate which is mainly due to trace contamination of cupricions. The enzymatic reaction is terminated by adding sodium azide solution prior to spectrometry.

Following is a method developed by Ravin (1961) and later on modified by colombo and Richterich (1964). According to these workers, ceruloplasmin catalyses the oxidation of the colourless p-phenylenediamine to be a bluish to violet coloured reaction product. The procedure is followed photometrically and the blank value is determined by inhibition of the enzyme wth sodium azide.

Reagents

1. Acetate buffer (0.43 M, pH 5.6)

134 ml of glacial acetic and 26.44 g sodium acetate (trihydrate) are dissolved in demineralized water and the volume adjusted to one litre . Stable indefinitely if frozen

2. Substrate solution (7.95 mM)

36 mg p - phenylenediamine dihydrochloride is dissolved in 25 ml of acetate buffer. The pH should be adjusted to 5.6 with a few drops of 0.1 N NaoH. The solution should be freshly prepared, as it is very sensitive to light and difficult to keep.

3. Sodium azide solution

460 mM grams for sodium azide dissolved in 100 ml of dimineralised water. Stable indefinitely.

Procedure

Mixture	T	B
Substrate solution, ml	1.0	1.0
Sodium azide solution, ml	_	0.2
Serum, ml	0.02	0.02
Incubate 15 minutes at 37°C		
Sodium azide solution, ml	0.2	_

Read absorbance after 15 minutes with photometer set at 546 nm against a water blank.

Calculation

mg ceruloplasmin/100 ml = 237 x [A(T)-A (B)]

where

A = Absorbance

T = Treatment

B = Blank

References

Colombo, J.P. and Richterich, R. (1964). *Schweiz. Med. Wschr.*, 94: 715

Fishmen, W.H. and Lerner, F. (1953). *J. Biol. Chem.*, 200: 89

Houchin, O.B. (1958). *Clin. Chem.*, 4: 519

Havin, H.A. (1961). *J. Lab. Clin. Med.*, 58 : 161

Richterich, R. (1969). *Clinical chemistry-Theory and Practice. English translation* S.Karger, Basel (Switzerland), pp 325.

Rice, E.W. (1961). *Clin. Chim. Acta*, 6 : 170

Karmen, A., Wroblewski, F. and La Due, J.S. (1955). *J. Clin Invest.*, 34: 126

King E.J. and Armstrong, A.R. (1934). *Canad. Med. Ass. J.*, 31: 376

King, J. (1965). *Practical clinical enzymology*, London. Von Nostrand.

Wilkinson, J.H. (1962). *An introduction to diagnostic enzymology*. Arnold, E. London.

Woodward, H.C. (1957). *J. Urol.*, 65 : 588

Wroblewski, F. and La Due, J.S. (1956). *Proc. Soc. Exptl. Biol and Med.*, 91: 569

Referencr fo further study

Mc Allister, R.A. (1970). *Enzymes and the determination of enzyme activity Butterworth*, London.

Chapter - 67

Column and Liquid Partition Chromatography

Celite Column Chromatography

(Method of Wiseman and Irvin, 1957)

Principle

Celite columns with an internal indicator have been developed for the quantitative separation of silage and rumen volatile fatty acids ranging from butyric to succinic. The aqueous phase employs minimal amounts of sulphuric acid to prevent retention of organic acids, sugar is added to the phase to increase elution resistance. Aqueous samples, 2 ml or less are added directly to a dry column cap. Eluting solvents are mixtures of acetone and petroleum ether. Single zone collections make possible a reduced number of titrations with increased accuracy. The column permits fairly wide separations of lactic acids, often difficult on silicic acid columns.

The method employs celite with alphamine red R as an internal indicator. A distinctive feature is the use of concentrated sugar solution as the stationary phase to resist leaching action of solvents.

Apparatus

1. Chromatographic tube with a fritted glass filter and delivery stopcock with an inside diameter of 18 mm and a length (top to stopcock) of 50cm is used. A filter, extra porous, is sealed in 2 cm above the stopcock,

2. Nitrogen gas cylinder with regulator valve to give 0 to 15 pounds per square inch pressure.
3. Tamping rod consisting of statinless steel rod (60 cm in length) silver soldered to the centre of the stainless steel disk, 16 mm in diameter.
4. Titration assembly, 25 ml burette with a two-way stopcock, gravity fed from a 4 litres polyethylene bottle provided with a carbondioxide adsorption tube for an air inlet.
5. Magnetic stirrer.

Reagents

1. *Celite analytical filter aid should contain SiO_2 97.46, Fe_2O_3 0.27, Al_2O_3 1.3, TiO_2 0.11, Cao 0.10, Mgo 0.26, alkalies (as Na_0O) 0.22 percent on ignited basis. This may be imported from M/s Celite Division, Johns-Manville, 22 E. 40th St., N.Y. 16, N.Y. (U.S.A)*
2. *Petroleum ether (AR, BDH) 60-80°C for chromatography.*
3. *Acetone, Distilled through a 50 cm vigreux column.*
4. *O-Kresolphthalein (3′, 3″ - Dimethylphenolphthalein indicator pH 8.2-9.8). Dissolve 100 mg indicator in 50 ml methanol and mix 2.6 ml N/10 NaOH and made up to 100 ml with isopropanol.*
5. *N/100 potassium hydroxide, Dissolve 1.4 gram potassium hydroxide in 10 ml distilled water and add to a mixture of 1.250 litre methanol and 1.250 litre isopropanol. In all 2.5 litre solution will be prepared.*
6. *N/100 oxalic acid. Dissovle 0.1575 gram oxalic acid in 250 ml isopropanol.*
7. *N/10 sulphuric acid, Dissolve 0.7 ml conc. Sulphuric acid (36 N) in 250 ml distilled water.*
8. *Cap material. Sodium sulphate 480 g, Celite 320 g and Ammonium sulphate 40 g.*
9. *Alphamine Red "R" indicator. Dissolve 0.4 g alphamine red "R" indicator in 100 ml distilled water.*
10. *Preparation of column material. Take in waring blender (electric run), 75 g celite, 15 ml 0.4 percent alphamine red "R" indicator, 0.5 ml N/10 sulphuric acid, 30 ml sugar (2 parts sugar and 1 part water). First add 500 ml petroleum ether acetone (1:1) and 250 ml (1:1) later on, mix thoroughly.*
11. *Sugar solution. Dissolve 500 g sugar in 250 ml distilled water.*

12. *Eluting solvents (method for two litre solution).*

PA1	*Acetone* 20	*Pet. ether* 1980
PA3	*Acetone* 60	*Pet. ether* 1940
PA15	*Acetone* 300	*Pet. ether* 1700
PA35	*Acetone* 700	*Pet. ether* 1300
PA50	*Acetone* 1000	*Pet. ether* 1000

13. *0.6 N H_2SO_4 (Sulphuric acid). Dissolve 17 ml sulphuric acid in one litre distilled water.*

14. *Volatile fatty acids standard. Dissolve following acids in 250 ml isopropanol.*

Acetic acid	*5.96 ml (625 mg)*
Propionic acid	*2.52 ml (250 mg)*
Butyric acid	*1.56 ml (150 mg)*
Valeric acid	*0.75 ml (75 mg)*
Lactic acid	*1.40 ml (175 mg)*

Note : These acids should be purified and of AR grade.

Procedure

1. Wash column thoroughly with PA 50.
2. Press cotton with tamping rod.
3. Keep 10-15 cm level of PA 50 in column and keep glass wool.
4. Fill column with column material and pack with stainless steel rod.
5. Add PA about 100 ml and press with 0.8 kilo pressure/cm^2 of nitrogen. Repeat this process twice at least.
6. Exactly 2 grams of rumen liquor and 0.5 ml of 0.6 N H_2SO_4 is mixed thoroughly with 4 grams cap material and put on the top of column.
7. Fill the column with PA_1 and press with nitrogen 0.2 kilo pressure/cm^2 of nitrogen.
8. Collect the elute in flask No.1.

9. Add PA_3 in column and press with nitrogen (0.02 kilo pressure/cm^2 or nitrogen).
10. Collect the elute in flask No.2.
11. Add PA_{15} in column and press with nitrogen (0.2 kilo pressure/cm^2) and collect the elute in flask No. 3.
12. Add PA_{35} in column and press with nitrogen (0.2 kilo pressure/cm2) and collect the elute in flask No.4.
13. Add PA_{50} in column and press with nitrogen (0.2 kilo pressure/cm^2) and collect the elute in flask No. 5.
14. Titrate the contents of flask No. 1, 2, 3,4 and 5, with N/100 potassium hydroxide using O-kresolphthalein (3′, 3″- Diemthyl phenolphthalein) indicator.

The chronology of events of elution of volatile fatty acids from the column is in the order-valeric, butyric, propionic, acetic, formic and lactic. Complete extraction of each from the column is judged by the movement of blue bands from the top to the bottom.

Factors for Volatile Fatty Acids

Where f is based on relationship $= \dfrac{\text{Molecular weight of acid}}{\text{Normality of acid}}$

Valeric	0.000102
Butyric	0.000881
Propionic	0.000740
Acetic Acid	0.000600

Unit = μ moles/ml or mEq/lit

$$= \frac{f \times a \times (\text{weight of sample} + 0.6 N\, H_2SO_4) \times 100}{1 \times \text{weight of sample}}$$

where

f = factor.

a = volume of N/100 KOH

Silica gel column chromatography

(Method of Bullen *et al.*, 1952)

Apparatus

Chromatography tube 12.15 mm internal diameter and 45 cm long with a constriction 5 cms from bottom to support a glass wool filter, test tubes 15 cms long, 1.5 cm diameter and microburette 10 ml capacity.

Reagents

Silica gel, thiopene free benzene, N-butanol, phenol red indicator, sodium hydroxide solution carbonate free (standard N/100).

Principle

This involves physical analytical separation procedure in liquid-liquid column chromatography. The separation of the various volatile fatty acids is achieved by the varying concentration of n-butanol (mobile phase). Silica gel acts an inert support. The volatile fatty acids get partitioned by the eluting liquid through column and the varying concentration of eluting butanol used separates out the volatile fatty acids depending upon their respective partition Coefficient. The difference in the partition co-efficients of the various constituents is exposed in the easy and distinct separation of butyric, propionic, acetic and lactic acids by using n-butanol in Benzene of 1%, 5%, 10% and 20%. After separating in separate containers, these various volatile fatty acids are estimated by titration with standard alkali solution.

Procedure

Preparation of column. Put a pinch of glass wool into the bottom of the chromatographic tube. Six groups of prepared silica gel is mixed with 4 ml of 0.5 N sulphuric acid in a morter. The resulting free flowing powder is stirred in washed benzene and added to the chromatographic tube. Allow slurry to settle down. Stir the upper portin occasionally during this process to assure uniform packing and levelled surface. Drain off benzene to about 5 cms above the silica gel column by air pressure.

Place approximately 1.5 gram of prepared silica gel powder in a morter and add 3 drops concentrated sulphuric acid, mix well, then add 1 ml of rumen liquor and mix well again. Place the powdery mixture into the column and drain off benzene to about 1 cm above silica gel column. Pass the following through one column under slight pressure in the order listed below:

A. 30 ml 1% butanol in benzene equilibrated with water.
B. 30 ml 5% butanol in benzene.
C. 40 ml 10% butanol in benzene.
D. 80-100 ml 20% butanol in benzene

The solvents are added just when the preceding solvent is 1 cm from top of silica gel in the column.

1% butanol in benzene = 29.7 + 0.3 = 30 ml
5% butanol in benzene = 28.5 + 1.5 = 30 ml
10% butanol in benzene = 27.0 + 3.0 = 30 ml
20% butanol in benzene = 24.0 + 6.0 = 30 ml

Collect all the effluent for each fraction in a separate conical flask and titrate with the standard sodium hydroxide (0.01 N) using phenol red solution as an indicator.

Calculations

The volume of standard sodium hydroxide used gives directly the milliequivalents of the various volatile fatty acids present in the rumen liquor. It is expressed as the milli-equivalents of the butyric, propionic, acetic and lactic acids present per ml of rumen juice taken for analysis.

Example

0.5 ml rumen liquor taken for analysis.

Titre value of 0.01 N NaOH in the case of individual VFA's.

Butyric	Nil
Propionic acid	6.8 ml
Acetic acid	0.41 ml
Lactic acid	0.56 ml

Therefore 1 ml rumen liquor will contain

Propionic acid	=	6.8 x 2	=	13.6 milliequivalent.
Acetic acid	=	0.41 x 2	=	0.82 milliequivalent.
Lactic acid	=	0.56 x 2	=	1.12 milliequivalent.

Application of Celite or Silica gel Column Chromatography to Silage Extracts

(Method of Wiseman and Irvin, 1957)

Fifty grams of finely chopped silage are tamped into a 4-ounce wide mouthed bottle provided with a tight-fitting plastic screw cap. The sample is covered with 50 ml of 0.6 N sulphuric acid and a crystal of thymol is added. The bottle is capped and stored in a refrigerator for a week. The contents are mixed and compressed with a stout flat headed glass rod so that the liquor can be drained into a plastic centrifuge tube. After being centrifuged the supernatant liquid is drained off in a bottle and stored for analysis. If 2 ml are taken for analysis, the equivalent dry matter is calculated from, or read from a graph of the equation.

$$\text{Dry matter aliquot} = \frac{2\text{x dry matter (\%)}}{200 - \text{dry matter (\%)}}$$

Smaller aliquotes may be desirable when individual organic acids exceed 50 micro-equivalent on the column, in which case correspondingly less cap material is used.

Chemical Parameter for Evaluating the Quality of Silage

(Standard of Breirem and Ulvesli, 1960)

pH Value	4.2
Lactic acid	1.5-2.5%
Acetic acid	0.5-0.8 %
Butyric acid	< 0.1 %
NH_3 - N as % of total N preferably not exceeding	5 - 8

Ion Exchange Chromatography

Ion exchange term is used to describe the exchange of ions between a solution and a solid insoluble material in contact with the solution. In order to make this possible, the solid material must contain ions which are available for exchange. In addition, an open mesh structure through which the solution can permeate is necessary to facilitate the exchange. Many solid material, including natural substances, have the ability to exchange ions and many artificial ion exchange materials have been developed. The ion exchange process is reversible and use is made of this fact in ion exchange chromatography. When a sample containing several ions of different electric charge is introduced at the top of an ion exchange column, the ion exchange rapidly with ions in the resin. If a suitable mobile phase is used, the samples ions are displaced into the solution again and then re-exchange on to the resin. Further displacement occurs and this process continues until the sample ions charge form the end of the column. If the various sample ions are held on to the resin to different extents than the time taken for them to pass through the column will be different and a separation will be achieved.

Both cationic and anionic exchange resins are available. Commonly used cationic exchange resins consist of divinyl benzens, cross-linked with polystyrene which has been sulphonated, and many anion exchanges a polymers containing amine or quaternary ammonium groups. The resin are supplied in bead from varying in size from 40 microns up to about 2.0 millimeters. The fine beads are used when high column resolving power is necessary, whereas the coarse beads find application in simpler separations such as the deionisation of water.

Table 1 : Common ion exchange resins

Permutit	Amberlite	Duolite	Dowex	Remarks
Cation exchange resin				
Zeo-Karb 215	IR-1	C-10	30	Strongly acidic
	IR-100	C-3	–	–
Zeo-Karb 225	IR-120	C-20	50	Strongly acidic
Zeo-Karb 226	IRC-50	–	–	Weakly acidic
Anion exchange resins				
De-Acidite E	IR-4B	A -2	–	Weakly basic
De-Acidite FF	IRA-400	–	1	Strongly basic
	IRA-410	–	2	
De-Acidite G	IR-45	–	–	Weakly basic
De-Acidite H	–	–	–	Weakly basic

Dowex chelating Resin A-1 is comprised of a styrene divinylbenzene copolymer matrix which are attached iminodiacetate active groups, It should be stored moist and in a salt form. As with conventional ion exchange resins, it is important not to allow A-1 to become dry since re-wetting a dry resin may result in excessive bead breakage. Dry resin should be wet first by a concentrated electrolyte and the solution solely diluted with water until the resin is again completely water swollen.

In recent years, the use of ion exchange materials other than ion-exchange resins of the "plastic" type have been increasingly employed in biochemistry. Following cellulose ion-exchangers are available in the market.

1. Triethylamino ethyl cellulose (TEAE)
2. Diethylamino ethyl cellulose (DEAE)
3. Carboxmethyl cellulose (CM)
4. Sulphoethyl cellulose (SE)
5. Sulphomethyl cellulose (SM)

Gel Filtration Chromatography

It is also known as permeation chromatography. It is based on the principle that different molecular species are often of different physical size. The gel permeation column is packed with a stationary phase in the form of a gel which contains pores of a specific size. As the sample is carried through the column bed by the carrier liquid sample molecules which are small enough to do so penetrate the pores in the packing gel to an extent depending on the molecule's size and shape. Large molecules do not penetrate the gel and are rapidly carried through the column by the solvent and in consequence are quickly eluted. The penetration of the gel by small molecules is a reversible process, and eventually these molecules will be eluted from the column in inverse order of their degree of gel penetration, i.e. in order of decreasing molecular size.

There are two main types of gel in common use. These are the hydrophilic gels which are used with aqueous solvents and the organophilic gels which are used with organic solvents. The most commonly used hydrophilic gels are those made from dextran cross linked with epichlorophdrin and sold under the trade name "Sephadex". The polymer pore size varies with the degree of cross linking and gels are available which are applicable to the analysis of polymers with molecular weights ranging from 100 up to 800,000. The hydrophilic gels are widely used in the analysis and separation of naturally occurring materials such as proteins and sugars and in the analysis of water soluble polymers such as polyethlene glycols. Sephadex LH 20 is used in the separation of polyethylene glycols.

Sephadex of the LH-series is an alkylated product with lipophilic as well as hydrophilic properties. Sephadex LH therefore swells in many organic solvents as well as in water. Sephadex is supplied in the form of minute beads. The bead form has considerable advantages, as it imparts good flow and separation properties to chromatographic materials. When all the molecules are eluted from the Sesphadex bed, the column is ready for another experiment.

The automatic regeneration is one of the advantage of gel filtration, the same column can in general be used for a large number of experiments.

Sephadex G-10 has a water regain value of 1 and sephadex G-200 has a water regain value of 20. The sephadex gels are insoluble in all solvents (unless the sephadex is chemically degraded). They are stable in water, salt solutions, organic solvents, alkaline and weakly acidic solutions. In strong acids the glycosidic linkages in the gel matrix are hydrolysed, However, sephadex can be exposed to 0.1 M HCL for 1-2 hours without noticeable effects, and in 0.02 M HCI sephadex is still unaffected after 6 months. Prolonged exposure to oxidising agents will affect the gel and should be avoided. Sephadex can be sterilized in the wet state by autoclaving for 40 minutes at 110°C without any changes in the properties of the gel. If dry sephadex is heated to more then 120°C, will start to caramelise.

One of the most striking properties of sephadex gels as chromatographic materials is their capacity for separating substances according to molecular size. For proteins, extensive investigations have shown that the elution volume of globular proteins are largely determined by their molecular weight. For instance gel filtration is often used to determine the contents of aromatic substances in a mixture, as aromatic substances are usually retarded on a column compared with aliphatic substances of similar molecular weight.

In some instances, gel filtration has proved to be a valuable technique for the determination of chemical equilibria. In the case of slow reactions, where the reactants and the products can be separated on a sephadex column, these substances can be quantitatively determined in the effluent, thereby establishing the position of the equilibrium, Gel filtration has also been applied to the estimation of reaction rates.

Liquid Partition Chromatography

(Liquid / liquid)

In liquid-liquid chromatorgraphy the stationary phase is often water and the mobile phase some solvent only slightly miscible with water. Often the mobile phase consists of a mixture of two or more solvents which together give the correct conditions for satisfactory separation.

If a compound A, is added to a system of two immiscible solvents in contact, A will distribute itself between the two solvents in a characteristic way. Under fixed conditions of temperature the concentration ratio of A in the two liquid phase will be constant and this constant is known as the partition coefficient. If a mixture of two compounds, A and B, which exhibit different partition coefficients, is added to a two phase liquid system, A and B will be distributed between the two phases in concentrations determined by their partition coefficients. The concentration of "A" relative to that of "B" in the solvent with the greater affinity for compound A will be enhanced compared with the original mixture composition. If the solvent with the greater affinity for A is removed from the system and shaken with more of the second liquid phase, the distribution process will be repeated and the relative concentration of A will further increase in the transferred liquid phase. In liquid/liquid partition chromatography these steps are carried out continuously as the mobile phase percolates through the column bed containing the stationary liquid phase. Provided that the partition coefficients of the sample components are sufficiently different a separation will be achieved. If the difference in partition coefficient is large. a short column only will be required fro separation, but if the difference is very small then a long column will be required. In such a situation it is often possible to employ a different combination of mobile and stationary liquid phase between which the sample components exhibit a greater difference in partition characteristics.

Fields of applications of liquid chromatography

The technique of liquid chromatography include the analysis of acids, alcohols, aldehydes, ketone, phenols, esters, hydrocarbons, polymers pesticides, lipids, vitamins, steroids, amino acids and carbohydrates etc.

Comparative polarity Table

Following is Tarppe (1940) and Strain (1942) systems for comparing the polarity of solvents.

Trappe (1940) system	Increasing polarity ↓	Strain (1942) system
Light petroleum		light petroleum 30 to 50°C
Cyclohexane		light petroleum 50 to 70°C
Carbon tetrachloride		light petroleum 70 to 100°C
Toluene		Carbon tetrachloride
Benzene		Cyclohexane
dichloromethane		Carbon disulphide
chloroform		Anhydrous ether
ether		anhydrous acetone
ethyl acetate		benzene
acetone		toluene
n-propanol		esters of organic acids
ethanol		1:2 dichloroethane
methanol		alcohols
		water
		pyridine
		organic acids

References

Breirem, K. and Ulvesli, O. (1960). *Herbage Abstracts,* 30: 1.

Bullen, W.A. Varner, J.E. and Burell, R.C. (1952). *Analyt. Chem.,* 24: 187.

Krishna, G. and Ekern, A. (1974a). Volatile fatty acid metabolism in sheep I. Volatile fatty acid production and availability of energy by using Isotope Dilution Technique. *Z. Tierphysiologie Tierernährung U, Futternuttelkde.* 33: 275-280.

Krishna, G. and Ekern, A. (1974b). Volatile fatty acid metabolism in sheep II. Studies on Kineties of volatile fatty acid pool as determined by Isotope dilution technique. *Z. Tierphysiologie Tierernährung U. Futtermittelkunde.* 33: 281-284.

Krishna, G. and Ekern, A. (1974c). Volatile fatty acid metabolism in sheep III. Effect of intra-rectal infusion of volatile fatty acid on the utilization of nutrients and some biochemical constituents, rectal temperature and pulse rate. *Z. Tierphysiologie Tierernährung U. Futtermittelkunde,* 33: 323-328.

Krishna, G. (1984). Possibilities of ensiling paddy straw and Agro Industrial byproducts for rearing crossbred calves in tropics. *World Review of Animal Production.* 20: 39-43.

Strain, H.H. (1942). *Chromatography adsorption analysis.* Intersci. Pub., N:Y:

Trappe, W. (1940). *Biochem. J.* 305: 150

Wiseman, H.G. and Irvin, H.M. (1957). *J. Agric. Food, Chem.,* 5: 213.

Text books Bulletins for further study

Done, J.N., Knox, J.H., Loheac, J. (1975). *Applications of high speed liquid chromatography.* John Wiley & Sons.

Hawk, G.L. (1979). *Biological/Biomedical application of liquid chromatography,* Marcel Dekker.

Huber, J.F.K. (1978). *Instruments for high performance liquid chromatography.* Elsevier.

Perry, S.G. *et al.* (1973). *Practical liquid chromatography.,* Plenum Press, USA.

Simpson, C.F. (1978). *Practical high performance liquid chromatography,* Heyden and Sons, Inc. USA.

Synder. L.R. and Kirkland, J.J. (1974). *Introduction to modern liquid chromatography* John Wiley & Sons. USA.

Chapter - 68

Conway Diffusion Technique (Method of Conway, 1957)

Principle

The use of boric acid as an ammonia absorbent was first introduced by winkle (1913-15). Conway and O'Malley (1942) used boric acid for ammonia absorption in their original micro diffusion technique.

The ammonia liberated in the outer chamber by alkali addition in the usual way is absorbed in boric acid mixture plus indicator in the central chamber (slightly reddish), the pH of this mixture being approximately 5 before absorption. During the ammonia absorption the pH of the mixture rises, and to upwards of 8.0 (the strength of the mixture being such as to prevent it rising further). After the required period, the fluid in the central chamber is titrated to a faint permanent reddish tint with standard acid. A mixture of methyl red and bromocresol green was found satisfactory to work as an indicator to assist in titration job.

It has been observed that ammonia is present at acid pH as the ammonium ion (HN_4^+) but at alkaline pH it is present as free ammonia. The diffusion of ammonia from the outer chamber to the central chamber can be broken down into three steps as suggested by Richterich (1969).

1. Liberation of ammonia from outer chamber.
2. Diffusion of ammonia from outer chamber to central chamber.
3. Absorption of ammonia through the surface of central chamber.

In step 3, the ammonia gas is absorbed and converted into ammonium ion. Richterich (1969) pointed out that partial pressure of the ammonia gas thus falls to zero creating a concentration gradient which permits an extremely rapid absorption of a sufficiently large surface area is provided

Conway (1957) tried the following releasing agent for liberatig ammonia from the testing sample.

Table 1 : Liberation of ammonia by addition of different anions and cations.

Releasing agent	Concentration	Relative rates of ammonia release (water = 100)
Water		100
NaoH	0.5 N	112
	20%	218
KOH	20%	241
$K_2C_2O_4$	Half saturated	141
K_2HPO_4	Half saturated	206
KF	Half saturated	265
K_2CO_3	Half saturated	294
KBO_4	Half saturated	318

Source : Conway. E.J. 1957. Microdiffusion analysis and volumetric error. 4th edn., Crossby and Lockwood, London.

Practical Application of Conway Diffusion Technique for Analysing Various Biochemical Constituents

Conway (1957) has standardised the various methods for analysing the following constituents.

1. Acetaldehyde
2. Acetone
3. Adenosine-monophosphate (AMP)
4. Adenosine-triphosphate (ATP)
5. Adenosine-diphosphate (ADP)
6. Ethanol
7. Amides

8. Amines
9. Ammonia
10. Bromide
11. Calcium
12. Carbonate
13. Chloride
14. Cyanide
15. Volatile fatty acids
16. Trimethylamine(TMA)
17. Urea
18. B-Hydroxy - amino acids.
19. Iodide
20. Isopropanol
21. Volatile ketones
22. Carbon monoxide
23. Methanol
24. Lactic acid
26. Nitrate
27. Phenol
28. Total nitrogen
29. Formaldehydrogenic steroide
30. Sulfide
31. Threonine
32. Urethane
33. Serum protein (albumin and globulin)

The author of this compendium has mentioned the techniques of ammonia and urea nitrogen, total non-protein (NPN), serum protein fractions (albumin and globulin) and trimethylamine (TMA) in this chapter.

Description of "Agla Micrometer Syringe outfit" used for Titration

This syringe outfit is manufactured by M/S Wellcome Reagents Ltd. England. In this syringe, mode of action of the device is such that the volume extruded is determined by the diameter of the plunge rather than by the internal diameter of the barrel. The complete revolution of micrometer head advances the plunger of the syringe by 0.5 mm., delivering a volume of 0.01 ml. The total graduated travel of the micrometer (50 revolutions of 25 mm) thus corresponds to a delivered volume of 0.5 ml. The peripheral scale of the micrometer head is divided into fiftieths of a revolution., each graduation on this scale thus corresponds to a volume of 0.0002 ml.

The convenient relationship between the micrometer reading M and the volume delivered in microlitres is given by

500-20 M = V microlitres

For example, the micrometer reading is 6.461, and add the syringe zeroed, the volume extruded at this point is given by 500-20 x 6.461= 370.78 microlitres.

Each syringe is tested at the Wellcome Research Laboratories. The required accuracy is such that with proper attention to detail the standard deviation of replication of deliveries of a volume as small as 0.01 ml should be approximately ± 0.00005 ml s.d.

Table 2 : Fractions of nitrogen in human plasma

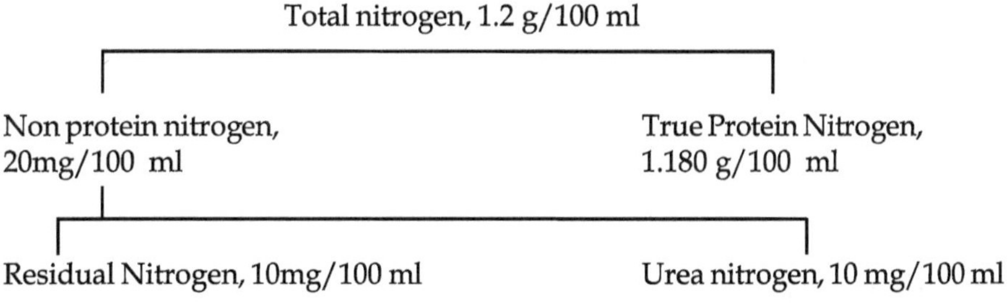

a. Amino nitrogen, 5 mg/100 ml
b. Uric acid nitrogen, 1 mg/100 ml
c. Creatinine nitrogen, 0.5 mg/100 ml
d. Creatine nitrogen, 0.2 mg/100 ml
e. Ammonia nitrogen, 0.1 mg/100 ml
f. Phenols
g. Bilirubin

Conversion Factors

1. Protein = Protein nitrogen X 6.54
   (Protein contain on the average 15% nitrogen)
2. Urea = Urea nitrogen X 2.14
3. Uric acid = Uric acid nitrogen X 3.0
4. Creatinine = Creatinine nitrogen X 2.69
5. Creatine = Creatine nitrogen X 3.12
6. Ammonia = Ammonia nitrogen X 1.22

Table 3 : Fractions of nitrogn in human urine

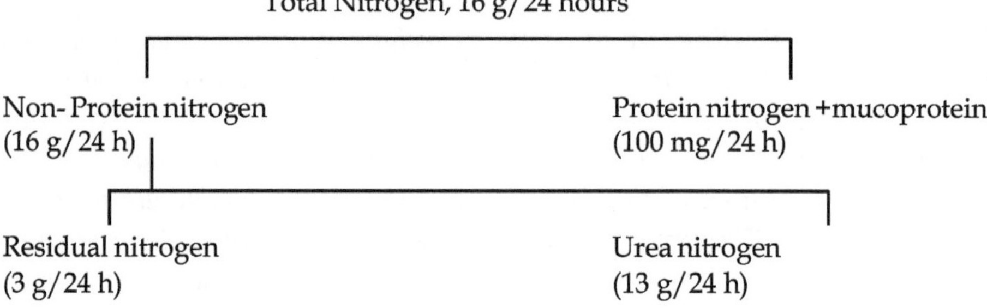

a. Creatinine nitrogen, 0.6 g/24 hrs
b. Uric acid nitrogen, 0.2 g/24 hrs
c. Ammonia nitrogen, 0.5 g/24 hrs
d. Amino acid nitrogen, 0.5 g/24 hrs
e. Hippuric acid nitrogen, 0.1 g/24 hrs

1. Protein = Protein nitrogen X 6.54
2. Urea = Urea nitrogen X 2.14
3. Creatinine = Creatinine nitrogen X 2.69
4. Uric acid = Uric acid nitrogen X 3.00
5. Ammonia = Ammonia nitrogen X 1.22
6. Hippuric acid = Hippuric acid nitrogen X 12.79

Ammonia nitrogen in rumen liquor, blood and feed sample

Reagents

1. *Boric acid. The strength depends somewhat on the range expected. Upto 300 μg NH_3 - N, 1 percent suffices. To make a litre of the reagent, 10 grams of the purest boric acid are introduced into a one litre flask, 200 ml alcohol are added, then about 700 ml distilled water. The boric acid is brought into solution add 10 ml of the mixed indicator (bromocresol green and methyl red) are added. On mixing, the whole is brought to the desired end-point colour of faint reddish, which usually requires the addition of a little alkali, and the mixture is made up to the mark.*

2. *Mixed indicator. This contains bromocresol green, 0.033 percent and methyl red 0.066 percent in alcohol. It keeps indefinitely.*

3. *N/10 HCI. Dissolve 8.845 ml conc. HCI in one litre distilled water, titrate it against N/10 NaOH (secondary standard) and N/10 oxalic acid (Primary standard).*

4. *Saturate potassium carbonate. Weigh 110 grams of K_2CO_3 in 100 ml distilled water. heat until dissolved.*
5. *Gum arabic fixative. To 10 parts by weight of powered gum acacia (also termed gum arabic) are added, 15 volume water, 5 volume glycerol and 5 volume saturated potassium carbonate. In preparing this fixative, water is added slowly to the powder, the mixture being ground in a large mortar to hasten the solution of the gum. The glycerol and carbonate are then added and stirred in. The mixture may then be used or poured into a large separating funnel and allowed to settle overnight, when the lower fluid can be separated easily from a somewhat frothy upper layer and stored in a stoppered vessel. In using a few drops are smeared over a glass lid or may be applied at the brim of glasslid.*
6. *Ammonia (NH_3-N) standard solution. Dissolve 0.471 g of pure ammonium sulphate in one litre ammonia free distilled water. Pipette 2 ml of this stock solution in a 100 ml volumetric flask and made upto mark with ammonia free distilled water. This will give a concentration (2 μ g/ml) of NH_3-N.*

Equipments

1. Conway Petridish

These are specially designed petridish which has two chambers and glass lid. In India such type of Conway petridish are available in the country.

2. Agla Micrometer syringe outfit

This syringe is used for titration purpose and manufactured by M/s Wellcome Reagents Ltd. (England).

Processing of Feed Sample

Weigh one gram sample in a test tube and add 10 ml ammonia free distilled water, cork it and keep it for overnight in an incubator at 39°C. Centrifuge the material in the test tube at 3000 rpm for 10 minutes, separate out the supernatant for estimation purpose.

Procedure

Pipette 1 ml boric acid in central chamber and deliver 1 ml posassium carbonate in the outer chamber. Smear gum fixative on the brim of lid. Measure one ml of rumen liquor or plasma or supernatant from test tube (containing feed sample) in the outer chamber. After one hour titrate with N/10 HCI, the central chamber contents using AGLA micro meter syringe outfit as designed specially for the purpose by Conway (1957).

Blank for Ammonia Nitrogen

Measure 1 ml ammonia free distilled water in the place of unknown sample aliquot, follow rest of the procedure as usual.

Calculation

Ammonia or urea nitrogen in 100 gram feed sample

Ammonia or urea nitrogen per ml extract =
R x A x 14 x 0.02 = U
R x 0.028 = U

U mg of ammonia or urea nitrogen per ml extract

Each gram of the sample corresponds to :

$\frac{10+0.1W}{W}$ (ml) extract

Therefore 100 g sample will corresponds to ;

$\frac{10+0.1W}{W}$ X 100 ml extract

where 10 is volume of distilled water added in 1 g of sample
0.1 = 10 % moisture in sample
W = Weight of sample in grams

Hence if U is mg of ammonia or urea nitrogen in 1 ml extract, the amount of ammonia or urea nitrogen in 100 gram of sample will be U X $\frac{10+0.1}{W}$ X 100 = Z .... Formula A

Finally the concentration of ammonia or urea nitrogen will be Z mg/100 gram sample

Example

1. Estimation of ammonia nitrogen in sample D

Moisture percent	=	9%
Weight of material taken	=	1 g
Reading of AGLA micro meter syringe	=	3.49 micro litre
Reading X 0.028	=	mg ammonia nitrogen in one ml extract
3.49 X 0.028		= 0.09772 mg ammonia nitrogen in 1 ml extract.

Apply formula A and use the above data.

0.09772 x 1009 = 98.59948 mg ammonia nitrogen per 100g sample.

= 0.09859948 g ammonia nitrogen per 100g sample

Result : Sample D contained ammonia nitrogen 0.09859948 g per 100 g dry matter.

II. Estimation of ammonia nitrogen in plasma samples from buffalo

Ammonia nitrogen = R x A x 14 x 0.02 x 100
(mg/100 ml) = R x 2.8

where

R = is reading of micrometer syring outfit.
A = is the normality of acid used in the titration

Factor = 0.02 is calibration constant of AGLA micrometer syringe outfit.

In the present case, suppose the value of R is 0.24, then ammonia nitrogen concentration will be

= 0.24 x 2.8
= 0.672 mg/100 ml

Result : The given sample of plasma contained 0.672 mg ammonia nitrogen /100 ml.

☞ **Note**

We may calculate ammonia by using relationship

Ammonia = Ammonia nitrogen x 1.22

III. Estimation of ammonia in rumen liquor samples from buffalo

Note: Use same formula as mentiond in the case of plasma. In the present case suppose the value of R is 3.685, then ammonia nitrogen concentration will be

= 3.685 x 2.8
= 10.318 mg

Result : The given sample of rumen liquor contained 10.318 mg ammonia nitrogen per 100 ml.

☞ **Note**

We may calculate ammonia by using relationship

Ammonia = Ammonia nitrogen X 1.22

General note

1. Cork the centrifuge tube containing sample and keep in the incubator at 39°C.
2. Apply a very thin layer of gum arabica on the brim of lid.
3. Immediately put lid after adding potassium carbonate solution.
4. Immediately put lid after adding urease in the outer chamber of Conway petridish
5. After titration, watch the permanent stay of pink colour, if colour disappears then add 1 drop N/10 HCI.
6. Washing of Conway petridish should be done very carefully with ammonia free distilled water and there should be no grease in the central chamber of petridish, otherwise boric acid will not be spread.
7. Testing of distilled water for the presence of ammonia could be done using Tashiro's indicator, if water remain light pink on adding indicator then it is ammonia free, if the colour of water is green then it contained ammonia.
8. In the case of meat and blood samples, use of 2 percent boric acid is recommended.
9. It is recommended that extract of feed samples should not be kept for more than 24 hours at 39°C.

Urea nitrogen in blood, rumen liquor, feed sample

Reagents

☞ **Note**

All the reagents are same which has been used in the case of ammonia estimation except urease phosphate mixture.

1. Preparatioin of urease-phosphate mixture

The glycerol extract of jack bean (Conway, 1957) has been found very satisfactory, it retains its activity for many months in the refrigerator. In the usual routine this is diluted ten times with an equal volume of phosphate solution before use. It has been experienced that incorporating the phosphate in the original preparation produced an extract which has very good keeping powers and filters quickly. The preparation is made as follow:

To 10 grams of jack bean meal, 20 ml of water is added and the mixture is agitated vigorously for about 15 minutes (a mechanical stirrer or shaker may be conveniently employed). 100 ml phosphate buffer at pH 7.4 (3 g anhydrous Na_2HPO_4) and 2 g anhydrous KH_2PO_4 in 100 ml water) and 20 ml glycerol is added. This mixture is shaken well, allowed to stand for a short time and the fluid is decanted on to a large folded filter paper. The mixture filters comparatively quickly and may then be cleared of traces of ammonia or stored directly. To clear solution from NH_3, 5 grams finely powdered permutit, washed with 2 percent acetic acid is added and allowed to settle, the acid is decanted and the permutit washed twice with distilled water. To the permutit is added the urease phosphate preparation, the mixture is well shaken for some time and allowed to settle when the clear fluid is decanted off and stored in the refrigerator. A small volume of this is diluted three times when required for a series of determinations.

2. Preparation of urease-phosphate enzyme using urease tablets.

a. Phosphate buffer is prepared as below

0.2 N $NaH_2PO_4.2H_2O$. (A) Dissolve 27.6 g Sodium dihydrogen phosphate in one litre ammonia free distilled water.

0.2 N $Na_2 HPO_4. 2H_2O$ (B) Dissolve 71.7 grams disodium hydrogen phosphate in one litre ammonia free distilled water.

pH 7 : A 39.0 ml] + ammonia free distilled
B 61.0 ml] water till 200 ml

Dissolve urease Tablets at the rate of 10mg/ml phosphate buffer.

3. Urea standard solution

Dissolve 5 grams reagent grade urea in water and dilute to one litre water: Pipette 2, 6, 8, 10, 12, 14, 16, 18 and 20 ml stock solution into 250 ml volumetric flasks and dilute it to volume with phosphate buffer. Dilution contain 0.2, 0.4, 0.6, 0.8, 1.0, 1.2, 1.4, 1.6, 1.8, and 2.0 mg urea/5 ml respectively.

Reference solution

Use standard solution containing 1 mg urea /5 ml as reference standard. Store at temperatue 24°C. This solution is stable for a week.

Procedure in the Case of Feed Sample

As mentioned previously in the case of ammonia estimation, feed sample is incubated at 39° C for overnight and centrifuged at 3000 rpm. Decant the supernatant using micro-pipette, Now measure 1 ml of supernatant using micro pipette in the outer chamber. In the central chamber measure 1 ml boric acid. Add 0.5 ml urease in the outer chamber. Incubate the contents of petridish at 39°C for $1\frac{3}{4}$ hrs. After $1\frac{3}{4}$ hrs incubation add 1 ml potassium carbonate in the outer chamber. Again incubate the contents of petridish for one hour at 39°C. Residual urea nitrogen will be liberated, then titrate the content of central chamber with N/100 HCI till the original colour of boric acid return to reddish pink, calculate the result as mentioned in the following example:

Example

Name of sample	- Sample "D"
Weight of sample "A" taken in the centgrifuge tube	= 1 g
Reading of AGLA micro-meter syringe outfit.	= 2.31
mg urea nitrogen in 1 ml extract	= Reading x 0.028 extract
mg urea nitrogen in 1 ml extract	= 2.31 x 0.028 = 0.06468

Apply formula "A" (See Ammonia-N calculation) and use the above data.

0.06468 X 1009	= 65.26212 mg urea-N/100 g
-do-	= 0.06526212 g urea N/100 g

The sample "D" contained 0.6526212 g/100 g urea nitrogen. If results are required in term of urea only then multiply by 2.14 as mentioned below:

Urea = 2.14 x urea nitrogen
= 2.14 x 0.06526212
= 0.1396564 g/100 g

The sample "D" contained 0.1396564 g urea per 100 g feed sample.

Note : Blank for urea estimation : Measure 1 ml ammonia free distilled water in the place of unknown sample aliquot and rest of the procedure is same.

Procedure in the case of serum and plasma urea nitrogen

Pipette 1 ml boric acid in the central chamber. Measure 1 ml urease-phosphate enzyme preparation in the outside chamber and add 1 ml serum or plasma simultaneously. Mix urease enzyme with the serum or plasma by tilting the conway petridish. Keep it in the incubator at 39°C for $1\frac{3}{4}$ hrs. After $1\frac{3}{4}$ hrs incubation, add 1 ml saturated potassium carbonate in the outer chamber. Again incubate the contents of petridish for one hour at 39°C, titrate content of central chamber using AGLA micro-meter syringe outfit filled with N/10 HCI. The results may be calculated as mentioned below:

Calculation

Estimation of urea nitrogen in plasma samples from buffaloes.

Urea nitrogen = R x A x 14 x 0.02 x 100
(mg/100 ml) = R x 2.8

where

R = is reading of micrometer syringe outfit

A = is the normality of acid used in the titration.

Factor 0.02 is calibration constant of *AGLA micro-meter syringe outfit.*

In the present case, suppose the value of R is 8.04 ml, then urea nitrogen concentration will be:

= 8.04 x 2.8

= 22.512 mg/100 ml

Result : The given sample of plasma contained 22.512 mg/100 ml.

Note : Blank for urea estimation: It is always advisable to run blank simultaneously with set of estimation. The micro-meter syrings reading is then subtracted from the previous recorded reading (in the case of unknown sample).

Fraction of proteins (albumin and globulin) in a sample of serum using Conway diffusion technique : Method.

Reagents

1. *Digestion mixture : The digest mixture is made of equal parts of concentrated sulphuric acid and saturated KHSO4 and contains about 0.2g SeO2 per 100 ml. (Copper sulphate may also be included, but not more than 0.1 g per 100 ml., as it tends to inhibit the rate of the subsequent ammonia release).*
2. *23 per cent sulphate (anhydrous) solution maintained in the incubator.*
3. *0.6 or 0.9 % NaCl*
4. *2 % boric acid reagent*
5. *40 per cent KOH*
6. *N/50 HCl*

Procedure

1 ml of the serum is pipetted into two conical flasks of about 50 ml capacity. Into the first is run 25 ml of 0.9 per cent NaCl.

Into the second flask is added 25 ml of warm 23 per cent (stored at 37°C) sodium sulphate solution. The stoppered flasks with the contents are mixed and placed in the incubator at 37°C for one and half and hours.

The contents of flask 2 are filtered. Five ml volume of each conical flask is introduced into 100 ml. Incinerating flasks, and 2.5 ml of the digest mixture is added (from a graduated 5 ml pipette.). Incinerate in the usual manner, with small funnel in neck of flask.

After incinerating, cool and add 25 ml water from a pipette to each and mix well.

Ammonia determination. One ml 2 per cent boric acid reagent is added to the central chambers of micro diffusion "units" and 1 ml of the final mixture is delivered in the outer chambers. The subsequent procedure is as before, release ammonia using 1 ml of 40 per cent KOH as the alkali. After 2 hours incubation, titrate with N/50 HCl from the Conway micro-meter syringe outfit.

Calculation

Multiply the number of large divisions of micrometer syringe outfit (minus blank) for the first mixture (without sodium sulphate) by 0.217 which gives the alubmin and globulin as g/100 ml.

The similar reading for the second mixture is multiplied by 0.209 which gives the albumin as g/100 ml.

Total non-protein nitrogen in blood using Conway-diffusion technique : Method.

De-proteinising

This is carried out by the method of Folin and Wu (1919). One part of blood is haemolysed in 7 parts of water and then treated successively with 1 part of 10 per cent sodium tungstate and 1 part of 2/3 N sulphuric acid. The mixture is vigorously shaken and allowed to stand until it has assumed a chocolate colour (about 15-20 minutes). It is then filtered or centrifuged.

Digestion

Into a 100 ml kjeldahl incinerating flask is pipetted 10 ml of the filtrate (corresponding to 1 ml blood or plasma) and 2 ml of the digest mixture is added. The water first boils off, and the incineration is carried on for about five minutes after dense anhydride fumes appear using a microburner, is then begum with a small funnel in the incinerating flask.

Ammonia Determination

After cooling, 10 ml of distilled water is pipetted into the flask and mixed with the remaining contents. One ml of the mixture is pipetted into the outer chambers of 2 or more "units" and 1 ml boric acid reagent is delivered in the central chamber of Conway petridish. As already described, 1 ml 40 per cent KOH is used to release the ammonia.

After two and half an hours incubation period, the contents of the central chamber is titrated with N/50 HCl from the AGLA micrometer syringe outfit.

Calculation

The number of large division used for the titration is multiplied by 3.08 and the result expresses the non-protein nitrogen per cent. (in the calculation it is assumed that 1 ml remains after incineration).

Total nitrogen in feeds and rumen liquor samples : Method

Conway diffusion technique (Conway, 1957) is quite successful in estimating total nitrogen (over 100 μg N) in the samples of feed and rumen liquor. Whe large number either determinations of total nitrogen are being carried out either of macro or micro kind, the micro diffusion principle, in conjunction with the Kjeldahl digestion, is of value in considerably diminishing the work in such serial determinations, and also for the all micro ranges increases the accuracy of the procedure.

In the incineration process the use of certain catalysts in excess should be avoided for example, copper sulphate, since it shows the absorption considerably when in comparatively high concentration. It may still be used when in small quantitites of 0.1 per cent solution. *Copper is not so good a catalyst as mercury, selenium, tellurium, titanium, or iron.*

For the alkalinisation of the digest or aliquot part thereof, saturated metaborate or 40 per cent KOH would appear the most suitable. With 40 per cent KOH the times for diffusion are about 25-30 per cent longer than with metaborate.

Saturated potassium metaborate and saturated potassium carbonate have practically the same effect in raising the ammonia tension of solutions, and hence increasing the absorption rate, but the carbonate cannot be used here owing to the high acidity of the digest.

Macro-Kjeldahl determinations

Example 1. Sample : Wheat flour

Incineration. 0.5 g of flour is weighed into a 300 ml Kjeldahl flask incinerating flask. 10 ml of the digest mixture is added and the mixture incinerated in the usual way with a small funnel in the top of the incinerating flask, somewhat longer than the usual clearing time of the fluid being allowed.

Digest mixture. The digest mixture is made of equal parts of concentrated H_2SO_4 and saturated $KHSO_4$ and contains about 0.2 gram SeO_2 per 100 ml (copper sulphate may be also included, but not more than 0.1 gram per 100 ml, as it tends to inhibit the rate of the subsequent ammonia release).

Ammonia determinations : Subsequently the mixture is cooled. 25 ml water is added cautiously and cooled under the tap. The mixture is now made up to 50 ml in a volumetric falsk, and 0.5 ml in duplicate is pipetted into the outer chamber of two or three "units" (No. 1). The pipetting may be very accurately and suitably done by means of a straight tube pipette taking about 10-20 seconds to deliver, and the final fluid blown out immediately after delivery with the tip touching the glass.

After pipetting the fluid, the "units" are allowed to remain on the bench for about five minutes (to allow escape of any volatile acid formed in the incineration), 1 ml of boric acid reagent which need be only roughly measured is run into the central chambers of the "units". Two ml of saturated potassium metaborate or 1 ml of 40 per cent KOH is added in the usual way after placing the lid with fixative in position, and the contents of the outer chamber mixed by rotation and left on the bench for one and half an hours. The contents of the central chambers are then titrated with N/50 HCl from the AGLA micrometer syringe outfit.

Calculation

The number of large divisions (each equal to 0.01 ml) required in the titration, is multiplied by 0.056 to give the nitrogen as gram per cent in the sample of flour.

Example 2. Sample : urine

Incineration : 2 ml of urine is pipetted into the incinerating flask from a straight tube pipette (a standard 2 ml pipette is also suitable). The pipette, about 15 to 20 cm long, should take about 10-20 seconds to deliver, the final amount being blown out gently with the tip against glass and rotating while blowing. Remaining procedure is same as given in *example 1.*

Ammonia determination : After the incineration as above the dilution is made to 200 ml and the ammonia determination made in the same way. The calculation is the same as for *example 1.*

Accuracy of the above macro-Kjeldahl determinations

It has been well established that the diffusion technique can give an accuracy as great as the macro-kjedahl conducted at the 25 to 50 ml titration level. With regard to the passage of the ammonia from the kjeldahl digest to the acid, it is obvious that the diffusion procedure is much less liable to error, and goes automatically without any observation being required during the process.

Trimethylamine (TMA) in Spoiled Flesh

Principle

Following chemical reactions may occur in spoiled flesh (Pearson, 1973).

1. Breakdown (deamination) of protein producing ammonia, indole, skatole, H_2S etc.
2. Formation of trimethylamine (TMA) from trimethylamine Oxide (TMO) due to reduction by bacteria.

   Lacitc acid + TMO Acetic acid + TMA + Water
3. Formation of dimethylamine (DMA) - precursor unknown.
4. Formation of ammonia from urea due to bacterial action

   $$\text{Urea + Water} \xrightarrow{\text{urease}} \text{Ammonia + Carbondioxide}$$
5. Spoilage of fat causing hydrolysis (FFA production) and oxidative and other forms of rancidity. Usually volatile bases (TVB or TVN = ammonia + amines) are often estimated as a group. In the case of fresh white fish, total volatile nitrogen is less than 20 mg per 100g, while in the case of spoiled white fish, it is more than 50g/ 100 g flesh.

On adding potassium carbonate solution to fish extract, volatile nitrogen is released, which diffuses into boric acid solution. The absorbed base is then titrated with acid. By using deproteinised juice and carrying out the diffusion below, say, 45°C, no additional breakdown of protein is possible. If formalin is added to the juice prior to the addition of alkali, the ammonia reacts to form hexamethylenetetramine and only the TMA diffuses over into the boric acid.

$$\text{Formalin + Ammonia} \longrightarrow \text{Hexamethylenetetramine + water.}$$

Reagents

1. *We use the same reagents which has been advised for ammonia estimation mentioned previously.*
2. *Formalin (AR grade).*

Preparation of Extract

Triturate thoroughly 2.5 grams of trichloroacetic acid with 50 g of minced fish (or meat) in glass mortar. Allow the mixture to stand for 30 min., then filter it, first on Buchner funnel (press the sample well down) and then using an ordinary funnel (Whatman No. 5 filter paper). Store the filtered extract at 0°C in a small screw caped bottle. Carry out estimations in duplicate together with a blank.

Procedure (TVN)

For estimating total volatile nitrogen (TVN), procedure is same which has been followed in the case of ammonia nitrogen.

Procedure (TMA)

Add 20 drops of the neutral formalin to the outer compartment of Conway dish and then deliver 1 ml fish extract and 1 ml saturated potassium carbonate and incubate at 36°C for one hour. Titrate with N/10 Hcl, the central chamber contents using AGLA micro-meter syringe outfit. Calculate the results as done in the case of ammonia nitrogen. We may use colorimetric method developed by Fernandez-Flores and Salwin (1968) for estimating ammonia nitrogen in fish sample.

References

Conway, E.J. and Malley, E.O. (1942). *Biochem. J.*, 36: 655.

Conway, E.J. (1957). *Microdifussion analysis and volumetric error*, 4th edn., Crossby, Lockwood and Son Ltd., London.

Fernandez-Flores, E. and Salwin, H. (1968). *J.Ass. Off. Analyst. Chem.*, 51 : 1109.

Folin, O. and Wu, H. (1919). *J. Biol.Chem.*, 38 : 98.

Krishna, G., Paliwal, V.K. & Yadav K.R. (1980). True protein and non protein fractions in Agro-Industrial Wastes/byproducts in Haryana State. *Haryana Agricultural Univ., J. Res.* 11: 458-462.

Krishna, G. (1979). A note on menace of urea adulteration in Indian Poultry feeds. *Poultry Guide.* 16: 59-62.

Pearson, D. (1973). *Laboratory techniques in food analysis.* First edn. Butterworths, London. pp 168.

Richterich, R. (1969). *Clinical chemistry - Theory and Practice,* English translation. S. Karger, Basel (Switzerland) pp 88.

Tiwari, S.P., Krishna, G. and Naresh Kumar, (1993). Nitrogen metabolism in growing male buffalo calves fed guarseed (*Cyamopsis Tetragonoloba* L.) and groundnut Cake. *Indian Vety. J.* 70: 519-523.

Winkler, (1913). *Angew. Chem.* 26 : 231.

Chapter - 69

Colorimetric Methods of Trace Element Analysis

Steps in the Estimation of Trace Elements

Estimation of trace elements in feeds and fodders and other biological materials involves the following steps :

1. Production of an acidic solution of the inorganic elements in the biological samples after removal of the organic matter by dry ashing or wet oxidation.
2. Removal or masking of interfering substances.
3. Determination of the selected elements, usually by using colorimetry.

Results of trace elements determinations are expressed as parts per million (ppm), mg/kg or μg/g dry matter.

Dry ashing procedure of biological samples is mentioned under chapter entitled, *"Atomic absorption Spectrophotometry"* of this Compendium.

Wet ashing (Oxidation) Procedure of wet oxidation of biological sample is mentioned in this compendium.

Copper in Biological Samples

(Method of Eden and Green, 1940 modified by Sandell, 1959)

At the Indian Veterinary Research Institute, Izatnagar (India), method proposed by Eden and Green (1940) modified by Sandell (1959) is followed for the estimation of copper in the biological materials. Author has used this method for his M.V.Sc. degree research work at IVRI, IZAT NAGAR (U.P.), India, (Krishna & Mahadevan, 1969).

Principle

Callan and Henderson (1929) discovered that when diethyldithiocarbamate is added to a solution of copper, a golden brown colour is produced. McFarlane (1932) found that the coloured copper salt could be rapidly and quantitatively extracted from aqueous solution by amyl alcohol and that the colour was intensified in the organic solvent. The colour complex is stable for at least two hours and the pH of solution has little effect on the colour intensity between pH 5.9 and 9.2. Iron gives a brown colour with the reagent and is the only substance in biological ash which is known to interfere significantly. However, when sodium pyrophosphate is added, iron pyrophosphate is formed and this complex does not react with carbamate, whereas the reactiontity of copper is unaffected. In this microestimation method of copper, amyl alcohol is used because ionisation of copper salt is depressed in the organic solvent, this intensifying the colour and so giving the reaction greater sensitivity.

The whole method is divided into four stages.

1. *Wet oxidation.*
2. *Deionisation*
3. *Colour development*
4. *Colour measurement*

Reagent

1. *Sulphuric acid AR*
2. *Perchloric acid, Baker's analysed (70%)*
3. *Nitric acid, AR*
4. *Sodium pyrophosphate 4% solution*
5. *Hydrochloric acid, AR*
6. *Ammonia (concentrated). Analar sp.gr. 0.980.*
7. *Amyl alcohol A.R.*
8. *Sodium diethyl dithiocarbamate*
9. *Standard copper solutions*

Preparation of reagents

Reagent No. 8 : Sodium diethyl-dithiocarbamate solution. 5 g sodium diethyl dithiocarbamate is dissolved in 100 ml distilled water. It may be heated at 60-70°C for half an hour to dissolve most of the carbamate when using, filter the solution and dilute a known volume of the solution with three times the volume of distilled water to give 0.5 % carbamate solution. Stock solution should be kept in dark.

Reagent No. 9 : Standard copper solution. 0.3928 gram pure copper sulphate (crystal) E. Merck showing no signs of fluorescence is dissolved in water, a drop of sulphuric acid being added to prevent the formation of basic copper sulphate on hydrolysis. The solution is made up to one litre (1 ml = 0.1μg Cu), 25 ml of the later solution is diluted further to 250 ml (giving 0.01μg Cu/ml) water.

Wet Oxidation : In the case of feeds and faeces, 1 gram sample is weighed in micro-kjeldahl flask and digested using procedure mentioned in this compendium.

In the case of blood, 5 ml of citrated blood is taken up in micro-kjeldahl flask and digested using procedure mentioned in this compendium.

In the case of water, about 1000 ml water is evaporated in large silica crucible on water bath, but at a time only 50 ml water is evaporated and in different lots, the required amount should be taken for the purpose. After this the dried residue is digested using the wet oxidation procedure.

In the case of milk, 10 ml aliquot is taken in the micro-kjeldahl flask and digested using the wet oxidation procedure mentioned in this compendium.

In the case of wet tissue, 1 to 5 grams of wet tissue is taken in the micro-kjeldahl flask and digested using the wet oxidation procedure mentioned in this compendium.

For urine the wet oxidation procedure has to be slightly modified becasue of the larger volume require to obtain sufficient copper for subsequent determination. 50 ml urine is measured into a 100 ml pyrex kjeldahl flask and about 3 ml nitric acid added and two glass beads to prevent bumping. Heating is carefully controlled to bring through the boiling point without undue frothing, and smooth boiling is continued over a low flame until the volume is reduced to about 2 ml. The flame is turned out and after cooling actual wet oxidation procedure is followed using 1 ml of sulphuric acid, 3 ml perchloric acid and a few ml nitric acid.

☞ Notes

In case of tissues and feeds rich in Ca and P and in case of faeces proceed as follows :

After digestion, add 5 ml distilled water in the kjeldahl flask, heat to dissolve, next add 10 ml of 4 per cent sodium pyrophosphate solution, shake, and then heat the flask for 20 minutes in a water bath to make the percipitate granular. Next filter through an acid extracted filter paper into a glass stoppered graduated cylinder. Wash the flask twice with 5 ml hot distilled water and the filter paper twice with 3 ml hot distilled water. Next add 2 ml ammonia and on cooling make up the volume equal to that of standard and proceed as before.

Transferring to Stoppered Cylinder

Before the stop of deionisation the digested material is transferred in a 50 ml glass stoppered cylinder. First 5 ml of glass distilled water is added to the flask and flask is gently warmed on the low burner flame for 1 minute and the digested material is filtered through 9 cm No. 42 filter paper into the glass stoppered cylinder and flask is washed thrice with 5 ml distilled water.

Deionisation

5 ml of 4 per cent sodium pyrophosphate is added in the kjeldahl flask and warmed on the low flame, cooled and transferred to a 50 ml glass stoppered cylinder, again 5 ml of 4 per cent sodium pyrophosphate is added and warmed, cooled and transferred to a 50 ml stoppered cylinder, finally flask is washed with 5 ml glass distilled water and washing transferred to the cylinder, after transferring the material completely in the cylinder, 5 ml of ammonia (Sp. gr. 0.880) is added, cylinders are shaken completely and kept for cooling upto 15 minutes, then the volume is made upto 50 ml.

Colour Development and Extraction

The digested and oxidised material is then quantitatively transferred to pyrex separating funnel washed with glass distilled water, and two washings of glass stoppered cylinder is done with 2 ml glass distilled water. 2 ml of 0.5 per cent recently filtered sodium diethyl dithiocarbamate is added with the help of a pipette and 7 ml amyl alcohol is added with the help of glass distilled water rinsed pipettes, the contents of the funnel is vigorously shaken for about 1 minute, yellow copper compound readily dissolved in the amyl alcohol and remains at the top, contents below the amyl alcohol layer is drawn out and comparison is done against blank and extinction is observed on the scale of Hilger Photoelectric colorimeter, amount of copper in μg/g or mg/kg, i.e. ppm is calculated by taking observation against optical density with the help of standard graph. 430 mμ filter paper of the colorimeter is used for taking the reading.

Blank 10 ml of glass distilled water is measured in the glass stoppered cylinder, 1 ml distilled sulphuric acid is added and further operations are same as we did with the other samples.

☞ **Notes**

1. *If vitreosil basins are used for evaporation of water then the basins are treated for the removal of copper as follows :*

   To each basin is added alcoholic solution of sodium acetate containing 1 gram of the salt, the latter is evaporated to dryness and ignited and basins are then allowed to stand for several days in 1:1 (HCl).

2. *Glass apparatus used must be cleaned first with vim or other cleaning powder and then with dilute Hcl and finally with distilled water.*

3. *A fresh solution of 0.5 per cent sodium diethyl-dithio-carbamate must be prepared by filtering through 42 No. filter paper.*

Cobalt in Biological Samples

(Method of Marston and Dewey, 1940 modified by Sandell, 1959)

Principle : Cobalt is extracted from ash solution with dithizone. Cobalt forms a red complex with sodium l-nitroso-2-naphthol-3. 6-disulphonate, nitroso-R salt, which is stable in boiling nitric acid. This last property makes possible a determination that is nearly specific for cobalt. Three moles of reagent combine with one of cobalt. This reaction furnishes a most sensitive method for the determination of traces of cobalt such in soils, plants and animal organs.

Equipments

1. Spectronic '20' or equivalent spectrophotometer.
2. Separating funnel.
3. Vitreosil crucible.

Reagents

1. *Nitroso-R salt (sodium - 1- nitroso-2-hydroxy naphthalene-3.6-disulphonate) 0.2% aqueous solution. This solution under goes no change for months if kept in the dark.*

2. *Standard cobalt stock solution. 0.0100% cobalt. Dissolve 0.040 grams of* $CoCl_2 . 6H_2O$ *in water, add 1 ml of concentrated HCl and dilute to 100 ml. From this solution prepare a more dilute one (10 micrograms of cobalt per millilitre).*

3. *Citric acid, 0.20 M. Dissolve 4.2 grams of the monohydrate citric acid in water and dilute to 100 ml.*

4. *Buffer solution. Dissolve 6.2 grams of boric acid, 35.6 grams of disodium phosphate dihydrate and 500 ml of 1N sodium hydroxide in a total volume of one litre.*

5. *Dithizone : Dissolve 0.5 gram dithizone in 600 to 700 ml* CCl_4 *. Filter into 5 litre separatory funnel containing 2.5 to 3.0 litres of 0.02 N* NH_4OH*, shake well, and discard* CCl_4 *layer, Shake with 50 ml portions of high grade* CCl_4 *until* CCl_4 *phase, as it separates, has pure green colour. Add one litre of* CCl_4 *and acidify slightly with HCl (1+1). Shake the dithizone into* CCl_4 *layer and discard aqueous layer. Store in cool, dark place, preferably in refrigerator.*

6. *Ammonium citrate solution. (40%) Dissolve 800 grams of citric acid in 600 ml of water and while stirring, add slowly 900 ml* NH_4OH*. Adjust pH to 8.5, if necessary. Dilute to two litres and extract with 25 ml portions of dithizone solution until aqueous phase stays orange and* CCl_4 *until all orange colour is removed.*

7. *Hydrogen peroxide, 30%*

8. *Concentrated sulphuric acid.*

9. *Concentrated nitric acid.*

10. *Concentrated hydrochloric acid.*

11. *Phenolphthalein, 1% alcoholic solution. Dissolve 1 gram in 95 per cent ethyl alcohol and dilute to 100 ml.*

12. *Ammonium hydroxide (1+1). Distill concentrated* NH_4OH *into equal volume of water.*

13. HNO_3 *and* H_2SO_4 *solution combine 45 ml concentrated nitric acid and 30 ml concentrated sulphuric acid.*

Procedure

1. Weigh 6 grams sample into a vitreosil crucible.

2. Ash at 500°C overnight, Cool, Dissolve ash with 3 ml conc. HCl and add 25 ml water. Evaporate two-third of solution. Add 15 ml water. Evaporate two-thirds of solution.

   Add 15 ml water. Evaporate one-half of solution. Filter into 25 ml volumetric flask and make to volume.

3. Transfer all or part of this solution to a 150 ml separatary funnel. Add 5 ml of the ammonium citrate solution and one drop phenolphthalein solution : adjust to pH 8.5 with citrate. Add 10 ml of the dithizone in CCl_4 and shake the solution for five minutes. Drain CCl_4 phase into 100 ml beaker. Repeat as many times as necessary, using 5 ml quantities

of dithizone solution and shaking five minutes each times Extraction is complete when aqueous phase remains orange and CCl_4 phase remains predominantly green.

4. Then add 100 ml CCl_4, shake five minutes, and combine with CCl_4 extract. Final 10 ml CCl_4 should be pure green. If not, extraction is incomplete and must be repeated.
5. Add 2 ml of HNO_3 and H_2SO_4 solution evaporate to dryness Cool. Add 20 ml water. Add 2 ml 30 per cent H_2SO_4 until solution is clear. Evaporate solution to 5 ml volume. Add 1 ml of citric acid solution and 1.2 ml of phosphate-boric buffer. The pH should be 8.0; if not, add more buffer until pH 8.0 is reached.
6. Add exactly 0.5 ml of nitroso-R salt solution, while strirring. Boil for one minute, add 1 ml of concentrated nitric acid, and again for exactly one minute.
7. Cool immediately in the dark and make up to 10 ml after transferring to volumetric flask. Observe the optical density of the solution at 420 millimicron. Compare the observed optical density to a standard cobalt curve ranging from 0 to 10 microgram cobalt per 10 ml final volume.

Calculations

Cobalt (mg per kg) on as fed basis.

$$= \frac{\text{Micrograms cobalt in sample}}{\text{Wt. of sample before ashing (grams)}}$$

Adjust to dry basis

$$= \frac{\text{Cobalt (mg/kg) on as fed sample}}{\text{dry matter \% of as fed sample}} \times 100$$

Manganese in Biological Samples

(Method of Strickland and Spicer, 1949; Waterbury *et al.*, 1952 modified by Sandell, 1959).

Principle : The colorimetric determination of manganese by oxidation to permanganate in acid solution is both sensitive and specific. Periodate oxidases managanous salts comerted smoothly to permanganate. The reaction is as follows :

$$2\ MN^{++} + 5IO^-_4 + 3H_2O = 2MnO^-_4 + 5IO^-_3 + 6H^+$$

Phosphoric acid decolourises ferric iron by complex formation, and its presence is desirable in any case since it prevents possible precipitation of periodate or iodates of manganese.

Equipments

1. *Spectronic "20"*
2. *Vitreosil crucibles.*

Reagents

1. *Concentrated sulphuric acid.*
2. *Concentrated nitric acid.*
3. *Phosphoric acid (85%).*
4. *Sodium or potassium periodate (meta).*
5. *Hydrofluoric acid (48%).*
6. *Standard manganese solution.*

Preparation of Standard Manganese Solution

Dissolve 0.5756 gram of dry potassium permanganate in about 50 ml of water in a beaker of suitable size. Add 40 ml of concentrated sulphuric acid and reduce the permanganate by careful addition of sodium metabisulphite solution until the manganese solution just becomes colourless. Oxidise the excess sulphuric acid in the hot solution by the addition of a little nitric acid. Cool and transfer the solution quantitatively to a 2 litre graduated flask. Make up the volume and store the solution in a glass stoppered reagent bottle. This solution contains 0.1 mg of manganese per millilitre.

Procedure

1. Weight 5 gram material in a conical flask and ash as per method mentioned below under 2.
2. Add 10 ml of 48 per cent hydrofluoric acid. This will prevent loss of manganese as insoluble silicate. Warm to dissolve, cool, add 10 ml concentrated sulphuric acid and evaporate under a fume hood until fumes of sulphuric trioxide come off. Transfer quantitatively to a 100 ml volumetric flask and dilute to volume. The ash may also be taken up directly in 10 ml concentrated nitric acid and dilute to volume.
3. The solution, ready for analysis (0.1 to 1.0 mg manganese), should contain 10 ml concentrated sulphuric or 15 to 20 ml nitric acid : and in addition, 5 to 10 ml of 85 per cent phosphoric acid in a volume of 100 ml. However, if the amount of manganese present is of the order of a few micrograms,

make the solution 2 N in sulphuric acid and add 20 mg of silver nitrate, in additon to phosphoric acid.

4. Add 0.3 gram of potassium meta-periodate, or equivalent amount of sodium meta-periodate for each 100 ml of solution. heat to boiling with stirring, and keep at or slighltly below the boiling point for 10 minutes for at least one hour for any small amounts of manganese and cool.

5. Dilute to volume and observe the optical density at 525 millimicrons (nm) in a spectrophotometer. Compare the observed optical density to a standard manganese curve ranging from 0.1 to 1.0 mg of manganese per 100 ml.

Calculations

$$\text{Manganese (mg/kg) on as fed basis} = \frac{\text{mg manganese in sample}}{\text{wt. of sample before ashing}} \times 1000$$

$$\text{Adjust to dry basis} = \frac{\text{manganese (mg/kg) on as fed basis}}{\text{dry matter \% of as fed sample}} \times 100$$

Iron in biological samples

Method of Woods and Mellon, 1941; Daniel and Harper, 1934; Powell and Taylor, 1954; Brown and Hayes, 1952; Venture and White, 1954; Peters *et al.*, 1939; Sandell, 1959).

Reagents

1. *Acetate buffer : Dissolve 16.6 grams of anhydrous sodium acetate (dried at 100°C in water, add 24 ml of glacial acetic acid) and dilute the mixture with water to 200 ml.*

2. *Hydroquinone solution : Dissolve 2.5 grams of hydroquinone in water, add 0.5 ml of concentrated HCI and dilute the mixture with water to 100 ml.*

3. *2.2′ Dipyridyl solution (0.1 per cent in water)*

4. *Standard iron solution (Formula 1). Dissolve 3.512 grams of Fe* $(NH4)_2(SO4)_2.6H2O$ *in water, add 2 drops of 5N HCl and dilute the mixture with water to 500 ml. Then, when required, dilute 10 ml of this solution to one litre (1 ml of solution contain 0.01 mg of Fe).*

   (Formula 2) : Dissolve 0.7022 gram of ferrous ammonium sulfate $(Fe\ SO_4\ (NH_4)_2\ SO_4\ 6\ H_2O)$ *in 100 ml of water, add 5 ml of concentrated sulphuric acid, warm slightly and add potassium permanganate solution*

(approximately 0.1 N) drop by drop until the solution shows a slight pink colouration. make up the volume to one litre in a graduated flask. Pipette 10 ml of this solution into a one litre graduated flask, add 10 ml of hydrogen peroxide solution and make up the volume with water. This solution contains one microgram of iron per millilitre.

Procedure

Clean a silica dish by heating HCl in it and then wash it thoroughly with water, taking precuations against contamination with metal from the tongs used. Ash a suitable amount of sample (e.g. 2-10 grams of feed sample) at 550°C. Add 2 ml of conc. HCl, cover the dish with a clock glass and place it on a water bath for 30 minutes. Carefully wash any drops of condensed water into the dish using a little water from a wash bottle.

Then transfer the ash solution down a rod, using several small volumes of water, into a 100 ml volumetric flask. Make up the volume to the mark with water, then mix and filter. To a boiling tube add 10 ml of filtrate (or smaller aliquot made up to 10 ml), 3 ml of acetate buffer, 2 ml of hydroquinone solution and 2 ml of 2, 2′-dipyridyl solution. Mix and measure the optical density of the solution in a 1 cm cell againsst water at 520 nm. Also perform a blank and compare both readings with the calibrating curve to obtain the concentration of iron in the original sample.

Preparation of Calibration Curve

To a series of boilng-tubes add 0, 0.5, 1.0, 1.5, 2.0, 3.0 and 4.0 ml volumes of the diluted standard iron solution (containing 0.01 mg ml-1 of Fe), dilute each to exactly 10 ml and add reagents as for the sample. Construct the calibration curve relating optical density at 520 nm to micrograms of Fe in each tube.

Serum Iron

(Method of Peters *et al.*, 1956)

Principle : Dilute hydrochloric acid and mercaptoacetic acid ($HSCH_2$ COOH) are added to serum to liberate all iron as the ferric iron. The protein is removed, by precipitation with trichloroacetic acid and the iron in the filtrate determined by formation of a coloured complex with buffered bathophenanthroline (4, 7-diphenyl-1, 10-phenanthroline).

Reagents

1. Iron-free distilled water and iron free glassware ordinary distilled water is redistilled in an all-glass still or passed through a deionizer to remove all traces of iron. Iron-free glassware (including syringes and bottles) is

an absolute necessity. Glassware is made iron-free by soaking in either 6 N nitric acid. 25 per cent hydrochloric acid, or a dichromate cleanig solution for 24 hours. The glassware is then rinsed thoroughly with tap water, then several times with distilled water, and finally with iron free water.

Glassware may be checked for iron contamination as follows :

Into the glassware to be checked, place 10 ml of water, 1 ml of concentrated hydrochloric acid, 0.1 ml of concentrated nitric acid, 3 ml 3 N sodium cyanide, and 2 ml isoamyl alcohol. Shake the mixture well and allow the two layers to separate. If iron is present, the isoamyl alcohol will become pink.

Table 1 : Conductivity values for water of different standards of purity. (Source : Russow, F. and Schneider, H. 1959. Arzneimittelforsch, **9 :** 525)

Form of Water	mho
Tap water	290
Distilled water	5
Double distilled water (Glass)	1
Double distilled water (Quartz)	0.5
Dimineralised water	0.2

2. 0.02 per cent bathophenanthroline solution

   Dissolve 0.080 gram of 4.7 diphenyl -1, 10-phenanthroline in 400 ml isopropyl alcohol. Store in an iron-free bottle.

3. 0.2 N hydrochloric acid. Transfer 4 ml of concentrated hydrochloric acid to 200 ml iron-free distilled water and dilute to 250 ml.

4. 30 per cent trichloroacetic acid.

   Dissolve 30 grams of trichloroacetic acid in enough distilled water to make 100 ml.

5. 40 per cent sodium acetate : Dissolve 40 grams of anhydrous acetate or 60 grams of hydrated sodium acetate in enough water to make 100 ml of solution.

Procedure

Into three iron-free test tubes place 2 ml iron free water (blank), 2 ml dilute iron standard (standard), and 2 ml clear, non-haemolysed serum (sample), respectively. Add 3 ml of 0.2N hydrochloric acid to all tubes and mix. Add 2 drops of mercaptoacetic acid, mix and let stand for 30 minutes at room temperature. Add slowly, with continuous mixing, 1 ml of 30 per cent trichloroacetic acid, stopper and mix thoroughly by inversion, and let the mixture stand at room temperature for 30 minutes. Centrifuge at 2500 rpm for 10 minutes. Remove 2 ml of the supernatant solution from each tube and place in a properly labelled photometer cuvette. To each cuvette add 0.25 ml 40 per cent sodium acetate solution and 1 ml of bathophenthroline solution. Mix by inversion and let stand for 30 minutes after which the material is read in a phtometer at 540 nm, zeroing the instrument with the blank.

Calculation

$$\frac{\text{Density of unknown}}{\text{Density of Standard}} \times 200 = \mu\text{g iron per 100 ml serum}$$

Serum Iron-binding Capacity

(Method of Ramsay, 1957)

The ability of serum to combine with iron is known as *Iron Binding Capacity* (IBC). Upon addition of small increments of iron a maximum is reached where no more iron will combine with the iron binding protein (also referred to as *transferrin* or *siderophilin*). The determination of serum iron content is a measurement of iron already bound to protein, while the determinatin of the iron bindig capacity is a measurement of the iron that can be bound by the same protein. The amount which can be bound in excess of the iron contents is sometimes referred to as latent or unsaturated iron-binding capacity (UIBC). The sum of the iron content and the UIBC is the total iron binding capacity (TIBC). Serum iron-binding capacity, unlike haemoglobin, is approximately the same in both sexes. In iron deficiency anemia, the serum iron is lowered and both the TIBC and UIBC are above normal with a resultant fall in the per cent saturation. In infection, both serum iron and TIBC will be lowered with no change in the per cent saturation.

High serum iron and normal TIBC values, with a resultant increase in the per cent saturation, are seen in refractory anemia, pernicious anemia, haemochromatosis, liver disease and transfusion haemosiderosis.

Principle

Excess ferric iron is added to the serum. On standing the siderophillin binds iron at every possible binding site. The unbound ferric iron is removed by adsorption on magnesium carbonate and the treated serum is analysed for iron content.

Reagents

1. *Ferric Chloride solution : Weigh 0.100 gram of ferric chloride to the nearest 0.001 gram and dissolve in a mixture of 10 ml of nitric acid and 40 ml of distilled water. Heat untill just boiling to bring the ferric chloride into solution, cool and transfer quantitatively to a clean, dry, iron free 100 ml volumetric flask and make up to the mark with iron-free distilled water. Dilute 5 ml of this standard to 100 ml with 0.005 N hydrochloric acid.*
2. *0.005 N hydrochloric acid : dilute 5 ml of 1 N hydrochloric acid to one litre with distilled water.*
3. *Light magnesium carbonate ($MgCO_3$).*

Procedure

Place 2 ml of clear, non haemolysed serum into a test tube, add 4 ml of ferric chloride solution, and mix well.

Let stand for 30 minutes at room temperature with occasional mixing. Centrifuge at 2000 rpm for five minutes. Remove 2 ml of the supernatant solution and proceed with the iron determination as directed above.

Calculation

$$\text{Total iron-binding capacity (TIBC)} = \frac{\text{Density of unknown}}{\text{Density of standard}} \times 200 \times 3$$

$$= \mu\text{g iron per 100 ml serum}$$

TIBC is also the total siderophillin (transferrin) content in 100 ml serum unsaturated iron-binding capacity (UIBC)

TIBC - serum iron = mcg.iron per 100 ml serum.

Per cent saturation of iron-binding protein (siderophillin)

$$= \frac{\text{Serum iron}}{\text{TIBC}} \times 100 = \text{per cent saturation}$$

Zinc

(Method of Cholak *et al.*, 1943 Modified by Sandell 1959)

Reagents

1. *Zinc free distilled water : obtained by redistilling double-distilled water in a pyrex still, is used throughout.*

2. *Ammonium hydroxide : The concentrated reagent is distilled into water which is chilled in an ice bath.*
3. *Hydrochloric acid : A volume of concentrate sulphuric acid is dropped into an equal volume of concentrate hydrochloric acid contained in a pyrex flask, by mean of a separating funnel, the stem of which extends to just below the surface of the hydrochloric acid. The hydrogen chloride evolved is carried by a delivery tube into water cooled in an ice bath. The strength of the zinc free acid thus prepared is obtained from standard tables, on the basis of its specific gravity and it is then diluted to a concentration of 0.2 N.*
4. *Ammonium citrate solution (40 per cent W/V) : 400 gram of ctric acid is dissolved in water, sufficient ammonium hydroxide is added to make the solution just alkaline to thymol blue and the volume is made upto to one litre with water. Before use, the quantity required for one day is placed in a large separating funnel diluted with an equal volume of water and shaken with a chloroform solution of di-β-napthylthicar-bazone untill the latter retains its original colour.*
5. *Carbamate solution (Sodium diethyldithiocarbamate) : 1.25 grams is dissolved in 100 ml of water. This solution must be made up freshly daily.*
6. *Extraction and standard Di-B-naphthyl-thicarbazone solution : For solution 1 (0 to 50 μg range) 20 mg of di-β-naphthylthicarbazone is dissolved in one litre of redistilled chlorofom containing 10 ml of absolute ethyl alcohol. For solution 2 (0 to 50μg range) 200 mg is dissolve in one litre of the same slovent. Both solutions should be stored in brown bottles in the refrigerator.*

   Note : Pyrex ware is used throughout. Before use, extraction funnel should be rinsed once with dilute nitric acid and several times with water. The separating funnels are of the squibb type, of 150 ml capacity and with graduations at 5 ml, 10 ml and all subsequent 10 ml, intrevals upto 100 ml. The 200 ml of glazed silica evaporating dish employed are immersed in dilute nitric acid (1 part of nitric acid, sp.gr. 1.42 to 1 part of water) when not in use.

Standard for Zn : Dissolve 4.3987g Zn SO4.7H2O in 0.1 N hydrochloric acid and dilute to one litre. This will be 0.1 per cent standard (1000 ppm).

For the determination, the sample consisting of weighed tissue or other material (10 to 20 g) or urine (100 ml) is placed in a 200 ml glazed silica evaporating dish. 10 ml of nitric acid is added and the samples is taken to dryness on a hot plate. The organic matter is destroyed by ignition in an electric muffle furnace maintained at 500°C, the complete destruction of organic matter being hastened, if necessary, by treating the ash with a little nitric acid from time to time, evaporating to dryness and replacing the dish in the furnace. (As little nitric acid should be employed as is consistant with rapid ashing, since it is not possible to free this reagent of zinc by distillation prior to its free). A blank analysis must therefore be run with each series of samples, to correct for the zinc in the reagent. The clean ash is taken up in a little hydrochloric acid and water.

The entire sample, or a suitable portion, is placed in a 150 ml separating funnel. To this are added 30 ml of 20 per cent ammonium citrate solution and 4 drops of 0.1 per cent aqueous solution of thymol blue, and the mixture is adjusted to pH 9.5 with ammonium hydroxide (sp.gr.0.9). Next 4 ml of carbamate solution (50 mg) is added and water to the 100 ml mark, and the *solution 1*. This will give an indication of the amount of zinc present less than 5μg giving a faint violet colour and amounts above 5μg giving deeper shades of red. Five ml of extraction *solution 2* is then added and the mixture again shaken for 1 minute. If the amount of zinc exceeds the 0 to 5μg range, extractions with 5 ml portions of the stronger solution are repeated until the last portion retains its original bluish green colour, each portion being drained into a second funnel before the next is added (small differences in colour are more readily discernible in the shaken mixture than in the small volume of the chloroform phase). The collected chloroform extracts are now washed with a 50 ml portion of water and drained into another funnel. The chemical Di-B-naphthylthio-carbazone present in the aqueous phase is removed by shaking the latter with one or two 5 ml portions of chloroform, which are also added to the washed chloroform phase. The chloroform solution (or a portion containing not more than 50μg of zinc) is now shaken with 50 ml of 0.2N hydrochloric acid, and after the phases have been allowed to separate the chloroform phase is discarded. The chemical complex di-B-naphthyl thiocarbazone is then removed from the hydrochloric acid by one or two washings with 5 ml portions of chloroform. The 0.2 N hydrochloric acid contains all of the zinc feed of copper, nickel, cobalt, iron, mercury, silver, phsphates and aluminium sulphates and most of the bismuth and may be used for either polarographic or colorimetric determination of zinc.

For the colorimetric determination, 45 ml of ammonium hydroxide solution (perpared from 50 ml of ammonium hydroxide, sp.gr.0.90, and water to one litre and stored in the refrigertor when not in use) and add 1 ml of carbamate (12.5 mg) are shaken with 5 ml of extraction solution 1, to remove any zinc that may have been taken up from the glass by the weak ammonia during storage. The extract is discarded and the ammonia solution is washed once with 5 ml of chloroform, which is also discarded. Any chloroform floating on the surface of the ammonia solution is allowed to evaporate, its removal is hastened by swirling the funnel and applying suction. The weak carbamate-ammonia mixture is then added to the funnel containing the 0.2 N hydrochloric acid extract of the zinc from which floating chloroform has been removed as just described. The contents of the funnel are mixed and the solution is shaken for 1 minute with 10 ml of the proper extraction solution (2 for the 0 to 50μg range and solution 1 for the 0 to 5μg range). For the estimation of 0 to 5μg of zinc, 5 ml of the extract is run quantitatively into a 25 ml glass stoppered cylinder and the volume made up to 25 ml with chloroform. A 2.5 cm cell is then filled and the optical density of the solution measured at either 550 or 650 mμ, when 0 to 50 μg range is used, 5 ml of the extract is diluted to 100 ml. with chloroform and the optical density of the solution measured with a 1 cm cell. The amount of zinc present is determined by reference to standard curves by carrying known amounts of zinc through the final colorimetric step.

References

Brown, E.G. and Hayes, T.J. (1952). *Anal.Chim.Aeta.,* 7 : 324.

Callan, T. and Henderson, J.A.R. (1929). *Analyst,* 54 : 650.

Cholak, J., Hubbard, D.M. and Burkey, R.E. (1943). *Ind. Eng. Chem. Anal.,* 15 : 754.

Daniel, H.A. and Harper, H.J. (1934). *J.Assoc.official.Agr. Chem.,* 17 : 286.

Eden, A. and Green, H.H. (1940). *Biochem. J.,* 34 : 1202.

Krishna, G. and Mahadevan, V. (1969). Effect of Copper Supplementation on growth and Utilization of nutrients in large white Yorkshire growing pigs. *Indian Vety. J.* 46: 320-329.

Krishna, G., Paliwal, V.K., Yadav, K.R. and Khirwar, S.S. (1981). Trace elements in Agro-Industrial byproducts and Wastes of Haryana State. *Indian J. Dairy Sci.* 34: 336-338.

Marston, H.R. and Dewey, D.W. (1940). Australian. *J. Expt. Biol and med.Sci.,* 18 : 343.

Mc Farlane, W.B. (1932). *Biochem.J.,* 26 : 1022.

Peters, C.A., Mac Masters, M.M. and French, C.L. (1939). *Ind. Eng.Chem.Anal.,* 11 : 502.

Peters, Givanniello,Apt, adn Rosss, (1956). *J.Lab. Clin.Med.,* 48 : 280.

Powell, R. and Taylor, C.G., (1954). Chemistry and Industry, London, pp 726.

Ramsay, W. (1957). *Clin. Chim.Acta,* 2 : 221.

Sandell, E.B. (1959). *Colorimetric determination of traces of metals.* 3 rd edition. Interscience publishers, Inc., New York.

Strickland, J.D.H and Spicer, G. (1949). *Anal. Chim.Acta,* 3 : 517.

Waterbury, G.R. Hayes, A.M. and Martin, D.S. Jr. (1952). *J. American Chem. Soc.,* 74 : 15.

Woods, J.T. and Mellon, M.G. (1941). *Ind.Eng.Chem.Anal.,* 15 : 551

Ventura, S. and White, J.C. (1954). *Analyst,* 79 : 39.

Annexures

Annexure-1 : Name of Chemicals, Molecular Formula and Molecular Weight

Name of Chemical	Molecular Formula	Molecular Weight
Acetamide	$CH_3.CO.NH_2$	59.07
Acetanilide	$C_6H_5NH.COCH_3$	135.17
Acetic acid (Glacial)	$CH_3.COOH$	60.05
Acetic anhydride	$(CH_3CO)_2\,O$	102.09
Acetyl chloride	$CH_3.COCl$	78.50
Acetone	$(CH_3)_2.CO$	58.08
Acetophenone	$C_6H_5.CO.CH_3$	120.15
Adipic acid	$(CH_2.CH_2.COOH)_2$	146.14
Aluminium acetate (Basic)	$Al(OH)\,(CH_3COO)_2$	162.08
Aluminium Chloride (anhydrous)	$AlCl_3$	133.34
Aluminium Nitrate	$Al\,(NO_3)_3$ + H2O	
	$Al\,(NO_3)_3$ (ExAl)	
Aluminium oxide (Active)	(Acidic)	-
Aluminium oxide (Active)	(Basic)	-
Aluminium oxide (Active)	(Neutral)	-
Aluminium Potassium Sulphate	$AlK\,(SO_4)_2.12H_2O$	474.39

Aluminium sulphate	$Al_2(SO_4)_3.16H_2O$	630.39
1-Amino-2-naphthol 4-sulphonic acid (purified)	$NH_2.C_{10}H_5$ (OH).SO_3H	239.25
3-Aminophenol (meta-Aminophenol)	$NH_2.C_6H_4.OH$	109.13
Ammonia Solution	NH_3	17.03
Ammonium hydroxide	NH_4OH	28% NH_3 in water
Ammonium acetate	$CH_3.COO.NH_4$	77.08
Ammonium Carbonate	$NH_4HCO_3+NH_2COO.NH_4$	30% Min.
Ammonium chloride	$NH_4.Cl$	53.49
Ammonium ceric sulphate	2 $(NH_4)_2.SO_4$ Ce $(SO_4).2H_2O$	632.56
Ammonium dichromate	$(NH_4)_2Cr_2O_7$	252.07
Ammonium dihydrogen Orthophosphate	$NH_4.H_2PO_4$	115.03
Ammonium Ferric sulphate (Iron Alum)	NH_4Fe $(SO_4)_2.12H_2O$	482.19
Ammonium Ferrous sulphate	$(NH_4)_2SO_4FeSO_4.6H_2O$	392.14
Ammonium Format	H.COO NH_4	63.06
Ammnonium molybdate	$(NH_4)_6MO_7O_{24}.4H_2O$	1235.95
Ammonium bicarbonate	NH_4HCO_3	79.06
di-Ammnonium hydrogen orthophosphate	$(NH_4)_2HPO_4$	132.06
Ammonium Nickel sulphate	$(NH_4)_2SO_4.NiSO_4.6H_2O$	395.00
Ammonium nitrate	NH_4NO_3	80.04
Ammonium sulphate	$(NH_4)_2.SO_4$	132.14
Ammonium sulphate (Ammonium Alum)	NH_4 $(SO_4)_2.12H_2O$ (Al)	455.33
Amyl alcohol	$C_5H_{11}OH$	88.15
Aniline	$C_6H_5.NH_2$	93.13
Anthrone	$C_{14}H_{10}O$	194.22
Anisole (Methoxy Benzene)	$CH_3.O.C_6H_5$	108.14
Barium acetate	$(CH_3.COO)_2Ba$	255.43
Barium carbonate	$BaCO_3$	197.35
Barium chloride	$BaCl_2.2H_2O$	244.28
Barium hydroxide	$Ba(OH)_2.8H_2O$	315.48
Barium Nitrate	Ba $(NO_3)_2$	261.35
Benzaldehyde	$C_6H_5.CHO$	106.13
Benzene (crystallizable)	C_6H_6	78.11
Benzene (Thiopene free)	C_6H_6	78.11
Benzoic acid	$C_6H_5.COOH$	122.12

Benzoyl chloride	$C_6H_5.COCl$	140.57
Benzyl alcohol	$C_6H_5.CH_2OH$	108.14
Benzyl chloride	$C_6H_5.CH_2CL$	126.59
2, 2′-Bipyridyl	$(C_5H_4N)_2$	156.19
Bismuth Nitrate	$Bi\ (NO_3)_3.5H_2O$	485.07
Biuret (carbamoylurea)	$NH_2CO\ NH\ CONH_2$	103.09
Boric acid	H_3BO_3	61.83
Butan-1-OL (n-Butyl alcohol)	$CH_3.(CH_2)_3.OH$	74.12
Butan-2-one (Ethyl Methyl Ketone)	$C_2H_5.CO.CH_3$	72.11
N-Butyl acetate	$CH_3.COO(CH_2)_3.CH_3$	116.16
Iso-Butyl methyl ketone	$(CH_3)_2/CH.CH_2.CO.CH_3$	100.16
Calcium acetate (dried)	$(CH_3.COO)_2Ca$	158.17
Cadmium iodide	CdI_2	366.21
Calcium carbonate	$CaCO_3$	100.09
Calcium chloride dihydrate	$CaCl_2.2H_2O$	147.02
Calcium hydroxide	$Ca\ (OH)_2$	74.09
Calcium Oxide (powder)	CaO	56.08
Calcium sulphate (anhydrous)	$CaSO_4$	136.14
Calcium sulphate (dihydrate)	$CaSO_4.2H_2O$	172.17
Carbon tetrachloride	CCl_4	153.82
Chloroacetic acid (Monochloroacetic acid)	$CH_2Cl.COOH$	94.50
Chlorobenzene	C_6H_5Cl	112.56
Chloroform	$CHCl_3$	119.38
Cholesterol (cholest-5-en-3-01)	$C_{27}H_{46}O$	386.64
Cholesterol monohydrate	$C_{27}H_{46}O.H_2O$	404.66
Cobalt chloride	$COCl_2.6H_2O$	237.93
Cupric chloride	$CuCl_2.H_2O$	170.48
Cupric Nitrate	$Cu\ (NO_3)_2.3H_2O$	241.60
Cupric sulphate	$CuSO_4.5H_2O$	249.68
Cuprous chloride	$CuCl$	98.99
Cyclohexane special for Spectroscopy	$CH_2.(CH_2)_4.CH_2$	84.16
1, 4-Dioxan	$CH_2.CH_2.O.CH_2.CH_2.O$	88.11
Diphenylamine	$(C_6H_5)\ 2NH$	169.23
Digitonin	$C_{56}H_{92}O_{29}$	1229.3
Dipotassium hydrogen phosphate anhydrous	K_2HPO_4	174.8
Disodium hydrogen phosphate anhydrous	Na_2HPO_4	141.98
Ether (Diethyl ether)	$C_2H_5O\ C_2H_5$	74.12

Ethylene diaminetetra acetic acid disodium salt, dihydrate	$C_1H_2.N(CH_2.COOH)$ $CH_2.COONa]_2.2H_2O$	372.24
Ethyl acetate	$CH_3.COO\ C_2H_5$	88.11
Ferric chloride	$FeCl_3.6H_2O$	270.32
Ferric nitrate monohydrate	$Fe\ (NO_3)_3,H_2O$	259.90
Fructose (B-D-Fructose) or levulose	$C_6H_{12}O_6$	180.16
Ferrous sulphate	$FeSO_4.7H_2O$	278.02
Formaldehyde solution	H.CHO	30.03
Glucose (Dextrose)	$(CHOH)_4.COH.CH_2OH$	180.16
Heparin : sodium, potassium, lithium ammonium salts	-	-
Hydrazimium sulphate	$NH_2.NH_2H_2SO_4$	130.12
Hydriodic acid	HI	127.91
Hydrochloric acid	HCl	36.46
Hydrofluoric acid	HF	20.01
Hydroxylammonium chloride	$HO.NH_3Cl$	69.49
8-Hydroxyquinoline (oxine)	$N.CH.CH{:}CH.C_6H_3.OH$	145.16
Lead nitrate	$Pb\ (NO_3)_2$	331.20
Magnesium chloride	$MgCL_2.6H_2O$	203.31
Magnesium sulphate	$MgSO_4.7H_2O$	246.48
Manganous chloride	$MnCl_2.4H_2O$	197.91
Mercuric chloride	$Hgcl_2$	271.50
Mercuric nitrate	$Hg\ (NO_3)_2$	342.64
Mercurous nitrate	$Hg_2\ (NO_3)_2.2H_2O$	561.22
Mercury (Metal)	Hg	200.59
Mercuric Oxide, red	HgO	216.61
Methanol	CH_3OH	32.04
2-Methylpropan-1-01 or iso-butyl alcohol	$(CH_3)_2.CH.CH_2OH$	74.12
Methylene blue (Methylthionine chloride)	$C_{16}H_{18}ClN_3S.3H_2O$	373.9
Nickel nitrate	$Ni\ (NO_3)_2.6H_2O$	290.81
Nickel sulphate	$NiSO_4.H_2O$	-
Nitric acid	HNO_3	63.01
Orthophosphoric acid	H_3PO_4	98.00
Perchloric acid	$HClO_4$	100.47
Petroleum ether 40-60°C	-	-
Petroleum ether 60-80°C	-	-
Phenol	C_6H_5OH	94.11
Potassium bromide	KBr	119.01
Potassium chloride	KCL	74.56

Pottasium chromate	K_2CrO_4	194.20
Potassium hydroxide	KOH	56.10
Potassium dichromate	$K_2Cr_2O_7$	294.19
Potassium dihydrogen orthophosphate	KH_2PO_4	136.09
Potassium ferricyanide	$K_3Fe(CN)_6$	329.26
Potassium ferricyanide	$K_4Fe(CN)_6 . 3H_2O$	422.41
Potassium hydrogen phthalate	$COOH.C_6H_4.COOK$	204.22
Potassium carbonate (anhydrous)	$K_2CO_3 . 1\frac{1}{2} H_2O$	165.23
Potassium iodate	KIO_3	214.00
Potassium iodide	KI	166.01
Potassium metaborate	KBO_2	81.8
Potassium periodate	KIO_4	230.00
Potassium permanganate	$KMnO_4$	158.04
Potassium sulphate	K_2SO_4	174.27
Potassium Thiocyanate	KSCN	97.18
Propan-2-Ol El	-	
or iso-propyl alcohol	$(CH_3)_2(CHOH)$	60.10
Pyridine	C_5H_5N	79.10
Silver Nitrate	$AgNO_3$	169.87
Sodium Acetate (Anhydrous)	$CH_3.COONa$	82.03
Sodium Acetate Trihydrate	$CH_3.COONa.3H_2O$	136.08
Sodium Bismuthate	$Na BiO_3$	279.97
Sodium Carbonate (anhydrous)	$Na CO_3$	105.99
Sodium chloride	NaCl	58.44
Sodium Cobaltnitrite	$Na_3CO(NO_2)_6$	403.94
Sodium dihydrogen Orthophosphate	$Na H_2PO_4.2H_2O$	156.01
Sodium Fluoride	NaF	41.99
Sodium Nitrite	$NaNO_2$	69.00
Sodium Thiosulphate	$Na_2S_2O_3.5H_2O$	248.18
Sodium Oxalate	$Na_2C_2O_4$	134.00
Sodium tungstate (hydrated)	$Na_2WO_4.2H_2O$	329.86
Sodium hydrogen carbonate	$NaHCO_3$	84.01
Sodium hydroxide	NaOH	40.01
Sodium hypochlorite	$NaClo, 5H_2O$	164.53
Sodium lactate	CH_3 CHOH COONa	112.06
Sodium sulfite	$NaSO_3$	126.06
Sodium tetraborate (Borax)	$Na_2B_4O_7, 10H_2O$	381.42
Sodium Pyrosulphite	$Na_2S_2O_5$	190.11
Sodium pyruvate	$C_3H_3O_3$ Na	110.11
Strontium chloride	$Sr Cl_2.6H_2O$	266.62

Starch	$(C_6H_{10}O_5)n$	165.15
Sucrose	$C_{12}H_{22}O_{11}$	342.30
Sulphanilic acid	$NH_2.C_6H_4.SO_3H$	173.19
Sulphamic acid (Ammonium salt)	$NH_2.SO_3.NH_4$	114.12
Sulphuric acid	H_2SO_4	98.08
(+) Tartaric acid	$(CHOH.COOH)_2$	150.09
Thiourea	$H_2NCS\ NH_2$	76.12
Tris (Tris (hydroxymethyl) amino-methane	$NH_2C\ (CH_2OH)_3$	121.14
Trisodium phosphate	$Na_3PO_4.12H_2O$	380.14
Trichloroethylene	$CHCl:CCl_2$	131.40
Trichloroacetic acid	CCl_3COOH	163.40
Triethanolamine	$(HOCH_2CH_2)_3\ N$	149.19
Triethanolamine hydrochloride	$(HOCH_2CH_2)_3N.HCI$	185.66
Tri-sodium citrate	$Na_3C_6H_5O_7.2H_2O$	294.10
Toluene	$C_6H_5.CH_3$	92.14
Urea	$NH_2.CO.NH_2$	60.06
Uric acid	$C_5H_4N_4O_3$	168.11
Veronal (5, 5-Diethyl-barbiturate)	$C_8H_{12}N_2O_3$	184.19
Veronal Sodium (Sodium 5, 5-diethylbarbiturate)	$C_8H_{11}N_2O_3Na$	206.18
Xylene	$C_6H_4.\ (CH_3)_2$	106.17

Annexure-2 : Melting and Boiling Points and Atomic Weights of the Elements

Based on the assigned relative atomic mass of $^{12}C = 12$

The following values aply to elements as they exist in materials of terrestrial origin and to certain artificial elements. When used with the footnotes, they are reliable to ± in the last digit, or ± 3 if that digit is in small type.

Name	Symbol	At.No.	At.Wt.	M.P.°C	B.P.C
Actinium	Ac	89	(227)	1050	3200 ± 300
Aluminium	Al	13	26.98154a	660.37	2467
Americium	Am	95	243	994 ± 4	2607
Antimony	Sb	51	121.75	630.74	1750
Argon	Ar	18	39.948b.c.d	-189.2	-185.7
Arsenic (gray)	As	33	74.9216a	817 (28atm)	613 (sub.)
Astatine	At	85	210	302	337
Barium	Ba	56	137.34	725	1640

Berkelium	Bk	97	247	-	-
Beryllium (5 mm)	Be	4	9.01218a	1278±5	2970
Bismuth	Bi	83	208.9808a	271.3	1560±5
Boron	B	5	10.81c.d.e.	2300	2550 (sub)
Bromine	Br	35	79.904	-7.2	58.78
Cadmium	Cd	48	112.40	320.9	765
Calcium	Ca	20	40.08	839±2	1484
Californium	Cf	98	(251)	-	-
Carbon	C	6	12.011 b.d	3550	4827
Cerium	Ce	58	140.12	798±3	3257
Cesium	Cs	55	132.9054c	28.40±0.01	678.4
Chlorine	Cl	17	35.453e	-100.98	-34.6
Chromium	Cr	24	51.996	1857 ± 20	2672
Cobalt	Co	27	58.9332	1495	2870
Copper	Cu	29	63.546c.d	1083.4±0.2	2567
Curium	Cm	96	(247)	1340±40	-
Dysprosium	Dy	66	162.50	1409	2335
Einsteinium	Es	99	(254)	-	-
Erbium	Er	68	167.26	1522	2510
Europium	Eu	63	151.96	822±5	1597
Fermium	Fm	100	(257)	-	-
Fluorine	F	9	18.99840a	-219.62	-188.17
Francium	Fr	87	223	27	677
Gadolinium	Gd	64	157.25	1311±1	3233
Gallium	Ga	31	69.72	29.78	2403
Germanium	Ge	32	72.59	937.4	2830
Gold	Au	79	196.9665 a	1064.43	2807
Hafnium	Hf	72	178.49	2227±20	4602
Helium	He	2	4.00260 b	-272.2[26 atm.]	-268.934
Holmium	Ho	67	164.9304 a	1470	2720
Hydrogen	H	1	1.0079b.d	-259.14	-252.87
Indium	In	49	114.82	156.61	2080
Iodine	I	53	126.9045 a	113.5	184.35
Iridium	Ir	77	192.2	2410	4130
Iron	Fe	26	55.84	1535	2750
Krypton	Kr	36	83.80	-156.6	-152.30±0.10
Lanthanum	La	57	138.905 b	920±5	3454

Lawrencium	Lr	103	(257)	-	-
Lead	Pb	82	207.2d.e	327.502	1740
Lithium	Li	3	6.941c.d.e	180.54	1347
Lutetium	Lu	71	174.97	1656±5	3315
Magnesium	Mg	12	24.305c	648.8±0.5	1090
Manganese	Mn	25	54.9380	1244 ± 3	1962
Mendelevium	Md	101	(256)	-	-
Mercury	Hg	80	200.59	-38.87	356.58
Molybdenum	Mo	42	95.94	2617	4612
Neodymium	Nd	60	144.24	1010	3127
Neon	Ne	10	20.179 c	-248.67	-246.048
Neptunium	Np	93	237.0482 b	640±1	3902
Nickle	Ni	28	58.71	1453	2732
Niobium (Columbium)	Nb	41	92.9064	2468±10	4742
Nitrogen	N	7	14.0067b.c	-209.86	-195.8
Nobelium	No	102	(254)	-	-
Osmium	Os	76	190.2	3045±30	5027±100
Oxygen	0	8	15.9994b.c.d	-218.4	-182.962
Palladium	Pd	46	106.4	1552	3140
Phosphorus	P	15	30.97376	44.1 (white)	280 (white)
Platinum	Pt	78	195.09	1772	3827±100
Plutonium	Pu	94	(244)	641	3232
Polonium	Po	84	210	254	962
Potassium	K	19	39.098	63.65	774
Praseodymium	Pr	59	140.9077a	931±4	3212
Promethium	Pm	61	(145)	1080	2460 (?)
Protactinium	Pa	91	231.0359a	<1600	-
Radium	Ra	88	226.0254	700	1140
Radon	Rn	86	(222)	-71	-61.8
Rhenium	Re	75	186.2	3180	5627 (est.)
Rhodium	Rh	45	102.9055	1966±3	3727±100
Rubidium	Rb	37	85.4678c	38.89	688
Ruthenium	Ru	44	101.07	2310	3900
Samarium	Sm	62	150.4	1072±5	1778
Scandium	Sc	21	44.9559	1539	2832
Selenium	Se	34	78.96	217	684.9±1.0

Silicon	Si	14	28.086d	1410	2355
Silver	Ag	47	107.868 c	961.93	2212
Sodium	Na	11	22.9898 a	97.81 ± 0.03	882.9
Strontium	Sr	38	87.62	769	1384
Sulphur	S	16	32.06 d	112.8	444.674
Tantalum	Ta	73	180.9479 b	2996	5425 ± 100
Technetium	Tc	43	98.9062	2172	4877
Tellurium	Te	52	127.60	449.5 ± 0.3	989.8 ± 3.8
Terbium	Tb	65	158.9254	1360 ± 4	3041
Thallium	TI	81	204.37	303.5	1457 ± 10
Thorium	Th	90	232.0381	1750	-4790
Thulium	Tm	69	168.9342	1545 ± 15	1727
Tin	Sn	50	118.69	231.9681	2270
Titanium	Ti	22	47.90	1660 ± 10	3287
Tungsten	W	74	183.85	3410 ± 20	5660
Uranium	U	92	238.029 bcd	1132.3 ± 0.8	3818
Vanadium	V	23	50.9414 bc	1890 ± 10	3380
Wolfram (see Tungsten)					
Xenon	Xe	54	131.30	-111.9	-107.1±3
Ytterbium	Yb	70	173.04	824±5	1193
Yttrium	Y	39	88.9059	1523±8	3337
Zinc	Zn	30	65.38	419.58	907
Zirconium	Zr	40	91.22	1852±2	4377

a Mononuclidic element

b Element with one predominant isotope (about 99 to 100% abundance)

c Element for which the atomic weight is based on calibrated measurements.

d Element for which variation in isotopic abundance in terrestrial samples limits the precision of the atomic weight given.

e Element for which users are cautioned against the possibility of large Variations in atomic weight due to inadvertent or undisclosed artificial isotopic separation in commercially available materials.

Most commonly available long-lived isotope.

In some geological specimens this element has a highly anomalous isotopic composition corresponding to an atomic weight significantly different from that given.

Annexure-3 : Average Composition of Milk of Different Species.

	Red Sindhi	Gir	Tharparkar	Sahiwal	Cross Bred	Murrah Buffalo	Surati Goat	Kathiawar Sheep
Sp.Gr. at 68°F	1.02941	1.02903	1.02936	1.02988	1.02927	1.03060	1.0307	1.03384
Fat %	4.90	4.73	4.55	4.55	4.50	6.56	4.50	6.04
Total solids %	13.66	13.30	13.25	13.37	13.12	15.75	13.50	16.30
S.N.F %	8.76	8.67	8.70	8.88	8.63	9.19	9.00	10.26
Lactose %	4.91	4.85	4.83	5.04	4.92	5.83	4.68	4.99
Total protein %	3.42	3.32	3.36	3.33	3.37	3.86	3.49	4.84
Ash %	0.70	0.66	0.68	0.66	0.67	0.70	0.77	0.81
Vitamin C mg/100 ml	2.54	2.56	2.43	2.65	2.45	2.81	3.51	5.50
Vitamin A (B.U./100ml)	148.9	138.4	145.0	135.0	139.7	175.6	137.4	189.7

Source : Singh, Harbans and Parnekar, Y.M. 1973. Cattle Wealth of India. Farm information unit, Directorate of Extension, Ministry of Agriculture, New Delhi

Annexure-4 : Total Protein of Serum or Plasma

Species	Sample	Value g/100 ml
Men		
Birth	Serum	6.2 ± 0.5
Adult	Serum	7.0 ± 0.4
Horse	Serum	7.1 ± 0.4
Cattle	Serum	6.2 ± 0.3
Calf	Serum	7.2 ± 0.1
Goat	Serum	7.5
Sheep		
Lamb (7-17 weeks)	Serum	6.5 ± 0.3
Ewe	Serum	7.5 ± 0.1
Pig	Serum	6.8 ± 0.4
Dog	Plasma	6.2 ± 0.6
Cat	Serum	7.1 ± 0.1
Guinea pig	Serum	6.2 ± 0.3
Rat	Serum	6.0 ± 0.2
Chicken		
Embryo (14 days)	Serum	0.9 ± 0.1
Chick (1 day)	Serum	2.1 ± 0.2
Pullet (13 weeks)	Serum	3.9 ± 0.5
Laying-early	Serum	4.6 ± 0.1
Laying-Late	Serum	4.0 ± 0.5

Annexure-5 : Conversion from Values (mg/100 ml) to mEq/L and Vice Versa.

Constituents	Conversion factor
Sodium	mg/100 ml ÷ 2.3 = mEq/L
Potassium	mg/100 ml ÷ 3.9 = mEq/L
Calcium	mg/100 ml ÷ 2.0 = mEq/L
Magnesium	mg/100 ml ÷ 1.2 = mEq/L
T CO_2	Vol % ÷ 2.2 m Eq/L
Chloride	mg/100 ml ÷ 3.5 = mEq/L
(Expressed as Nacl)	
Phosphorus	mg/100 ml ÷ 1.7 = mEq/L
Sulphate	mg/100 ml ÷ 1.6 = mEq/L
Protein	gm/100 ml ÷ 0.41 = mEq/L

Source : Long, Cl. 1961. Biochemists, Handbook., E.&F.N. Spon Ltd., London, pp. 841.

The unit of measures of electrolytes is the milliequivalent (mEq) which express the chemical activity, or combining power, of a substance relative to the activity of 1 mg of hydrogen, Thus, 1 mEq is represented by 1 mg hydrogen, 23 mg of Na, 39 mg of K, 20 mg of Calcium and 35 mg of chloride

$$m\,Eq/L = \frac{(mg/L) \times Valence}{Formula\ Wt.}$$

$$mg/L = \frac{(m\,Eq/L) \times Formula\ Wt.}{Valence}$$

N.B. Formula Wt. = Atomic or Molecular Wt.

Milliosmols

The mEq is roughly equivalent to the milliosmol (mOsm), the unit of measure of osmolarity or tonicity. Normally, the body fluid compartments each contain about 280 m Osm of solute per litre.

Annexure-6 : Iron in Blood.

Species	Sample	Value (μg/100 ml)
Man		
Adult	Serum	130 ± 5.2
		330 ± 4.9 (Iron binding capacity)
Mother at parturition	Serum	98 ± 6.7
		470 ± 15.3 (Iron binding capacity)
Infant cord blood	Serum	173 ± 6.9
		259 ± 10.5 (Iron binding capacity)
Adult	Cell	104 (mg/100g)
Newborn	Cell	99 (mg/100g)
Foetus	Cell	95 (mg/100g)
Cattle		
Adult	Serum	162.4 ± 18.1
Pregnant	Serum	150 rising to 204
Calves (milk only)	Serum	81.5 ± 14.3
Calves at weaning	Serum	195.3 ± 18.8
Sheep	Plasma	193.7
		334 ± 18 (Iron binding capacity)
Pig		
Adult	Cell	100 (mg/100g)
Newborn	Cell	87 (mg/100g)
Foetus	Cell	80 (mg/100g)
Rat		
4 months	Serum	245 ± 59
11 months	Serum	160 ± 34

Source : Long, Cl. 1961. Biochemists handbook, E and F.N. Spon Ltd., London, pp. 882

Annexure-7 : Manganese in Blood.

Species	Sample	Value (μg/100 ml)
Man		
Man	Blood	12 ± 6
	Plasma	4 ± 3
	Cell	8 ± 6
Cattle		
Lactating	Blood	6.6 ± 2.03
	Serum	2.5 ± 3.0
Rabbit	Serum	4.8 ± 3.5

Source : Long, Cl. 1961. Biochemists Handbook, E.&F.N. Spon Ltd., London, pp. 883

Annexure-8 : Zinc in Blood.

Species	Sample	Value (μg/100 ml)
Man	Blood	880 ± 200
	Plasma	300 ± 160
	Cell	1440 ± 270
Cattle	Blood	319 ± 34
Cat	Blood	438
Rabbit		
Adult	Plasma	248 ± 62
Rat	Blood	636
Pig	Plasma	75 ± 10
	Cell	740 ± 100

Source : Long, Cl. 1961. Biochemists Handbook, E.F.N. Spon Ltd., London, pp. 882

Annexure-9 : Proportions of VFA (Molar basis) in the Rumen of Sheep

Diet	Acetic	Propionic	Isobutyric	n-butyric	Iso-valeric	n-Valeric
Dried grass	55-69	16-26	0.5-1.4	7.6-11.9	0.8-1.9	0.7-1.5
Grass silage	53-72	15-25	1.3-2.6	7.4-10.7	1.9-3.2	0.6-2.3
Hay	78-81	13-19	0.4-0.6	2.4-2.9	0.2-0.3	0.3-0.5
Hay + maize	41-56	18-35	0.2-0.5	8.9-28.9	0.3-1.8	0.3-3.7
Hay + maize + peanut	41-60	26-34	0.9-2.4	10.1-24.1	0.9-24.1	1.6-3.5

Source : Swenson, M.J. 1977. Duke's physiology of domestic animals 9th Edn. Cornell University Press, pp. 261.

Annexure-10 : Proportions of Volatile Fatty Acids with Different Numbers of Carbon Atoms in the Rumen (calculated as a percentage of the total VFA on a molecular basis)

Ratio	No. of carbon atoms			
	C_2	C_3	C_4	C_5
High roughage with low concentrate	65-95	16-20	12	3
Low roughage with high concentrate	52-61	17-30	10-18	3-5

Source : Swenson, M.J. 1977. Duke's physiology of domestic animals 9th Edn. Cornell University Press, pp. 260.

Annexure-11 : Usual Ranges of some Chemical Constituents of the Blood of Mature Domestic Animals.

Species	SERUM			
	Total cholesterol mg/100 ml	Calcium mEq/L	Phosphate mEq/L	Chloride mEq/L
Cow	50-230	4.5-6	2-5.2	80-100
Sheep	100-150	4.5-6	2-5.2	95-110
Goat	55-200	4.5-6	2-5.2	100-125
Pig	100-250	4.5-7.5	3.2-5.2	95-110
Horse	75-150	4.5-7.5	1.3-3.2	95-110
Dog	125-250	4.5-5.5	1.3-2.6	105-120
Chicken (laying)	125-200	8.5-19.5	4-6.4	110-120
Chicken (Non laying)	125-200	4.5-6.0	2.6-5.2	110-120

Source : Swenson, M.J. 1977. Duke's physiology of domestic animals 9th Edn. Cornell University Press, pp. 260.

Annexure-12 : Usual Ranges of some Chemical Constituents of the Blood of Mature Domestic Animals.

Species	Whole blood (mg/100 ml)						
	Glucose	Total NPN	Urea nitrogen	Uric acid	Creatinine	Amino acid nitrogen	Lactic acid
Cow	40-70	20-40	6-27	0.05-2	1-2	4-8	5-20
Sheep	30-50	20-38	8-20	0.05-2	1-2	5-8	9-12
Goat	45-60	30-44	13-28	0.3-1	1-2	-	-
Pig	80-120	20-45	8-24	0.05-2	1-2	8	-
Horse	55-95	20-40	10-20	0.9-1	1-2	5-7	10-16
Dog	80-120	17-38	10-20	0.0-0.5	1-2	7-8	8-20
Chicken (laying)	130-290	20-35	0.4-1	1-7	1-2	4-9	20-98
Chicken (Non laying)	130-260	23-36	0.4-1	2	1-2	5-10	47-56
Man*	88.3±6.7	25.7±6.5	32.1±3.4	2.5±0.4	3.9±0.5	5.8±0.5	19±12

Source : Swenson, M.J. 1977. Duke's physiology of domestic animals 9th Edn. Cornell University Press, pp. 28.

*** Glucose**

Infant 1 day 56.7 ± 16.4 Infant 6 days 67.1 ± 12.5

Annexure-13 : Total Lipids in Blood Samples.

Species	Sample	Value (mg/100ml)
Man		
Birth	Plasma	198 ± 80
Non-pregnant	Plasma	617 ± 75
Pregnant	Plasma	900 ± 130
Cattle, Cow	Serum	331 ± 55
Dog	Serum	679 ± 95
Cat	Plasma	376 ± 110
Rabbit	Plasma	243 ± 89
Guinea pig	Plasma	169 ± 34
Rat	Plasma	230 ± 31
Chicken (Male)	Blood	428 ± 45
Immature (Female)	Blood	446 ± 62
Laying	Blood	1689 ± 900

Source : Long, Cl. 1961. Biochemists Handbook, E.F.N. Spon Ltd., London.

Annexure-14 : Distribution of Blood VFA's Between Cells and Plasma.

Species	Sample	Total VFA (m.moles/lit)	Molecular proportions of VFA's		
			Formate	Acetate	Propionate
Sheep	Cells	0.77	13	84	3
	Plasma	1.03	4	94	2
	Whole blood	0.96	7	90	3
Ox	Cells	0.54	11	89	0
	Plasma	0.80	9	91	0
	Whole blood	0.74	5	95	0
Sheep	Washed cells	0.24	52	48	0
	Whole blood	1.04	24	75	1

Source : Annison, E.F. 1951 b Biochem.J., **58 :** 670.

Annexure-15 : Total Volatile Fatty Acids in Blood.

Species	Sample	Value (mg/100ml)
Man	Blood	1.68
Horse	Blood	3.34
Cattle		
Calf 1 week	Blood	1.8 ± 0.6
	Blood	6.0 ± 1.5
	Blood	5.36
Goat	Blood	6.08
Sheep		
Pre-feed	Blood	2.59
5 hrs. after feed	Blood	6.30
	Plasma	5.81
Dog	Blood	1.81
Cat	Blood	1.91
Rabbit	Blood	7.05

References

Annison, E.F. (1954). *Biochem. J.*, 58 : 670.

Mc Carthy and Kesler, (1956). *J. Dairy Sci.*, 39 : 1280.

Annexure-16 : Ammonia in Blood.

Species	Sample	Value (μg/100ml)
Man	Blood	96.5 ± 3.2
Cattle, winter feed	Blood	41.6 ± 13.4
Sheep	Blood	130 ± 0.50

Source : Long, Cl. 1961. Biochemists Handbook, E.&F.N. Spon Ltd., London, pp. 841.

Annexure-17 : Proportion of Individual Volatile Fatty Acids.

Species	Sample	Value (% of total by wt.)		
		Formic	Acetic	Propionic
Man	Blood	24	75	1
Horse	Blood	25	71	4
Cattle	Blood	16	83	1
Goat	Blood	16	83	1
Sheep (Pre-feed)	Blood	17	81	2
5 hr after feed	Blood	10	88	1
	Plasma	3	94	2
Dog	Blood	35	61	4
Cat	Blood	38	57	5
Rabbit	Blood	14	83	3

Source : Annison, E.F. (1954). Biochem.J., 58 : 670.

Annexure-18 : Ascorbic Acid in Blood.

Species	Sample	Value (mg/100ml)
Man		
Age 16-39 Male	Blood	0.82 ± 0.14
Female	Blood	1.02 ± 0.18
Age 40-59 Male	Blood	0.59 ± 0.32
Female	Blood	0.48 ± 0.29
Age 75-79 Male	Blood	0.35 ± 0.10
Female	Blood	0.41 ± 0.17
	Plasma	0.69 ± 0.15
Horse	Serum	1.30 ± 0.41
Cattle, lactating	Plasma	0.53
Sheep	Serum	1.30 ± 0.25
Pig	Serum	2.04 ± 0.39
Chicken : Adult	Serum	2.45 ± 0.32
Immature	Serum	2.23 ± 0.44
Adult	Blood	2.22 ± 0.64
Rat	Serum	1.05 ± 0.39

Annexure-19 : Carotenoids and Vitamin A in Blood.

Species	Sample	Value (μg/100 ml)	
		Vitamin A	Total carotenoids
Man	Plasma	54 ± 3	120 ± 10
Horse	Serum	12.1 ± 3.8	9.7 ± 3.8
Cattle			
Lactating	Plasma	37 ± 4	362 ± 127
Calves	Plasma	16.5 ± 5.4	-
Sheep			
Adult	Serum	33.8 ± 7.2	9.5 ± 2.5
	Plasma	27.6 ± 7.6	-
Pig	Serum	25.2 ± 4.9	7.5 ± 3.3
Rabbit	Plasma	65	-
Rat	Serum	24.4 ± 6.9	2.0 ± 0.5
Chicken			
Adult	Serum	32.0 ± 20.9	142 ± 101
Immature	Serum	53.4 ± 13.9	867 ± 316

Source : Long, Cl. 1961. Biochemists, Handbook, E & F.N. Spon Ltd. London, pp 865.

Annexure-20 : Folic Acid in Blood.

Species	Sample	Value (µg/100ml)	
		Value A	Total carotenoids
Man	Blood	0.09 ± 0.03	3.8 ± 0.24
	Plasma	< 0.05	4.0 ± 0.83
Cattle	Blood	0.19 ± 0.15	2.5 ± 0.44
	Plasma	<0.05	2.0 ± 0.19
Calf	Blood	0.05	-
Sheep	Blood	< 0.02	4.6 ± 0.8
Rabbit	Blood	0.46	19.4
Pig	Blood	0.66 ± 0.23	2.6 ± 0.47
Chicken	Blood	0.87 ± 0.41	3.1 ± 0.69

Source : Long, Cl. 1961. Biochemist's Handbook, E.&F.N. Spon Ltd. London, pp. 867.

Annexure-21 : Calcium in Blood.

Species	Sample	Value (mg/100ml)
Man	Serum	9.26 to 10.30
5 day infant	Serum	7.40 ± 0.90
Horse	Serum	12.4 ± 0.58
Cattle	Serum	11.08 ± 0.67
At parturition	Serum	8.7
Sheep	Serum	12.16 ± 0.28
Goat	Serum	10.30 ± 0.7
Cat	Serum	8.22 ± 0.97
Dog	Serum	10.16 ± 2.04
Rabbit	Plasma	7.68 ± 1.30
Rat	Serum	12.10 ± 0.98

Source : Long, Cl. 1961. Biochemist's Handbook, E.&F.N. Spon Ltd. London, pp.

Annexure-22 : Chloride in Blood.

Species	Sample	Value (mg/100ml)
Man		
Adult	Blood	246 to 303
New born	Serum	385 ± 6
Foetus	Serum	378 ± 4
Monkey	Blood	321 ± 28
Cattle	Serum	385 ± 44
Sheep	Plasma	367 ± 9.8
Pig (Adult)	Serum	371 ± 14
Dog	Plasma	373 ± 17
Rabbit	Plasma	354 ± 22
Cat	Serum	705 ± 29
Rat	Plasma	371 ± 14

Annexure-23 : Magnesium in Blood.

Species	Sample	Value (mg/100ml)
Man	Blood	3.82
Horse	Blood	4.0 ± 0.62
Cattle	Blood	2.4 ± 0.32
Sheep	Blood	3.3 ± 0.13
Pig	Blood	6.4 ± 0.78
Rabbit	Blood	5.4 ± 0.74
Dog	Serum	2.1 ± 0.3
Goat	Blood	3.7 ± 0.65
Rat	Blood	5.5 ± 0.39
Mouse	Blood	10.3
Chicken	Blood	5.0 ± 0.26

Source : Long, Cl. 1961. Biochemist's Handbook, E.&F.N. Spon Ltd. London, pp. 875.

Annexure-24 : Phosphorus (Inorganic) in Blood.

Species	Sample	Value (mg/100ml)
Man	Blood	3.2
	Plasma	3.33 ± 1.14
Monkey	Blood	3.60
Horse	Blood	2.1 to 2.2
Cattle	Blood	6.7-8.5
	Serum	5.56 ± 1.56
Goat	Blood	6.8-8.4
Sheep	Blood	5.4 ± 1.0
Pig	Blood	6.9-7.3
Dog	Blood	3.2
Cat	Serum	6.40 ± 1.17
Rat	Blood	5.6
Chicken	Blood	2.4-5.0

Annexure-25 : Phosphorus (Organic) in Blood.

Species	Sample	Value (mg/100ml)
Man	Cell	55.0
Monkey	Cell	56.6
Horse	Cell	44.9-50.9
Cattle	Cell	10.8
Goat	Cell	10.8-11.8
Sheep	Cell	15.4
Pig	Cell	95.0-98.7
Dog	Cell	52.1
Cat	Cell	19.4-20.2
Rat	Cell	66.8
Mouse	Cell	84.1-85.8
Chicken	Cell	86.5-95.2

Source : Long, Cl. 1961. Biochemist's Handbook, E.&F.N. Spon Ltd. London, pp. 877.

Annexure-26 : Sulphur in Blood.

Species	Sample	Sulphur	Sulphate		
		Total	**Organic**	**Inorganic**	**Conjugated**
Man	Plasma	2.97 ± 0.39	1.79 ± 0.40	0.99 ± 0.08	0.19 ± 0.10
Cattle	Plasma	5.64	1.20	3.44	1.00
Pig	Plasma	3.88	1.80	1.89	0.19
Rabbit	Plasma	7.05 ± 0.810	1.65 ± 0.39	4.98 ± 0.88	0.42 ± 0.35
Rat	Plasma	3.85 ± 0.10	1.52 ± 0.10	2.17 ± 0.12	0.20 ± 0.08

Source : Long, Cl. 1961. Biochemist's, Handbook, E & F.N. Spon Ltd. London, pp 880.

Annexure-27 : Copper in Blood.

Species	Sample	Value (μg/100ml)
Man	Blood	93.9 ± 2.2
	Plasma	116 ± 14
	Serum	114.6 ± 12.2
Female, late pregnancy	Blood	239 ± 49
Cattle		
Adult	Blood	115 ± 31
Calf	Plasma	79 ± 24
Sheep	Blood	101 ± 96
Pig	Blood	138 ± 15.2
	Plasma	110 ± 42.0
Guinea pig	Blood	50 ± 0.6
Chicken	Blood	23 ± 0.8
Duck	Blood	35 ± 0.7
Turkey	Blood	23 ± 0.7

Source : Long, Cl. 1961. Biochemist's, Handbook, E & F.N. Spon Ltd. London, pp 881

Annexure-28 : Iodine (Protein Bound and Total) in Blood.

Species	Sample	Value (μg/100ml) Protein bound	Total
Man	Serum	5.7 ± 0.83	7.0 ± 0.7
Monkey	Serum	3.59 ± 1.08	-
Cattle	Plasma	3.53 ± 0.25	4.61 ± 0.64
0-2 days old	Plasma	13.7 ± 5.0	-
Sheep	Serum	3.84 ± 1.22	-
Pig	Serum	3.08 ± 1.12	-
Dog	Serum	3.0	29 ± 18
Rabbit	Serum	2.16 ± 0.48	-
Rat	Plasma	3.5 ± 0.1	3.4 ± 0.1
Mouse	Serum	3.8	-
Chicken	Serum	1.03 ± 0.47	-
	Plasma	-	7.2 ± 2.3
Duck	Serum	1.26 ± 0.04	-

Source : Long, Cl. 1961. Biochemist's, Handbook, E & F.N. Spon Ltd. London, pp 882

Annexure-29 : Serum Lipoprotein and Its Composition

Species	Lipoprotein (mg/100 ml)	Protein content %	Lipid constituents as % by weight of total lipid**			
			Phospho-lipid	Free Cholesterol	Cholesterol-ester	Trigly-ceride
Man	A*	16	15	6	22	19
	B*	33	4	1	4	1
	C*	59	14	1	9	4
Dog	A*	24	3	1	2	6
	B*	35	7	1	3	2
	C*	50	40	4	23	8
Rat	A*	18	6	2	5	13
	B*	33	15	3	11	0
	C*	52	22	2	17	4
Chicken	A*	17	9	3	8	15
	B*	42	3	1	2	1
	C*	51	31	3	13	11

Source : Hillyard et al. 1955. J. Biol. Chem., 214 : 79

* Fractions A, B and C correspond to Albumin, Bilirubin and Cholesterol.

** "Total lipid" is that present in fraction A, B and C.

Annexure-30 : Free Amino Acid Nitrogen in Blood.

Species	Sample	Value (μg/100ml)
Man		
Infant	Blood	6.2 ± 1
Adult	Blood	5.8 ± 0.5
Cattle		
Calf	Blood	9.3 ± 0.6
Beef	Blood	7.3
Lactating	Serum	5.6 ± 0.6
Sheep	Blood	9.2 ± 0.5
Rabbit	Plasma	6.8
Rat	Blood	8.9
Chicken		
5 weeks	Plasma	8.4 ± 1.2
Laying	Plasma	8.0 ± 0.3

Source : Long, Cl. 1961. Biochemists, Handbook, E & F.N. Spon Ltd. London, pp 846

Annexure-31 : Non-protein Nitrogen in Blood

Species	Sample	Value (μg/100ml)
Man		
0-5 days	Blood	40.6 ± 8.0
Adult	Plasma	23.7 ± 6.5
Cattle		
Calf	Blood	41.0 ± 3.6
	Serum	21.5 ± 1.0
	Serum	28.3 ± 3.3
Sheep	Blood	37 ± 2
	Serum	34
Cat	Blood	40.2 ± 6
Rat	Blood	38.9
Chicken	Blood	33.3

Source : Long, Cl. 1961. Biochemist's, Handbook, E & F.N. Spon Ltd. London, pp 845

Annexure-32 : Normal Values of Serum Glutamic Oxalacetic Transaminase (SGOT) in Various Domestic Animals.

Species	Comment	SGOT activity (Sigma-Frankal units/ml Mean)
Bovine	Bull, 1-97 week	23.7 ± 17.3
	Cows, 2-10 year	43.8 ± 5.7
	Calves, 7-27 days	23.6 ± 3.7
Canine	5 year	22.4 ± 5.2
Equine	Unexercised, not in training	
	1 year	186 ± 52
Feline	1 month	19.0
Ovine	10 week	<81
Porcine	1-3 year	31.1
Gallus domesticus	6 months	370 ± 186

Source : Kaneko, J.J. and Cornelius, C.E. 1971. Clinical biochemistry of domestic animals. 2nd Edn. Academic Press, New York pp 167.

Annexure-33 : Normal Values for Serum Electrolytes (mEq/L).

Species	Determination	Range
Dog	Sodium	141.1-152.3
	Potassium	4.37-5.65
	Chloride	105.2-114.8
Cat	Sodium	147-156
	Potassium	4.0-4.5
	Chloride	117-123
Ox	Sodium	132-152
	Potassium	3.9-5.8
	Chloride	97-111
Horse	Sodium	132-146
	Potassium	2.4-4.7
	Chloride	99-109
Sheep	Sodium	139-152
	Potassium	3.9-5.4
	Chloride	95-103
Swine	Sodium	135-150
	Potassium	4.4-6.7
	Chloride	94-106
Man	Sodium	135-155
	Potassium	3.6-5.5
	Chloride	98-109

Source : Kaneko, J.J. and Cornelius, C.E. 1971. Clinical biochemistry of domestic animals. 2nd Edn. Academic Press, New York pp 95.

Chapter - 70

Standard Units of Measure and Weight Used in Analytical Work

Unit of Length

A metre (m) is taken from the international prototype metre at the International Bureau of weights and measures; at 32°F. (0°C) = 39.37 inches (in.) = 3.280833 feet (ft.) = centimetres (Cm.). A centimetre (Cm.) = 10 millimetres (mm.) = 10,000 microns (μ) = 0.337 inch (in.) or 10^{-4}cm. A millimetre (mm.) = 1,000 microns (μ) = 0.03937 inch. A micron (mμ) = 1,000 milli-microns (μ) = 3.937×10^{-5} inch. A milli-micron (mμ) = 0.001 micron or 10^{-7} cm. A foot (ft.) = 0.3048006 metre (m.) = 30.48006 centimetres (Cm.) = 12 inches (in.)., inch = 2.5 cm. An inch (in.) = 2.539998 centimetres (Cm.) = 25.39998 mm = 25,399.98 microns (μ).

1. Angstrom unit (A) = 10^{-8} cm
2. Fermi = 10^{-13} cm
3. Yard = 3 feet = 91.4 cm

Unit of Capacity

A litre (1) is the volume occupied by the mass of 1 kg of pure water at 4°C under barometric pressure of 760 millimetres = 0.26417762 gallon (gal.) = 0.035316 cubic foot (cu.ft.) = 61.025 cubic inches (cu.in.) = 1.05671 quarts (qt.) = 2.1134 pints (pt.) = 33.8147 fluid ounces (oz.fl.) = 1000.027 cubic centimetres (cc) = 1,000 millilitres (ml.)

A millilitre (ml.) = 0.0338147 fluid ounce (oz.fl.) = 0.001 litre (l)

= 1.000027 cubic centrimeter (cc.)

A cubic centimetre (cc. or cm^3) = 0.0010567 quart (qt.) = 0.033814 fluid ounce (oz. fl.) = 0.99997 ml.

A gallon U.S. (gal.) = 231 cubic inches (cu.in) = 3.785332 litres (1) = 3785.4 cubic centimetres (cc). = 3785.332 ml.

A fluid ounce (oz. fl.) = 0.0625 pint (pt.) = 0.0295729 litre (l) = 29.5737 cubic centimetre (cc) = 29.5729 millilitres (ml).

Unit of Weight or Mass

A kilogram (kg) is taken from the international prototype kilogram at the International Bureau of Weights and Measures = 2.02046223 pounds (avoirdupois) (lb. av.) = 35.273957 ounces (avoirdupois) (oz. av.) = 1, 000 grams (g).

A gram (g) = 0.0352739 ounce (avoirdupois) (oz. av.) = 1,000 milligrams (mg).

A milligram (mg) = 3.52739×10^{-5} ounce (avoirdupois) (oz.av.)

= 0.001 gram (g) = 1,000 microgram (μg or gamma)

A microgram (μg or gamma) = 0.001 milligram (mg)

A pound (avoirdupois) (lb. av) = 16 ounces (avoirdupois) (oz. av.) = 0.4535924 kilogram (kg) = 453.5924 grams (g)

An ounce (avoirdupois) (oz. av.) = 0.0625 pound (avoirdupois) (lb. av.) = 28.349527 grams (g).

1 Kilogram (kg) = 2.205 pounds

1 pound (lb) = 453.592 grams

1 long ton =1016 kilograms

Unit of area

1 barn (b) = 10^{-24} cm^2

1 millibarn (mb) = $10^{-27} cm^2$

1 microbarn (μb) = 10^{-30} cm^2

Unit of Time

Number of seconds in 1 day = 86,400

Number of seconds in 1 week = 6.048×10^5

Number of seconds in 365 days = 3.156×10^7

Unit of Surface

1 square inch = 6.45 sq.cm.

1 square foot = 0.09 sq. metre

1 square yard = 0.84 sq. metre

1 acre = 4050 sq. metres

We may use exponential notation as 1×10^3 in the place of the figure 1,000 and correspondingly 1×10^{-3} instead of 0.001 or 1/1000.

In metric system, metre is the primary standard of length.

Table 1 : Basic units of length

Unit	Symbol	Definition	Snonym	Symbol
Metre	m			
Millimetre	mm	1×10^{-3} m		
Micrometre	µm	$1 \times 10^{-6} = 1 \times 10^{-3}$ mm	Micron	µ
Nanometre	nm	$1 \times 10^{-9} = 1 \times 10^{-6}$ mm $= 1 \times 10^{-3}$ µm	Millimicron	mµ
Picometre	pm	1×10^{-12} m $= 1 \times 10^{-9}$ mm 1×10^{-6} µm $= 1 \times 10^{-3}$ nm	Micromicron	µµ

Table 2 : Basic units of weight

Unit	Symbol	Definition	Snonym	Symbol
Kilogram	kg			
Gram	g	1×10^{-3} kg		
Milligram	mg	1×10^{-6} kg $= 1 \times 10^{-3}$ g		
Microgram	µg	1×10^{-9} kg $= 1 \times 10^{-6}$ g 1×10^{-3} mg	gamma	r
Nanogram	ng	1×10^{-12} kg $= 1 \times 10^{-9}$ g 1×10^{-6} mg $= 1 \times 10^{-3}$ µg		mµg
Picogram	pg	1×10^{-15} kg $= 1 \times 10^{-12}$ g = 1×10^{-9} mg $= 1 \times 10^{-6}$ µg $= 1 \times 10^{-3}$ ng		

Table 3 : Basic units of volumes

Unit	Symbol	Definition	Snonym	Symbol
Litre				
Millilitre	ml	1×10^{-3} litre		
Microlitre	µl	1×10^{-6} litre = 1×10^{-3} ml	cubic millimetre	cmm mm^3
			Lambda	λ
Nanolitre	ml	1×10^{-9} litre = 1×10^{-6} ml = 1×10^{-3} µl		
Picolitre	pl	1×10^{-12} litre = 1×10^{-9} ml = 1×10^{-6} µl = 1×10^{-3} nl		

In litreature, wavelengths are usually expressed in terms of length units. The wavelentghs of visible light lies between 400 and 760 nanometre. Measurements in the region of the infrared (i.e. above 760 nm) are conveniently given in units of microns. On few occasions, wavelengths are given in Ångstrom units (Å). In general, one Å corresponds to 0.1 nm. Thus, for example 500 nm is equal to 5,000 Å. The wavelength of maximum transmission of a filter is often given to two significant figures. Similarly the addition of a zero after the two figures gives the wavelengths of maximum transmissin in nm, filter number 40 has a transmission band at 400 nm.

The gamma (r) which means 0.001 mg, it has been replaced by the microgram (µg).

Generally the unit of volume measurement in the metric system is the litre, which defined as the volume occupied by one kg of water at the temperature of greatest density (3.98°C) under normal atomospheric pressure (one atomosphere = 760 Torr). This volume is not identical to the cubic decimetre which is a unit of space. One litre equals 1.000028 cubic decimeters. *One lambda (λ) is equal to 0.001 ml and this unit was introduced by Kirk,* similarly unit cubic millimetre (ccm, mm^3) was introduced by Sahli. Twenty-two microlitres (ul) are therefore the same as 0.022 millilitre (ml) or 22 cubic millimeters (cmm, mm^3) or 22 lambda (λ).

One Mole = molecular weight (or corresponding atomic weight) in grams. The molecular weight can be calculated from the molecular formula by addition of the atomic weights. We may derive the following units.

Table 4 : Molar units

Unit	Symbol	Definition
Mole	Mole	
Millimole	m mole	1×10^{-3} mole
Micromole	µ mole	1×10^{-6} mole

Actually word "mole" should not be confused with the concentration unit "molar". Usually the expression in most experimental investigations is the unit of moles per 1,000 ml, i.e. molarity. A molar solution contains one mole in 1,000 ml. Simultaneously, a millimolar solution contains one m mole and a micromolar solution one μ mole per litre. One millilitre of a solution contains one mmole. In mentioning weight data the word "mole" itself and the expressions "millimole" and "micromole" should always be written out in full, while describing concentration data, however, "molar" may be noted as "m". In general, molarity is defined as the number of moles per litre of solution, simultaneously, molality is defined as the number of moles per kilogram of the solvent.

In biochemistry, we almost always deal with small amounts and low concentration, we use units which are smaller by the factor of 1000; they are the millimole (m mole), for amounts, and the millimole per litre (mM), for concentrations. The next smaller unit is μm (micromolar = 10^{-6} M). Concentrations of solutes in tissues are best expressed as micromoles per gram (μ moles/gm) of fresh weight. Care should be taken not to use the abbreviation of concentration mM (= millimolar) incorrectly for millimoles, which are amounts. In the older published literature, concentrations are often expressed as mg/100 ml; this has been called completely incorrectly "milligram per cent" and has been abbreviated as mg%. In the case of electrolytes, it is frequently advantageous to take into account the valence of the ions and to express amounts in equivalents or milliequivalents. The equivalent weight is the atomic or molecular weight divided by the valence of the ion. In the case of calcium, for example, 1 milliequivalent equals 40.1 mg divided by 2 (the atomic weight of calcium is 40.1), which is electrochemically equivalent to 1 milliequivalent of sodium or 23 mg. Concentrations are measured by the unit milliequivalent per litre, which is abbreviated as mEq/litre.

Temperature

°C = 5/9 (°F-32), °F = 9/5 °C + 32

Energy

1 calorie = 1 small calorie (cal) = 4.184 joules

4.184 Joule = One Calorie

4.184 Kilojoules = one Kilocalorie

1 Kilojoule (KJ) = 0.239 Kcal

1 Kilocalorie (kcal) = 1large calorie (Cal) = 1000 calories

1 megacalorie (Mcal) = 1000 kilocalories

One horse power (hp) = 10.692 Kcal energy output/min.

One foot pound (ft 1b) = 0.000324 Kcal

International Federation for clinical chemistry and International union of Pure and applied chemistry have approved system International "d" unit's (SI units) for expressing the results of analyses and these units have been fully described by Dybkaer and Jorgensen (1967).

Table 5 : Prefixes denoting multiples and submultiples of SI units (Dybkaer and Jϕrgensen, 1967)

Factor	Name	Symbol	Factor	Name	Symbol
10^{12}	tera	T	10^{-3}	milli	m
10^{9}	giga	G	10^{-6}	micro	μ
10^{6}	mega	M	10^{-9}	nano	n
10^{3}	kilo	K	10^{-12}	pico	p
10^{2}	hecto	h	10^{15}	femto	f
10^{1}	deca	da	10^{-18}	atto	a
		10^{-1}	10^{-1}	deci	d
		10^{-2}	10^{-2}	centi	c

Table 6 : The change of present normal blood (human subjects) constituents values to SI units (Dybkaer and Jϕrgensen, 1967)

Constituent	Present normal Values	Converstion factor	Normal values in SI units
Na^+	136 to 149 mEq/l	1.00	136 to 149 mmol/l
K^+	3.8 to 5.2 mEq/l	1.00	3.8 to 5.2 mmol/l
cl^-	100 to 107 mEq/l	1.00	100 to 107 m mol/l
HCO^-_3	24 to 30 mEq/l	1.00	24 to 30 m mol/l
Urea	15 to 40 mg/100 ml	0.166	2.5 to 6.6 m mol/l
Creatinine	0.1 to 1.4 mg /100 ml	88.4	9 to 124 μ mol/l
Uric acid	2 to 7 mg/100 ml	0.0595	0.12 to 0.42 m mol/l
Triglycerides	60 to 140 mg/100 ml	0.0113	0.68 to 1.58 m mol/l
Cholesterol	170 to 250 mg/100 ml	0.0259	4.4 to 6.5 m mol/l
Total protein	6.5 to 7.9 g/100 ml	10.0	65 to 79 g/l
Albumin	3.5 to 5.5 g/100 ml	10.0	35 to 55 g/l
Ca^{++}	4.5 to 5.5 mEq/l	0.500	2.25 to 2.75 m mol/l
Inorg. P.	1.5 to 2.5 mEq/l	0.500	0.75 to 1.25 m mol/l
Mg^{++}	1.4 to 1.8 mEq/l	0.500	0.7 to 0.9 m mol/l
Billirubin total	0.1 to 0.8 mg/100 ml	17.1	2 to 14 μ mol/l
Glucose	64 to 97 mg/100 ml	0.0555	3.6 to 6.2 mol/l
Standard bicarbonate	23 to 28 mEq/l	1.0	23 to 28 m mol/l
Base excess	-3 to +3 mEq	1.0	-3 to +3 m mol/l
Iron	110 to 130 μg/100 ml	0.179	20 to 23 μ mol/l
T_1 BC	250 to 400 μg/100 ml	0.179	45 to 72 μ mol/l
PBI	4 to 8 μg/100 ml	78.8	316 to 630 n mol/l

Carotene Conversion

(NRC, 1971)

International standards for vitamin A activity as related to vitamin A and beta carotene are as follows :

1 IU of vitamin A	=	1 USP unit
	=	Vitamin A activity of 0.300 μg of crystalline vitamin A alcohol, which corresponds to 0.344 μg of vitamin A acetate or 0.550 μg of vitamin A palmitate

Beta Carotene is the standard for provitamin A.

1 IU of vitamin A	=	0.6 μg of beta carotene
1 mg of beta carotene	=	1667 IU of vitamin A (Rat)
1 mg of beta carotene	=	500 IU of vitamin A (Pig)
1 mg of beta carotene	=	400 IU of vitamin A (Ruminant)
IU of vitamin A activity (%)	=	24
Factor for converting carotene to vitamin A	=	4.17
Rats and Chicks	=	Carotene is converted to vitamin A with an efficiency of 50%.
Cattle	=	Carotene is converted to vitamin A with an efficiency of 12%.

References

Dybkaer, R. and Jϕrgensen, K. (1967). Quantitites and units in clinical chemistry. Copenhagen, Munksgaard, Denmark.

National Research Council, (1971). No. 3. Nutrient requirements of dairy cattle, 4th revised edition, National Academy of Sciences, Washington, D.C.

Chapter - 71

Sampling and Processing of Biological Samples

Blood Sampling

Blood samples shall be taken in the early morning hours before offering any diet to human subjects or ration to livestock. The syringe and needle should be autoclaved, needle should be free from any blockage etc. In the case of ruminants, blood sample is taken directly from jugular vein, while in swine, blood sample is drawn from ear vein, while in human subjects, blood is taken from prominent vein on the inner surface of the yellow usually the (medium basilic). The container (test tube etc.) should be dried and autoclaved. We should separate plasma (from anticoagulent mixed blood) and serum from ordinary blood by centrifugation immediately. *We should remember by heart that blood samples should not be kept in deep freezer, because there are chances of haemolysis as well as an abnormal distribution of certain ions and enzymes between the cells and the serum*. We should never force the blood through the needle as such type of practice may result in extensive hemolysis. We should discard first few drops of blood, while taking sample. We should prepare protein free filtrate immediately. Protein-free filtrate may be kept in a much better way than whole blood or plasma.

Separation of Plasma

Plasma is a colourless fluid portion of blood in which the corpuscles are suspended. We should mix anticoagulant with the blood before the start of clotting. Anticoagulants may interefere with thrombin formation or with calcium availability. It is better to have thin film over the inner surface of the tube (collecting vessel). The thin film promotes quick solubility and mixing with the added blood.

Following anticoagulants are usually recommended for separating plasma.

	Anticoagulant	Quantitity required (mg/ml)
1.	Heparin	0.2
2.	Ethylenediamine tetraacetic acid (EDTA)	1.0
3.	Oxalates of lithium, sodium, potassium and ammonium	1 to 2
4.	Sodium citrate	5
5.	Sodium fluoride	10

General Anticoagulant for Use in the Clinical Laboratories

Dissolve 3 grams ammonium oxalate and 2 grams potassium oxalate in water and dilute to 250 ml. Pipette 0.05 ml of this solution for each ml of blood to be received in a container (small test tube or bottle), put in a film and dry in an incubator at 37°C or in a vacuum desiccator.

We should remember that the addition of anticoagulant may interfere with the analysis, e.g. heparin in the estimation of acid phosphatase, and EDTA or oxalate in calcium estimation. It has been observed that lithium heparin tubes are suitable for electrolyte estimation, which can be prepared by using 10 to 20 iu/ml of blood. Fluoride-oxalate tubes for glucose estimation should contain 1 mg of sodium fluoride and 3 mg of neutral potassium oxalate per ml of blood. To prepare such type of anticoagulant, dissolve 12 g of potassium oxalate and 4 g sodium fluoride in 200 ml of water and adjust to pH 7.4. *We may keep plasma in a refrigerator or cold room at 2 to 4°C for a few days if necessary. Samples required for enzyme assay should be kept in deep freeze at -20°C. Sometimes thymol is mixed with sodium fluoride (1 mg + 10 mg) for effective control microbial growth in stored blood samples. Try to keep the blood samples at room temperature and centrifuge immediately so as to avoid haemolysis.*

Separation of Serum

Serum is a colourless fluid portion of blood remaining after clotting and removal of corpuscles. *It differs from plasma in that the fibrinogen has been removed.*

Deliver the blood directly into a collecting vessel without anticoagulant, blood should be allowed to clot at room temperature. We should try to detach the clot from the walls of the tube by carefully using a broomstick (sterilised). Immediately centrifuge the blood samples at 2000 rpm and remove the supernatant serum with a rubber bulb pipette. If centrifuge is not available, keep the blood collecting vessel in a slanting position and let it be allowed in the same position overnight. Next day suck out the serum using rubber bulb pipette. We should not allow serum to come in contact with clott for a long time, because some of the cells in clott disintegrate and serum could not be used for estimating potassium and alkaline phosphatase. Serum for calcium estimation should be kept in glass test tubes. According to Hall and Whitehead (1970) serum calcium is adsorbed rapidly on to polystyrene containers (analyser cups) though this may be prevented if they are protected from loss of carbon dioxide and placed immediately in the refrigerator at 2 to 4°C.

Choice of Serum / Plasma in analytical Work

We may use serum/plasma for analysing biochemical constraints but following choice may be considered.

Biochemical constraint	**Sample**
Acid phosphatase	Serum
Alkaline phosphatase	Serum
Bicarbonate	Plasma
Bilirubin	Serum (keep in dark)
Calcium	Serum
Chloride	Plasma
Cholesterol	Serum
Creatinine	Serum
Fibrinogen	Plasma
Glucose	Blood
	Plasma
Iron	Serum
Lactate dehydrogenase	Serum
Lipids	Serum
Magnesium	Serum
Oxygen, pH	Blood
Phosphate	Serum
Potassium	Plasma
Protein	Serum
PBI	Serum
Sodium	Plasma
Urea	Plasma
	Serum
Uric acid	Serum

Wootton (1974) has given in detail about the perparation of serum and plasma and Oser (1954) has discussed the practical points while serum and plasma samples in the analytical work.

We should keep in mind that haemolysis is one of the important source of error, therefore all the possible percautions should be taken to avoid the haemolysis. To use heparin as an anticoagulant, dissolve 300 mg of ammonium heparinate (corresponding to 30,000 units) in 20ml of demineralised water. Use 50 micro litres (75 units) or this solution per ml of blood. This solution is then dried at 90-100°C. We may keep the tubes stable indefinitely. We should not keep whole blood for a longer time even at 4°C. We should only transport plasma in vials packed in a ice in thermos flask. Bacterial may grow in unfrozen samples if kept longer than 24 hours. A thymol fluoride mixture (10 mg sodium fluoride + 1 mg thymol/mg of blood) may be used as a bacteriostat. However freezing or lyophilization is a best procedure for preserving the serum or plasma samples.

Walford *et al.* (1956) analysed plasma for several biochemical constituents, they observed that only non-protein nitrogen, glucose and alkaline phosphatase showed significant alteration, further no alteration in the concentration of albumin, globulin, total protein, urea, uric acid, creatinine, cholesterol, Bilirubin, chloride, amylase, acid phosphatase was observed. Leverly and Jennings (1950) recorded no change in total protein, albumin, chloride and urea after preservation for a long time in the frozen state. Strumina (1952) studied the changes in several constituents for ten years in both dried and frozen plasma, he observed albumin and globulin remain unchanged, prothrombin activity decreased slightly after five years, but electrophoretic analysis showed surprisingly small changes. According to Hersey *et al.* (1963) lyophilized preparations are best for enzyme assay.

Preparing Protein free Filtrate in Blood Samples

(Method of Folin and Wu, 1919)

Principle

Long back, Folin and Wu (1919) proposed a system of analysis which requires only about 10 ml of blood for the quantitative determination of a series of constituents including non-protein nitrogen, urea, creatine, creatinine and uric acid. The proteins of the blood are removed most frequently by tungstic acid or trichloroacetic acid and different non-protein nitrogen fractions are analysed in the filtrate. The heavy metal acids are unstable and is therefore prepared by the interaction of sodium tungstate and sulphuric. In general, 1 ml of blood, plasma or serum will yield about 6 ml of filtrate (1:10 dilution) which is sufficient for atleast two of the determinations.

Reagents

1. Sodium Tungstate (10% solution)

Dissolve 100 grams of reagent grade carbonate free sodium tungstate in water and dilute to one litre.

2. Sulphuric Acid (2/3rd Normal)

Weigh 35 grams of concentrated sulphuric acid in a small tared, beaker, diluted to one litre with water and mix, check by titration against standard alkali by titration and adjust if necessary. The 2/3 N acid is intended to be equivalent to the sodium tungstate, so that when equal volumes are mixed substantially, the whole of the tungstic acid is set free without the presence of an excess of sulphuric acid. The liberated tungstic acid is taken up almost quantitatively by the blood proteins, to yield a filtrate which is only slightly acid.

Procedure

Transfer a measured quantity of blood to a flask having a capacity atleast 15 times that of the volume taken. For each volume (A ml) of blood taken, add from a burette exactly 7 volume (7xA ml) of water and mix. Add one volume (A ml) of 10 per cent sodium tungstate solution and mix. Finally, add slowly and with shaking one volume (A ml) of two thirds normal sulphuric acid. Stopper the flask and shake it. Only a few bubbles should form as a result of this shaking if all the proteins have been precipitated. Allow to stand for 10 minutes. The colour of the mixture should change from red to dark brown. If this change in colour does not occur, the coagulation is incomplete, usually because too much oxalate is present. In such an emergency the sample may be saved by adding 10 per cent sulphuric acid, drop by drop with shaking, until there is no foaming and the dark colour has set in. Pour the mixture on a dry folded filter paper large enough to hold it all. Cover the funnel with a watch glass to minimise evaporation. Collect the filtrate in a clean dry container. If the first few drops of filtrate are not absolutely clear, return this portion to the funnel and replace the receiver with a fresh one. Allow to filter until as much filtrate as possible has been obtained.

Blood filtrate prepared by this method represent a 1:10 dilution of the sample that is, 1 ml of filtrate corresponds to 0.1 ml of the original material.

☞ **Note**

This method is recommended by Oser (1954) for preparing protein free filtrate of blood.

Rumen Liquor Sampling

In cattle, there is a well marked stratification of both solids and liquid in the rumen (Pearson and Smith, 1943; Smith, Sweeney, Rooney, King and

Moore, 1956, Lampila and Poijarvi, 1959), but in sheep perhaps not to the same extent (Mc Donald, 1952, Hyden, 1961). Inert substances added to the rumen of sheep or cattle take at least an hour to become thoroughly mixed with the contents (Emery *et al.*, 1958, Gray, Jones and Pilgrim, 1960, Hyde'n 1961). When volatile fatty acids labelled with ^{14}C have been added to the rumen of cattle or sheep, the specific activities, particularly of the acid derived from the one which was added, have shown wide fluctuations lasting for some times (Sheppard, Forbes and Johnson, 1959, Gray *et al.*, 1960, Krishna and Ekern, 1974a,b,c). Inadequate mixing may well have been an important cause of those fluctuations. Time required for mixing in the rumen can sometimes be shortened by using some means for mechanical mixing, e.g., the pumping devices of Sutherland, Ellis, Reid and Murray (1932). Those devices, by alerting the environment, will have some effect on the rumen micro-organisms and their metabolism, the magnitude of any such effect is not yet known, but seems unlikely to be large. Mixing may also be helped by some such procedure as spraying an added solution relatively evenly throughout the rumen (Hyde'n, 1961).

Drawing Rumen Liquor Through Fistula

Weller *et al.* (1967) have developed an apparatus for continuous automatic sampling from the rumen of sheep. The principle of this apparatus is that up-stroke of a syringe sucks rumen fluid through a special four-way cock. The stop-cock is turned through 90° and the contents of the bore ejected into the collecting vessel. The stop-cock is against turned through 90° and the down-stroke of the syringe returns the excess fluid to the rumen. This completes the cycle, which is repeated throughout the sampling period. They have used this automatic device in their study, main advantage of this apparatus is that draw equal volumes (0.5 ml) of fluid at intervals of one minute. The rumen liquor was passed into a collecting vessel containing 350 g magnesium sulphate in 200 ml water. The collected contents were stirred continuously, and tests showed that no change took place in the VFA during the holding of composite sample. No doubt, this is a versatile and accurate technique to collect homogenous sample of rumen liquor round the clock.

A simple technique to draw rumen liquor samples followed by Krishna and Ekern (1974a,b,c) at the Agricultural University of Norway, ÅS-NLH (Norway) is recommended under Asian conditions. A cycle pump having a reverse valve is attached with plastic tube about 30 mm in diameter. This tube has several 9 mm holes in the terminal two inch portion. This tube is attached with two empty glass bottles wrapped with a woolen cloth. One bottle receive the rumen liquor is filtered through Terylene cloth (Westen and Hogan, 1967). This filtered rumen liquor is delivered into a glass bottle (under anaerobic conditions) containing mercuric chloride solution or thymol 10% (W/V) dissolved in isopropanol and stored at -20°C in a deep freezer. The rumen liquor samples are drawn at 0, 2, 4, 6 and 8 hrs after offering full day allocated complete ration to the ruminants.

Krishna and Ekern (1974a,b,c) have fed equally divided ration at an every hour interval during day and night for studying diurinal variation in the volatile fatty acids production rate using radio-isotope dilution technique. This technique was adopted by them so as to create conditions of homogenous mixing in the rumen. Troelsen (1971) emphasized that rumen liquor should be collected into a prewarmed thermos container so as to minimise the thermal and atmospheric shock to the microflora. We should always remember that conditions should be anaerobic one during all the steps of collecting rumen liquor. If the fluid is not perpared for use at once (within 10 minutes or so) after its collection, it should be aerated by a stream of CO_2, and placed in an incubator or a thermobath at 39°C.

Drawing Rumen Liquor Samples by Aspiration Through Stomach Tube

In this technique, esophageal probang is used for taking out the rumen liquor samples. It is very difficult to use this technique for repeated collections, therefore this is not adopted in most of the research stations.

Drawing Rumen Liquor Samples by Evacuating the Rumen Contents

This technique was followed by Troelsen (1971) at the Swift current Research Station, Saskatchewan (Canda) for taking rumen liquor from the donor animals. In this technique, rumen liquor sample is taken by inverting the sheep on a specially constructed table, removing the fistula plug, and placing the collection vessel under the fistula. Ocassionally it is necesary to use a long handled spoon to remove solid pockets of digesta obstructing the flow. The rumen liquor was filtered through a wire guaze (60 mesh).

General Recommendations

It is advisable to follow the technique as adopted by Krishna and Ekern (1974a,b,c) to collect the rumen liquor followed at the Agricultural University of Norway, ÅS-NLH, Norway.

Preparation of Protein Free Filtrate in Rumen Liquor
(Method of Pearson and Smith, 1943)

Deliver 10 ml rumen liquor in 100 ml volumetric flask, add 50 ml N/6 sulphuric acid and transfer the mixture to a 500 ml volumetric flask, add 50 ml 10 per cent sodium tungstate and made up the volume up to the mark with N/6 sulphuric acid. After standing for at least 24 hours, the mixture is filtered and an aliquot of the filtrate is taken for analysis of non-protein nitrogen fractions. It has been experienced that rumen liquor could remain in 10 ml volumetric flask with sulphuric acid for atleast two days before it is made up to 500 ml and after that any time between 24 and 48 hours could elapse before filtration.

Sampling Urine

We should collect cumulative 24-hour sampling so as to minimise the variations in the biochemical constituents. It is advisable to add preservative so that unstable substances may be perserved and the growth of bacteria is prevented. Toluene or Thymol (10% w/v in Isopropanol) are cheaper and better preservatives, which may be used to keep the excretory products in a stable form.

References

Emery, R.S., Smith, C.K. and Lewis, T.R. (1958). *J. Dairy Sci.*, 41: 647.

Folin, O. and Wu, H. (1919). *J. Biol. Chem.*, 38: 98.

Gray, F.V., Jones, G.B. and Pilgrim, A.G. (1960). *Austral. J. Agric. Res.*, 11: 383.

Hall, R.A. and Whitehead, T.P. (1970). *J. Clin. Path.*, 23: 323.

Hersey, M.G., Hartwell, K. adn Dos, R.P. (1963). *Clin. Chem.*, 9: 557.

Hyde'n, S. (1961). Kungl. Lantbrukshogs K. *Ann.*, 27: 51.

Krishna, G. and Ekern, A. (1974a). Z. *Tierphysiol., Tierernahrg. U. Futtermittelkde.*, 33: 275.

Krishna, G. and Ekern, A. (1974b). Z. *Tierphysiol., Tierernahrg. U. Futtermittelkde.*, 33: 281.

Krishna, G. and Ekern, A. (1974c). Z. *Tierphysiol., Tierernahrg. U. Futtermittelkde.*, 33: 323.

Krishna, G. Razdan, M.N. and Ray, S.N. (1977). Studies on energy and protein requirements of Zebu (*Bos Indicus*). Z. *Tierphysiologie* und *Tierernährung und Futtermittelkde.* 38: 281-284.

Krishna, G., Razdan, M.N. and Ray, S.N. (1976). Effect of different planes of nutrition on heat and methane production in dry cows. *Ind. J. Exptl., Biol.* 14: 710-711.

Krishna, G., Razdan, M.N. and Ray, S.N. (1977). A note on effect of seasonal variation on the nuitrient metabolism in lactating cows. *Indian J. Dairy Sci.* 30: 68-70.

Krishna, G., Razdan, M.N. and Ray, S.N. (1978). Assessment of Calorific value of dairy cows ration in tropical / subtropical region of India (Short Communication). *Indian J. Dairy Sci.* 31: 385-387.

Lampila, M. and Poijarvi, I. (1959). *Maataloust Aikakausk.*, 31: 315.

Levey, S. and Jennings, E.R. (1950). *Amer. J. Clin. Path.*, 20: 1059.

Mc Donald, I.W. (1952). *Biochem. J.*, 51: 86.

Oser, B.L. (1954). *Hawk's Physiological Chemistry.* 14th edn. McGraw Hill Book Co., London, pp 1017.

Pearson, R.M. and Smith, J.A.B. (1943). *Biochem. J.*, 37: 142-148.

Smith, P.H., Sweeney, H.C., Ronney, J.R., King, K.D. and Moore, W.E.C. (1956). *J. Dairy Sci.*, 39: 494.

Sheppard, A.J., Forbes, R.M. and Johnson, B.C. (1959). *Proc. Soc. Exp. Biol. Med.*, 101: 715.

Strumia, M. M., Mc Grawn, J.J. and Heggestad, G.E. (1952). *Amer J. Clin. Path.*, 22: 313.

Sutherland, T.M., Ellis, W.C., Reid, R.S. and Murray, M.G. (1962). *Brit. J. Nutrition,* 16: 603.

Troelsen, J.E. (1971). *Outline of procedure for in vitro digestion of forage samples.*, Bulletin, Research Station, Swift Current, Saskatchewan (Canada).

Walford, R.L., Sowa, M. and Daley, D. (1956). *Amer. J. Clin. Path.*, 26: 376.

Weller, R.A., Gray, F.V., Pilgrim, A.F. and Jones, G.B. (1967). *Aust. J. Agric. Res.*, 18: 107.

Weston, R.H. and Hogan. J.P. (1967). *Aust. J. Agri. Res.*, 19: 419-32.

Wooton, I.D.P. (1974). *Micro-analysis in Medical Biochemistry*, 5th edn., Churchill Livingstone, London, pp 35.

Chapter - 72

Calcium in Biological Materials

Estimation of Calcium in Feeds, Fodders and Faeces

(Titrimetric method of AOAC, 1965)

Principle

When a solution containing calcium is treated with ammonium oxalate, all the calcium present is precipitated as calcium oxalate, The precipitate on treatment with sulphuric acid dissolves, forming calcium sulphate liberating free oxalic acid which is quantitatively estimated by titration against standard N/10 potassium permanganate solution to arrive at the calcium content present in the given solution. The reactions which take place are given below:

$$(NH_4)_2C_2O_4 + (CH_3COO)_2Ca \rightarrow \underset{\substack{\text{Calcium oxalate} \\ \text{(white percipitate)}}}{CaC_2O_4} + CH_3\ COONH_4$$

When calcium oxalate reacts with dilute sulphuric acid, oxalic acid and calcium sulphate is formed.

$$CaC_2O_4 + H_2SO_4 \rightarrow Ca\ SO_4 + (COOH)_2$$

We should remember that calcium is precipitated at about pH4 (to prevent interference by phosphate) as the oxalate, which is dissolved in sulphuric acid and the liberated oxalic acid is titrated with standard potassium permanganate solution in the presence of sufficient volume of dilute sulphuric acid.

We should also know that sufficient volume of dilute sulphuric acid should be added otherwise known turbidity of manganous oxide may be formed.

$$2\ KMnO_4 + 3\ Mn\ SO_4 + 7\ H_2O \rightarrow K_2SO + 2H_2SO_4 + 5\ MnO_2H_2O$$

(Brown percipitate)

$$2\ KMnO_4 + 2\ H_2O \rightarrow K_2O + 2MNO_2.H_2O + 3O$$

(Brown precipitate)

In this case last drop of $KMnO_4$ acts as a self indicator.

Reagents

1. *Hydrochloric acid: 25 ml of concentrated hydrochloric acid diluted to 100 ml.*
2. *Methyl red indicator: Dissolve 0.15 g of methyl red in 500 ml of rectified spirit (95 per cent by volume)*
3. *Ammonium hydroxide solution 50 per cent (v/v)*
4. *Dilute Ammonium hydroxide solution 2 per cent (v/v)*
5. *Ammonium oxalate solution saturated.*
6. *Concentrated sulphuric acid specific gravity 1.84.*
7. *Standard potassium permanganate solution 0.1 N.*
8. *Stock calcium standard solution*

   Place 2.497 g of dry calcium carbonate into an evaporating dish. Dissolve in a minimal amount of 6 N hydrochloric acid, and evaporate to dryness on a steam bath. Dissolve the residue ($CaCl_2$) in sufficient distilled water to make 100 ml.

   Working standard : Dilute 1 ml of stock calcium standard to 100 ml with 1.4 N sodium chloride. This solution contains 0.1 mg calcium per ml.

Procedure

Weigh accurately about 1 g of the material in a silica basin and ignite at 600°C ± 20°C in a muffle furnace to carbon-free ash. Boil the ash in 40 ml of hydrochloric acid and a few drops of nitric acid. Transfer to a 250 ml graduated flask. Cool, dilute to the mark and mix thoroughly and filter through a dry fluted filter paper. The clear solution is to be used also for the determination of phosphorus.

Transfer a 25 ml aliquot of the solution prepared as above to a 400 ml beaker, dilute to about 100 ml with water and add two drops of methyl red indicator so that the colour of the solution is pink (pH 2.5 to 4.0). Dilute to about 150 ml, bring to the boil and add slowly, with constant stirring, 10 ml of hot ammonium oxalate solution. If the red colour of the solution changes to orange or yellow, add dilute hydrochloric acid dropwise until the colour again changes to pink. Leave overnight to allow the precipitate to settle. Filter the supernatant liquid through an ashless whatman filter paper No. 44 and wash the precipitate thoroughly with dilute ammonium hydroxide solution. Place the paper with the precipitate in the beaker in which precipitation was carried out and add a mixture of 125 ml of water and 5 ml of concentrated sulphuric acid. Heat to a temperature between 70° and 90°C and titrate with the standard potassium permanganate solution until the first slight pink colour is obtained.

Calculation

Calcium (on moisture free basis) per cent by weight (g/100g)

$$= \frac{R \times 0.002 \times \text{volume of extract made} \times 100}{w \times \text{Aliquot taken}}$$

where

R = volume of 0.1 N $KMnO_4$ used in titration

W = Weight of material (g) on dry matter basis

General factors

(Calcium)	1 ml 0.1 N permanganate = 0.00 2004 g Ca
(Calcium carbonate)	1 ml 0.1 N permanganate = 0.00 5004 g $CaCO_3$
(Calcium Oxide)	1 ml 0.1 N permanganate = 0.00 2804 g CaO

Interconversion factors

Mineral conversion	**Multiply by**	**Reciprocal multiply by**
Calcium to calcium oxide	1.4	0.714
Calcium to calcium carbonate	2.5	0.400

Example : Sample A

R	= 28.5 ml
W	= 1.9112 g
Volume of extract made	= 250 ml
Aliquot taken	= 25 ml

Substituting these values in the above formula

$$= \frac{28.5 \times 0.002 \times 250 \times 100}{1.9112 \times 25}$$

= 29.82 per cent (g/100g) calcium.

Result : The given sample contained 29.82 g/100 g calcium

☞ Notes

1. *Wash the filter paper with very dilute ammonia solution until the filtrate no longer gives a precipitate on addition of dilute nitric acid and silver nitrate solution.*
2. *To check whether the precipitate is free from oxalate, collect half a test tube full of the filtrate, acidify with a few drops of conc. sulphuric acid and heat the test tube. Add only one drop of N/10 $KMnO_4$ solution. Pink colour persisting, shows absence of oxalate.*
3. *In the place of methyl red, we may add bromocresol green to the filtrate and make it just alkaline with dilute ammonia. Acidify the solution with dilute acetic acid and then add 0.5 ml of glacial acetic acid. Heat the solution to boiling and slowly add 10 ml of saturated ammonium oxalate solution. Then add dilute ammonia to the hot solution until it becomes yellow-green (pH 3.8) and allow it to stand for at least 4 h (preferably overnight).*
4. *Keep the filter paper outside the beaker in a separate petridish and boil the contents of beaker just before titration. At the time of appearing light pink colour, put back the filter paper and proceed further with titration job till the faint pink colour appears permanently.*
5. *Calcium can be titrated with EDTA, provided precuations are taken against interfering ions. Flame photometry or Nephelometry may be used for the assay of calcium.*

☞ Note

This method was standardised long back by Talapatra et al. (1940) under tropical conditions. Indian Standards Institution (1975) has adapted this method under IS: 7874 (Part II) for use in Asian subcontinent regions and same method has been followed by the Indian Standards Institution BIS (1968) under IS : 1664 for analysing calcium in mineral mixtures for supplementing cattle feeds.

Estimation of Calcium in Blood

Introduction

There is no calcium in the corpuscles. The total calcium may be fractioned with suitable methods into three fractions. They are (1) non-diffusible calcium (thought to be bound to protein) and diffusible calcium which may be separated into (2) ionizable and (3) non-ionizable fractions. Most of the anticoagulants for blood act by reaction with calcium. Serum from clotted blood is ordinarily used for analysis., heparinised plasma may also be used.

Method I (Titrimetric method of clark and Collip, 1925)

Principle

Calcium is precipitated directly from the serum as oxalate and the latter is titrated with potassium permanganate. After washing out the excess of reagent, the oxalate of the precipitate is titrated by oxidising it with permangante in acid solution.

Procedure

Introduce into a graduated 15 ml centrifuge tube, 2 ml of clear serum, 2 ml of distilled water and 1 ml of 4 per cent ammonium oxalate solution. Mix thoroughly mixing is aided by holding the tube at the mouth and giving it a circular motion by tapping the lower end. The centrifuge tube should have an outside diameter of 6 to 7 mm at the 0.1 ml mark. Allow to stand for overnight. Again mix contents. Centrifuge for about five minutes at 1500 revolutions per minute. Carefully pour off the supernatant liquid and while the tube is still inverted, let it drain in a rack for 5 minutes, resting the mouth of the tube on a pad of filter paper. Wipe the mouth of the tube dry with a soft cloth. Stir up the precipitate and wash the sides of the tube with 3 ml of diluted ammonia (2 ml of concentrated ammonia to 98 ml of water) directed in a very fine stream, from a wash bottle. Centrifuge the suspension and drain again as before. Add 2 ml of approximately normal sulphuric acid (28 ml of concentrated acid to a litre) by blowing it from a pipette directly upon the precipitate so as to break up the material and facilitate solution. Place the tube in a boiling water bath for about 1 minute. Titrate with 0.01 normal potassium permanganate to a definite pink colour which persists for at least 1 minute. If necessary during the courseof the titration, warm the tube by placing in a water bath kept at 70°C to 75°C. A microburette graduated in 0.02 ml should be used.

Calculation

One ml of 0.01 N $KMnO_4$ is equivalent to 0.2 mg calcium. $(a\text{-}b) \times 0.2 \times \frac{100}{2}$ = mg calcium/100 ml serum or (a - b) x 10 = mg Calcium / 100 ml serum

Where

a = Volume of 0.01 N $KMnO_4$ used in the titration of unknown sample.

b = volume of 0.01 N $KMnO_4$ used in the titration of blank (2 ml of approximately normal sulphuric acid).

Method II (Colorimetric method of Trinder, 1960).

Principle

Trinder (1960) has described the use of naphthalhydroxamic acid as a precipitating agent which is so efficient that only a small excess of the reagent is required. This means that it is unnecessary to wash the precipitate to remove excess reagent and a very convenient and accurate method results.

Reagents

1. *Calcium reagent* : Dissolve 250 mg of naphthalhydroxamic acid by warming in 100 ml of water containing 5 ml of ethanolamine and 2 g of tartaric acid. Add 9 g of sodium chloride dissolved in 500 ml of water and dilute to one litre with water. If a precipitate forms, filter through a Whatman No. 40 or 43 paper.
2. *EDTA solution* : 2 g of disodium EDTA per litre in 0.1 N - sodium hydroxide.
3. *Colour reagent* : Dissolve 60 g of ferric nitrate ($Fe(NO_3)_3 \cdot 9H_2O$) in 500 ml of water, add 15 ml of concentrated nitric acid and dillute to one litre with water.
4. Calcium standard (5 mEq/L). Dissolve 125 mg of dry calcium carbonate in 40 ml of 0.1 N-hydrochloric acid and dilute to 500 ml with water.

Procedure

1. Centrifuge tubes of 12 to 15 ml capacity are used.
2. *Test* : Pipette 0.2 ml of serum or plasma into a centrifuge tube. Add 5 ml of calcium reagent and mix.
3. *Standard.* 0.2 ml of caclium standard (m Eq/L) and 5 ml of calcium reagent.
4. Blank, 5 ml of calcium reagent.
5. Allow the tubes to stand at room temperature for 30 minute. Centrifuge the tubes at 3500 rpm and decant the supernatant fluid carefully by slowly inverting the tubes and immediately placing them to drain mouth down wards on a pad of filter paper, without returning them to the upright position. After 5 minutes, wipe the mouths of the tubes and add 1ml of EDTA solution. Shake to suspend the precipitate, cover the mouth

of the tube with an aluminium cap or a marble and warm in a boiling water bath for 10 minutes with occasional mixing to ensure complete solution of the precipitate. Cool, add 3 ml of colour reagent and mix. Compare the colours at 450 nm using an Ilford 622 blue or chance 0B 10 filter.

$$\text{Serum Calcium (mEq/l)} = \frac{T - B}{S - B} \times 5$$

(To convert the result into mg/100 ml, multiply by 2).

where

T = Test solution

S = Standard solution

B = Blank

References

AOAC, (1965). *Official methods of analysis of the Association of Official Agricultural Chemists*, 10th edn, AOAC, Benjamin Frankling Station, Washington, D.C., pp 340.

Clark, E.P. adn Collip, J.B. (1925). *J. Biol. Chem.*, 63 : 461.

Indian Standards Institutiion, (1968). *Specification for mineral mixtures for supplementing cattle feeds (first Revision), IS : 1664*, ISI, Manak Bhavan, New Delhi 1.

Indian Standards Institution, (1975). *Animal feeds and feeding stuffs, method of tests for : Part II. Minerals and trace elements* (BIS). IS : 7874. ISI, Manak Bhavan, New Delhi 1.

Krishna, G. (1973). Studies on energy and protein requirements for milk production in Indian Dairy Animals. Ph.D. Thesis, NDRI, Karnal (Haryana), Agra University Agra, U.P. (India).

Oser, B.L. (1954). *Hawk's physiological chemistry*, 14th edn. McGraw Hill Book Co., London, pp 1133.

Talapatra, S.K., Ray, S.C and Sen, K.C. (1940). *Indian J. Vet. Sci.*, 10 : 243.

Trinder, P. (1960). *Analyst.*, 85 : 889.

Wootton, I.D.P. (1974). *Microanalysis in medical biochemistry*, 5th edn. Churchill. Livingstone, London, pp 68.

Chapter - 73

Phosphorus in Biological Materials

Estimation of Phosphorus in Feeds, Fodders and Faeces

(Titrimetric method of AOAC, 1965)

Principle

Metaphosphates and pyrophosphates are converted to the orthophosphate, which is treated at 65-70°C with excess of molybdate in the presence of nitric acid. When acid solutions of phosphates are heated with ammonium molybdate, the phosphoric acid is precipitated as yellow ammonium phosphomolybdate $(NH_4)_3$ PO_4 (Mo03)12 $2HNO_3.H_2O$. Impurities like molybdic oxide, if happened to be formed any, goes into solution. The yellow precipitate formed reacts quantitatively with standard alkali, the excess of which is back titrated with acid.

Reagents

1. Concentrated nitric acid (specific gravity 1.42).
2. Nitric acid (1:1) a mixture of equal volumes of concentrated nitric acid and water.
3. Ammonium Molybdate stock solution. Take 200 grams of powdered ammonium molybdate in a stoppered graduated cylinder of 1000 ml capacity, add to it 800 ml of water and shake well for 25 minutes to

dissolve the ammonium molybdate. Add gradually 25 per cent (W/V) ammonium hydroxide solution till the solution is clear (about 100 to 140 ml ammonium hydroxide may be required). Avoid adding excess of ammonia. Make up the volume to one litre. If necessary, filter the solution through a fluted filter paper and stock this solution.

4. Dilute nitric acid 2 per cent (W/V).
5. Potassium nitrate solution 3 per cent (W/V).
6. Standard sodium hydroxide solution (N/7).
7. Standard nitric acid (N/7).
8. Phenolphthalein indicator solution. Dissolve 0.1 gram of phenolphthalein in 100 ml of 60 per cent (W/V) rectified spirit.

Procedure

Preliminary ashing. Weigh accurately about 5 grams of the material in a silica basin. Slowly ash at a temperature below 600°C. Fixing agents may be necessary if the feed is high in phosphorus and does not contain sufficient amounts of calcium carbonates. If a fixing agent is to be used, add 5 ml of calcium acetate solution to the material, dry on a waterbath and then in an oven and ash the material slowly over a Bunsen burner or in a muffle furnace.

Extraction. Moisten the dry ash slowly with water taking care that no particle is blown off. Transfer the ash with water, to a beaker of 150 ml capacity. Add 5 ml of concentrated nitric acid to the basin and a little water and transfer the same to the beaker. Again rinse the basin with 5 ml of nitric acid (1:1) and transfer to the beaker. Finally, rinse the basin with hot water and transfer the washings to the beaker. Boil the contents of the beaker for a few minutes and filter into a 250 ml graduated flask. Wash the residue on the filter paper with hot water until the filtrate is free from acid. Cool and then make up the volume to 250 ml with water.

Precipitation. Take a 50 ml aliquot in a 150 ml beaker. In a dry beaker prepare ammonium molybdate solution by pouring into it, quickly and simultaneously, 10 ml of ammonium molybdate stock solution and 10 ml of concentrated nitric acid, or take 10 ml of concentrated nitric acid first in the beaker and into this pour quickly 10 ml of ammonium molybdate solution, whirling the beaker during addition. Pour this freshly prepared clear liquid quickly into the beaker containing the aliquot and stir.

The temperature developed in the molybdate solution is sufficient to precipitate all the phosphorus present in the aliquot. Under no circumstances the phosphomolybdate precipitate should be heated either on a water-bath or directly over a burner to avoid precipitation of molybdic anhydride.

Filtration and washing. Allow the precipitate to stand overnight and then filter through a disc of whatman filter paper No. 42 in a Gooch crucible by suction, or through a 9 cm whatman filter paper No. 42 over an ordinary funnel. (In case of urgency, the precipitate may be filtered off after two to three hours). As far as possible, the precipitate should not be transferred but only the supernatant liquid should be passed through. When the supernatant liquid is decanted off, wash the precipitate twice with dilute nitric acid and, then with potassium nitrate solution, until the washings are free from acid. If ordinary funnel and filter paper are used, freedom from acidity may be tested by collecting sufficient filtrate in a test-tube to which a few drops of phenolphthalein indicator solution and one drop of the standard sodium hydroxide solution have been added. If the pink colour appears with one drop of the standard alkali, the precipitate is free from acid.

Titration. Transfer the precipitate with the filter paper back to the beaker in which precipitation is carried out. Add sufficient quantity of N/7 sodium hydroxide solution from a burette just sufficient to dissolve the precipitate and then add 5 ml in excess. See that no yellow precipitate sticks to the filter paper. Note the total volume of the N/7 sodium hydroxide solution added. Add about 10 drops of phenolphthalein indicator solution and titrate the excess of alkali with the N/7 nitric acid.

Calculation

Phosphorus (g/100 g) on dry matter basis

$$= \frac{(N-H) \times 0.0001925 \times 100 \times 250}{\text{Wt. of material on dry matter basis} \times \text{aliquot}}$$

In this formula, factor is based on the hypothesis :

1 ml of N/7 NaOH = 0.0001925 g of phosphorus

where,

N = Volume of N/7 NaOH used in the titration.

H = Volume of N/7 HNO_3 used in the titration.

Conversion factors

Mineral conversion	Multiply by	Reciprocal multiply by
Phosphorus to phosphoric acid	2.29	0.436

Example

Sample - N

N = 25.0 ml

H = 19.9 ml

Wt. of material on dry matter basis = 9.005 g

Aliquot = 50 ml

$$=\frac{(25.0-19.9)\times 0.0001925\times 100\times 250}{9.005\times 50}$$

= 0.054 g p/100 g on dry matter basis

Result : The sample W contained 0.054 g phosphorus/100 g on dry matter basis

Precautions

1. Avoid the formation of molybdic acid at the time of adding mixture of concentrated nitric acid and 20 per cent Ammonium molybdate.
2. The glass rod should not touch the wall and bottom of the beaker, when stirring to avoid the molybdic acid formation.
3. There must be no gap in the filtration process.
4. Tap water flow must be continued at the time of removal of gooch crucible from the suction flask.
5. The phosphorus must be in the form of the orthophosphate. This can be ensured by boiling the solution with nitric acid.
6. We may use 0.5 N NaOH and 0.5 N HCl for titration purpose, but in this case factor will be as below.

   1 ml 0.5 N NaOH = 0.001544 g P_2O_5

☞ Note

This method was standardised long back by Talapatra et al., (1940) under tropical conditions. Indian Standards Institution (1975) BIS, has adapted this method under IS : 7874 (Part II) for use in Asian subcontinent regions and same method has been followed by the Indian Standards Institution (1968) BIS under IS : 1664 for analysing phosphorus in mineral mixtures for supplementing cattle feeds.

Estimation of Phosphorus in Feeds, Fodders and Faeces

(Colorimetric method of Donald *et al.*, (1956)

Principle

The method is based on *Mission's reaction,* in which the phosphorus present as the orthophosphate reacts with a vanadate-molybdate reagent to produce a yellow-orange complex, the optical density of which is measured at 420 nm. The original method was developed by Donald *et al.* (1956) and later on evaluated by Park and Dunn (1963).

Reagents

1. *Standard stock solution : Containing 0.1 mg P in 1 ml is made from either 1.1246 gram K_2HPO_4 or from 0.8788 gram KH_2PO_4 dissolved and diluted with distilled water to 200 ml.*
2. *Nitric acid. Concentrated nitric acid diluted with water 1:2.*
3. *Ammonium vanadate : 2.5 grams ammonium vanadate is dissolved in about 500 ml boiling water. After cooling, 20 ml concentrated nitric acid is added, then diluted to 1000 ml with water.*
4. *Ammonium molybdate : 50 grams ammonium molybdate or 70 grams sodium molybdate is dissolved in about 800 ml water at about 50°C. After cooling the solution is diluted to 1000 ml with water. The reagents 2,3 and 4 are mixed in ratio 1:1:1, and in the order given.*

The mixture is almost indefinitely keepable in a brown coloured glass stoppered bottle.

The phosphorus factor : Aliquots of standard (*reagent 1*) are diluted in 100 ml volumetric flasks to about 50 ml, then 30 ml of the reagent mixture is added and finally water is added to the mark. After mixing, stay for 10 minutes, optical density, is read by 450 nm in a 1 cm cuvette.

$$fp = \frac{\text{mg P in standard solution}}{\text{optical density}}$$

where,

fp = factor is on 100 g basis.

Procedure

5-10 grams dried or predried material or equivalent fresh sample is ashed at 550-600°C. The ash is moistened with water, 10 ml concentrated hydrochloric acid is added and then taken to dryness on a hot plate. This is repeated twice, and then taken to dryness on a hot plate. This is repeated twice, and then taken to dryness on a hot plate. This is repeated twice, and the dry residue heated again for a short time in the oven at 550°C. The silicates are also filtered. 10 ml diluted HNO_3 (1:2) is added, and boiled for 5-10 minutes in the crucible, it is diluted with water and made up to 250 ml in a volumetric flask. Finally, the solution is filtered, and from filterate an aliquot, is taken for analysis. About 25-50 ml aliquot is necessary. The aliquot is diluted to about 50 ml in the 100 ml volumetric flask, then proceed as for the standard.

☞ Note

Samples poor in ash, may be added 20 ml 5 per cent magnesium acetate before reduction in the furnace. The ash solution is then, however, made invalid for the simultaneous determination of Ca and Mg.

Calculation

Estimating P in the given sample

Sample	- W
Volume of standard	= 9 ml
Concentration of phosphorus in 9 ml	= 0.9 mg
O.D. of standard	= 0.260

$$pf = \frac{\text{Concentration of P in standard}}{\text{O.D. of standard}}$$

$$pf = \frac{0.9}{0.260} = 3.461$$

$$P, g/100g = \frac{\text{Vol. of extract made x factor x O.D. of unknown x 100}}{\text{Wt. of material on dry matter basis x Aliquot x 1000}}$$

Volume of extract made	= 250 ml
Factor	= 3.461
O.D. of unknown	= 0.276
Wt. of material on dry matter basis	= 4.544 grams
Aliquot	= 25 ml

Substituting these values in the above formula

$$P, g/100 = \frac{250 \times 3.461 \times 0.276 \times 100}{4.544 \times 25 \times 1000}$$

= 0.210 g/100 g

Result : The given sample W contained phosphorus 0.210 g/100 g.

Estimation of Inorganic Phosphorus in Blood

(Colorimetric method of Fiske and Subba Row, 1925)

Principle

Phosphomolybdic acid and phosphotungstic acid are easily reduced forming solutions which are coloured intensely blue. Various reducing agents may be used and, as a result, a number of colorimetric methods have been developed. Phosphate may be determined after it reacts with molybdic acid to form phosphomolybdic acid which is then reduced by some reducing agent. In the method described below reducing agent 1,2,4 - amino naphtholsulphonic acid (ANS) has been used to develop blue colour. It has main limitation that the rate of reduction of phosphomolybdate is slow and its use require at least 45 minutes for the development of maximal absorbances.

Reagents

1. *Trichloroacetic acid (10%) : Dissolve 10 grams of reagent grade trichloroacetic acid in water and dilute to 100 ml.*

2. *Sulphuric acid (10 N) : Carefully add 450 ml of concentrated sulphuric acid to 1300 ml of water. To check, dilute 10 ml of this solution to 100 ml in a volumetric flask, mix, and titrate a 10 ml portion with standard 1 N sodium hydroxide. From the titration results, adjust the original solution if necessary to make it exactly 10 N.*

3. *Molybdate solution : Dissolve 25 grams of reagent grade ammonium molybdate in about 200 ml of water. In one litre volumetric flask place 300 ml of 10 N sulphuric acid. Add the molybdate solution and dilute with washings to one litre with water. Mix, it is stable indefinitely.*

4. *Aminonaphtholsulphonic acid reagent : Place 195 ml of 15 per cent sodium bisulfite solution (see below) in a glass stoppered cylinder. Add 0.5 gram of 1,2,4- aminonaphtholsulphonic acid. Add 5 ml of 20 per cent sodium sulphite (see below). Stopper and shake until the powder is dissolved. If solution is not complete, add more sodium sulfite, one ml at a time, with shaking, but avoid an excess. Transfer the solution to a brown glass bottle and store in the cold. This solution is usable for about four weeks, if kept as described.*

5. *Sodium bisulphite (15%) : To 30 gram of reagent grade sodium bisulphite in a beaker add 200 ml of water from a graduated cylinder. Stir to dissolve, and if turbid allow to stand well-stoppered for several days and filter, Keep well stoppered.*

6. *Sodium sulphite (20%) : Dissolve 20 gram of reagent grade anhydrous sodium sulphite in water, dilute to 100 ml and filter if necessary. Keep well stoppered.*

7. *Standard phosphate solution : Dissolve exactly 0.351 gram of pure dry monopotassium phosphate in water and transfer quantitatively to a one litre volumetric flask. Add 10 ml of 10 N sulphuric acid, dilute to the mark with water and mix. This solution contains 0.4 mg of phosphorus in 5 ml. It is stable indefinitely.*

Procedure

To 8 ml of 10 per cent trichloroacetic acid solution in a small flask, add slowly, with mixing, 2 ml of whole blood, serum or plasma. Stopper, shake and filter through a low ash filter paper. Transfer 5 ml filtrate to a cylinder or other container graduated at 10 ml, and add 1 ml of the molybdate. Mix, add 0.4 ml of aminonaphthol-sulphonic acid reagent and again mix. Dilute to the mark, mix and allow to stand five minutes. Transfer a portion of the coloured solution to a suitable container and read in the photometer at 660 to 720 mμ. Set the photometer to zero density with a blank prepared by treating 5 ml of 10 per cent trichloroacetic acid with one ml of molybdate solution and 0.4 ml of aminonaphtholsulphonic acid reagent, followed by water to a volume of 10 ml. Establish the density of a standard phosphate solution as follows : Transfer 5 ml of the stock phosphate standard, containing 0.4 mg of P, to a 40 ml volumetric flask, make up to volume with 10 per cent trichloroacetic acid, and mix. Transfer 5 ml of this dilute standard containing 0.04 mg of phosphorus, to a suitable container, add one ml of molybdate solution and 0.4 ml of aminonaphtholsulphonic acid reagent, dilute to 10 ml with water and mix. Allow to stand five minutes and determine the density in the photometer, whose zero is set with a blank as described above.

Calculation

$$\frac{\text{Density of unknown}}{\text{Density of standard}} \times 0.04 \times 100 = \text{mg inorganic P/100 ml blood, plasma or serum}$$

To permit the covering of a greater range of phosphate concentration, the amount of sample taken for protein precipitation may be reduced e.g., one ml (or 0.5 ml) of whole blood, serum or plasma is treated with 10 per cent trichloroacetic acid at a final volume of 10 ml and 5 ml of filtrate taken for analysis as described. If this is done, the calculation is the same except that the final result is multiplied by two (or 4, if 0.5 ml of sample is taken).

The colour obtained in this procedure shows little change between 5 and 20 minutes after adding the aminonaphthol-sulphonic acid reagent, and the agreement with Beer's law is excellent, permitting calculation of results in terms of the density of a simultaneously prepared standard and eliminating the necessity for a calibration curve.

Note : To avoid the effects of glycolysis in shed blood, the serum should be separated from the cells as promptly as possible.

Estimation of inorganic phosphorus in blood
(Colorimetric method of Gomori, 1942)
Principle

This method is the modification of Fiske and Subba Row (1925) procedure. In this case reducing agent, elon is used which is oxidised to quinone.

Reagents

1. *Trichloroacetic acid (10%)*
2. *Sulphuric acid (10 N) : Pour 282 ml of concentrated sulphuric acid into 600 ml of water. Cool and make up to one litre.*

3. *Molybdate-sulphuric reagent : Mix one part of a 7.5 per cent solution of sodium molybdate ($Na_2MoO_4.2H_2O$), 1 part of 10 N sulphuric acid and 2 parts of water.*
4. *Reducing solution : Dissolve 1 g of methyl-p-aminophenol sulphate (elon) in 100 ml of a 3 per cent solution of sodium bisulfite.*
5. *Stock standard phosphate solution (5 ml = 0.4 mg P) : Dissolve 0.351 grams of pure monopotassium phosphate in water. Transfer quantitatively to a litre volumetric flask, add 10 ml of 10 N sulphuric acid, dilute to the mark and mix. The standard may be kept indifinitely.*

Procedure

Transfer to a dry Erlenmeyer flask 20 ml of 5% trichloroacetic acid. Add, while rotating the flask gently, 5 ml of blood or plasma or serum. Stopper the flask, shake vigorously a few minutes. Filter through ashless whatman paper. Measure 5 ml of the filtrate into a tube graduated at 10 ml. Add 2 ml of molybdate sulphuric reagent and after mixing, deliver 1 ml of the reducing solution. Dilute to the mark and mix. At the same time prepare a standard by transferring 5 ml of standard phosphate solution (containing 0.4 mg of phosphorus) to a 10 ml volumetric flask and add about 60 ml of water, 20 ml of molybdate-sulphuric reagent and 10 ml of reducing solution. Dilute the contents of the flask to the mark and mix. After 15 minutes, read the standard and unknown in a photometer which has been set at zero using a solution prepared as described for the standard but with water in place of the standard solution. Use a red filter. Calculate the mg. of phosphorus per 100 ml and millimoles per litre.

☞ Note

Dryer et al. (1957) have modified the original Fiske and Subba Row (1925) method by using a different reducing agent-semidine hydrochloride (N-phenyl-p-phenylenediamine) in the place of ANS (1,2,4-aminonaphtholsulphonic acid).

Estimation of Available Phosphorus in Poultry Feeds

(Colorimetric method of Fiske and Subba Row, 1925., AOAC, 1965)

Introduction

The value of phosphorus in poultry nutrition is dependent upon the form in which it is present in the diet. Phosphorus from cereal sources in the form of phytates and it is relatively unavailable to poultry. For optimum results it appears that at least 0.4 to 0.5 per cent of the total phosphorus in the diet, and probably all of it, should be from non-cereal sources. Inorganic phosphorus is much more readily available and good sources are fish meal, meat and bone meal, steamed bone flour and anhydrous dicalcium phosphate. The term *"available phosphorus"* is used to refer to the *"inorganic phosphorus"*. All the phosphorus from animal sources, and a maximum of 40 per cent of that from cereal and vegetable protein sources, may be regarded as being "available phosphorus" in the formulation of poultry diets. *As per Indian Standards Institution (1992) BIS recommendations, requirement of available phosphorus in the chicken feeds is about 0.5 per cent by mass.*

Reagents

1. Aminonaphtholsulphonic acid

Place 195 ml of 15 per cent sodium bisulhite solution in a glass stoppered cylinder. Add to it 0.5 g of 1,2,4-aminonaphtholsulphonic acid and 5 ml of 20 per cent sodium sulfite solution. Stopper the cylinder and shake, well to dissolve the powder. If the powder is not dissolved completely and more sodium sulphite solution, 1 ml at a time, with shaking, but avoid excess. Transfer the solution to a brown coloured glass bottle and store in the cold. The solution, if stored as just mentioned, may be used for about four weeks.

2. Sodium bisulphite solution - 15 per cent (W/V)

Weigh accurately 30 g of sodium bisulphite in a beaker and add 200 ml of water. Stir to dissolve, and if the solution is turbid, allow to stand and then filter. Keep the solution in a brown coloured stoppered bottle.

3. Sodium sulphite solution - 20 per cent (W/V)

Dissolve 20 g anhydrous sodium sulphite in water and dilute to 100 ml, if necessary, filter the solution. Keep the solution in a brown coloured stoppered bottle.

4. Calcium chloride solution - 10 per cent (W/V)

Saturate this solution with calcium hydroxide at pH 8.8.

5. Calcium chloride solution - 20 per cent (W/V)

6. Hydrochloric acid dilute

7. Molybdate I

Dissolve 25 g of reagent grade ammonium molybdate in about 200 ml water. Place in a one litre volumetric flask, 500 ml of 10 N sulphuric acid and add to it the molybdate solution. Dilute to one litre with water. Mix well, the solution keeps stable indefinitely.

8. Molybdate II

Dissolve 25 grams of reagent grade ammonium molybdate in about 200 ml of water. Place in a one litre volumetric flask, 300 ml of 10 N sulphuric acid and add to it the molybdate solution. Dilute to one litre with water. Mix well. The solution keeps stable indefinitely.

9. Phenolphthalein indicator solution

Dissolve 0.1 g of phenolphthalein in 100 ml of 95 per cent (W/V) ethyl alcohol.

10. Standard phosphate solution

Prepare standard solution in a similar way as mentioned under Fiske and Subha Row (1925) method or Gomori (1942) method.

11. Sulphuric acid - 10 N

Add carefully 450 ml of concentrated sulphuric acid to 130 ml of water. To check, dilute 10 ml of this solution to 100 ml in a volumetric flask, mix and titrate a 10 ml portion of this solution with standard 1 N sodium hydroxide solution. From the titration results, adjust, if necessary, the normality of the original solution to make it exactly 10 N.

12. Trichloroacetic acid - 5 per cent (W/V)

Dissolve 5g of the reagent grade trichloroacetic acid in water & dilute to 100ml.

Apparatus

Photoelectric Colorimeter.

Procedure

Weigh accurately about 20 g of the ground material and transfer into a 250 ml beaker. Add 100 ml of trichloroacetic acid (maintained at about 5°C) and stir occasionally for 15 minutes. Allow it to stand for 2 hours.

Transfer the contents to a 250 ml graduated flask and make up the volume to the mark with trichloroacetic acid (maintained at about 5°C). Stir the contents of the flask thoroughly and allow to stand for 30 minutes. Filter about 120 ml of the supernatant liquid and transfer 100 ml of the filtrate to a 250 ml beaker. Neutralize with the sodium hydroxide solution using phenolphthalein as indicator. Add to it 2 ml of calcium chloride solution and allow it to stand at room temperature for 10 minutes. Centrifuge the precipitate and wash with a small volume of water containing the calcium chloride solution. Filter and wash. Place the funnel containing the filter paper and the precipitate on an empty 100 ml volumetric flask. Dissolve the precipitate with dilute hydrochloric acid, wash the filter paper, and then make up the volume of the filtrate to the mark.

Transfer 5 ml of the filtrate to a 10 ml graduated cylinder and add to 1 ml of the molybdate II reagent. Shake thoroughly and add 0.4 ml of the aminonaphtholsulphonic acid reagent and mix again. Make up the volume to the 10 ml mark with water, mix, and allow the contents to stand for five minutes.

For developing colour in the standard solution, transfer 5 ml of the standard phosphate solution, containing 0.4 mg phosphorus, to a 100 ml volumetric flask and add 50 ml of water. Add 10 ml of molybdate I reagent. Mix thoroughly and add 4 ml of aminonaphtholsulphonic acid reagent. Dilute with water to the 100 ml mark, mix well and allow the contents of the flask to stand for five minutes. Compare the standard against itself in the colorimeter before taking a reading of the unknown solution. If the colour of the unknown is particularly strong, repeat the reading of the unknown a few minutes later, to make sure that the maximum colour development has taken place.

Take the reading of both unknown and standard sample at 660 to 720 mμ in a photoelectric colorimeter. Calculate the percentage of the available phosphorus in the material from the reading of the colorimeter.

Note : This method has been adapted by the Indian Standards Institution (1979) under IS : 1374, BIS for analysing poultry feeds for available phosphours. As per AOAC (1965) recommendations, available P_2O_5 can be calculated by subtracting citrate insoluble P_2O_5 from total P_2O_5.

Estimation of Organic Phosphorus in Feeds, Fodders and Faeces

(Volumetric method AOAC, 1965)

Introduction

Many of the biochemical reactions that occur in living cells involves the participation of phosphate esters at some stage, and a very large number of these compounds have been isolated from plant, animal and microbial sources. It is possible to divide the phosphate esters of biological importance into several groups, and compounds belonging to three of these, the inositol phosphates, the nucleic acids and the phospholipids. *Salts of myo-inositol hexaphosphate (phytic acid)*, are common constituents of plant materials, and occur principally in the seeds, which are the usual source of commercial phytin, the calcium-magnesium salt. *Phytic acid is a very stable substance, most of whose salts (phytates), with the exception of those of the alkali metals, are only sparingly soluble in water.* The insolubility of the ferric salt in hydrochloric acid has been used to distinguish inositol hexaphosphate (IHP) from other phosphate esters and orthophosphate, and as a basis for estimation in plant extracts. Phosphate esters are strong acids with pK values of about 1 and 6 for the first and second dissociation, and are readily adsorbed by anion exchange resins. Smith and clark (1952) were the first to describe a method for the separation of IHP from orthophosphate and lower phosphate esters of inositol by ion-exchange chromatography. The lipids containing phosphorus, the phospholipids or phosphatides, can be divided into distinct groups, one of the most important being the glycerophosphatides which are present in plants, animals and micro-organisms.

Milk consist organic (36%) and inorganic (64%) phosphorus. Out of 36% organic phosphorus, acid soluble phosphorus is 21% and acid insoluble phosphorus is 15 per cent. Further in the case of 64 per cent inorganic phosphorus, 34 per cent is acid soluble phosphorus and rest 30 per cent is acid insoluble phosphorus.

Reagent

1. Magnesium nitrate solution

Dissolve 8 g MgO in HNO3 (1+1), avoiding excess acid., add little MgO in excess, boil, filter from excess MgO and dilute to 100 ml.

2. Molybdate solution

Dissolve 100 g MoO_3 in mixture of 144 ml NH_4OH and 271 ml water. Cool, and pour solution slowly, stirring constantly, into cool mixture of 489 ml HNO_3 and 1148 ml water. Keep final mixture in warm place several days or until portion heated to 40°C, deposits no yellow precipitate. Decant solution from any sediment and keep in known coloured glass bottle.

Procedure

Transfer 1 gram sample to about 140 ml porcelain crucible, add 3 ml of the Mg $(NO_3)_2$ solution, and mix well, using small glass rod. Clean rod with small piece of filter paper and place in crucible. Drive off most of moisture by drying in oven at 100°C about two hour, transfer to cold muffle, and ignite at 550°C to white or grey ash (6-8 hr). Cool, cover with watch glass, take up with 10 ml HCl (1+4), and add 5 ml HCl. Rinse watch glass and evaporate to dryness on steam bath. Add 5 ml Hcl and 50 ml water, heat 15 minutes on steam bath, filter into 100 ml volumetric flask, cool and dilute to volume. Pipette 50 ml into 300 ml erlenmeyer, neutralise to litmus paper with NH_4OH, make just faintly acid with nitric acid, dilute to 75-100 ml, add about 15 g NH_4NO_3 and proceed as below.

Generally in the case of materials containing large quantities of organic matter for example cottonseed meal, it is best to add first about 5 ml HNO_3 and then the H_2SO_4. Boil with 20-30 ml H_2SO_4 in 200 ml flask, adding 2-4 grams $NaNO_3$ or KNO_3 at beginning of digestion and small quantity after solution is nearly colourless, or adding nitrate from time to time in small portions. When solution is colourless, cool, add 150 ml H_2O, and boil few minutes. Before adding the $NaNO_3$ or KNO_3, let mixture digest, at gentle heat if necessary, until violence of reaction is over.

Pipette, into beaker or flask, aliquot corresponding to 0.4 g sample for P_2O_5 content of sample < 5%, 0.2 g for 5-20%, 0.1 g for > 20%. Add 5-10 ml HNO_3, depending on method of solution (or equivalent in NH_4/NH_3), then add NH_4OH until precipitate that forms dissolves only slowly on vigorous stirring, dilute to 75-100 ml, and adjust to 25-30°C. If sample does not give precipitate with NH_4OH as test of neutralization, make solution slightly alkaline to litmus paper with NH_4OH and then slightly acid with HNO_3 (1+3). Add 20-25 ml acidified molybdate solution for P_2O_5 content <5%, 30-35 ml for 5-20%, and enough molybdate solution to insure complete precipitation for <20%. Place solution in shaking or stirring apparatus and agitate 30 minutes at room temperature, decant at once through filter and wash precipitate twice by decanting with 25-30 ml portions water, agitating thoroughly and allowing to settle. Transfer precipitate to filter and wash with cold water until filtrate from two fillings of filter yields pink colour on adding phenolphthalein and 1 drop of the standard alkali, add few drops of phenolphthalein, and titrate with the standard acid. Report the result as per cent P_2O_5.

Estimation of Organic Phosphorus (Lipid phosphorus) in Egg

(Method of Bagnall and Smith, 1945)

Principle

Egg contains a relatively high porportion of organic phosphorus. It has been observed that organic phosphorus may be extracted successfuly by an organic solvent (Manley and Lobley, 1948). *In the following method 95 per cent alcohol is used for extracting organic phosphorus.* We may follow colorimetric method using vanadomolybdate reagent (Donald *et al.*, 1956) or titrimetric method of AOAC (1965) for estimating quantity of organic phosphorus in the extracted solvent.

Procedure

Weigh 20 g of sample in an oil flask, add 100 ml of 95% alcohol and attach a water reflux condenser. Heat the mixture in a boiling water bath for 6 h and allow it to stand overnight. Filter it through a Buckner or, preferably, a Hartley funnel. Wash the residue with a small volume of 95 per cent alcohol. Retain the filtrate (A) Return the residue in the funnel to the flask and place reextract it by heating it under reflux again with 100 ml of 95 per cent alcohol. Then filter the mixture as before and add the filtrate to the previous filtrate–A.

Place a silica basin on a boiling water bath and pour the combined filtrate into it in small portions until it is evaporated to dryness. Gently ignite the residue, then warm and stir the ash with 5 ml of dilute nitric acid, add 5 ml of water and filter the mixture into a 100 ml volumetric flask, B. Wash the filter with a small volume of water. Return the filter paper to the dish, ignite it, then warm and stir the ash with 2 ml of dilute nitric acid, add 3 ml of water, filter the mixture into B and wash the filter with a small volume of water. Dilute the cooled combined filtrate with water to the 100 ml mark, mix and pipette 50 ml of the solution into another 100 ml volumetric flask. Add a small piece of indicator paper, neutralise the solution with ammonia of sp.gr.0.880, make it just acidic with dilute nitric acid, add 25 ml of vanadomolybdate reagent, dilute the solution to the mark with water, mix and measure the optical density at 420 nm (Donald *et al.*, 1956). If, as is usual, the reading falls outside the range of the calibration graph, take a different volume of solution for determining the phosphate, such as the phosphomolybdate volumetric method (AOAC, 2965) can be used.

References

AOAC, (1965). *Official methods of analysis of the Association of Official Agricultural chemists,* 10th edn., Benjamin Franklin Station, Washington, D.C. pp. 11-15, pp. 193-194.

Bagnall, D.J.T. and Smitt, A. (1945). *Analyst, Lond.,* 70:211.

Donald, R., Schwehr, E.W. and Wilson, H.N. (1956). *J. Sci. Food Agric.,* 7:677.

Dryer, R.L., Jammes, A.R. and Routh, J.I. (1957). *J. Biol. Chem.,* 225:177.

Fiske, C.H. and Subha Row, Y. 1925). *J. Biol. Chem.,* 66:375.

Gomori, G.A. (1942). *J. Lab. Clin. Med.* 27: 955-960.

Indian Standards Institution, BIS. (1968). *Specification for mineral mixtures for supplementing cattle feeds* (First Revision). IS : 1664, ISI, Manak Bhavan, New Delhi - 1.

Indian Standards Institution, BIS. (1975). *Animal feeds and feeding stuffs, methods of tests for.* Part II. *Minerals and trace elements.* IS : 7874. ISI, Manak Bhavan, New Delhi-1.

Indian standards Institution, BIS, (1979). *Specifications for poultry feeds (Third Revision),* IS: 1374, Indian Standards Institution, Manak Bhavan, New Delhi-1.

Manley, C.H. and Labley, H. (1948). *Analyst, Lond.* 73:30.

Park, P.F. and Dunn, D.E. (1963). *J.A.O.A.C.,* 46:836.

Smith, D.H. and Clark, F.E. (1951). *Soil Sci.* 72:353.

Talapatra, S.K., Ray, S.C. and Sen, K.C. (1940). *Indian J. Vet. Sci.,* 10:243.

Tewatia, B.S. and Krishna, G. (1991). Fodder tree leaves as Animal Feed IV. Proximate Composition, Major and Minor minerals, carotene and tocopherol in fodder tree leaves of arid and semiarid zones. *The J. of the Remount and Veterinary Corps.* 30: 177-183.

Chapter - 74

Magnesium and Sulphur in Biological Materials

Estimation of Magnesium in Feeds, Fodders and Faeces

(Gravimetric method - AOAC, 1965)

Principle

Evaporation of calcium free filtrate is carried out to drive off ammonium chloride and nitric acid is added to decompose ammonium salts, which is then subsequently driven off by evaporation. $NH_4Cl + HNO_3 = HCl + NH_4NO_3$ (driven off). Sodium citrate in solution yields citric acid which has got a tremendous effect on aluminium and iron in that the citric acid keeps these materials in solution.

At neutrality, first the normal magnesium phosphate is formed, which is then turned to magnesium ammonium phosphate, which on incineration gives rise to magnesium pyrophosphate ($Mg_2P_2O_7$).

Procedure

Measure 25 ml. of calcium free filtrate in a beaker and evaporate it to dryness on a hot plate, after adding 30 ml of conc. HNO_3, again dry, 5 ml. of conc. hydrochloric acid is added, followed by addition of 100 ml. distilled water and 5 ml of 10 per cent sodium citrate and 10 ml of 10 per cent ammonium phosphate solution or enough to precipitate all the magnesium.

Concentrated ammonia (1+4) is added drop by drop with constant and thorough stirring using, policeman till the precipitate becomes granular which was allowed to stand overnight for setting. Next day the filtration is started and the precipitate is washed with cold (1+10) ammoniated water as ordinary distilled water should not be used in this case because precipitate is soluble in it. After completing the washings, filter paper along with the precipitate is transferred to a previously weighed vitreosil crucible and then kept in a hot air oven to dry. Process the precipitate as per standard procedure of gravimetric analysis. Separate the precipitate on glazed paper using pigeon feather. the filter paper is completely ashed in the crucible and precipitate is transferred from glazed paper into the crucible. Incinerate both filter paper and precipitate at 900-950°C for four hours in muffle furnace. Incinerated precipitate is magnesium pyrophosphate ($Mg_2P_2O_7$) chemically.

Precautions

1. The precipitate should be washed with cold (1:10) ammonia solution and not by distilled water.
2. The weight of the filter paper ash should be subtracted from the weight of precipitate.

Calculation

Name of Sample A

1. Weight of oven dried vitreosil basin = 24.9374 g
2. Weight of oven dried vitreosil basin and ignited magnesium pyrophosphate = 24.9447 g
3. Weight of filter paper ash = 0.00057 g
4. Weight of ignited magnesium pyrophosphate = 0.00730 g
5. Actual weight of magnesium pyrophosphate after ignition = 0.00673 g
6. Weight of substance taken on dry matter basis = 9 g
7. Volume of extract made = 250 ml
8. Aliquot taken = 25 ml

Per cent of magnesium present in the sample

$$= \frac{\text{Actual wt. of ignited Mag. pyrophosphate x 0.21839 x vol. made x 100}}{\text{Wt. of substance on dry matter basis x aliquot}}$$

$$= \frac{0.00673 \times 0.21839 \times 250 \times 100}{9 \times 25}$$

Result

Sample A : Contained 0.1633 g magnesium per 100 g sample.

Estimation of magnesium in blood

(Colorimetric method of Denis, 1922)

Principles

Magnesium is found constantly in small amount in blood, being distributed about equally between cells and plasma. Plasma or serum is ordinarily used for analysis, usually after the calcium has been precipitated to prevent interference in the analysis. Most methods proposed depend upon the precipitation of magnesium as phosphate, followed by colorimetric phosphate analysis. After removal of calcium as oxalate the magnesium is precipitated as magnesium ammonium phosphate and the latter is estimated by a colorimetric phosphate determination. In the present case, Fiske-Subba Row phosphate method (1925) is used. This method was standardised by Denis (1922) and mentioned in detail by Oser (1954).

Procedure

Reagents

Most of the reagents preparation has been mentioned under Fiske and Subba Row (1925) method recommended for serum inorganic phosphorus estimation.

Magnesium standard solution

Dissolve 0.560 g of pure dry monopotassium phosphate in water to make 1000 ml. Add a few drops of chloroform to prevent growth of molds. Dilute 10 ml of this stock solution to 100 ml.

1 ml = 0.01 mg of magnesium

Precipitate the calcium from two ml of serum as in the procedure for calcium in serum. After centrifuging, pipette three ml of the supernatant fluid into a 15 ml graduated centrifuge tube and add with stirring 0.5 ml of a 5 per cent solution of ammonium phosphate containing 5 ml of concentrated NH_4OH. let stand overnight. Centrifuge, siphon off the supernatant fluid and wash the tube with 5 ml of a mixture of one part of concentrated NH_4OH (sp.gr. 0.9) and two parts of water. Centrifuge and siphon off wash liquid. Repeat the washing second and third time and then wash finally with 5 ml of 75 per cent alcohol containing 10 ml of concentrated NH_4OH per litre. Siphon off again and let stand in a warm place until the ammonia has evaporated. To the residue in the centrifuge tube add one ml of the molybdate solution used in the Fiske-Subba Row phosphate method (1925) and tap to dissolve. When dissolved, add 5 ml of water and set aside. Prepare a standard by placing one ml of the molybdate solution in a second graduated tube and adding three ml of the standard phosphate solution (equivalent to 0.03 mg of magnesium) plus two ml of water. Prepare a blank by placing one ml of molybdate solution plus five ml of water in a third graduated tube. When all the tubes are ready, add to each 0.4 ml of aminonaphtholsulphonic acid reagent, followed immediately by water to the 10 ml mark. Mix and allow to stand 5 minutes before reading. Set the photometer to zero density at 660 mμ with the blank.

Calculation

$$\frac{\text{Density of unknown}}{\text{Density of standard}} \times 0.03 \times \frac{100}{102} = \text{mg magnesium per 100 ml serum}$$

The characteristics of the colour and the conditions of photometric measurement are the same as for the determination of inorganic phosphate. At 660 mμ, the standard has a density of approximately 0.500 in a 1 cm cuvette. Since this standard corresponds to a serum magnesium content of 2.5 mg per cent, up to 5 mg per cent may be accurately determined under these conditions. For higher values, or for measurement at a greater depth of solution, add 2 ml of molybdate solution to unknown, blank, and standard instead of the 1 ml specified (use the same 3 ml portion of standard) followed by water in each case to about 12 ml, then add 0.8 ml of aminonaphthol-sulphonic acid reagent and water to a 20 ml final volume. There is no change in the calculations. Colour development at a greater dilution is recommended rather than the analysis of a smaller portion of serum because it is not known whether or not precipitation of magnesium in this procedure will be quantitative at conditions other than those specified.

Sulphur in Feeds, Fodders and Faeces

(Gravimetric method of AOAC, 1965)

Reagents

1. *Magnesium nitrate. Dissolve 950 g P free magnesium nitrate in 500 ml of distilled water and dilute to one litre.*
2. *Barium chloride (10%)*

Apparatus

1. Hot plate
2. Muffle furnace

Procedure

Weigh 1 gram sample into large procelain crucible. Add 7.5 ml magnesium nitrate solution, so that all the material comes in contact with solution. It is important that enough magnesium nitrate solution be added to ensure complete oxidation and fixation of sulphur present. For larger samples and for samples with high sulphur content, proportionally large quantities of this solution must be used. Heat on electric hot plate (180°C) until no further action occurs. Transfer crucible while hot to muffle furnace and let it remain at low heat (≤500°C) until charge is thoroughly oxidized (No black particles should remain, if necessary, break up charge and return to muffle). Remove crucible from muffle and let cool. Add water, then HCl in excess. Bring solution to boil, filter, and wash thoroughly. If preferred, transfer solution to 250 ml volumetric flask before filtering and dilute to volume with water.

Dilute 100 ml filtered solution to 200 ml with distilled water test with litmus paper if sufficient acid is present then it will turn from blue to red, if sufficient acid is not present then add 0.5 ml hydrochloric acid to make the solution acidic, heat to boiling and add 10 ml 10 per cent barium chloride solution dropwise with constant stirring, continue boiling about five minutes and allow to stand five hours or longer in warm place. Decant liquid through ashless filter paper, ignited and weighed gooch crucible. Add 15-20 ml boiling water to precipitate, transfer to filter, and wash with boiling water until filtrate is chloride free. Dry precipitate and filter, ignite, and weigh as $BaSO_4$.

Factor = Weight of precipitate x 0.1374.

Calculation

Example

Name of Sample B

1. Weight of oven dried crucible = 17.9507 g
2. Weight of oven dried crucible + $BaSO_4$ precipitate + ignited filter paper = 17.9586 g
3. Weight of filter paper ash = 0.00057 g
4. Weight of BaSO4 precipitate and ignited filter paper = 0.0079 g
5. Weight of ignited BaSO4 precipitate = 0.00733 g
6. Weight of substance taken on dry matter basis = 0.9 g
7. Volume of extract made = 250 ml
8. Aliquot taken = 100 ml

Per cent of sulphur present in the sample.

$$= \frac{\text{Wt. of ignited } BaSO_4 \text{ ppt} \times 0.1374 \times \text{volume made} \times 100}{\text{Wt. of substance on dry matter basis} \times \text{aliquot}}$$

$$= \frac{0.00733 \times 0.1374 \times 250 \times 100}{0.9 \times 100}$$

= 0.279 g/100 g

Result : The sample B contained sulphur 0.279 g per 100 g.

Sulphur in Feeds, Fodders and Faeces

(Colorimetric method of AOAC, 1965 modified by Johnson *et al.*, 1970)

Principles

The sample is added magnesium nitrate and then combusted in a furnace oven. All the organic sulphur is then transferred to sulphate, which is then precipitated with barium chloride in a strongly acid solution. Barium sulphate is a fine precipitate and during short periods stay, evenly dispersed in the solution. Turbidity is then measured at 450 nm in a 1 cm cuvette.

Reagents

1. *Magnesium nitrate solution : 500 mg $(NO_3)_2$ $6H_2O$ is dissolved in 700 ml water, diluted to 1000 ml*
2. *Hydrochloric acid : diluted 1:1*
3. *Acid mixture : 50% acetic acid + 25% nitric acid + concentrated phosphoric acid ratio in 5:5:1.*
4. *Barium chloride 40/50 mesh.*
5. *Stabiliser : 2-2 dihydroxy di-n-propyl-ether + ethanol in ratio 55:45*
6. *Sulphur stock standard : 0.3844 $MgSO_4.7H_2O$ is dissolved in water and diluted to 1000 ml. One ml of stock standard is equivalent to 0.05 mg sulphur.*

The sulphur factor

Aliquots within the range 0.15 to 0.80 mg are added to 50 ml volumetric flasks, 11 ml reagent 3 (acid mixture) is added together with water to give 42 ml altogether. Now 1 grams barium chloride is added and made to dissolve by cautious swirling and turning of the flask. Then 8 ml stabilizer is added and then water to make volume up to the mark. After 30 minutes the reading is made in a spectrophotometer.

Procedure

Two grams finely ground sample is weighed into a porcelain crucible and soaked with 20 ml magnesium nitrate. The content is dried on a hot plate, raising the temperature oven 48 hours to 200°C. The final heating is applied to furnace at 550-600°C, for one hour. In this way a white and soluble ash is obtained. Twenty ml dilute hydrochloric acid and then 50 ml distilled water is added. The dish is heated on the hot plate to facilitate dissolution, and the acid solvent is transferred to 150 ml volumetric flask, diluted and an aliquot is proceeded as for the standard.

☞ Note

Protein rich or fatty materials may be pretreated with 2 x 5 ml concentrated nitric acid to avoid puffing.

Calculation

Estimating sulphur in the given sample

Sample	=	W
Volume of standard	=	2 ml
Concentration of sulphur in 2 ml	=	0.1 mg
O.D. of standard	=	0.0735

$$Sf = \frac{\text{Concentration of sulphur in standard}}{\text{O.D. of standard}}$$

$$Sf = \frac{0.1}{0.0735} = 1.36$$

$$S, g/100g = \frac{\text{Vol. of extract made x factor x O.D. of unknown x 100}}{\text{Wt. of material on dry matter basis x aliquot x 1000}}$$

Volume of extract made	=	100 ml
Factor	=	1.36
O.D. of unknown	=	0.102
Wt. of material on dry matter basis	=	1.9 grams
Aliquot	=	5 ml

Substituting these values in the above formula

$$= \frac{100 \times 1.36 \times 0.102 \times 100}{1.90 \times 5 \times 1000}$$

= 0.146 g/100 g

Result : The given sample W contained 0.146 g/100 g sulphur.

Estimation of Sulphur in blood

Of the total sulphur of whole blood, part is present at the inorganic sulphate ion, another part is in the form of various non-protein organic compounds which may be present (glutathione, ergothioneine etc.), most of which are found chiefly in the red cells, and the remainder is represented by the sulphur containing amino acids of the proteins present.

Total sulphur is determined by complete oxidation of organic matter, followed by estimation of inorganic sulphate present. The colorimetric method mentioned in the case of feed may be followed.

Estimation of Inorganic Sulphate in Urine

(Titrimetric method of Rosenheim and Drummond, 1914)

Principle

The sulphate is precipitated as benzidine sulphate. Because of the slight dissociation of benzidine, the salt may be titrated with phenolphthalein as if it were free sulphuric acid. Note that both hydrogens of the sulphuric acid are titrated.

Reagent

Benzidine solution

Grind 4 grams of benzidine to a fine paste with 10 ml of water, wash into a flask with 500 ml of water, add 5 ml of concentrated hydrochloric acid and make up to 2 litres. 150 ml of this solution is sufficient to precipitate 0.1 g of sulphuric acid.

Procedure

Introduce 25 ml urine and a small piece of congo red paper 4-5 mm square into a 250 ml Erlemeyer flask, and treat with 2 N hydrochloric acid, a drop at a time, until the reaction is distinctly acid to the congo red paper. 1 to 2 ml of dilute acid is usually sufficient. Add 100 ml of benzidine solution (0.2%) and allow the precipitate to settle for 10 minutes. Filter on a small paper and wash with water saturated with benzidine sulphate by pouring small amounts of the filter. Continue to wash until the top edge of the filter and the drops of filtrate are neutral to litmus. Transfer the filter paper and precipitate to the original flask with about 50 ml of water and titrate at the boiling point with 0.1 N sodium hydroxide after the addition of a few drops of phenolphthalein. Calculate the grams of sulphate sulphur in the 24 hour sample.

Estimation of total sulphate

The esters of sulphuric acid (commonly called ethereal sulphates) are hydrolysed by boiling with acid. The "total sulphate" is then determined as described in the previous method.

Place 25 ml of urine in a 250 ml flask and acidify to congo red paper with dilute hydrochloric acid. Cover with a watch glass and boil gently for 30 minutes adding water if necessary. Allow to cool and proceed as directed under inorganic sulphates. The difference between the two determinations represents ethereal or conjugate sulphate.

Estimation of Total Sulphur in Urine

(Titrimetric method of Benedict, 1909)

Principle

All of the sulphur of the urine is oxidised to sulphate by heating with copper nitrate and potassium chlorate, 50 grams, add distilled water to make 1 litre. A determination of the sulphur in the reagent should be made.

Procedure

To 10 to 20 ml of urine in a small porcelain evaporating dish, add 5 to 10 ml of Benedict's sulphur reagent and evaporate on the water bath or over a free flame just below the boiling point. When the mixture is dry, increase the heat gradually until it blackens fuses and is finally heated to dull redness. Continue heating for 10 minutes. Allow to cool and dissolve in 10 to 20 ml of 2N hydrochloric acid using a little heat if necessary. Evaporate the solution to dryness, dissolve the residue in water and proceed as directed under inorganic sulphate.

The difference between the quantities of total sulphur and the sulphur estimated as total sulphate represents "neutral sulphur".

Estimation of organic sulphur

Both direct and indirect methods have been used for measuring total organic sulphur. In the direct methods of Vinokurov (1937) and Evans and Rost (1945) biological samples were pre-extracted with sodium chloride and alcohol, or water and hydrochloric acid, respectively, and the sample residues oxidised with hydrogen peroxide. The sulphate released was precipitated as the barium salt and taken as a measure of organic sulphate. Values obtained in this way are likely to be low, principally due to incomplete oxidation of organic matter by the peroxide treatment (Puri and Sarup, 1937), but also in some cases to a slight loss of organic sulphur in the initial extracts (Williams & Steinbergs, 1959).

More commonly, the organic sulphur is measured by the difference between the total sulphur and the inorganic sulphate, although the latter may be difficult to estimate if insoluble forms are present. In many cases where the bulk of the sulphur is known to be in organic combination total sulphur values have been used in calculating the composition of the organic matter. Significant correlations have been found between the carbon and sulphur or nitrogen and sulphur contents of samples of the organic matter (Donald and Williams, 1954; Walker and Adams, 1958; Williams and Steinbergs, 1958; Williams and Scott, 1960 and Freney, 1961).

Cysteine which is an organic form of sulphur is converted into sulphate in the following way.

Cysteine → cystine → cystine disulfoxide → cysteine sulfinic acid → cysteic acid → sulphate.

Cystine and methionine contain the element sulphur in their make up and are sometimes referred to as the sulphur bearing amino acids.

References

AOAC, (1965). *Official methods of analysis of the Association of official agricultural chemists*, 10th edn., AOAC, Benjamin Franklin Station, Washington, D.C.

Benedict, S.R. (1909). *J. Biol. Chem.*, 6: 363.

Denis, (1922). *J. Biol. Chem.*, 52:411 cited Oser, B.L. 1954.

Donald, C.M. and Williams, C.H. (1954). *Austral. J. Agr. Res.*, 5: 664.

Evans, C.A. and Rost, C.O. (1945). *Soil Sci.*, 59: 125.

Fiske, C.H. and Subba Row, Y. (1925). *J. Biol. Chem.*, 66: 375.

Freney, J.R. (1961). *Australian J. Agril. Res.* 12: 424.

Johnson, W.H., Goodrich, R.D. and Meiske, J.C. (1970). *J. Anim, Sci.*, 31: 1003-1009.

Oser, B.L. (1954). *Hawk's physiological Chemistry*, 14th edn. McGraw-Hill Book Co., London, pp. 1138.

Puri, A.N. and Sarup, A. (1937). *Soil Sci.*, 44: 87.

Rosenheim, O. and Drummond, J.C. (1914). *Biochem. J.*, 8: 143.

Vinokurov, M.A. (1937). *Pedology*, 32: 493.

Walker, T.W. and Adams, A.F.R. (1958). *Soil Sci.*, 85: 307.

Williams, C.H. and Steinberg, A. (1958). *Australian J. Agr. Res.*, 9: 483.

Williams, C.H. Williams, E.G. and Scott, N.M. (1960). *J. Biol. Sci.* 11: 334.

Chapter - 75

Total Volatile Fatty Acids in Blood, Rumen Liquor & Silage Samples

TVFA Estimation in Blood

(Method of Friedemann, 1938 modified by Mc Anally, 1944)

A method for the determination of volatile fatty acids in various biological materials has been described by Friedemann (1938) which is said to be applicable to blood, then the blood is added to dilute sulphuric acid, then sodium tungstate solution and solid magnesium sulphate are added and the whole is steam distilled.

Reagents

1. *Saturated magnesium sulphate solution to which has been added 2.5 per cent by volume of concentrated sulphuric acid.*
2. *0.01 N KOH.*

Method

To one volume of oxalated blood, four volumes of water are added and then pipette five volumes of the acid magnesium sulphate solution. After standing a few minutes, the precipitate is filtered off and a clear colourless filtrate is obtained. An aliquot of the filtrate (equivalent to one-tenth its volume of blood) is taken for the distillation. The apparatus recommended by

Markham (1942) is used. Adjust the pH 3 with the help of 10 N NaOH to minimise the interfering effects of other substances such as pyruvic and lactic acids and chloride which are partially steam volatile under acid conditions. The Markham (1942) steam distillation apparatus with steam generator and connections, mounted on a retort stand is used for distillation purpose (Fig. 1).

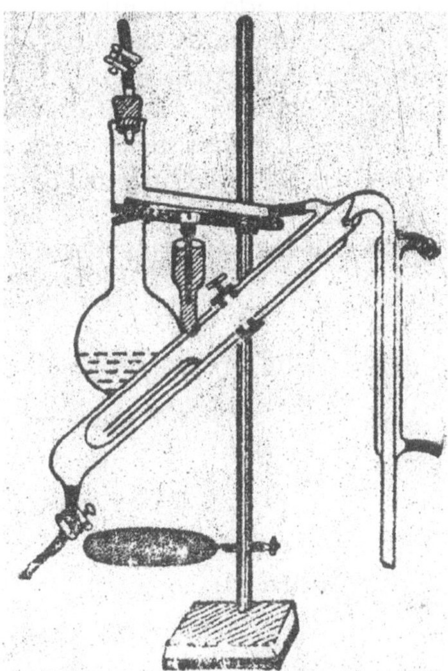

Fig. 1 : Markham (1942) steam distillation apparatus

Distillation is allowed until the volume in the receiver flask is reached up to 150 ml. The time taken for distillation does not appear to effect the results. The distillates are aerated for 3 minutes with CO_2 free air and, while the aeration is continued, the acid in the distillate is titrated against 0.01 N KOH added from a burette, whose tip passes through a rubber bung directly into a titrating flask.

Calculation

TVFA concentration in blood sample =

Volume of N/100 KOH used in sample – Vol. of N/100 KOH used in blank

= Net reading of N/100 KOH used in titration

= Total VFA (m.moles/litre)

TVFA Estimation in Rumen Liquor

(Method of Mc Anally, 1944 modified by Annison, 1954)

Procedure

Rumen contents are strained through muslin cloth, deproteinised with an equal volume of N-H_2SO_4 saturated with $MgSO_4.7H_2O$. Measure 5 ml rumen liquor in a centrifuge tube and add 5 ml saturated magnesium sulphate solution (containing 2.5 per cent concentrate sulphuric acid) keep overnight and centrifuge at 2000 r.p.m., decant the supernatant. Adjust the pH of filtrate to pH 3 with the help of 10 N NaOH. Distil 5 ml of supernatant solution in a Markham still (Markham, 1942) and collect the distillate upto 150 ml in the receiver flask and titrate with 0.02 N NaOH under CO_2 free conditions using phenolphthalein as indicator and calculate the result as mentioned below. Run blank sample with distilled water simultaneously.

Calculation

Rumen liquor TVFA (μ moles/ml or mEq/lit.)

$$= \frac{a \times b \times 1000}{\text{Volume of rumen liquor}}$$

where

a = Volume (ml) of alkali used in titration

b = Strength of alkali (0.02 N NaOH)

☞ **Note**

Long back (olmsted et al., 1929, Kromann et al., 1967) have developed methods for steam distillation of the lower volatile fatty acids from a saturated salt solution. These methods may also be followed, if facilities exists in the laboratory.

TVFA Estimation in Silage Extract

(Method of Mc Anally, 1944 modified by Annison, 1954)

Apparatus & reagents (same as used in the case of rumen liquor).

Procedure

Weigh 10g fresh silage in a 250 ml capacity beaker. Mix 80 ml distilled water, macerate it in a blender and filter using Whatman filter paper No.1, made up the volume upto 100 ml. Measure 5 ml of silage extract in a 50 ml capacity conical flask and add 5 ml saturated magnesium sulphate solution, keep overnight and centrifuge at 2000 rpm, decant the supernatant. Adjust the pH of filtrate to pH 3 with the help of 10 N NaOH. Later on follow the same procedure as recommended in the case of rumen liquor. Run blank sample with distilled water simultaneously.

Fresh silage TVFA (g/100g)

$$= \frac{\text{a x b x volume of silage extract made}}{\text{Wt. of fresh silage taken x Aliquot of extract taken}}$$

where

a = Volume of alkali used in titration

b = Strength of alkali (0.02 N NaOH)

References

Annison, E.F. (1954a). *Biochem. J.*, 57:400.

Friedemann, T.E. (1938). *J. Biol. Chem.*, 123: 161.

Kromann, R.P., Meyer, J.H. and Stielau, W.J. (1967). *J. Dairy Sci.*, 50:73.

Krishna, G., Czerkawski, J.W. and Breckenridge, Grace, 1986. Fermentation of various preparations of spent hops (*Humulus lopulus* L.) using the Rumen simulation Technique (RUSITEC). *Agricultural Wastes*. 17: 99-117.

Markham, R. (1942). *Biochem, J.*, 36:790.

Mc Anally, R.A. (1944). *J. Exp. Biol.*, 20:130.

Olmsted, W.H., Whitaker, W.M. and Duden, C.W. (1929). *J. Biol. Chem.*, 85:109.

Paliwal, V.K. Mandal, A.B., Yadav, K.R. Singh, N. and Krishna, G. (1989). Effect of culled guar seed (*Cyamopsis tetragonoloba* L. Taub) vis-a-vis protected guar meal on rumen metabolic profile and blood biochemical constituents in growing buffalo calves. *Indian Vety. Journal*. 66: 149-153.

Chapter - 76

Bacterial and Protozoal Fractions in Rumen Liquor

Separation of Bacteria and Protozoa

(Method of Czerkawski, 1975)

Rumen contents are obtained just before and two hours after feeding from sheep that had been given an experimental ration. The samples of rumen contents are strained through gauze and fractioned by sedimentation and centrifugation to give preparations of mixed protozoa (PR), large bacteria (LB) and small bacteria (SB). Whole particulate matter is also isolated by centrifugation at 20000g. The detail steps are mentioned in the flow chart given below.

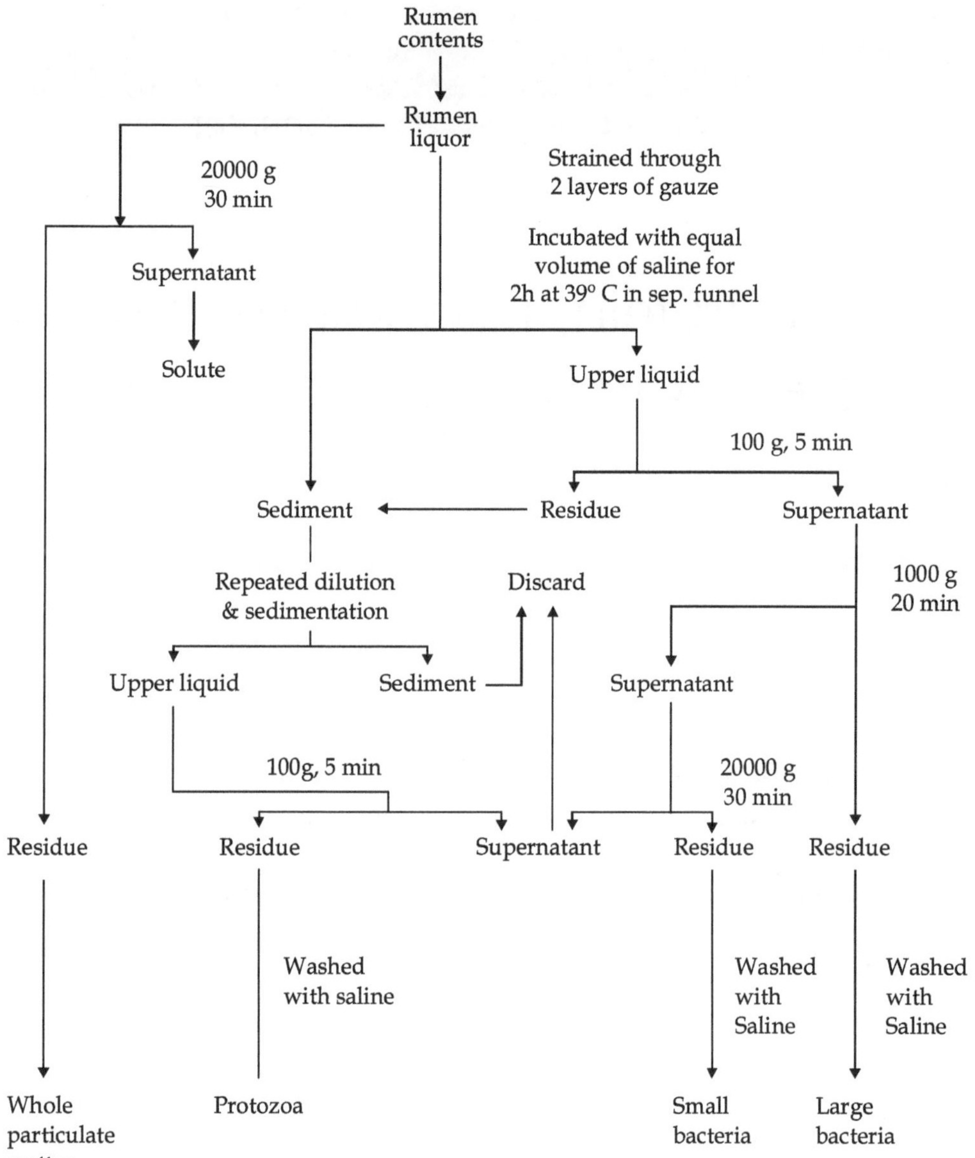

Source : Czerkawski, J.W., 1975, Proc. Nutr. Soc., 34:62A.

Reference

Czerkawski, J.W. (1975). *Proc. Nutr. Soc.*, 34:62A.

Krishna, G., Czerkawski, J.W. and Breckenridge, Grace, (1986). Fermentation of various preparations of spent hops (*Humulus lupulus* L.) using the Rumen simulation Technique (RUSITEC). *Agricultural Wastes.* 17: 88-118.

Chapter - 77

Total Protein, Lipoprotein and Protein Nitrogen Components

Total Protein in Tissue Extract or Blood, Serum or Plasma

(Method of Folin-Ciocalteu, 1927 modified by Lowry *et al.*, 1951)

Principle

A deep blue dye is formed when protein is treated with the phenol reagent of Folin ciocalteu. The extraordinary sensitivity of the method is due to the fact that two colour reactions are taking place simultaneously.

a. The biuret reaction of peptide bonds with copper in alkaline solution.

b. A reduction of phosphomolybdic acid and phosphotungstic acid by the aromatic amino acids, tyrosine and tryptophan, present in the protein.

Reagents

1. Phenol reagent of Folin-ciocalteu, 1 N

The stock solution is stable indefinitely in the dark, the commercial solution is more economical than solutions prepared in the laboratory. To prepare the working solution, 1 ml of the commercial preparation is titrated with 0.1 N sodium hydroxide against phenolphthalein and the normality is calculated. The reagent is then diluted to obtain a 1N solution. The working solution should also be kept in a dark bottle.

2. Sodium carbonate solution

0.189 M (2%) : 2g anhydrous sodium carbonate is dissolved in 100 ml distilled or dimineralised water, can be kept indefinitely at room temperature.

3. Copper sulphate, 0.04 M (1%)

1g of copper sulphate (Cu SO_4, $5H_2O$) is dissolved to 100 ml with dimineralised water. Stable indefinitely.

4. Potassium sodium tartrate solution

0.071 M (2%) 2g of potassium sodium tartrate (KNa $C_4H_4O_6$, $4H_2O$) is dissolved to 100 ml with dimineralised water stable indefinitely.

5. Standard protein solution

A commercial solution of known protein concentration is diluted with 0.154 M (0.9%) sodium chloride solution to produce a final protein concentration of 0.1 g/ 100 ml is present.

6. Folin working solution

0.5 ml copper sulphate solution and 0.5 ml potassium sodium tartrate solution are thoroughly mixed and diluted to 50 ml with sodium carbonate solution. The reagent cannot be kept and must be freshly prepared for each set of analyses.

Procedure

Additions	T	B	S
Folin Working solution, ml	2.0	2.0	2.0
Analytical sample, ml	0.1	-	-
Dimineralised water, ml	-	0.1	-
Standard solution, ml	-	-	0.1

Reagent is best added to the solution in a stream, preferably with automatic pipette. Mix well and wait 10 minutes.

Phenol reagent, ml	0.2	0.2	0.2

Mix well, Read the extinction at 578 nm against water not sooner than 30 minutes and not later than 60 minutes after mixing.

Calculations

$$C(A)\ \text{mg/100ml} = \frac{A(T) - A(B)}{A(S) - A(B)} \times c(S)$$

☞ Notes

1. *The method is relatively nonspecific, besides proteins and peptides, the colour reaction is also given by tyrosine, tryptophane, phenols, uric acid, guanine and xanthine. The colour intensity differs significantly with different proteins.*

2. *Zak and Cohen (1961) have recently described a stable Folin working solution which gave constant results and could therefore also be used in the Auto-Analyzer. Preparation 100ml 20% sodium carbonate and 10ml 10N sodium hydroxide are added to 250 mg of copper EDTA dissolved in water. The resulting solution is diluted to 100ml with dimineralised water.*

β-Lipoprotein (Turbidimetric Measurement by the Method of Burstein and Samaille, 1959)

Introduction

The unsaturated fatty acids and Lysolecithin bind with serum Albumin and the other phospholipids with lipoprotein. As is shown in the following Table 8.1, considerable differences in relative lipid and protein composition of the four main lipoprotein classes exist. α-lipoproteins, closely followed by the β-lipoproteins have the highest phospholipid content, whilst pre β-lipoproteins and chylomicrons are relatively poor in phospholipids.

Table 1 : Characteristics of lipoproteins

Parameters	**α-lipoprotein High density lipoprotein**	**β-lipoprotein Low density lipoprotein**	**Pre β-lipo protein very low density lipoprotein**	**Chylomicrons**
Protein	49%	32%	2-13%	1%

Principle

The β-lipoproteins of human serum are selectively precipitated by heparin in the presence of calcium chloride at reduce ionic strength. The content of β-lipoproteins in non-lipemic serum can easily be evaluated by measurement of the absorbance (turbidity) in the long wavelength range before and after the addition of calcium chloride.

Reagents

1. *Calcium chloride solution, 25 mM : 368 mg of calcium chloride dissolved in dimineralised water and the volume made upto 100 ml. It should be kept frozen.*

2. *Sodium chloride heparin solution 1 ml 1% heparin solution and 4 ml of physiological sodium chloride solution are mixed and kept frozen.*

Procedure

Mixtures	B	T
Calcium chloride, ml	1.0	1.0
Distilled water, ml	0.02	-
Heparin solution, ml	-	0.02
Serum, ml	0.02	0.02

Allow to stand 5 minutes at room temperature. Measure the absorbance between 640-650 nm against distilled water.

Calculation

The results are given directly in absorbance :

1. Turbidity of the serum

$$A = B \times = \frac{EV}{TV},\ A = B \times 52$$

2. β-lipoprotein content
   A = (T-B) x 52

Normal values

1. *Turbidity* : 0-0.1 (N=100)
2. *β-lipoproteins* : 4.0-10.0 (N=150)

☞ Note

Plasma cannot be used, test should always be used on fasting serum. Determination should be carried out on the day of collection of blood samples.

Reagents

Albumin and globulin in serum or plasma

(Method of Wong, 1923 modified by Kingsley, 1940)

In serum, total protein consists for the most part of albumin and globulins. Plasma also contains fibrinogen. The liver synthesises albumins, fibrinogen and a portion of globulins. Gamma globulins are produced in the lymphoplasmic reticulum. The chief functions of the plasma proteins are concerned with water binding and transport. Furthermore, they serve as buffers and protective colloids.

Principle

Total proteins are determined in serum or plasma by a micro-Kjeldahl method employing direct nesslerization, making the appropriate correction for non protein nitrogen. Fibrinogen in plasma is determined by isolation as fibrin, followed by digestion and direct nesslerization. Albumin is determined by analysis of the fluid remaining after precipitating the globulin fraction with 23 per cent sodium sulphate solution. Globulin in serum is estimated by substracting the albumin from the total protein content; in plasma by subtracting albumin and fibrinogen from total protein.

1. 23 per cent sodium sulphate solution. Dissolve 230 grams of anhydrous reagent grade sodium sulphate in 600-700 ml of water by warming and stirring. While still warm transfer to a one litre volumetric flask, dilute with water to the mark and mix. Transfer to a clean bottle and place in the incubator or water bath at 37°C. Keep at this temperature at all times, stoppered to prevent evaporation, since some of the salt will crystallize out if kept at room temperature.
2. 1:1 Sulphuric acid : Pour slowly and with stirring 1 volume of concentrated sulphuric acid into 1 volume of water. Cool, and keep stoppered to prevent absorption of ammonia from the air.
3. Persulphate solution. Shake about 8 grams of reagent grade nitrogen-free potassium persulphate in a glass-stoppered bottle with about 100 ml of water. The undissolved excess settles to the bottom and helps to keep the solution saturated even though there is gradual decomposition. Keep in the refrigerator, shake briefly and allow to settle before using, and prepare fresh every few weeks.

Method I

To one ml of serum or plasma in a 50 ml centrifuge tube add exactly 30 ml of 23 per cent sodium sulphate solution. Stopper and mix by inversion. Add about 5 to 10 ml of ether, again stopper and shake vigorously. Centrifuge for about 10 minutes, capping the tube to prevent loss of ether. After centrifuging, the precipitated globulins should form a compact layer below the ether and above the clear albumin solution. Slant the tube and insert a pipette of narrow bore, and with the mouthpiece closed by the finger, along the side of the tube post the packed globulin layer into the clear fluid below. Fill the pipette with the fluid and transfer to a dry test tube, wiping off any precipitate adhering to the outside of the pipette before discharging its contents. Use one ml of this for digestion as described below. If a centrifuge is not available, the mixture may be poured onto a retentive filter (such as Whatman No. 50) and covered with a watch glass to prevent evaporation. If the first portions of filtrate are not clear, return to the filter. Use one ml of the clear filtrate.

Into a pyrex test tube (graduated at 35 and 50 ml) place 1 ml of the solution to be analysed. Add 1 ml of 1:1 sulphuric acid and a quartz chip or a few glass beads. Digest over a microburner as described for the determination of non protein nitrogen until excess water has been driven off, the solution darkens, and white fumes appear. When the tube is nearly full of dense fumes, cover the mouth of the tube with a watch glass and reduce the flame or raise the tube so that the mixture boils gently. Continue boiling for three minutes. Remove the burner and allow to cool for one minute. Add to the tube contents, drop by drop, 0.5 ml of persulphate solution. Replace the burner, tap the tube to start boiling if necessary, and continue boiling until clear. Cool and dilute with water. The blank tube contains water, acid and persulphate as described for the standard.

Total protein in the serum or plasma may be estimated by Micro Kjeldahl procedure as described in this compendium (Volume I). The method of Lowry and Hunter (1945) may also be used to estimate total protein in the serum or plasma.

Total non protein nitrogen (NPN) may be estimated in the protein free filtrate by following the method of Folin and Denis (1916) modified by Wong (1923) or Conway diffusion (1957) technique as mentioned in volume II of this compendium.

Calculations

Total protein and albumin are calculated directly, as follows.

$$\left(\frac{\text{Density of unknown}}{\text{Density of standard}} \times 0.15 \times \frac{100}{V}\right) - \text{NPN} \times \frac{6.25}{1000} \times \text{gram, protein per 100ml}$$

Where V represents the actual volume of serum or plasma used in the determination; NPN represents the non-protein nitrogen content in mg per cent, as determined in a separate analysis. For total protein V = 0.02; for albumin V = 0.0323.

Globulin = Total protein — (Albumin + Fibrinogen) in the case of plasma; for serum globulin = Total protein — Albumin.

Non-Protein Nitrogen in Blood

(Method of Folin and Denis, 1916 modified by Wong, 1923)

Reagents

1. *Dilute sulphuric acid (50 per cent V/V) : Gradually pour 50 ml of nitrogen free concentrated sulphuric acid into a 300 ml flask containing 50 ml of distilled water, keeping it cool under the tap.*

2. *Saturated Potassium persulphate :The persulphate used should be nitrogen free as shown by a blank test. Shake about 7 g of potassium persulphate with 100 ml of water in a bottle. The undissolved crystals are left in the bottle and serve to keep the solution saturated even though some of the persulphate decomposes.*
3. *Gum Ghatti : Weigh about three grams of gum ghatti (tears, not powder) in a double gauze bag and place in 100 ml water overnight. Remove the bag, squeezing it gently. Filter the water solution through cotton cloth. Refilter if precipitate appears on standing.*
4. *Nessler's solution : Dissolve 50 g of mercuric iodide and 35 g of potassium iodide in 50 ml of water. Dilute to 400 ml with water. dissolve 100 grams of NaOH in 500 ml of water, add 3 grams of sodium citrate and cool the solution thoroughly. Mix the two solutions with constant shaking. A slight precipitate forms at once and increases slowly on standing. Allow it to settle and decant the clear solution. As the amount of alkali influences the colour development the amount used in the standard and unknown must be the same. Be sure that the solutions are cooled to 20°C before Nessler's solution is added.*
5. *Nessler's solution with extra akali : One volume of the above Nessler's solution is mixed with 2 volumes of 10% sodium hydroxide. The extra alkali serves in this analysis to neutralise the sulphuric acid of the digest.*
6. *Standard Ammonium sulphate solution : Prepare a stock solution by dissolving 0.472 gram of dried ammonium sulphate in distilled water and make the volume upto 1 litre. This makes a standard solution, each ml of which contains 0.1 mg of nitrogen.*

Procedure

Deliver 5 ml of the protein free blood filtrate (containing 0.2-0.3 mg N) in a dry test tube marked at 35 ml and at 50 ml., add 1 ml of 50% sulphuric acid, introduce a quartz pebble to prevent bumping and boil vigorously over a micro burner until the characteristic dense fumes begin to fill the tube. This usually occurs in 3 to 7 minutes. When the fumes nearly fill the tube turn down the flame so that the material is just kept boiling, close the mouth of the tube with a watch glass and continue boiling very gently for 2 minutes. Remove the burner and a low to cool for one minute. Take off the watch glass and add 2 drops of saturated potassium persulphate with a fine pipette or dropper. Replace the burner and continue the boiling until the digestion mixture becomes colourless. Stop the boiling about 15 seconds after the re-appearance of the white fumes, the test tube being covered with a watch glass during this period. Allow to cool 70-90 seconds, then add 20-25 ml of distilled water. Cool to room temperature under the tap and dilute with distilled water to the 25 ml mark.

In another similar pyrex test tube, measure exactly 2 ml of standard ammonium sulphate solution containing 0.1 mg of nitrogen per ml. Add 1 ml of the 50 per cent sulphuric acid and dilute to the 35 ml mark with distilled water. Now add to both the standard and unknown, 2 drops of gum ghatti and 15 ml "Nessler's solution with extra alkali". Insert a clean rubber stopper, mix and read in a photometer which has been adjusted to "zero" with a blank made as follows.

To 45 ml of distilled water containing 2 drops of gum ghatti, add 5 ml of Nessler's solution. Use the green (54) filter.

Calculate mg of total NPN per 100 ml of blood.

The method may be used for nitrogen determinations in various biological materials. The time of boiling and the amount of persulphate to be added very depending upon the type of material which is being digested.

☞ Note

Non protein nitrogen (NPN) may be estimated by digesting protein free filtrate and later on following micro kjeldahl method described in this compendium (Volume I).

Method : Estimation of total protein, albumin and globulin in serum (Biuret reagent method of Weichselbaum, 1946; and Gornall *et al.*, 1949).

Principle

The principle of the total protein determination according to the biuret reaction is based on the property that compounds containing at least two peptide bonds (-CO-NH-CO-NH), in an alkaline medium will give a violet colour complex with copper salts. The intensity of this violet colouration is a measure of the quantity of total protein present in the serum examined and can be determined colorimetrically at 545nm. The most simple compound giving a positive reaction is biuret ($NH_2CONHCONH_2$), which is formed by heating urea.

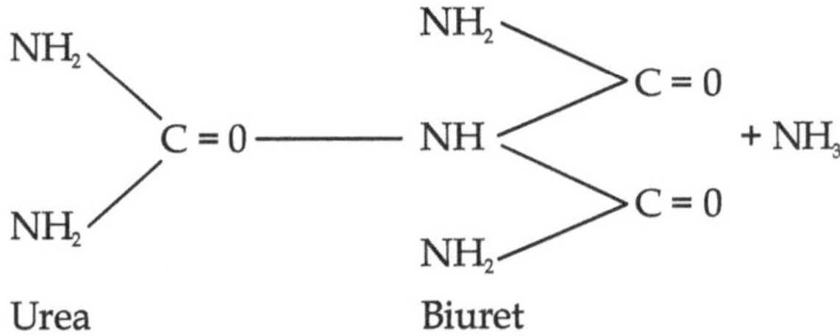

The biuret reaction is specific for peptides, polypeptides and proteins. Other nitrogen containing compounds, such as ammonia, amino acids, uric acid, urea and creatinine do not react. The colour which is formed depends on the structure of the compound, proteins give a purple violet colour, proteases, peptones and peptides give a salmon coloured compound, whereas gelatine give a blue coloured complex. There is no correlation between the colour formed (absorption optimum) and the molecular extinction coefficient are practically the same for the various proteins; this is why the biuret reaction gives good results even when strongly pathological sera are analysed. the method described permits the estimation of total protein, albumin and globulin on a single serum sample. The method is described by Oser (1954).

Reagents

1. *Sulphate-sulphite solution : Place 208 grams of sodium sulphate and 70 grams sodium sulphite in a 1000 ml heat-resistant volumetric flask. Add 2 ml of concentrated sulphuric acid to 900 ml of water in a second container. Transfer the acidified water without delay to the flask containing the salts, stirring until solution has occurred. Dilute to the mark and store in glass stoppered bottles above 25°C.*

2. *Biuret stock solution : Dissolve 45 grams of sodium potassium tartrate in approximately 400 ml 0.2 N sodium hydroxide. Add 15 grams copper sulphate ($CuSO_4.5H_2O$) and continue stirring until this is completely dissolved. Add 5 grams potassium iodide and dilute to 1000 ml with 0.2 N sodium hydroxide.*

3. *Biuret working solution : Dilute 200 ml of stock biuret solution in 1000 ml with 0.2 N sodium hydroxide containing 5 grams potassium iodide per litre.*

4. *Tartrate - Iodide blank solution : Dissolve 9 grams of sodium potassium tartrate in sufficient 0.2 N sodium hydroxide solution containing 5 grams potassium iodide per litre to make 1000 ml of solution.*

5. *Standard serum : Obtain a pooled lot of normal serum. Determine the total protein content of a portion by micro-Kjeldahl as described in volume I of this compendium. Divide into 2 ml portions and freeze these portions individually. As required for analysis, using one sample each time an analysis is made.*

Procedure

Transfer 7.5 ml of sulphate-sulphite reagent into a standard test tube 18 x 120 mm. Add slowly, with continuous stirring, 0.5 ml of serum. Stopper and mix by inversion. Remove 2 ml of the mixture and add it to 5 ml of biuret reagent in a cuvette. Set this aside until completion of the albumin/globulin separation. Add 3 ml of anhydrous, reagent grade ethyl ether to the tube containing the remainder of the sulphate-sulphite mixture, stopper, shake exactly 40 times in 20 seconds, and centrifuge the mixture at 2000 rpm for 5 to 10 minutes. Remove 2 ml of the bottom layer from the separated, centrifuged mixture and place in a cuvette. This is best accomplished by tilting the tube and inserting the pipette down the lower side holding one finger over the pipette until it is well into the lower layer. This will prevent the ethereal solution from entering the pipette. Add 5 ml of biuret solution. Prepare a serum blank by mixing 2 ml of serum suspension (0.5 ml serum plus 7.5 ml sulphate-sulphite reagent) with 5 ml of the tartrate-iodide blank solution. Prepare a biuret blank by mixing 2 ml of sulphate-sulphite reagent with 5 ml of biuret reagent. The standard is prepared by mixing 0.5 ml of the standard serum with 7.5 ml of the sulhate-sulphite reagent and taking 2 ml of this mixture and mixing with 5 ml of biuret reagent. No further treatment of the standard is necessary.

Place all tubes containing biuret reagent into a water bath at 30° to 37°C for 10 minutes. Cool at room temperature for 5 minutes and read in a photometer at wavelengths from 540 to 565 mμ, zeroing the instrument with the biuret blank.

Calculation

1. Total protein

$$\frac{\text{Density of unknown} \mid \text{Density of serum blank}}{\text{Density of standard} \mid \text{Density of std. blank}} \ \text{g\% protein in standard}$$

= g total protein per 100 ml serum.

2. Albumin

$$\frac{\text{Density of unknown (after ether)} \mid \text{Density of unknown blank}}{\text{Density of std.} \mid \text{Density of std. blank}} \ \text{g\% protein std.}$$

= g albumin/100 ml serum

3. Globulin

Total protein – albumin = grams globulin per 100 ml serum.

Upto 11 grams per cent of total protein may be determined accurately under the conditions described. For higher values use 1 ml portions instead of 2 ml portions, plus 1 ml of water, and multiply the results by 2.

Method II

Estimation of albumin using HABA

(Lindstad, P. 1973)

Reagent

Stock HABA solution. Dissolve 0.1 gram HABA (2-4 hydroxyazobenzene) – benzoic acid in phosphate buffer (5.81 g KH_2PO_4 and 8.6 g Na_2 HPO_4. $12H_2O$ mixed in 1000 ml distilled water).

Method

Take 0.1 ml serum and 3 ml stock HABA solution. After 10 minutes take the reading using spectrophotometer at 510 mμ compare the reading against standard bovine albumin and blank (0.1 ml ammonia free distill water + 3 ml stock HABA solution).

Prepare bovine albumin standard in 0.9 per cent sodium chloride solution.

Estimation of Globulin in Serum

(Method 1 - Lindstad, 1973)

Reagent

Zinc sulphate solution. Dissolve 250 mg zinc sulphate in 1000 ml distilled water.

Procedure

Mix 0.05 ml serum with 1 ml demineralised distilled water in a test tube, add 5 ml zinc sulphate reagent. Keep the test tube for one hour in water bath at 22-23°C, read at 650 mμ, using spectrophotometer. Multiply the observation by two and then final result is obtained.

Method III

(Weichselbaum, 1946 and Gornall, 1949)

Principle

Serum γ-globulin is precipitated by the addition of a mixture of ammonium sulphate and sodium chloride. The precipitate is dissolved in normal saline solution and the protein in suspension determined by development of the blue biuret colour reaction.

Reagents

1. *Ammonium sulphate solution : To approximately 700 ml of distilled water in one litre volumetric flask add 195 grams of reagent grade ammonium sulphate and 20.3 grams of reagent grade sodium chloride. Dissolve by mixing and*

make up to about 995 ml. Adjust the pH to 6.4 by means of concentrated ammonium hydroxide or sulphuric acid and dilute to one litre with distilled water.

2. *Working biuret solution : Dilute 100 ml of stock biuret solution to 1 litre with 0.2 sodium hydroxide containing 5 grams of potassium iodide per litre.*
3. *Albumin standard solution : The number of peptide bonds per gram of protein is the same for all pure protein. The intensity of the blue complex formed with the biuret reagent is dependent on the number of peptide bond present. Therefore, any pure protein can be used as a standard for the determination of any other protein by the biuret reaction. Prepare standard with 0.9 per cent sodium chloride having concentration of about 0.0015 gram protein per ml. Avoid vigorous shaking as this will cause foaming.*

Procedure

Place 5.7 ml of the ammonium sulphate solution into a 12 to 15 ml conical centrifuge tube. Carefully mix the reagent with 0.30 ml clear, non haemolysed serum. Stopper, gently invert (do not shake) the tube 6 times, and place in an ice bath for 15 minutes. Centrifuge the cold mixture at 3000 rpm for 10 minutes and discard the clear supernatant fluid. Repeat the centrifugation and discard any additional supernatant fluid. Dry the inner surface of the tube with absorbent paper or cloth and add 2 ml 0.9 per cent sodium chloride to the residue. Agitate the mixture gently until the precipitate dissolves. Add 5 ml of the working biuret solution and let the mixture stand at room temperature for 10 minutes. Read at 555 mμ, zeroing the photometer with a mixture of 2 ml of 0.9 per cent sodium chloride and 5 ml working biuret solution. Mix 2 ml of the albumin standard with 5 ml of the working biuret solution and let the mixture stand at room temperature for 10 minutes. Read in the same manner as the serum.

Calculation

The concentration of the standard times the aliquot of the standard divided by the serum sample volume equals one; therefore:

$$\frac{\text{Density of unknown}}{\text{Density of standard}} = \text{g, } \gamma \text{ globulin per 100 ml serum}$$

II. Amino acid Nitrogen in Blood, Plasma and Serum

(Method of Folin, 1922 and Denielson, 1933)

Principle

The colour developed by the reaction between aminoacids and B-naphthoquinone-4-sulphonic acid in alkaline solution is the basis of this method. This principle was evolved by Folin (1922). The method was considerably improved by Denielson (1933) and the time required for a determination was reduced by Sahyun (1938), who suggested heating to develop the colour. The procedure is described by Oser (1954).

Reagents

1. *10 per cent sodium tungstate : Dissolve 100 grams reagent grade, carbonate free $Na_2WO_4.2H_2O$ in water and dilute to one litre and mix. This can be used for a period not exceeding 3 weeks.*
2. *0.667 NH_2SO_4 : This should be standardised.*
3. *Amino acid standard : Weigh 0.268 gram dry glycine and 0.525 gram dry glutamic acid; dissolve in water and transfer with washings to a 500 ml volumetric flask. Add 35 ml N Hcl and 1 gram sodium benzoate. Add water to dissolve and dilute to mark with water and mix. This standards contains 0.2 mg N/ml. It is stable indefinitely. To prepare working standard, transfer 3 ml of standard to 100 ml volumetric flask and dilute to the mark with water and mix. This standard contains 6 μg N/ml and is usable for one week, if kept in the cold.*
4. *0.25% phenolphthalein in 95% ethanol.*
5. *0.1 N NaOH.*
6. *1 per cent borax solution : Dissolve 10 grams sodium tetraborate, $Na_2B_40_7$. $10H_2O$ in water and dilute to one litre with water, mix stable indefinitely.*
7. *B-Napthoquinone-4-sulphonic acid : Solution. Dissolve 0.25 gram beta-naphthoquinone-4-sulphonic acid in a water and dilute to 50 ml, mix. Prepare immediately before using, discard remaining solution.*
8. *Acid-formaldehyde solution : Four volumes of a solution made by diluting 11.3 ml of 40 per cent formaldehyde to one litre with water is mixed with three volumes of 1.5 N hydrochloric acid and one of glacial acetic acid.*
9. *0.05 M sodium thiosulphate solution : This need not be standardised. Dissolve 12.4 grams of crystalline sodium thiosulphate in water, dilute to one litre with water and mix. usuable indefinitely.*

☞ **Notes**

With the exception of the dilute standard and the Beta-naphthoquinone-4-sulphonic acid solutions, all the above reagents could be kept indefinitely.

1. *For the determination, a tungstic acid filtrate of whole blood or plasma is prepared as follows :*

   a) For whole blood, mix 7 volume of water, 1 volume 10% sodium tungstate and 1 volume 2/3 N H_2SO_4.
2. *Place 9 ml protein precipitation solution into 15 ml conical bottom centrifuge tubes.*
3. *Add 1 ml whole blood, plasma or serum. Stopper and shake. Only a few bubbles should form as a result of this shaking if all the proteins have been precipitated. let stand for 10 minutes. The colour of the mixture in the case of whole blood should change from red to dark brown. Centrifuge or filter to obtain clear filtrate.*
4. *Transfer 3 ml protein free filtrate in duplicate to test tubes with a capacity of at least 20 ml and graduated at 10 ml. Place 2, 3 and 4 ml of the working amino acid standard in duplicate into similar test tubes. Blank tubes are prepared using ammonia free distilled water. Add 1 drop of 0.25 per cent alcoholic phenolphthalein to each tube.*
5. *Adjust each tube to permanent pink colour using 0.1 N NaOH. Please do not add excess NaOH.*
6. *Dilute contents of each tube to 10 ml with water, mix.*
7. *Add 2 ml borax solution, mix.*
8. *Add 1 ml freshly prepared naphthoquinone reagent and mix immediately.*
9. *Place tubes immediately into a boiling water bath for 10 minutes.*
10. *Place tubes in cold water bath for 5 minutes.*
11. *Add 1 ml acid-formaldehyde solution and mix immediately.*
12. *Add 1 ml 0.05 M sodium thiosulphate and mix immediately.*
13. *Allow to stand 10 to 30 minutes and read colour intensity at 480 mμ, setting colorimeter at zero OD (100% T) with the blank tube.*
14. *Amino acid standards should read as follows with the Spectronic-20 at 480 mμ.*

Amino acid standard	Tube cuvette (OD)	Automatic cuvette (Transmittancy)
2 ml	0.176-0.194	65.5-69.0
3 ml	0.261-0.289	53.7-57.0
4 ml	0.352-0.388	42.6-46.2

☞ Notes

1. *The protein precipitation solution should be checked with Nessler's reagent to make sure if it is free of ammonia.*

2. *Off the possible interferring substances, glutathione is the main one. Since it is found primarily in the corpuscles, interferrence is minimised if plasma or serum is used. Uric acid at a concentration of 1 mg/100 ml gives colour equivalent to 0.1 mg amino acid N/100 ml, sulfonamides also gives a coloured reaction.*

3. *For acceptable precision, the following are important*
   a) Adjusting to equal volume (Step 7).
   b) Immediate mixing (Steps 9, 12 and 13).

Table 2 : The following chart can be used to determine amino acid nitrogen concentration per 100 ml sample. Standards should read within the range shown before this chart is used. Blank tubes are used to adjust colorimeter to 100% transmittancy.

% T	0.0	0.1	0.2	0.3	0.4	0.5	0.6	0.7	0.8	0.9
37	10.7	10.4	10.1	0.99	0.96	9.93	9.90	9.88	9.85	9.82
38	9.79	9.76	9.74	9.71	9.68	9.66	9.63	9.61	9.59	9.56
39	9.53	9.51	9.48	9.45	9.43	9.40	9.38	9.35	9.33	9.30
40	9.28	9.26	9.23	9.21	9.18	9.15	9.13	9.11	9.08	9.06
41	9.03	9.01	8.98	8.96	8.93	8.90	8.88	8.85	8.82	8.80
42	8.78	8.75	8.73	8.70	8.68	8.66	8.64	8.61	8.58	8.56
43	8.54	8.51	8.49	8.47	8.45	8.43	8.40	8.38	8.35	8.33
44	8.81	8.28	8.26	8.24	8.22	8.20	8.17	8.15	8.12	8.10
45	8.08	8.05	8.03	8.01	7.9	7.97	7.94	7.92	7.90	7.88
46	7.86	7.83	7.81	7.79	7.77	7.75	7.72	7.70	7.68	7.66
47	7.64	7.62	7.60	7.58	7.56	7.54	7.51	7.49	7.47	7.45
48	7.43	7.41	7.39	7.37	7.35	7.33	7.30	7.28	7.26	7.24
49	7.22	7.20	7.18	7.16	7.14	7.12	7.10	7.08	7.06	7.04
50	7.02	7.00	6.98	6.96	6.94	6.92	6.90	6.88	6.86	6.84
51	6.82	6.80	6.78	6.76	6.74	6.72	6.70	6.68	6.66	6.64
52	6.62	6.60	6.58	6.56	6.54	6.52	6.50	6.48	6.47	6.45
53	6.43	6.41	6.39	6.37	6.35	6.33	6.31	6.29	6.28	6.26
54	6.24	6.22	6.20	6.18	6.16	6.14	6.13	6.11	6.09	6.07
55	6.05	6.03	6.02	6.00	5.98	5.96	5.94	5.92	5.91	5.89
56	5.87	5.85	5.83	5.82	5.80	5.78	5.77	5.75	5.73	5.71
57	5.69	5.67	5.65	5.64	5.62	5.60	5.59	5.57	5.56	5.54
58	5.52	5.50	5.48	5.47	5.45	5.43	5.42	5.40	5.38	5.36
59	5.34	5.32	5.31	5.29	5.28	5.26	5.25	5.23	5.21	5.19

60	5.17	5.16	5.14	5.13	5.11	5.09	5.08	5.06	5.04	5.02
61	5.00	4.99	4.97	4.96	4.94	4.92	4.91	4.89	4.88	4.86
62	4.84	4.83	4.81	4.80	4.78	4.76	4.75	4.73	4.72	4.70
63	4.68	4.67	4.65	4.64	4.62	4.60	4.59	4.57	4.56	4.54
64	4.52	4.51	4.49	4.48	4.46	4.44	4.43	4.41	4.40	4.38
65	4.36	4.35	4.33	4.32	4.30	4.28	4.27	4.26	4.24	4.23
66	4.21	4.20	4.18	4.17	4.15	4.13	4.12	4.10	4.09	4.07
67	4.05	4.04	4.02	4.00	3.99	3.98	3.96	3.95	3.93	3.92
68	3.90	3.88	3.87	3.85	3.84	3.83	3.81	3.80	3.78	3.77
69	3.76	3.74	3.73	3.71	3.69	6.68	3.66	3.65	3.64	3.62
70	3.61	3.59	3.58	3.56	3.55	3.54	3.52	3.51	3.50	3.48
71	3.47	3.46	3.44	3.43	3.41	3.40	3.38	3.37	3.35	3.34
72	3.33	3.31	3.30	3.29	3.28	3.26	3.25	3.24	3.22	3.20
73	3.19	3.18	3.16	3.15	3.14	3.12	3.11	3.10	3.08	3.06
74	3.05	3.03	3.02	3.00	2.99	2.98	2.90	2.95	2.94	2.93
75	2.91	2.90	2.89	2.87	2.86	2.85	2.84	2.82	2.81	2.79

References

Burstein, M. and Samaille, J. (1959). *Ann. Biol. Clin.*, 17:23.

Conway, E.J. (1957). *Microdiffusion analysis and volumetric error*, 4th edn., Crossly, Lockwood and Son Ltd., London.

Danielsen, I.S. (1933). *J. Biol. Chem.*, 101:565.

Folin, O. and Denis, W. (1916). *J. Biol. Chem.*, 26:473.

Folin, O. (1922). *J. Biol. Chem.*, 51:393.

Folin, O. and Ciocalteu. (1927). *J. Biol. Chem.*, 73:627

Gornall, A.G., Bardawill, C.J. and David, M.M. (1949). *J. Biol. Chem.*, 177: 751.

Kingsley, (1940). *J. Biol. Chem.*, 133:731.

Lindstad, P. (1973). Personal communication.

Lowry, O.H. and Hunter, T.H. (1945). *J. Biol. Chem.*, 159 : 465.

Lowry, O.H., Rosenbrough, N.J., Farr, A.L. and Randall, R.J. (1951). *J. Biol. Chem.*, 193 :265.

Oser, B.L. (1954). *Hawk's physiological chemistry*, 14th edn. Mc Graw-Hill Book Co., London, pp 1048, pp 1083.

Sahyun, M. (1938). *J. Lab. Clin. Med.*, 24 : 548.

Tiwari, S.P. and Krishna, G. (1986). Rumen nitrogen metabolism in growing buffalo calves fed guar seed and ground nut cake. *Indian J. Animal Production*. 18: 18-22.

Tiwari, S.P., Krishna, G. and Naresh Kumar, (1993). Nitrogen metabolism in growing male buffalo calves fed guar seed (*Cyamopsis Tetragonoloba* L.) and groundnut cake. *Indian Vety. J.* 70: 519-523.

Tiwari, S.P., Krishna, G. and Naresh Kumar, (1994). Effect of feeding guar seed (*Cyamopsis Tetragonoloba* L.) on certain blood biochemical constituents in male buffalo calves. *Indian J. Dairy Sci.* 47: 702-703.

Weichselbaum, T.E. (1946). *Ann. J. Clin. Pathol. Tech. Sect.,* 10 : 4D

Wong, S.Y. (1923). *J. Biol. Chem.,* 55 : 431.

Zak, B. and Cohen, J. (1961). *Clin. Chim. Acta.,* 6 : 665.

Chapter - 78

Pepsin Digestibility of Human and Animal Food

(Method of AOAC, 1965)

Pepsin Digestibility of Food

Principle

Solvent extracted samples are digested for 16 hour with warm acid solution of pepsin under constant agitation. Insoluble residue is centrifuged, dried and weighed and analysed for protein ; or filtered, washed and analysed for protein.

Apparatus

1. *Centrifuge* : Capable of at least 1750 rpm with conical bottom tubes of 150 ml capacity. If necessary, solution may be centrifuged in 50 ml tubes.
2. *Agitator* : or water bath with shaking device and having temperature controlling unit.
3. Glass fiber filter paper.

Reagents

1. *Pepsin solution : 0.2% pepsin (activity 1:10, 100) in 0.075 N Hcl. Prepare dilute Hcl by diluting 6.1 ml Hcl to one litre with water. Add protein just before use, stirring until completely dissolved.*
2. *Alcohol : Denaturated is satisfactory.*

3. *Filter aid* : Diatomaceous earth type such as Hyflo Super-cel (Johns-Manville) or acid treated asbestos

Extraction

Method I

Weigh 1 g sample into thimble and extract for one hour with ether at condensation rate of 3-4 drops/second (If soxhlet is used, top of thimble should extend above siphon tube to avoid loss of solid particles). If paper containing sample is totally submerged in siphon cup, sample must be completely wrapped in paper. Observe ether extract to detect that no solid particles are carried into solvent beaker. If approximate fat content is desired, evaporate ether, dry and weigh residue. Remove paper from sample container or cup and let dry at room temperature. For guidance, we may refer the method compiled in volume I.

Unfold and brush defatted sample quantitatively into digestion bottle, avoiding contamination by brush bristles or filter paper fibers.

Method II

Stir 1 g sample thoroughly with 10 ml ether in 15 ml centrifuge tube and centrifuge for 5 minutes at 1750 rpm or greater. Decant ether and repeat extraction with three 5 ml portions ether. If approximate fat content is desired, combine ether extracts, evaporate, dry and weigh residue.

Pepsin Digestion

Transfer defatted sample quantitatively to 200 ml capacity conical flask and fix in a water bath clamps or agitator clamps having a continuous shaking arrangements. Add 150 ml freshly prepared pepsin - Hcl solution, prewarmed to 42-45°C. Stopper bottle, incubate the contents of flask with continuous shaking at 45°C for 16 hours duration.

Treatment of Residue

Transfer contents of agitator container to centrifuge tube and centrifuge 5 minutes at 1750 rpm or greater. If 150 ml tube is unavailable, centrifuge in 50 ml portions, collecting entire residue in same tube. Decant supernatant, rinse agitator bottle twice with 15-20 ml portions warm H_2O and add rinse H_2O to residue in tube. Stir well, centrifuge, and decant wash water. Wash residue once more with warm water and twice with alcohol. Resuspend residue in 5-10 ml alcohol and filter quantitatively with gentle suction through weighed No. 4 gooch crucible containing glass fiber filter paper or asbestos prepare crucible by inserting filter paper or asbestos washing twice with warm water and twice with alcohol with gentle suction. Dry in oven for 30 minutes at 100-110°C, cool and weigh). Wash indigestible residue with alcohol and suck dry. Dry in oven 30 minutes at 110°C, cool, weigh and calculate indigestible residue. Transfer residue and filter pad quantitatively to Kjeldahl flask and estimate crude protein as per method compiled in volume I of this compendium.

Calculation

Pepsin digestible crude protein = 100- pepsin indigestible crude protein

References

AOAC, (1965). *Officinal methods of analysis of the Association of official Agricultural Chemists. 10 th edn.*, AOAC, Benjamin Franklin Station, Washington, D.C. pp 330.

Chapter - 79

Antitryptic Activity of Human and Animal Food (Legume)

(Method of Kunitz, 1947 modified by Kakade *et al.*, 1969)

Introduction

Casein has been widely used as a substrate for measuring the trypsin inhibitor activity of natural trypsin inhibitors such as those which occur in Soybeans and other legume. The most common method employing casein is the one originally described by Kunitz (1947) which involves the spectrophotometric determination of the breakdown products produced by a given concentration of trypsin in the presence and absence of the inhibitor. On the other hand, the tryptic hydrolysis of a synthetic substrate such as benzoyl-DL-arginine-p-nitroanilide (BAPA), first introduced by Erlanger *et al.* (1961), does follow a zero order reaction, and one obtains, within broad limits, a linear relationship between the quantity of p-nitroaniline released and the concentration of the active enzyme. Although BAPA has been used for assaying the antitryptic activity of soybean fractions (Sambeth *et al.*, 1967).

Principle

The casein digestion method of Kunitz (1947) for the measurement of trypsin inhibitor activity of soybean extracts has been modified to obtain more accurate and reproducible results. The modification involved the use of 2 per cent casein (instead of 1 per cent) and the mathematical transformation of absorbance readings (A) at 280 mμ. The use of the synthetic substrates, benzoyl-DL-arginine-p-nitroanilide (BAPA), proved to be a convenient and reliable method of assaying trypsin inhibitor activity provided one takes into account the competitive nature of the inhibition. The latter effect could be largely compensated for by extrapolating the trypsin activity, expressed as trypsin units inhibited per ml extract, to zero concentration of the inhibitor. Although a series of soybean samples could be ranked in the same relative order of inhibitor activity by using either casein or BAPA, the quantity of trypsin inhibited was consistently higher when BAPA was employed as the substrate.

Method I (Trypsin Inhibitor Activity Using Casein Substrate)

Reagents

1. *Phosphate buffer (0.1 M, pH 7.6) : Dissolve 23.3 grams $Na_2HPO_47H_2O$ and 1.8 grams $NaH_2PO_4H_2O$ in 900 ml water. The pH is adjusted to 7.6 and the final volume is made up to one litre.*
2. *Casein solution (1 or 2 per cent) : 1 or 2 grams of casein is suspended in 80 ml of the phosphate buffer and completely dissolved by heating on a steam bath for 15 minutes. The solution is cooled, made to 100 ml with buffer and stored in the refrigerator, when not in use.*
3. *Stock trypsin solution : 4 to 5 mg of accurately weighed trypsin is dissolved in 100 ml 0.001 M Hcl. This solution be stored in the refrigerator for 2 to 3 weeks without appreciable loss in activity. The concentration of trypsin (mg/ml) may be determined by multiplying the absorbance of the trypsin solution at 280 mμ by the factor (0.65).*

Procedure

Samples of legume seeds are ground in a Wiley mill to pass through a 100 mesh screen and extracted with 10 ml of petroleum ether (B.P. 60 to 70°C) at room temperature. One gram of meal is suspended in 19 ml water, and the pH of the suspension is adjusted to pH 7.6. After mechanical shaking for one hour, the suspension is centrifuged and 1 ml of the supernatant is diluted to 50 ml with phosphate buffer. The protein content of the diluted extract is determined by the method of Lowry *et al.* (1951).

0.2 to 1.0 ml of the stock trypsin solution is pipetted into a triplicate set of test tubes (one set for each level of trypsin) and the final volume of each tube is adjusted to 2 ml with the phosphate buffer. The tubes are set in a water bath at 37°C. To one of the triplicate tubes is added 6 ml 5 per cent (w/v) trichloroacetic acid, this tube serve as a blank; 2 ml of the casein solution, previously brought to 37°C, is added to each tube. The tubes are allowed to remain at 37°C for exactly 20minute, at which time the reaction is allowed to stop by adding 6 ml of 5 per cent trichloroacetic acid to the experimental tubes. After standing for one hour at room temperature, the suspension is filtered, and the absorbance of the filtrate is measured at 280 mμ against the blank.

When assaying samples of processed soybean preparations in which the trypsin inhibitor activity may be partially destroyed, the original extract may be used directly or should be diluted to the point where 1 ml produces an inhibition of atleast 80%. The amount of protein extracted by this procedure will depend on the physical properties of the soybean product being examined. In view of the uncertainity that may attend the extractibility of the protein, it may at times be advisable to express the trypsin inhibitor activity on the basis of the protein content of the extract.

Trypsin inhibitor activity : 0.2 to 1.0 ml aliquots of the soybean extract are pipetted into a triplicate set of test tubes (one set for each level of extract), and the volume is brought to 1.0 ml with the phosphate buffer ; 1 ml of the stock trypsin solution is added to each tube, and the tubes are placed in the water bath at 37°C. The remainder of the procedure is the same as described in the paragraph.

Expression of activity

One trypsin unit (TU) is arbitrarily defined as an increase of 0.01 absorbance units at 280 mμ in 20 minutes per 10 ml of the reaction mixture under the conditions set forth herein. Trypsin inhibitor activity is defined as the number of trypsin units inhibited (TUI).

Method II (Trypsin Inhibitor Activity Using BAPA Substrate)

Reagents

1. *Tris buffer : (0.05 M, pH 8.2) containing 0.02 M $CaCl_2$; 6.05 grams, tris-(hydroxymethyl) aminoethane (Sigma) and 2.94 grams $CaCl_2.H_2O$ are dissolved in 900 ml water. The pH is adjusted to 8.2 and the volume is brought to one litre with water.*

2. *BAPA solution : 30 mg BAPA. Hcl is dissolved in 1 ml dimethylsulfoxide and diluted to 100 ml with the tris buffer prewarmed to 37°C. Care should be taken to dissolved all of the BAPA in dimethylsulfoxide since traces of undissoled crystals may cause precipitation to occur upon standing. The BAPA solution is freshly prepared daily and kept at 37°C while in use.*

3. *Trypsin solution (See casein method).*

Procedure

Method is same as described under casein procedure except that water is used to make the 1:50 dilution of the original soybean extract or (legume seed extract). Protein may precipitate upon the addition of 30 per cent acetic acid when dilutions of less than 1:50 are employed. In this case the solutions should be filtered prior to reading the absorbance.

0.2 to 1.0 ml of the stock trypsin solution is pipetted into a triplicate set of test tubes, and the volume is made upto 2 ml with water. The test tubes are placed in a water bath at 37°C ; 1 ml of 30 per cent acetic acid is added to one of the triplicate tubes to serve as a blank. To each tube is then added 7 ml BAPA solution, previously warmed to 37°C., and exactly 10 minutes later, the reaction is terminated by adding 1 ml of 30 per cent acetic acid to each of the experimental tubes. After thorough mixing the absorbance of each solution is measured at 410 mμ against the appropriate blank.

0.2 to 1 ml of the soybean extract is pipetted into a triplicate set of test tubes and final volume adjusted to 1 ml with water ; 1 ml of the stock trypsin solution is added to each of the tubes, which is then assayed as described in the previous paragraph.

One trypsin unit (TU) is arbitrarily defined as an increase of 0.01 absorbance units at 410 mμ per 10 ml of the reaction mixture under the conditions defined herein. *Trypsin inhibitor activity is defined as the number of trypsin units inhibited (TUI).*

References

Erlanger, B.F., KoKowsky, N. and Cohen, W. (1961). *Arch. Biochem., Biophys.,* 95 : 271.

KaKade, M.L., Simons, N. and Liener, I.E. (1969). *Cereal Chem.,* 46 : 518.

Kunitz, M. (1947). *J. Gen., Physiol.,* 30 : 291.

Lowry, O.H., Rosebrough, N.J., Farr, A.L. and Randall, N.J. (1951). *J. Biol. Chem.,* 193 : 265.

Sambeth, W., Nesheim, M.C. and Serafin, J.A. (1967). *J. Nutr.,* 92 : 479.

Chapter - 80

Polyethylene Glycol (PEG) in Biological Materials

(A turbidimetric method of Hyden 1955)

PEG Estimation

Introduction

Polyethylene glycol (PEG) is used as a marker for the estimation of rumen water volume and ruminant digestion studies (Hyden and Ekman, 1953). Long back, Hyden (1955) developed a turbidimetric method which is described below :

Principle

When trichloroacetic acid is added to a solution of PEG, a turbidity is produced, which can be measured photo-electrically. The intensity of the cloud, which consists of finely divided oily droplets, is increased in the presence of barium ions. Protein and sulphate must be completely removed from the sample before the addition of the trichloroacetic acid reagent. Sulphate is precipitated with barium chloride and the proteins are removed essentially according to Samogyi (1945). The method has been developed for determination of PEG in ruminal and abomasal fluids, but it has been tried with other biological materials too.

Reagents

1. *Trichloroacetic acid, 30 per cent w/v with 5 per cent barium chloride. The solution is filtered.*

2. *Barium hydroxide, 0.3 N*
3. *Barium chloride 10 per cent w/v*
4. *Zinc sulphate, 5 per cent w/v solution of Zn* $SO_4 \cdot 7H_2O$.

Pretreatment of biological samples

In a solution free from protein and sulphate the lowest concentration of PEG possible to determine is 0.0125 mg/ml. When an interfering substances are removed from a sample, the dilution of the sample must be balanced accordingly. For samples containing from 0.2 mg of PEG/ml, the following procedures are suitable.

1. Rumen fluid, urine, saliva and plasma

1-2 ml of the sample (if necessary strained through muslin or centrifuged) are pipetted into an Erlenmeyer flask, and in the order given, 10 ml distilled water, 1 ml barium chloride, 2 ml barium hydroxide and 2 ml zinc sulphate are added. The mixture is shaken after each addition and allowed to stand five minutes before filteration.

2. Abomasal fluid

The sample is centrifuged and to 1-2 ml of the supernatant, are added 10 ml distilled water, 3 ml barium hydroxide and 2 ml zinc sulphate. The mixture is shaken and allowed to stand as above before filteration.

3. Omasal and intestinal contents, faeces etc.

A weighed amount of the sample is macerated in water and diluted to an extent depending on the PEG concentration and the character of the sample. After mixing and standing for equilibration it is strained through muslin or centrifuged. To an aliquot (e.g. 5 ml) of the extract are added 1 ml barium chloride, 2 ml barium hydroxide and 2 ml zinc sulphate at above.

Procedure

4 ml of the perfectly clear filtrate (diluted if necessary), containing (0.05) 0.1-0.7 mg PEG are pipetted into a 25 ml Erlenmeyer flask. 4 ml of the trichloroacetic acid reagent are added, and the contents are quickly and carefully mixed. The solution is transferred to a cuvette and the turbidity is measured photoelectrically after exactly 5 minutes.

The method is worked out specially for PEG compounds with mean molecular weights of 3000-4000. After some slight modifications, it can be used for other compounds at least within the range 1500-6000. It is possible to determine from 0.05 to 0.7 mg of PEG in 4 ml filtrates. In the determination of 0.3 to 0.6 mg of PEG, the coefficient of variation is about 0.7 percent.

References

Hyden, S. (1955). *Kungl. LantbruKshoskolans Annaler*, 22: 139.

References for further study

Shaffer, C.B. and Critchfield, F.H. (1947). *Anal. Chem.*, 19:32.

Sperber, I., Hyden, S. and Ekman, J. (1953). *Ann. Agr. Coll. Sweden*, 20:337.

Chapter - 81

Estimation of Chloride in Biological Samples

Chloride Determination

I. Titrimetric Method of Estimating Salt in Fish Meal

(Modified AOAC, 1965 method)

Principle

The salt content is calculated as sodium chloride from the content of water solubles chlorides. The chlorides are dissolved in water and directly precipitated by titration with a silver nitrate solution using potassium chromate as an indicator.

Reagents

1. *0.1 N silver nitrate solution : Dissolve slightly more than theoretical quantity of* $AgNO_3$ *(equiv. Wt, 169.87) in halogen free water and dilute to volume. Thoroughly clean glassware, avoid contact with dust, and keep prepared solution in amber glass bottles away from light. Standardize the solution against 0.1 N NaCl containing 5.844 gram of pure dry NaCl/litre.*
2. *Potassium chromate solution (5 per cent) : Dissolve theoretical quantity of* K_2CrO_4 *in halogen free distilled water and keep this solution in a dark brown coloured bottle.*
3. *Carrez solution*

Carrez solution I and II are prepared as given below :

a) *Carrez I.* 23.8 g zinc acetate $(CH_3COO)_2$ Zn. $2H_2O$ and 3g glacial acetic acid diluted in water made up to 100 ml.

b) *Carrez II.* 10.6 potassium ferrocyanide K_4Fe (CN)6. $3H_2O$ is dissolved in water and made up to 100 ml.

Apparatus

Shaker rotating at a rate of 30-40 times a minute.

Procedure

a) *Preparation of solution.* About 5g of the fish meal is accurately weighed and washed quantitatively into a flask with warm water making a total volume of not more than 250 ml., adding 5 ml of *Carrez I* solution and shake, add 5 ml of *Carrez II* solution, then shake for 30 minutes in a shaker and filter. The residue is washed until chloride free.

b) *Determination.* To the solution prepared as mentioned in (a), 1 ml of K_2CrO_4 is added and from a burette the 0.1 N silver nitrate solution is added with a continuous shaking of the beaker till the first precipitable pale red salmon colour appears.

It is advisable to use a diffuse or indirect light during the titration.

Calculation

1 ml of 0.1 N $AgNO_3$ = 0.005845 g of NaCl

$$= \frac{\text{ml } 0.1\text{N } AgNO_3 \times 0.1 \times 0.585}{5}$$

= % Sodium Chloride

Mineral conversion

$$\text{Chlorine to sodium chloride} = \frac{\text{Multiply by}}{1.65} \quad \frac{\text{Reciprocal}}{0.607} \text{ (multiply by)}$$

II. Chloride in Blood or Serum or Plasma

(Modified method of Van Slyke, 1923)

Principle

Blood serum is digested with silver nitrate and nitric acid. The chloride is precipitated as silver chloride and can be determined by titrating the excess of silver nitrate with standard ammonium thiocyanate solution.

Reagents

1. *Standard silver nitrate solution 0.15 N : Dissolve 25.5 grams of silver nitrate in about 400 ml of water, transfer to a one litre volumetric flask and make up to the mark.*

2. *Standard Ammonium thiocyanate solution : Dissolve approximately 8 grams of ammonium thiocyanate in water and make up to one litre. Standardize against standard silver nitrate, and dilute to make it exactly 0.1 N. Dilute this solution 5 times with distilled water to prepare 0.02 N solution.*

3. *Ferric Alum Indicator : Prepare a 0.05 M solution of ferric alum (48 grams per litre).*

Procedure

Transfer 1 ml of serum to a large test tube (29 x 200 mm), add 1 ml of standard silver nitrate solution and mix by shaking. After standing 2 or 3 minutes, add 3 ml of concentrated nitric acid, washing down the sides of the tube. Cover with a small funnel to act as a condenser and heat over a small flame until frothing ceases and then boil gently for 10 or 15 minutes. The solution should be water clear and light yellow. Cool thoroughly, add 6 ml of ferric alum solution and titrate with 0.02 N ammonium thiocyanate solution. 0.04 ml of the thiocyanate solution is necessary to produce a strong red colour in the volume used. Therefore subtract the 0.04 ml excess from the amount of thiocyanate used in the titration. Calculate mg of chloride and mg of sodium chloride per 100 ml of serum as milliequivalent per litre.

Chloride in Serum

(Mercurimetric titration method of Schales and Schales, 1941)

Principle

In this method chloride ions in acid solution are titrated with mercuric nitrate, forming undissociated mercuric chloride. The violet colour with excess mercury ion is obtained with indicator "*diphenyl-carbazone*".

Reagents

1. *Indicator : 100 mg of diphenylcarbazone per 100 ml in alcohol. Store in a brown bottle in the cold and it will be better if a fresh solution is prepared at the time of analysis.*

2. *Mercuric nitrate solution : Dissolve 3 grams of mercuric nitrate in 500 ml of water. Add 20 ml of 2 N-nitric acid and make to one litre with water.*

3. *Standard sulphuric acid (N/12)*

This can be prepared as per methods mentioned in volume I of this compendium.

4. *Sodium tungstate solution. 10 grams of sodium tungstate ($Na_2 WO_4 . 2H_2O$) per 100 ml in water.*
5. *Standard sodium chloride solution (10 mEq/L).*

   Dissolve 585 mg of pure dry sodium chloride per litre in water.

Procedure

Deliver in centrifuge tube, 4 ml of N/12 sulphuric acid, 0.5 ml of plasma and 0.5 ml of sodium tungstate solution, mixing well after each addition. Centrifuge at 2000 rpm, measure 2 ml of supernatant (= 0.2 ml of plasma) into a 25 ml capacity centrifuge. Add 4 drops of indicator and titrate with mercuric nitrate solution from 2 ml microburette, shaking manually during the addition. At the end point (a violet colour), mercuric nitrate solution should be added in 0.01 ml instalment with the tip of burette under the surface of the liquid. Simultaneously measure 2 ml of standard (10 m Eq/l) and proceed as in the case of unknown sample.

Calculation

Plasma chloride :

$$(\text{mEq/L}) = \frac{\text{Volume of mercuric nitrate sol. (Test)}}{\text{Volume of mercuric nitrate sol. (Standard)}} \text{x100}$$

☞ Notes

1. *Do not use polyethylene containers and rubber stoppers. Use only glass containers with glass stoppers.*
2. *We may analyse plasma/serum samples without prior deproteinisation, unless the serum is heavily jaundicad. After removal of protein fraction, the end-point colour tends towards blue, while in the presence of protein end point colour is violet. However the results are nearly same.*
3. *We should try to complete the estimations within two hours after the drawing of blood. If due to unaviodable circumstances, estimation could not be done immediately, then plasma should be separated as quickly as possible from the red blood cells.*

III. Chloride in Serum

(Colorimetric method of Baginski *et al.*, 1958; Itano *et al.*, 1959 modified by Barney and Bertolacini, 1957)

Principle

Intensely violet-red chloranilic acid from the insoluble mercury chloranilate in amounts equivalent to the chloride formed in acid solution.

The colour intensity is directly proportional to the chloranilic acid concentration between 490 and 550 nm.

Reagents

1. *Sulphuric acid, 0.1 N. Prepare this solution as per methods compiled in volume I of this compendium.*
2. *Chloride standard, 0.1 N (100 mEq/1000 ml). Dissolve 7.455 grams potassium chloride in one litre demineralised water.*
3. *Chloride reagent suspension. Dissolve 1 gram of mercury chloranilate in 100 ml 0.1 N sulphuric acid. The mixture should be mixed well before use and pipetted quickly.*

Procedure

Mixture (Centrifuge tubes)	**T**	**RB**	**S**
1. Sulphuric acid, 0.1 N ml	2.0	2.0	2.0
2. Serum, ml	0.02	-	-
3. Demineralised water, ml	-	0.02	-
4. Standard solution, ml	-	-	0.02
5. Chloride reagent suspension, ml	1.0	1.0	1.0

Shake the tubes for few minutes and then centrifuge. Read the absorbance of the supernatant between 490 and 550 nm against distilled water. Colour is stable.

Calculation

$$\text{mEq/Litre} = \frac{A(T) - A(RB)}{A(S) - A(RB)} \times 100$$

where

A = Absorbance reading
RB = Reagent blank reading
S = Standard reading

IV. Chloride in Serum and Plasma

(Method of Cotlove *et al.*, 1958, 1961)

Principle

A constant current is passed through the sample solution mixed with reagent between two silver electrodes. The constant current generator reduces hydrogen ions of the solution at the generator cathode to hydrogen gas which escapes and oxidises the generator mode to silver ions at a constant rate, which enters solution. Silver ions thus liberated combines with chloride ions present in the solution and silver chloride is precipitated. During the titration period, the digital read out is up dated approximately every 250 m/Sec. When all chloride ions have been free, silver ions begin to appear and solution conductivity changes. This change is detected by a pair of silver sensing electrodes and the readout is stopped, displaying the result directly in mEq per litre. Another sample is again added to same reagent solution and the test cycle can be repeated. The display is held until next test cycle starts.

Apparatus

Chloride meter - This instrument is being manufactured by ELICO (P) Ltd., Hyderabad (500018), India under trade name, *"Elico Chloride Meter"* Model EE-34. The instrument is comprised of two units :

a) Titration head

b) Processor, control and display unit

a) It contains two silver titration electrode and two silver end points detector electrode; an automatic stirrer with associated circuitry and cable connection to main unit.

b) It comprises of a constant current generator end point detector, digital display.

Reagents

1. *Acid buffer : To a one litre volumetric flask add, approximately 200 ml of deionised water. 46 ml of glacial acetic acid (B.P. grade). Add 3 ml of concentrated nitric acid (Sp. gr. 142) and make upto the mark with deionised water.*

2. *Gelatin indicator : Add the following chemicals to one litre deionised water.*

   Gelatin, 6 grams

   Thymol blue water soluble, 0.1 gram

   Thymol reagent grade crystals, 0.1 gram

   The above solution should be heated and stirred gently until clear. It is recommended that the gelatin solution be dispensed into glass bottle and refrigerated, but not frozen. The gelatin should be liquified after refrigeration.

3. *Standard solution (100 mEq/l). Dissolve 5.845 grams of dried sodium chloride (AR grade) in one litre deionised water and make upto the mark with deionised water.*

Procedure

Fill the beaker with approximately 25 ml of 40 per cent nitric acid. Place the beaker on platform and dip the electrode into the solution. Press "Cond" switch. Raise the electrode and remove the beaker. Empty the nitric acid and wash it. Fill it again with distilled water. Place the beaker on the platform and dip the electrodes. Press "Cond" switch and "Cond" cycle for few times. Every time "Blank" will be displayed. Raise the electrode and remove the beaker. Take a fresh distilled water.

Wash the beaker thoroughly with distilled water. Take 35 ml of acid buffer and add 0.5 ml of gelatin indicator solution. Place the beaker containing the acid buffer and gelatin indicator (reagent solution) on the titration head platform, dip the electrode into the solution. Add 0.1 ml of 100 mEq/litre standard. Press "Cond" switch. These cycle conditions the acid buffer by retaining the amount of silver ions into acid buffer, which is detected by the sensing electrode at the end point. The reading will be probably high and should be disregarded. Omission of this step will lead to erroneous results.

Add further 0.1 ml of 100 mEq/litre standard to the beaker without removing the electrodes, Press "Cond" switch. Disregard the reading.

Add further 0.1 ml of 100 mEq/litre standard solution to the beaker without removing electrodes. Press "Titrate" switch. The reading indicated should be 100 mEq/litre ± 2 mEq/litre.

If the reading for 100 mEq/litres standard deviate more that 2 per cent, check the standard is deteriorated, otherwise adjust the calibrate potentiometer, so as to read 100 mEq per litre to be within ± 2 per cent. This adjustment is rarely required. Pipette 0.1 ml of sample into the beaker containing reagent (acid buffer and gelatin solution), press "Titrate" switch. When the mEq/litre lamp appear, read the results directly in mEq/litre (chloride).

Pipette a new sample directly into the beaker without removing electrode. After 8 to 10 samples have been titrated, it is necessary to wash the electrode with distilled water and wipe then with a soft cloth. This procedure can be repeated until the "Rep Sol" light comes on after titrating 2000 mEq chloride per litre in the reagent. Change the reagent solution.

When a series of test are completed, the instrument should be switched off and electrodes lowered into a beaker containing deionised water. This prevents the formation of salt deposits on the electrodes.

Precautions

1. Prevent the exposure of drawn blood to air (with loss of CO2) before separating serum.
2. The presence of free sulphydryl sulphide in the titration solution produced a negative initial amperometric current and load to erroneous high results due to combination of these anions with silver ions.
3. Avoid contact of reagent solution or sample with rubber stoppers or tubing. Since aqueous solution, especially if alkaline, extract sulphydryl groups from rubber, therefore use glass wares only in the analytical work.
4. Fouling of the electrode can cause electro chemical imbalance which will affect both of these functions. Always make sure that the electrodes are cleaned and conditioned and the mounting base is free from accumulated salts.
5. Pipetting error is very common, we should deliver the correctly measured solutions in the container, otherwise erroneous results may be obtained.

Instrument check

1. Lower the electrode assembly and connect the two front titration electrodes together with a piece of wire.
2. Switch the instrument "on" and press "cond" switch, then
   a) The digital display should reset to zero
   b) The "Cond" lamp should comes on
   c) The stirrer should start
   d) After a delay of 5 seconds, the digital read out should update a count for every 250 mEq.
   e) After 999 counts, "OVRG" light should come on
   f) After next 999 counts i.e. 2000 counts from start, Repeat solution light should comes on
   g) When the two titration and electrodes are disconnected, the counting and stirrer should stop and "El-up" light come on.

References

AOAC, (1965). *Official methods of analysis of the Association of Official Agricultural chemists.* 10th Edn. AOAC. Benjamin Franklin Station, Washington, D.C. pp. 273.

Baginski, E.S., Williams, L.A., Jarkowski, T.L. and Zak, B. (1958). *J. Clin. Path.*, 30: 559.

Cotlove, E. and Nishi, H.N. (1961). *Clin. Chem.*, 7: 285.

Cotlove, E., Trantham, H.V. and Bowman, R.L. (1958). *J. Lab. Clin. Med.*, 51: 461.

Itano, M., Williams, L.A. and Zak, B. (1959). *J. Clin. Path.*, 32: 213.

Schales, O. and Schales, S.S. (1941). *J. Biol. Chem.*, 140: 879.

Van Slyke, D.D. (1923). *J. Biol. Chem.*, 58: 523.

Chapter - 82

Methods for Detecting Adulteration in Animal Feeds and Human Foods

Adulteration Detection

I. Detection of Castor Husk in Oil Cakes and Oil Seed Meals (Method of ISI, (BIS), IS: 10165-1982)

Principle

The method is based on the fact that castor husk is not bleached under the conditions which cause the bleaching of almost all other materials of vegetable origin likely to be present in an oilcake. The method consists of the treatment of the material with dilute alkali and acid solutions followed by treatment with bleaching powder solution and the isolation of the unbleached castor husk.

Apparatus

White photographic dish

Reagents

1. *Sodium hydroxide, 5 per cent (m/v)*
2. *Dilute hydrochloric acid, 5 per cent (m/v)*
3. *Bleaching powder solution, 5 per cent (m/v)*

Procedure

Take three separate 100g portions of the material and boil for 30 minutes with one litre of sodium hydroxide solution. Filter through muslin, boil again for 30 minutes with one litre of dilute hydrochloric acid and filter. Digest the residue for a period, depending on the type of cake, with the solution of bleaching powder. When bleaching is complete, filter off the solution. Spread the bleached residue in a thin layer, under water, in a white photographic dish. Remove any black pieces and examine microscopically. After identification, compare the pieces with portions of castor husk which have undergone the above treatment. Castor husk has a characteristic structure, the sharp angled black pieces of husk showing a distinctive pitted surface, when examined in reflected light under a microscope.

II. Detection of Mahua Cake in Oil Cakes and Oilseed Meals (Method of ISI, IS: 10165-1982)

Principle

The method is based on the fact that the toxin saponin (Mowrin) gives a typical colour test when extracted.

Apparatus

Extraction Tube 150 x 13 mm with a taper tip having an internal diameter 1.5 mm.

Reagents

1. *Antimony Trichloride solution. Dissolve 125 grams of antimony trichloride in 300 to 400 ml of chloroform. Add 5 g of calcium chloride and filter while hot. Dilute the filtrate to 500 ml with chloroform.*
2. *Rectified spirit 95 per cent (v/v)*

Procedure

Take 10 grams of the finely ground material in the extraction tube. Tap it to pack it well. Pour rectified spirit into the tube so as to soak, the sample. Collect the first drop of the extract on a whatman No. 1 Filter paper of about 10 cm diameter. Dry and then wash by placing 2 to 3 drops of distilled water in the centre of the dried spot. Dry the filter paper completely. Dip the paper in a beaker containing antimony trichloride solution, and dry it on a spirit lamp or a burner. Care shall be taken not to over heat the paper, which will be evident by its charring. Appearance of a pink colour after heating for five minutes indicates the presence of Mahua oilcake.

III. Detection of Rice hulls in Rice bran and Rice (Method of AOAC, 1965)

Apparatus

Microscope

Reagent

Chloral hydrate solution (1+1)

Procedure

Grind small portion of well-mixed sample until it passes through 60 No. sieve. Weigh 4 mg on slide ruled with parallel lines 1/20" apart or transfer to ruled slide after weighing. Add just enough chloral hydrate solution (1+1) to fill in under cover-glass, which, preferably, should be square (about 22 mm). After placing cover-glass, warm gently, but do not boil, to eliminate starch masses and clear tissues. Count particles of hull tissue, using microscope at about 90 x magnification. High refraction and yellowish green colour of hull particles help distinguish small pieces not easily recognised by their structure. (To avoid duplicate counting, disregard particles that extend over upper line of strip). Compare results with those obtained on standard containing known quantities of hulls.

IV. Detection of Oat hulls in Oats and Oat feeds (Method of AOAC, 1965)

Apparatus

Sintered glass crucible

Reagents

Hydrochloric acid (AR) concentrated

Procedure

Place in one litre beaker 800 ml water and 2 g sample, previously ground to pass through sieve having circular openings 1 mm diameter. Stir vigorously to obtain centrifugal effect, let stand 5 min., and decant supernatant carefully, retaining so far as possible all hull particles. Repeat procedure several times until supernatant becomes clear, or nearly so, and then transfer residue with aid of 150 ml water to 300 ml beaker. Add 5 drops HCl and boil 2 minutes., stirring constantly. Transfer to original beaker with aid of 500 ml water, stir, and let stand until supernatant is clear. Siphon off liquid with 3-4 mm bore rubber tubing, using pinch clamp to control flow so that practically all liquid is removed. (Tilting beaker also helps to obtain this result). If deposit forms on standing, siphon again. Transfer hulls with aid of H_2O to filter paper, wash several times with alcohol, and dry to constant weight at room temperature. When dry, carefully remove hulls from paper, using small stiff brush if necessary, and weigh. (Weighed sintered glass crucible may be used instead of filter paper).

Weight of hulls x 50 = per cent hulls in sample.

V. Detection of Grit in Poultry and Similar Feeds (Method of AOAC, 1965)

Apparatus

Glass petridish

Reagent

Chloroform, AR grade

Procedure

Place 2 g prepared sample, thoroughly mixed, in about 30 ml evaporating dish. Add about 5 ml $CHCl_3$ and mix gently with glass rod until liquid contacts entire sample. Brush particles down into the $CHCl_3$ with 25 mm circular or square cover glass, use glass to skim off or pull floating material over top of dish, taking care not to dip cover-glass deep enough to disturb grit at bottom of dish. After skimming until surface of $CHCl_3$ is nearly clearly, slowly pour supernatant into second evaporating dish. Wash sides of dish with few ml more $CHCl_3$ and repeat skimming and decanting operation until no floating particles remain (10-15 ml $CHCl_3$). When only grit remains, let last traces of $CHCl_3$ evaporate spontaneously, and weigh.

Weight of residue x 50 = per cent grit.

After weighing, examine residue for impurities. Also pour out $CHCl_3$ washings collected in second dish and observe whether any grit has been transferred to it during process.

If sample contains NaCl, remove from grit by washing with water. *Identify bone in grit by charring*. If pelleted feeds or feeds containing molasses are being examined, disintegrate in cold water and dry with alcohol or ether.

VI. Detection of Cyanogenetic Glucosides in Feeds and Similar Materials (Method of AOAC, 1965)

Reagents

1. *Picric acid, 1%*
2. *Sodium carbonate, 10%*

Procedure

Prepare sodium picrate paper by dipping strips of filter paper into 1 per cent picric acid solution and drying, then dipping into 10 per cent sodium carbonate solution and drying. Store these papers in stoppered bottle. Place small quantity of testing material in test tube. Insert piece of the moist sodium picrate paper in tube, taking care that it does not come in contact with material. Add few drops $CHCl_3$ and stopper tube tightly. The sodium picrate paper gradually turns orange, then brick red, if testing materials contains cyanogenetic glucosides.

☞ **Note**

This test is delicate, and rapidity of change in colour depends upon quantity of free HCN present.

VII. Detection of Hydrocyanic Acid Formed by Hydrolysis of Glucosides in Beans (Method of AOAC, 1965)

Acid Titration Method

Apparatus

Kjeldahl flask

Reagents

1. *Silver nitrate, 0.02 N*
2. *Nitric acid*
3. *Potassium thiocyanate, 0.02 N*

Acid Titration Method

Procedure

Place 10-20 grams sample, ground to pass No. 20 sieve, in 800 ml Kjeldahl flask, add 100 ml water and macerate at room temperature keep for two hour. Add 100 ml water and steam distill, collecting distillate in 20 ml 0.02 N $AgNO_3$ acidified with 1 ml HNO_3. Before distillation, adjust apparatus so that tip of condenser dips below surface of liquid in receiver. When 150 ml has passed over, filter distillate through gooch; and titrate excess $AgNO_3$ in combined filtrate and washings with 0.02 N KCNS, using Ferric alum indicator.

One ml 0.02 N $AgNO_3$ = 0.54 mg HCN.

Alkaline Titration Method

Procedure

Place 10-20 g sample, ground to pass No. 20 sieve, in 800 ml Kjeldahl flask, add about 200 ml water, and let stand 2-4 hour (Autolysis should be conducted with approximate completely connected for distillation). Steam distill, collect 150-160 ml distillate in NaOH solution (0.5 gram in 20 ml water), and dilute to definite volume.

To 100 ml distillate (it is preferable to dilute to 250 ml and titrate 100 ml aliquot) add 8 ml 6 N NH_4OH and 2 ml 5% potassium iodide solution and titrate with 0.02 N $AgNO_3$, using microburette. End point is faint but permanent turbidity and may be easily recognised, especially against black background.

1 ml 0.02 N $AgNO_3$ = 1.08 mg HCN

VIII. Detection of Urea Adulteration in Animal Feeds

Weigh 1 gram testing material in a centrituge tube, add 10 ml distilled water, keep overnight at room temperature, centrifuge next day at 2000 rpm. Take out the supernatant liquid in another centrifuge tube, estimate urea by following distillation method as compiled in volume II of this compendium or by Conway diffusion technique (Conway, 1957) as mentioned in volume II of this compendium.

Krishna (1979) tested 12 samples of fish meal pertaining to Gurgaon (Haryana) region, out of these 12, eight samples were found adulterated with urea containing 0.945 to 3.050 g/100g, while in normal fish meal samples, the concentration of urea ranged from 0.080 to 0.405 g/100g. Therefore, we should be cautious, while testing animal feeds sample for total nitrogen, since some business personnel try to increase total nitrogen content by sprinkling urea solution as it has been experienced by author of this adulteration in his laboratory at CCS-HAU, Hisar (Haryana), India.

References

AOAC, (1965). *Official methods of analysis of the Association of official Agricultural chemists.* 10th Edn. AOAC. Benjamin Franklin Station, Washington, D.C. pp. 339-341.

Conway, E.J. (1957). *Microdiffusion analysis and volumetric error,* 4th edn., Crossby, Lockwood and Son Ltd., London.

Indian Standards Institution, BIS, (1982). *Indian Standard Specification for Decorticated Sunflower Oilcake as Livestock Feed Ingredient.* IS: 10165-ISI, Manak Bhavan, New Delhi-1.

Krishna, G. (1979). *Poultry Guide,* 16: 59.

Chapter - 83

Urease Activity in Legume Seeds and Their Byproducts

Urease Activity Determination

(Method of Schram and Aines, 1959)

All the legume seeds and their byproducts are very rich in urease activity which may be responsible for an appreciable loss of urea nitrogen on long duration storage. Therefore it is necessary to estimate urease activity in legume seeds and their byproducts.

Reagents

1. *Dimethyleaminobenzaldehyde solution (DMAB). Dissolve 16 g DMAB in 1 litre 95% ethyl alcohol and add 100 ml concentrated hydrochloric acid (Stable one month).*
2. *Pyrophosphate buffer. Dissolve 233 g* $Na_4P_2O_7$*.* $10H_2O$ *in approximately 980 ml distilled water. Add 3 ml of conc. Hcl and then dropwise further Hcl until the pH of the buffer is 7.7 to 7.8. Dilute to one litre.*
3. *Buffered urea solution. Dissolve 0.4 g urea in one litre pyrophosphate buffer (Stable one week).*
4. *Zinc Acetate solution. Dissolve 22 grams zinc acetate* $2H_2O$ *in distilled water, add 3 ml of glacial acetic acid and dilute to 100 ml.*

5. *Potassium Ferrocyanide solution.* Dissolve 10.6 grams K_4 Fe (CN)6 $3H_2O$ in distilled water, and dilute to 100 ml.
6. Charcoal

Apparatus

1. Water bath at 40°C, capable of maintaining temperature within ± 1°C, with shaking device.
2. Conical flasks, 125 ml
3. Volumetric flasks, 25 ml
4. Spectrophotometer

Method

Weigh accurately 1 g of soybean meal into a conical flask and add 50 ml of the buffered urea solution. Incubate in water bath for 30 minutes exactly at 40°C with shaking. Remove from water bath and quickly add 0.5 ml each of conc. HCl, ferrocyanide solution and zinc acetate solution and 0.1g of charcoal. Shake for 15 minutes and filter. If the filtrate is coloured, repeat the procedure using more charcoal. Pipette 10 ml aliquots of the filtrate and the DMAB solution into a 25 ml volumetric flask and make up to volume with distilled water. Make up also a reagent blank (10 ml DMAB made up to 25 ml with water) and a urea blank (10 ml buffered urea solution and 10 ml DMAB made up to 25 ml with water). Prepare a standard curve by pipetting aliquots of buffered urea solution from 2 to 12 ml into 25 ml volumetric flasks, adding 10 ml of DMAB and making upto volume. Mix flasks well, stand in water bath at 25°C for 10 minutes and then read at 430 mμ. Calculate urease activity as mg/litre.

Reference

Schram, G. and Aines, P.D. (1959). *J. Am. Oil. Chem. Soc.*, 36: 1-3.

Chapter - 84

Lactic Acid in Biological Samples

Lactic Acid Determination

(Colorimetric Method of Barker and Summerson, 1941)

I. Method for Blood / Plasma

Principle

In this method, glucose and other interfering material of the protein free blood filtrate is removed by the Van Slyke-Salkowski method of treatment with copper sulphate and calcium hydroxide. A part of the resulting solution is heated with concentrated sulphuric acid to convert lactic acid to acetaldehyde, which is then determined by reaction with p-hydroxydiphenyl in the presence of copper ions.

Reagents

1. *Copper sulphate (20 per cent) : Dissolve 400g of* $CuSO_4.5H_2O$ *in about 1 litre of water with the aid of heat, cool, dilute to 2 litres, and mix. Stable indefinitely.*
2. *Copper sulphate (4 per cent) : Dilute 1 volume of 20 per cent copper sulphate solution to 5 volumes with water and mix. Store in a bottle fitted with a stoper carrying a 1 ml pipette which delivers approximately 20 drops per ml. If this is done, 1 drop may be used instead of the 0.05 ml portion as mentioned in the procedure.*
3. *Calcium hydroxide, powder : It should be of AR grade.*

4. *Sulphuric acid, concentrated : It should be of AR grade and iron free. We should use burette, while dispensing at the time of analysis.*
5. *p-Hydroxydiphenyl Reagent : Dissolve 1.5 grams of p-hydroxydiphenyl in 10 ml 5 per cent sodium hydroxide solution, plus a little water, by warming and stirring, and dilute to 100 ml with water. Store in a brown bottle fitted with a stopper and pipette capable of delivering 20 drops per ml.*
6. *Standard Lactic acid solution. Dissolve 0.213 gram of pure dry lithium lactate in about 100 ml of water in a litre volumetric flask, add about 1 ml of concentrated sulphuric acid, dilute to the mark with water and mix. This solution contains 1 mg of lactic acid in 5 ml and is stable indefinitely if kept in the refrigerator. To prepare the working standard, dilute 5 ml of stock standard to 100 ml in a glass-stoppered volumetric flask with water and mix. This solution contains 0.01 mg of lactic acid per ml. It is advisable to prepare fresh standard solution at the time of analysis.*

Procedure

1. Prepare protein free filtrate (whole blood, plasma) with either tungstic acid or trichloroacetic acid at a 1:10 dilution following Folin and Wu (1919) method as mentioned under chapter entitled, *"Sampling and processing of biological samples" volume I of this compendium.*
2. Deliver 2 ml of the protein free filtrate, representing 0.2 ml of blood, to a centrifuge tube graduated at 10 ml.
3. In a second similar tube, place 5 ml of standard lactic acid solution, containing 0.01 mg of lactic acid per ml.
4. In a third tube place a little water; this is a blank, and serves to control the small amount of colour yielded by the reagents alone. To each tube add 1 ml of 20 per cent copper sulphate solution and dilute to 10 ml mark with water.
5. Add 1g of powdered calcium hydroxide to each tube, stopper, and shake vigorously until the solids are uniformly mixed.
6. Allow to stand for one-half hour, repeating the shaking at least once in the interim.
7. Centrifuge down the precipitate, and transfer duplicate 1 ml portions of the supernatant from each tube to thoroughly clean and dry test tubes having an internal diameter of 18 to 23 mm. To each tube add 0.05 ml of 4 per cent copper sulphate solution, followed by 6 ml of concentrated sulphuric acid from a burette.
8. The sulphuric acid should be added drop by drop at first, mixing the contents of the tube well during the addition. The contents of tube become hot, it is not necessary to cool the tube.

9. After the acid has been added to all the tubes, place then upright in boiling water for 5 minutes, then transfer the tubes to cold water (preferably running) and cool to 20°C or below.
10. When the contents of the tubes are sufficienty cool (but not before) add 0.1 ml of the p-hydroxydiphenyl reagent, drop by drop, to each tube.
11. The reagent precipitates out on entering the concentrated acid, it is mixed throughout the solution as quickly and uniformly as possibly by using test tube shaker.
12. When the reagent has been added, place the tubes in a beaker of water at 30°C and allow to stand for 30 minutes or longer.
13. Redisperse the precipitated reagent at least once during this period.
14. Finally place the tubes in vigorously boiling water for exactly 90 seconds, remove, and cool in cold water to room temperature. Transfer the coloured solution to centrifuge tubes and determine the optical density at 560 mμ, using water for setting the photometer at zero density.

Calculation

Note down the optical density with blank sample. Subtract this value from the average of standard and unknown to obtain their true densities. Since the 1 ml portion of copper-lime supernatant used for colour development contain 0.005 mg of lactic acid in the case of the standard, and this represents 0.02 ml of original blood in the unknown (i.e., a dilution of 50), the calculation in this case is as follows :

$$\frac{\text{Density of unknown}}{\text{Density of standard}} \times 0.005 \times 50 \times 100$$

= mg lactic acid per 100 ml blood

☞ Notes

1. *Generally blank colour is ordinarily about 10 per cent of the standard colour.*
2. *We may vary the volume of aliquots of filtrate depending upon the concentration of lactic acid. Lactic acid upto 60 mg per cent may be estimated accurately.*

II. Method for Silage Samples

Reagents and procedure is same as in the case of blood/plasma samples.

Process the silage samples as given below

Weigh 10 gram of freshly taken silage samples in a beaker. Add about 50 ml distilled water, transfer the contents of beaker in a homogeniser, macerate the contents for 10 minutes. Filter the content of homogeniser in a 100 ml capacity volumetric flask using fine glass wool. Make up the volume with water upto mark. Measure 1 ml of silage extract in 10 ml graduated centrifuge tube in duplicate. Add 7 ml distilled water, 1 ml of 10 per cent sodium tungstate, 1 ml of two-thirds normal sulphuric acid. Shake the centrifuge tube thoroughly and make up the volume upto 10 ml. The dilution will be 1:10. Wait for about 15 minutes and then centrifuge the contents of tube at 3000 rpm for 15 minutes. Transfer the supernatant in a separate centrifuge tube and proceed with the same procedure as mentioned in the case of blood/ serum.

Calculation

1 ml of lactic acid standard contains 0.01 mg of lactic acid.

$$= \frac{\text{OD of unknown sample}}{\text{OD of standard sample}} \times 0.01 \times 11$$

= Lactic acid (g/100g fresh silage)

Example

OD of unknown sample = 0.699

OD of standard sample = 0.032

$$= \frac{0.699}{0.032} \times 0.01 \times 11$$

= 2.409 g lactic acid per 100 g fresh silage

III. Method for Tissues

Procedure for lactic acid estimation in tissue extract is same as mentioned in the case of blood or plasma. However precautions should be taken to avoid postmortem changes in lactic acid content in tissues. This could be achieved by prompt freezing of tissues in solid carbon dioxide or by proper treatment with acid to destroy enzyme systems present. *It is advisable to estimate lactic acid in fresh unpreserved tissues immediately for getting accurate analytical results.*

References

Barker, S.B. and Summerson, W.H. (1941). *J. Biol. Chem.*, 138: 55.

Folin, O. and Wu, H. (1919). *J. Biol. Chem.*, 38: 98.

Chapter - 85

Chemical Analysis of Milk

Analysis of Milk

Preparation of Samples

Before withdrawing portions for analytical determinations, bring the sample to a temperature of 26 to 28°C and mix throughly by pouring gently into a clean dry receptacle and back, until a homogenous mixture is assured. If lumps of cream do not completely disappear, warm the sample to about 40°C, mix throughly, then cool to 26 to 28°C. In case a measured volume is required in a determination, bring the temperature of the sample to about 27°C before pipetting. All samples shall be allowed to stand for three to four minutes after mixing to allow air bubbles to rise ; the sample bottle shall then be inverted three or four times immediately prior to taking the milk for analysis. *If a sample is curdled, excessively churned or decomposed, the sample should not be taken up for analysis.*

Total Solids

(Gravimetric method of AOAC, 1965)

Apparatus

1. Flat bottomed evaporating aluminium moisture dish (7-8 cm diameter and 2.5 cm deep) with lid
2. Water bath
3. Desiccator

Principle

On drying the milk, the water is lost leaving the residue behind.

Procedure

1. Prepare the milk sample as mentioned previously.
2. Weigh the clean aluminium cup containing about 15-20 g of fine sand (30-90 mesh).
3. Transfer about 10 ml of milk into aluminium dish and weigh again.
4. Put the dish on a boiling water bath for about 30 minutes to dry up the contents.
5. Remove the dish, wipe the bottom and keep the dish with the lid by its side in a well ventilated oven at 98° to 100°C for about 3 hours.
6. Cool in a desiccator to room temperature and weigh.
7. Record the weight. Repeat the process of heating, cooling and weighing till there is no further change in the weight.

Observations

1. Weight of dish containing sand = x, g
2. Weight of dish containing sand + milk = y, g
3. Weight of milk taken = (y-x) g
4. Weight of dish + sand + residue after drying = z, g
5. Weight of residue of milk = (z-x), g

Calculation

The precentage of total solids in milk

$$= \frac{(z - x) \times 100 \times 100}{(y - x) \times 25}$$

Total Nitrogen

(Method of AOAC, 1965)

We may estimate total nitrogen in milk following the macro-Kjeldahl/ micro-Kjeldahl method mentioned in volume I of this compendium or by Conway diffusion technique (Conway, 1957). Volume II of compendium.

In the case of human milk where less quantity is available, it would be advisable to follow up Conway-diffusion technique, where only 5 ml milk aliquot will be enough for estimating total nitrogen. Conway-diffusion technique is a more simple and accurate technique and in a day twenty four samples analysis could be completed without any problem.

To convert nitrogen into crude protein, multiply by the factor 6.38.

True Protein
(Method of AOAC, 1965)

Reagent

Trichloroacetic acid solution - 15 per cent by volume.

Procedure

Pipette 10 ml of the prepared sample into a 50 ml tared graduated flask and weigh accurately. Dilute to the mark with trichloroacetic acid solution and mix immediately. When the precipitate has settled, leaving a clear supernatant liquid, filter on a dry 9 cm filter paper (Whatman No. 40 or its equivalent) into a dry flask. Wash the precipitate on the filter paper twice with the trichloroacetic acid solution.

Determine the nitrogen in the washed precipitate and paper by usual procedures mentioned in volume I of this compendium.

Casein
(Method of AOAC, 1965)

Casein should be determined in fresh milk or nearly fresh milk. If it is not possible to make this determinationwithin 8 hours, add 2.5 parts of formaldehyde to 2500 parts of milk and keep the sample in a cool place.

Reagents

1. *Acetic acid 10 per cent by volume.*
2. *Sodium acetate solution 1 N.*

Procedure

Pipette, and accurately weigh, 5 ml of the prepared sample into a 100 ml beaker. Add 50 ml of water at about 40°C and 0.5 ml of acetic acid and mix the contents of the beaker. After 10 minute, add 0.5 ml of sodium acetate solution and mix again. Allow the contents of the beaker to cool to about 20°C (30 minutes) and decant through 9 cm Whatman filter paper. Wash the precipitate with water three times, and by decantation, transfer it to the paper and wash it twice on the paper. (Preserve the filtrate for the determination of albumin).

Determine the nitrogen in the washed precipitate by usual procedures mentioned in volume I of this compendium.

Albumin
(Method of AOAC, 1965)

Reagents

1. Sodium hydroxide solution 10 per cent W/V.
2. Dilute acetic acid 1:9 by volume.

Procedure

Exactly neutralise the filtrate obtained in case in estimation with sodium hydroxide solution. Add 0.3 ml of dilute acetic acid, and heat on a steam bath until the albumin is completely precipitated. Collect the precipitate on an acid-washed filter and ash with cold water. Determine the nitrogen by the procedures mentioned in volume I of this compendium. The results will be in terms of percentage of albumin.

Non Protein Nitrogen
(Method of Folin and Wu, 1919)

Procedure

Precipitate milk protein using Trichloroacetic acid (TCA) or tungstic acid as per method suggested by Folin and Wu (1919) and estimate nitrogen in the filtrate as per method mentioned in volume I of this compendium.

Fat by Gerber Method
(Method of ISI, 1977, IS : 1224)

Principle

When a definite quantity of sulphuric acid and amyl alcohol are added to a definite volume of milk, the proteins will be dissolved and the fat globules will be set free which remains in liquid state due to heat produced by the acid. On centrifugation fat being lighter will be separated on top of the solution.

Apparatus

Gerber centrifuge, Gerber butyrometers for milk (0-10% scale with 0.1 per cent mark), hot water bath maintained at 65° ± 2°C. 10 ml-automatic tilt measure for acid, 1 ml-automatic tilt measure for amyl alcohol, 11 ml pipette, Butyrometer stoppers, Butyrometer stand, cotton wool.

Reagents

Gerber sulphuric acid density 1.807 to 1.812 g/ml at 27°C corresponding with a concentration of sulphuric acid from 90 to 91 per cent byweight. Amyl alcohol 95 per cent of clear, colourless liquid shall distil between 130° to 132°C, density to 0.805 g/ml at 27°C.

Procedure

1. Take 10 ml of Gerber sulphuric acid from automatic measure into the butyrometer.
2. Pipette out 11 ml of the well mixed sample of milk and transfer it to the butyrometer carefully without allowing it to mix with the acid. This is done by allowing the jet of milk from the pipette to hit the inside wall of the butryrometer by holding the pipette in a slanting manner and resting the tip end on the mouth of the butyrometer.

3. With the help of automatic pipette add 1 ml amyl alcohol to the above butyrometer.
4. Tighten the stopper and mix the content by shaking the butyrometer at a 45° angle until all the curd has been dissolved.
5. Keep the butyrometer in the water bath at 65° ± 2°C for five minutes.
6. Place the butyrometer in the centrifuge and balance the machine. Centrifuge for five minutes (1000-1200 rpm).
7. After centrifuging, keep the butyrometer in the water bath at 65° ± 2°C for five minutes.
8. Adjust the fat column within the scale on butyrometer and take the reading.

Observation

Record the fat precentage and note down in the practical record book.

☞ Notes

1. *Care must be taken not to wet the neck of the butyrometer while adding sulphuric acid, milk and amyl alcohol.*
2. *The test must be repeated if particles of curd are observed.*

Fat by Roese - Gottlieb Method

(Method of AOAC, 1965)

Equipments

1. Well ventillated electrically heated oven (98° - 100°C).
2. Evaporating dish, porcelain or metallic.
3. Weighing bottle
4. Dropper
5. Flask 100 ml.

Reagents

1. *Concentrated ammonia solution* (sp. gr. 0.88).
2. *Ethyl alcohol 95 to 96% v/v.*
3. *Diethyl ether sp. gr. 0.720, peroxide free.*
4. *Light petroleum ether - boiling range 40° - 60°C.*
5. *Mixed solvent-prepared by mixing equal volumes of diethyl ether and light petroleum.*

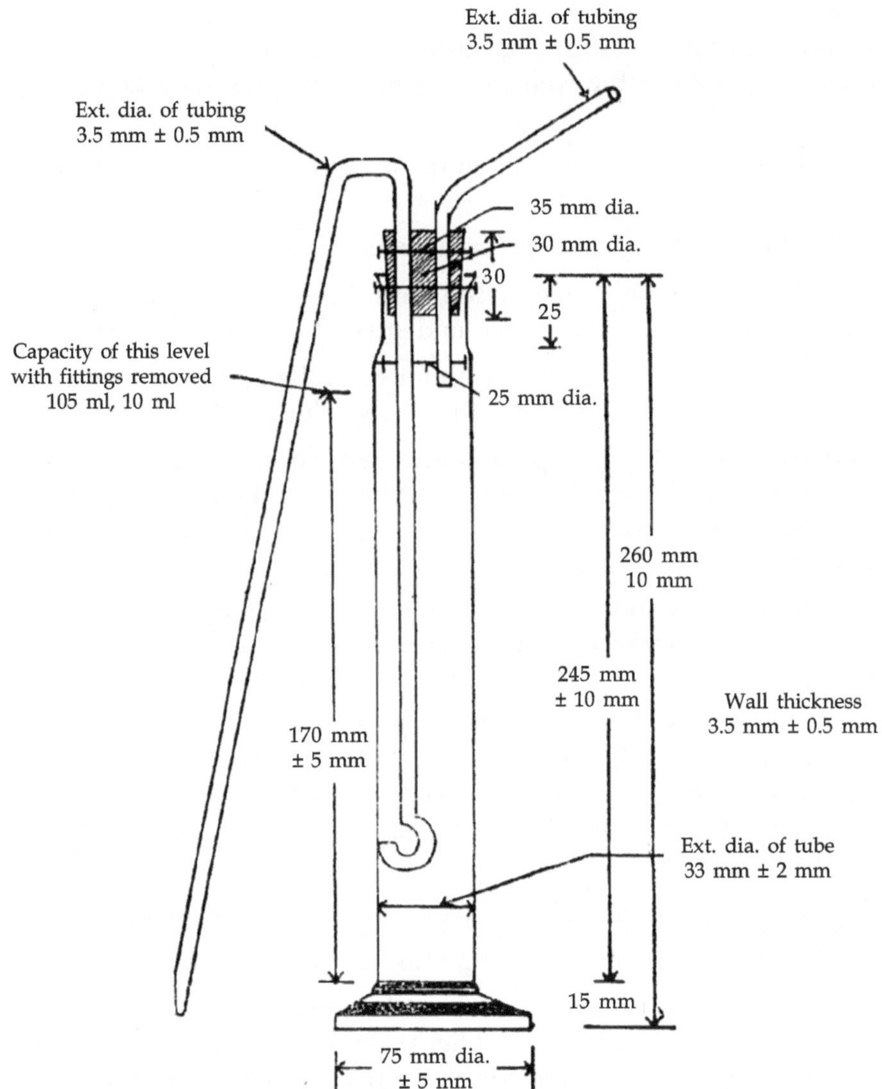

Fig. 1 : Fat extraction tube with syphon by Roese Gottlieb method.

Principle

To effect a quantitative separation of fat from milk, it is necessary to break up the protective film surrounding the fat globule by using suitable agents. Ammonia brings about break up of the protective layer and addition of alcohol facilitates the passage of fat globules from the aqueous phase to the solvents. The mixed solvent, petroleum and diethyl ether being non-miscible with water, effects a food extraction of fat from the non-fatty solids in the solution.

Procedure

1. Weigh accurately by difference using a weighing bottle with a dropper about 10 grams of the well mixed sample of milk into the extraction tube.
2. Add 1 ml of concentrated ammonia and mix well by gentle swirling motion.
3. Add 10 ml of alcohol and again mix well.
4. Add 25 ml of diethyl ether, close the tube with the cork (or stopper) which sould be wet with water, and shake vigorously for one minute.
5. Remove the cork, wash the cork and neck of the tube with 25 ml of light petroleum ether in such a way that the washings run into the tube.
6. Replace the cork (or stopper) again wetted with water and shake vigorously for 30 seconds. Allow the tube to stand until the etheral layer is clearly separated from the aqueotts layer, (Usually for not less than 30 minutes).
7. Remove the cork and insert the siphon fitting so adjusted for length that the inlet is 2 to 3 mm above the interface between the etheral and aqueous layers, and transfer the etheral layer to a flask.
8. Add 5 ml of mixed solvent to the extraction tube, using it to wash the siphon fitting which is raised sufficiently to permit washing without complete removal, and also, to wash the inside of the tube. Lower the fittings and transfer the solvent, without shaking to the above mentioned flask.
9. Repeat this operation with a further 5 ml of mixed solvent.
10. Wash the tip of the siphon fitting into the flask with mixed solvent.
11. Remove the siphon fitting and repeat the extraction of the milk residue, using 15 ml of ether and 15 ml of light petroleum. Repeat the subsequent operation as before, use the ether to wash the inner limit of the siphon fitting during its removal from the tube.
12. Finally repeat the extraction once more with 15 ml each of diethyl ether and petroleum.
13. Distill carefully the solvent from the flask.
14. Dry the residual fat in the oven at 98° to 100°C for one hour.
15. Cool the flask to room temperature in a desiccator and weigh it.
16. Repeat heating, cooling and weighing until successive weighings do not differ by more than 1 mg.

17. Extract completely the fat from the flask by repeated washings, with light petroleum ether allowing any sediment to settle before each decantation, dry the flask in the oven, cool and weigh as before. The difference in weights before and after the petroleum extractions, subject, if necessary, to a correction for the blank described below is the weight of fat present in the weight of milk taken.
18. Conduct a blank determination using the specified quantities of reagents throughout plus a similar weight of distilled water in place of the milk, and deduct the value found, if any, from the apparent weight of fat. A flask similar to that used to collect the fat from the milk sample, should also be used in case of the blank and should be subjected to heating, cooling and weighing treatments as in the case of original experiment.

Observations

1. Weight of weighing bottle with milk before transfer = W_1 g
2. Weight of weighing bottle with the remaining milk after transfer = W_2 g
3. Weight of the flask with dried fat = W_3 g
4. Weight of the flask after removal of fat = W_4 g
5. Weight of fat present in the flask used for the blank experiment (if any) = a, g

Calculations

Weight of milk taken for analysis = $(W_1 - W_2)$

Weight of fat obtained after deduction of the balnk value = $(W_3 - W_4 - a)$ g

Percentage of fat in the milk $= \dfrac{(W_3 - W_4 - a)}{(W_1 - W_2)} \times 100$

Lactose by the Volumetric Method of Lane-Evnon

(Method of ISI, 1961, IS : 1479)

Principle

Lactose solution reduces quantitatively alkaline cupric salt solution on boiling to red cuprous oxide; from the amount of copper salt reduced the quantity of lactose is calculated.

Reagents

1. *Fehling solution : Prepared by mixing immediately before use, equal volumes of solutions (A) and (B).*

   Solution (A) : Dissolve 173 grams of Rochelle salt (KNa $C_4H_4O_6$, $4H_2O$) and 50 grams of sodium hydroxide in water. Dilute to 500 ml, allow to stand for two days, and filter through prepared asbestos.

   Standardisation of Fehling solution : Pipette 5 ml or 12.5 ml of each of the solutions (A) and (B) into a flask of 300 to 400 ml capacity. The quantity of copper taken will differ significantly between the two methods of pipetting, and the method used shall be followed consistently during standardisation and determination. Prepare a standard solution of pure lactose of such concentration that more than 15 ml and less than 50 ml will be required to reduce all the copper. The titre may be calculated as follows :

$$\frac{\text{Factor}}{\text{mg lactose in 1 ml}}$$

   Add almost the whole of the lactose solution required to effect reduction of all the copper, so that not more than 0.5 to 1.0 ml is required later to complete titration. Heat to cold mixture to boiling on wire gauze and maintain in moderate ebullition for two minutes, lowering the flame sufficiently to avoid bumping. Without removing flame, add 2 to 5 drops of one per cent aqueous methylene blue solution and complete the titration within a total boiling time of about three minutes, by small additions of sugar solution, to the point of decolorisation of the indicator.

   Multiply the titre by the number of milligrams in one millilitre of the standard solution to obtain the factor. Compare with the tabulated factor (Table 16.1) to determine correction, if any, to be applied to the Table 16.1. Small deviations from the tabulated factors may arise from variations in individual procedure or composition of reagents. If only approximate results (within one per cent) are required, the standardisation may be ommitted provided specifications of the analysis are rigidly observed.

2. *Methylene blue : one per cent (w/v) solution in water.*
3. *Pure lactose*
4. *Acetic acid : 10 per cent solution*

Procedure

1. Take 25 ml of milk with a pipette into a 500 ml conical flask.
2. Dilute the milk with distilled water to about 200 ml.
3. Add about 3.75 ml of 10 per cent acetic acid solution and boil.

4. Cool, transfer quantitatively to a 250 ml volumetric flask and make up the volume to mark with distilled water.
5. Filter through a dry filter paper, discard the first few ml of the filtrate and collect the rest in a dry conical flask.
6. Fill the burette with this filtrate.
7. Pipette 5 ml each of Fehling solution A and B into 250 ml conical flask.
8. Make a preliminary titration by adding the filtrate containing lactose, from the burette, 1 ml at a time, to the Fehling solution kept boiling till the blue colour changes to red.
9. Take another 10 ml of Fehling A and B and add to in cold almost the whole volume of the filtrate required for reduction in step B, so that no more than 0.5 to 1 ml of it will be required for complete titration.
10. Heat the above mixture to boiling and maintain a moderate ebullition for 2 minutes; lower the flame if necessary to avoid bumping.
11. Add about 5 drops of methylene blue indicator to the boiling mixture and complete the titration within a total boiling time of three minutes by additions of 4 to 6 drops of the filtrate. The end point is indicated by the change of blue colour to colourless supernatant.
12. Repeat the titration to get values within 0.1 ml.

Observations

Record the titre values in the usual tabular form.

Calculations

1. Volume of milk filtrate required for complete reduction of 10 ml of Fehling solution = V ml
2. Find out from the table given the lactose in mg for V ml = W mg

   V ml of filtrate = W mg lactose

   250 ml of filtrate = $\frac{W}{V} \times 250$ mg lactose

   = 25 ml milk
3. Weight of lactose present in 100 ml of milk = $\frac{W}{V} \times 250 \times \frac{100}{25}$ mg

Table 1 : Factors for Fehling solution to be used in connection with the Lane Lynon General method.

Titre	10 ml Fehling solution	
(1)	(2) Anhydrous Lactose $C_{12}H_{22}O_{11}$	(3) Hydrated Lactose $C_{12}H_{22}O_{11}H_2O$
15	64.90	68.30
16	64.80	68.20
17	64.80	68.20
18	64.70	68.10
19.	64.70	68.10
20	64.60	68.00
21	64.60	68.00
22	64.60	68.00
23	64.50	67.90
24	64.50	67.90
25	64.50	67.90
26	64.50	67.90
27	64.40	67.80
28	64.40	67.80
29	64.40	67.80
30	64.40	67.80
31	64.40	67.80
32	64.40	67.80
33	64.40	67.80
34	64.40	67.90
35	64.50	67.90
36	64.50	67.90
37	64.50	67.90
38	64.50	67.90
39	64.50	67.90
40	64.50	67.90
41	64.60	68.00
42	64.60	68.00
43	64.60	68.00
44	64.60	68.00
45	64.70	68.10
46	64.70	68.10
47	64.80	68.20
48	64.80	68.20
49	64.80	68.20
50	64.90	68.30

Specific gravity of milk by a specific gravity lactometer calibrated for use at 15.6°C (60°F)

(Method of ISI, 1961, IS : 1479)

Apparatus

1. Specific gravity lactometer calibrated for use at 15.6°C (60°F).
2. 250 ml capacity cylinder suitable to float the given lactometer.
3. Enamel tray for spillage.
4. Thermometer with range 0° - 50°C.
5. 400 ml beaker.
6. Thermostatic water bath adjusted at 15.6°C.

Principle

The principle involved in measuring the specific gravity or density by a lactometer is that a floating object sinks until it has displaced a weight of fluid equal its own weight. The greater is the volume of the displaced fluid the smaller is the density of the fluid the lower the lactometer reading. A lactometer reading of 32° denotes a specific gravity of 1.032. The determination should be made at about 60°F (15.6°C) and the lactometer reading corrected by adding or subtracting 0.1° for every degree F above or below that temperature. *Total solids content of milk are related to its fat percentage and specific gravity. The relationship is given to fair accuracy by the Richmond's formula.*

Procedure

1. Adjust the temperature of the milk sample as near to 15.6°C (not below 10°C or above 21°C) as possible.
2. Mix gently by pouring several times from one vessel to another, avoiding incorporation of air or foam formation.
3. Pour sufficient milk into the glass cylinder to allow the lactometer to float freely and the stem of the lactometer to be seen clearly.
4. Place the lactometer in the milk and allow it to come to a constant level.
5. Read the lactometer as soon as it assumes a constant level.
6. Record the lactometer reading and temperature of the milk.
7. Take another reading by flapping the top of the stem of the lactometer gently and when it again assumes the constant level.
8. Take the average of two readings and get from the standard Table the corrected value at 15.6°C.

Table 2 : Corrections to be applied to specific gravity lactometer for correcting specific gravity to 15.6ºC (60ºF)

Temperature Degrees°F	Quevenne degrees of specific gravity observed 25	26	27	28	29	30	31	32	33	34	35	36	Temperature Degrees°C
	Corrections to reduce specific gravity to 60°F SKIM												
40	1.5	1.5	1.5	1.6	1.7	1.7	1.9	2.0	2.0	2.1	2.2	2.3	4.40
41	1.4	1.4	1.4	1.5	1.6	1.7	1.8	1.9	2.0	2.0	2.1	2.2	5.00
42	1.4	1.4	1.4	1.5	1.5	1.6	1.7	1.8	1.9	2.0	2.1	2.1	5.56
43	1.3	1.3	1.3	1.4	1.4	1.5	1.6	1.7	1.8	1.9	2.0	2.0	6.11
44	1.2	1.2	1.3	1.3	1.3	1.4	1.5	1.6	1.7	1.8	1.9	1.9	6.67
45	1.2	1.2	1.2	1.3	1.3	1.4	1.5	1.6	1.6	1.7	1.8	1.8	7.22
46	1.1	1.1	1.2	1.2	1.2	1.3	1.4	1.5	1.6	1.7	1.7	1.7	7.78
47	1.0	1.1	1.1	1.2	1.2	1.3	1.4	1.5	1.5	1.5	1.6	1.6	8.33
48	1.0	1.0	1.0	1.1	1.1	1.2	1.3	1.4	1.4	1.4	1.5	1.5	8.89
49	0.9	0.9	0.9	1.0	1.0	1.1	1.2	1.3	1.3	1.3	1.4	1.4	9.44
50	0.9	0.9	0.9	1.0	1.0	1.0	1.1	1.1	1.2	1.2	1.3	1.3	10.00
51	0.8	0.8	0.8	0.9	0.9	0.9	1.0	1.0	1.1	1.1	1.2	1.2	10.56
52	0.7	0.8	0.8	0.8	0.8	0.9	0.9	1.9	1.0	1.0	1.1	1.1	11.11
53	0.6	0.7	0.7	0.7	0.7	0.8	0.8	0.8	0.9	0.9	1.0	1.0	11.67
54	0.5	0.6	0.6	0.6	0.6	0.7	0.7	0.7	0.7	0.7	0.8	0.9	12.22
55	0.4	0.5	0.5	0.5	0.6	0.6	0.6	0.6	0.6	0.7	0.7	0.7	12.78
56	0.4	0.4	0.4	0.4	0.4	0.4	0.5	0.5	0.5	0.5	0.6	0.6	13.33
57	0.3	0.3	0.3	0.3	0.3	0.3	0.4	0.4	0.4	0.4	0.5	0.5	13.89
58	0.2	0.2	0.2	0.2	0.2	0.2	0.2	0.3	0.3	0.3	0.3	0.3	14.44
59	0.1	0.1	0.1	0.1	0.1	0.1	0.1	0.1	0.1	0.1	0.2	0.2	15.00
60	25	26	27	28	29	30	31	32	33	34	35	36	15.56

SUBSTRACT FROM READING

61	SUBSTRACT FROM READING	0.1	0.1	0.1	0.1	0.1	0.1	0.1	0.1	0.1	0.1	0.1	0.1	16.11
62		0.2	0.2	0.3	0.3	0.3	0.3	0.3	0.3	0.3	0.3	0.3	0.3	16.67
63		0.3	0.3	0.4	0.4	0.4	0.4	0.4	0.4	0.5	0.5	0.5	0.5	17.22
64		0.4	0.5	0.5	0.5	0.5	0.5	0.5	0.6	0.6	0.6	0.6	0.6	17.78
65		0.5	0.6	0.6	0.6	0.7	0.7	0.7	0.8	0.8	0.8	0.8	0.8	18.33
66		0.6	0.7	0.7	0.7	0.8	0.8	0.8	0.9	0.9	0.9	0.9	1.0	18.89
67		0.7	0.8	0.8	0.8	0.9	0.9	1.0	1.0	1.0	1.0	1.1	1.1	19.44
68		0.9	1.0	1.0	1.0	1.1	1.1	1.1	1.1	1.2	1.2	1.2	1.2	20.00
69		1.0	1.1	1.1	1.1	1.2	1.2	1.2	1.3	1.3	1.3	1.3	1.4	20.56
70		1.1	1.2	1.2	1.2	1.3	1.3	1.4	1.4	1.5	1.5	1.5	1.6	21.11
71		1.2	1.3	1.3	1.4	1.4	1.4	1.5	1.5	1.6	1.6	1.7	-	21.67
72		1.4	1.4	1.4	1.5	1.5	1.6	1.6	1.7	1.7	1.8	1.8	-	22.22
73		1.5	1.5	1.6	1.7	1.7	1.8	1.8	1.9	1.9	2.0	2.0	-	22.78
74		1.6	1.7	1.7	1.8	1.9	1.9	2.0	2.1	2.1	2.2	2.2	-	23.33
75		1.8	1.8	1.9	1.9	2.0	2.1	2.2	2.3	2.3	2.4	2.4	-	23.89
76		1.9	1.9	2.0	2.0	2.1	2.2	2.3	2.4	2.4	2.5	2.6	-	24.44
77		2.0	2.0	2.2	2.2	2.3	2.4	2.4	2.5	2.6	2.7	-	-	25.00
78		2.2	2.2	2.2	2.3	2.4	2.5	2.6	2.7	2.8	2.9	-	-	25.56
79		2.3	2.3	2.4	2.4	2.5	2.6	2.7	2.8	3.0	3.0	-	-	26.11
80		2.4	2.4	2.5	2.6	2.7	2.8	2.9	3.0	3.1	3.2	-	-	26.67
								SKIM						
		25	26	27	28	29	30	31	32	33	34	35	36	

Observations

1. Lactometer readings

   A. ....

   B. ....

   Average ....

2. Temperature of milk
3. CLR = observed lactometer reading ± correction factor.

Calculations

$$\frac{CLR}{1000} + 1 = \text{sp.gr. of milk}$$

Richmond's formula for the calculation of total solids (TS) and solids not fat (SNF) using lactometer reading

$$\text{Percentage of total solids} \quad \frac{CLR}{4} + (1.2 \times F) + 0.14$$

$$\text{Percentage of solids not fat} \quad \frac{CLR}{4} + (0.2 \times F) + 0.14$$

where

F = Fat percentage

CLR = Corrected lactometer reading

Specific Gravity Using Density Hydrometer at 20°C.

(Method of British Standards Institution, BS 734 : 1959)

The density of milk is measured by a specially calibrated hydrometer covering the appropriate range of specific gravity from 1.025 to 1.035, which for simplicity are marked as 25-35°C.

Procedure

1. Warm the milk sample to 40°C and maintain at this temperature for 5 minutes.
2. Remove the sample bottle and mix the contents by rotating and inverting the bottles taking care to avoid the formation of air bubbles and froth.

3. Cool the sample approximately to 27°C. Invert the sample bottle two or three times and then pour enough milk into the glass cylinder, taking care to avoid formation of air bubbles, so that some milk overflows when the hydrometer is inserted.
4. Insert the hydrometer gently and allow it to come to rest.
5. Note the reading of the hydrometer corresponding to the level of liquid surface of the milk, keeping eye in level with the surface of the liquid.
6. Note the temperature of the milk immediately after the hydrometer is taken (Temperature correction may be made as given in Table).
7. Convert the observed density hydrometer reading at 27°C to the corrected value to 20°C making use of Table.

Precuations

If the milk is freshly drawn, it should be prewarmed to 40°C and then cooled to 20°C. This is necessary as the density changes during the first few hours (Rechnagel's phenomenon).

Aged milk do not require such preparation.

Observations

1. Density hydrometer readings

   A ....

   B ....

   Average ....
2. Temperature of milk ....

Table 3 : Correction (C) to density hydrometer readings to give the density of milk at the temperature of observation.

Temperature of observation 0°C	Correction
17	+3
19	+2
21	+2
23	+1
25	+1
27	0
29	-1
31	-1
33	-2
35	-2
37	-3

Table 4 : Corrections to be applied to density hydrometer readings taken at temperatures other than 20ºC (or 68ºF) to obtain the density of milk at 20ºC (or 68ºF)

Temperture 0°C	Percentage fat in sample					
	0	2	4	6	8	10
30.0	+27	+28	+29	+30	+32	+33
29.5	+26	+27	+28	+29	+30	+30
29.0	+24	+25	+26	+27	+28	+29
28.5	+22	+23	+24	+25	+26	+27
28.0	+21	+22	+23	+24	+25	+26
27.5	+19	+20	+21	+22	+23	+24
27.0	+18	+19	+20	+20	+21	+22
26.5	+17	+17	+18	+19	+20	+21
26.0	+15	+16	+17	+17	+18	+19
25.5	+14	+15	+15	+16	+17	+17
25.0	+12	+13	+14	+14	+15	+16
24.5	+11	+12	+12	+13	+14	+14
24.0	+10	+10	+11	+11	+12	+12
23.5	+9	+9	+9	+10	+10	+11
23.0	+7	+8	+8	+8	+9	+9
22.5	+6	+6	+7	+7	+7	+8
22.0	+5	+5	+5	+6	+6	+6
21.5	+4	+4	+4	+4	+5	+5
21.0	+2	+2	+3	+3	+3	+3
20.5	+1	+1	+1	+1	+2	+2
20.0	0	0	0	0	0	0
19.5	-1	-1	-1	-1	-1	-2
19.0	-2	-2	-3	-3	-3	-3
18.5	-3	-4	-4	-4	-4	-5
18.0	-4	-5	-5	-5	-6	-6
17.5	-5	-6	-6	-7	-7	-8
17.0	-6	-7	-7	-8	-9	-9
16.5	-7	-8	-9	-19	-10	-11
16.0	-8	-9	-10	-11	-12	-13
15.5	-9	-10	-11	-12	-13	-14
15.0	-10	-11	-12	-13	-15	-16

Calculation

Observed ± correction factor

Richmond's formula for the calculation of total solids (TS) and solids not fat (SNF) using Density hydrometer reading.

$T = 0.25\ D + 1.21\ F\ +0.66$

$SNF = 0.25\ D + 0.21\ F + 0.66$

where

T = percentage of total solids

SNF = Percentage of non-fatty solids (solids non fat)

D = 1000 (d-l)

d = Density of the milk sample at 20°C

F = percentage of fat

Total Ash in Milk

(Method of AOAC, 1965)

Apparatus

1. Dish - platinum or silica
2. Desiccator
3. Chemical balance
4. Muffle furnace

Principle

Milk contains soluble substances containing salts like the phosphate, citrates, sulphates, chlorides and bicarbonates of calcium, magnesium, potassium, sodium etc. Heating milk at higher temperature decompose organic matter and soluble inorganic salts are left behind in the form of ash.

Procedure

1. Heat the dish in order to remove any moisture from it.
2. Cool the dish in a desiccator to room temperature and weigh it accurately.
3. Weigh quickly and accurately about 10 grams of milk in the weighed dish.
4. Evaporate the sample to dryness on a water bath, avoid spurting of the milk by using a thin glass rod drawn to a point and remove any particle adhering to the rod into the dish.
5. Keep the evaporated milk sample in a muffle furnace at temperature not more than 55°C until the ash is free from carbon.
6. Cool in a desiccator to room temperature and weigh quickly.

Observations

1. Weight of empty dish = W,g
2. Weight of dish with milk = W_1, g
3. Weight of dish after ashing = W_2, g
4. Weight of milk taken = W_1 - W, g
5. Weight of ash = W_2 - W, g

Calculation

$$\text{Percentage of ash by weight} = \frac{W_2 - W}{W_1 - W} \times 100$$

Gross energy of milk

If bomb calorimeter is available in the laboratory then acutal gross energy of milk may be estimated by using bomb calorimeter as per method mentioned in volume I of this compilation when there is no bomb calorimeter available then approximate gross energy of milk may be estimated using the following factors published by Mitchell (1962). These factors could be used both in human and animals milk.

Mitchell's Factor

1. Gross energy of butterfat = 9.11 kcal/g
2. Gross energy of protein = 5.86 kcal/g
3. Gross energy of lactose = 3.76 kcal/g

The total value of all the three multiplied observations will indicate gross energy (kcal/100 g of milk).

Gaines and Overman (1938) Formula for Calculating Gross Energy of Milk Using fat Percentage

kcal/kg milk = 304.8 + 114.1 f

where f

is the percentage of fat in the milk

☞ **Note**

Milk with 4 percent fat has a calorific value of 750 kcal/kg, while Krishna (1973). reported value of 760 kcal/kg.

References

AOAC, (1965). *Official methods of analysis of the Association of official agricultural chemists,* 10th edn., AOAC, Benjamin Franklin Station, Washington, D.C.

British Standards Institution, (1959). *Density Hydrometers for use in milk,* BS 734, BSI, London.

Conway, E.J. (1957). *Microdiffusion analysis and volumetric error, 4th edn.,* crossby, Lockwood and Son Ltd., London.

Folin, O. and Wu, H. (1919). *J. Biol. Chem.,* 38 : 98.

Gaines, W.L. and Overman, O.R. (1938). *J. Dairy Sci.,* 21 : 261.

Indian Standards Institution, (1961). *Diary Industry, methods of test for* : Part II. Chemical analysis of milk. IS 1479. ISI. Manak Bhavan, New Delhi (India).

Indian Standards Institution, (1977). *Fat, determination by the Gerber method.* Part I Milk (first revision). IS 1224. ISI, (BIS) Manak Bhavan, New Delhi (India).

Krishna, G. (1973). Studies on energy and protein requirements for milk production in Indian dairy animals, Ph.D. Thesis, NDRI, Karnal, (Haryana). Agra University, Agra, India.

Krishna, G., Razdan, M.N. and Ray, S.N. (1977). Studies on energy and protein requirements of Zebu (*Bos Indicus*). *Z. Tierphysiologie und Tierernährung und futtermittelkde.* 38: 281-284.

Krishna, G., Razdan, M.N. and Ray, S.N. (1977). Effect of seasonal and nutritional variations on the quality and quantity of milk produced by Zebu cows in the tropical/ subtropical region of India. *The Indian J. Nutr. Dietetics.* 14: 173-181.

Krishna, G., Razdan, M.N. and Ray, S.N. (1973). "Dairy Search" formula for the estimation of Calorific value of milk in *Bos Indicus* in the tropical/subtropical region. International Research Communication System (73-11) 32-49-4.

Mitchell, H.H. (1962). *Comparative nutrition of man and domestic animals,* Vol. 1. Academic Press, USA, pp 596.

References for further study

Davies, J.G. (1959). *Milk testing,* 2nd edn., Diary Industries Ltd. 9 Gough sq., London, E.C. 4.

Eckles, C.H., Combs, W.B. and Macy, H. (1943). *Milk and milk products.* 3rd edn., Mc Graw Hill Book Co., Inc. New York and London.

Ganguli, N.C. (1974). *Milk proteins,* Indian Council of Agricultural Research, New Delhi.

Jenness, R. and Patton, S. (1959). *Principles of Dairy Chemistry.* Ist edn., John Wiley Sons, Inc. New York.

Lyons, J. and O'shea, M.J. (1950). *Commercial methods of testing milk and milk products,* Ist edn. Cork university press, Oxford, B.H. Blackwell Ltd.

Mc Kanzie, H.A. (1970). *Milk protein chemistry and molecular biology*. Academic Press, New York.

Srinivasan, M.R. and Ananta Krishnan, C.P. (1964). *Milk products of India*. ICAR, New Delhi (India).

Walter, W.G. (1967). *Standard methods for the examination of dairy products.* Twelth edition, American Public Health Association, Inc. 1740, Broadway, New York, N.Y. 10019.

Chapter - 86

Quality Control in Feed and Mineral Mixture Processing Industries : A Vision

Quality Assurance Methods

Adulteration in animal and human foods has become common feature in the country, therefore we should be cautious while selecting animal/human feed ingredients.

The author of this compendium has developed. *"Animal Feed Testing Kit"* based on novel cud liquor enzyme complex (innovation certified by ISA, International Search Authority - Patent office, Vienna), registered with WIPO (Geneva). This method is described in detail in this chapter and Patent application is field at Indian Patent Office Delhi.

Now-a-days, animal feed is being adulterated with extraneous materials viz, *Saw dust, Ric hulls, sand* and *Silica, Castor husk, oat hulls* and *urea* (higher than 01 percent limit on dry matter basis).

Every consumer whether human being or animal, want eatable materials of purest quality having no adulteration. Profit making business personnel try to earn maximum money by way of adulteration, without thinking in terms of adverse effects on health. Any commodity whether ice cream, baby food, cattle feed or poultry feed should be checked thoroughly before releasing in the market for sale. While purchasing any eatable materials from local market, emphasis should not be given on the lowest price, but weightage should be given to quality which is coinciding with an Intrenational standard.

It has been experienced that good quality control of both raw materials and finished products is even more necesasry for feed manufacturers in the less developed countries than for their counterparts in the developed world. In the developing contries very less or negligible emphasis is being given to quality control programme. Government of India has fixed up the responsibilities on Indian Standards Institution (BIS) and Agmark Grading scheme organised by the Ministry of Agriculture and Irrigation, India, to maintain the quality control programme for screening human preserved food materials, animal feeds, edible oils, ghee and butter etc.

Factors affecting quality of ingredients

1. *The presence of non edible items, e.g. silica or any harmful constraints.*
2. *Changes in nutrient content.*
3. *The extent of grinding and freshness.*
4. *Storage conditions which can lead to infestations, over-heating (browning) and rancidity.*
5. *The presence of toxins, pathogenic organisms and other harmful substances.*

Cockerell *et al.* (1975) have emphasised that the following legislation may be regulated for making quality control programme successful.

1. To protect the purchasers of mixed feeds from fraud, by laying down regulations for the description and testing of feeds. Such regulations normally specify the information which must be given to the customer with regard to the nutritive value and nature of the feed, and lay down procedures for ensuring that feeds meet their stated specifications.
2. To restrict the presence of substances in feeds which could be harmful to persons eating the products of animals which had consumed the feed. Regulations in this regard relate to naturally occuring toxic constituents of feeds, growth promoting additives and medicaments.
3. To ensure that the feed is appropriate in composition and nutritive value for the particular class of animal for which it is intended. For example, if a feed is described as a poultry starter feed, it should be of sufficient nutritive value and acceptability to produce a satisfactory rate of growth and efficiency of feed conversion in chicks. Such requirements are met by laying down minimum requirements for the nutritive value of feeds marketed for consumption by different classes of animals.

Only a few developing countries have so far enacted legislation on animal feeds, *particularly Indian has not approved any legislation so far in relation to adulteration of animal feeds*. There is an urgent need of strict measure to prevent the adulteration of animal feeds with extraneous matters. There are a number of factors which have to be borne in mind when assessing the suitability of various raw materials as ingredient of compound feeds, the first and probably the most important being that of protein and energy content in relation to price. The quality of protein and the mineral and vitamin contents must also be considered in addition to, in certain cases, the presence of substances which may limit usage e.g. excessive fiber, toxic substances or components which may result in low palatability. *Now-a-days, in most of the developing countries non conventional resources (NCR) are being used which lacks in palatability and interfering materials like tannins and glucosides may depress the utilisation of nutrients which thereby resulted in retarding the developments of body mass. Actual energetic values (ME/NE) of NCR based on Respiration chamber studies are not available in the country, research is required to fill up the gap of information.*

Preliminary Inspection

Cockerell *et al.* (1975) have described the importance of preliminary inspection in the quality control programmes. When any raw material received at mill, whould be looked at carefully for evidence of wetting, the presence of deleterious substances such as stones and dirt or other materials, and of storage pests.

Evidence of damage of feed ingredients which has previously occured should be noted. Immediately after arrival of consigment in the mill, moisture should be estimated, any consigment containing more than 13 per cent moisture should not be taken into store until after drying, otherwise there are chances of fungal infestation which may be responsible for producing harmful mycotoxin and may lead to deterioration in the normal health of animals and human subjects.

Sampling

This is a very important stage in the quality control programme. Sampling should be carried out very carefully as there is little point in analysing materials in the laboratory if the results obtained do not give an adequate representation of the composition of the whole material from which the samples was drawn.

Cockerell *et al.* (1975) reported minimum limits of sampling raw materials as mentioned below:

Size of consignment	% of bags to be sampled
2-20 bags	20%
20-60 bags	10%
60-200 bags	7%
200-500 bags	5%
500-1000 bags	4%
More than 1000 bags	3%

Samples of less than 100 kg consisting of as little as one bag should be sampled so as to produce as representative a sample as possible weighing at least 0.75 kg.

Similar materials received in bulk require samples to be taken in accordance with the size of the consignment as specified below:

Size of consignment	Number of samples
Less than 1 ton (t)	4
1-2 tons	6
2-5 tons	10
5-10 tons	15
10-25 tons	25
25-50 tons	40
50-100	60

For each additional 10 t in excess of 100 t, 2 Nos of samples should be drawn.

The samples taken either from individual bags or from different portions of the bulk consigment should be bulked together, thoroughly mixed and reduced in size by quartering or using a sample divider, to between 1 and 2 kg in weight.

Very coarse materials such as oil cakes require a slightly different sampling procedure, in which pieces are selected from different parts of the whole quantity as follows :

Size of consignment	No. of pieces
Less than 2 tons	5
2-5 tons	10
5-50 tons	15
50-100 tons	25
For each additional 20 tons in excess of 100	2

The pieces selected should be ground thoroughly mixed and the sample reduced in size to between 1 and 2 kg as outlined above.

Cockerell *et al.* (1975) have reported that liquid feed like molasses should be sampled in accordanec with the plan for baggase consignments, outlined above. Bulk tanker delivery of molasses can be sampled by removing portions from the top, middle and bottom of the tank. The samples taken from individual drums or tanks should be thoroughly mixed and reduced in size to 1 to 2 kg, if necessary.

Normal Tests Required in Quality Control Programmes

Weende proximate analysis should be carried out in the case of animal feeds and fodders and human foods. Proximate composition indicates possible constraints on usage due to the presence of excessive content of cellulosic materials, oil or mineral matter. Those ingredients found rich in total ash should be resorted to fractionisation into insoluble and soluble ash. The amount of acid insoluble ash is a good guide to the amount of sand or other dirt which may be present. *Free fatty acids* and *iodine value* should be estimated in order to detect adulteration of any other oil cakes. Normal tests for the detection of *castor husk* or *Mahua cake* in animal feeds should be carried out.

a. Indian Standards Instituion (BIS) Specification for Cattle Feed

In India, Indian standards Instiution (BIS) has played an important role to fix up standard as mentioned below for compounded cattle feed.

I.	Moisture	10%
II.	Crude protein	20%
III.	Crude fiber	13%
IV.	Acid insoluble ash	4%
V.	Digestible crude protein	14-16%
VI.	Total digestible nutrients	68-74%

Sources : Indian standards Institution, (BIS), 1979. Compound feeds, cattle (Third revision) IS : 2052, ISI, (BIS) New Delhi

b. Indian standards Institution specification for poultry feed

For taking the maximum output from poultry in terms of meat or egg production it is necessary that poultry feed should be manufactured as per ISI, (BIS) specifications, which are given below in Table 1.

Table 1 : BIS Requirements for chicken feeds IS 1374 : 1992 (Fourth Revision)

S.No.	Characteristic	Requirements for					
		Broiler Starter Feed	Broiler Finisher Feed	Chick Feed	Growing Chicken Feed	Laying Chicken Feed	Breeder Layer Feed
1.	Moisture % by mass, Max	11	11	11	11	11	11
2.	Crude protein	23	20	20	16	18	18
3.	Acid insoluble ash % by mass, max	3	3	4	4	4	4
4.	Salt (NaCl) % by mass, Max	0.6	0.6	0.6	0.6	0.6	0.6

BIS Requirements for chicken feeds to be declared (on dry matter basis)

S.No.	Characteristic	Requirements for					
		Broiler Starter Feed	Broiler Finisher Feed	Chick Feed	Growing Chicken Feed	Laying Chicken Feed	Breeder Layer Feed
1.	Calcium % by mass, Min	1.2	1.2	1	1	3	3
2.	Available Phosphorus % by mass, Min	0.5	0.5	0.5	0.5	0.5	0.5
3.	Lysine % by mass, Min	1.2	1.0	0.9	0.6	0.65	0.65
4.	Methionine % by mass, Min	0.50	0.35	0.3	0.25	0.30	0.30
5.	Metabolizable energy (Kcal/kg), Min	2800	2900	2600	2500	2600	2600

BIS Requirements for minerals, fatty acids, amino acids and vitamins in chicken feed

S.No.	Characteristic	Requirements for					
		Broiler Starter Feed	Broiler Finisher Feed	Chick Feed	Growing Chicken Feed	Laying Chicken Feed	Breeder Layer Feed
1.	Manganese, mg/kg	90	90	90	50	55	90
2.	Iodine, mg/kg	1	1	1	1	1	1
3.	Iron, mg/kg	120	120	120	90	75	90
4.	Zinc, mg/kg	60	60	60	50	75	100
5.	Copper, mg/kg	12	12	12	9	9	12
6.	Vitamin A, IU/kg	6000	6000	6000	6000	8000	8000
7.	Vitamin D3, IU/kg	600	600	600	600	1200	1200
8.	Thiamin, mg/kg	5	5	5	3	3	3
9.	Riboflavin, mg/kg	6	6	6	5	5	8
10.	Pantothenic acid, mg/kg	15	15	15	15	15	15
11.	Niacin, mg/kg	40	40	40	15	15	15
12.	Biotin, mg/kg	0.2	0.2	0.2	0.15	0.15	0.20

13.	Vitamin B12, mg/kg	0.015	0.015	0.0150	0.01	0.01	0.01
14.	Folic acid, mg/kg	1	1	1	0.5	0.5	0.5
15.	Choline, mg/kg	1400	1000	1300	900	800	800
16.	Vitamin E, mg/kg	15	15	15	10	10	15
17.	Vitamin K, mg/kg	1	1	1	1	1	1
18.	Pyridoxine, mg/kg	5	5	5	5	5	8
19.	Linoleic acid g/100 g	1	1	1	1	1	1
20.	Methionine + Cystine, g/100 g	0.9	0.7	0.6	0.5	0.55	0.55

Source : BIS (ISI) 1992. Nutrient requirements of Poultry, Bureau of Indian Standards Manak Bhawan, Delhi. IS : 13574.

Table 2 : Nutrient Requirements of broilers as percentage of units per kilogram of diet (90% dry matter), NRC, 1994, USA.

Nutrient	Unit	3-6 Weeks	6-8 Weeks
Crude protein	%	20	18
Arginine	%	1.10	1.00
Glycine+serine	%	1.14	0.97
Histidine	%	0.32	0.27
Isoleucine	%	0.73	0.62
Leucine	%	1.09	0.93
Lysine	%	1.00	0.85
Methionine	%	0.38	0.32
Methionine+ Cystine	%	0.72	0.60
Phenylalanine + tyrosine	%	1.22	1.04
Proline	%	0.55	0.46
Threonine	%	0.74	0.68
Tryptophan	%	0.18	0.16
Valine	%	0.82	0.70
Fat			
Linoleic acid	%	1.00	1.00
Calcium	%	1.00	1.00
Chlorine	%	0.15	0.12
Magnesium	mg	600	600
Nonphytate phosphorus	%	0.35	0.30
Potassium	%	0.30	0.30
Sodium	%	0.15	0.12
Trace Minerals			
Copper	mg	8	8
Iodine	mg	0.35	0.35

Iron	mg	80	80
Manganese	mg	60	60
Selenium	mg	0.15	0.15
Zinc	mg	40	40
A	IU	1500	1500
D3	ICU	200	200
E	IU	10	10
K	mg	0.50	0.50
Water Soluble Vitamins			
B_{12}	mg	0.01	0.007
Biotin	mg	0.15	0.12
Choline	mg	1000	750
Folacin	mg	0.55	0.50
Niacin	mg	30	25
Pantothenic acid	mg	10	10
Pyridoxine	mg	3.5	3.0
Riboflavin	mg	3.6	3
Thiamin	mg	1.80	1.80

Nutrient Requirements of Immature Leghorn Type Chickens as Percentages or Units per Kilogram of Diet, NRC - 1994, USA

Nutrient	Unit	White Egg Laying Strains				Brown-Egg Laying Strains			
		0-6 wk	6-12 wk	12-18 wk	18 wk to first egg	0-6 wk	6-12 wk	12-18 wk	18 wk to first egg
Energy		**2850**	**2850**	**2900**	**2900**	**2800**	**2800**	**2850**	**2850**
Crude protein	%	18.00	16.00	15.00	17.00	17.00	15.00	14.00	16.00
Arginine	%	1.00	0.83	0.67	0.75	0.94	0.78	0.62	0.72
Glycine + serine	%	0.70	0.58	0.47	0.53	0.66	0.54	0.44	0.50
Histidine	%	0.26	0.22	0.17	0.20	0.25	0.21	0.16	0.18
Isoleucine	%	0.60	0.50	0.40	0.45	0.57	0.47	0.37	0.42
Leucine	%	1.10	0.85	0.70	0.80	1.00	0.80	0.65	0.75
Lysine	%	0.85	0.60	0.45	0.52	0.80	0.56	0.42	0.49
Methionine	%	0.30	0.25	0.20	0.22	0.28	0.23	0.19	0.21
Methionine + cystine	%	0.62	0.52	0.42	0.47	0.59	0.49	0.39	0.44
Phenylalanine	%	0.54	0.45	0.36	0.40	0.51	0.42	0.34	0.38
Phenylalanine + tyrosine	%	1.00	0.83	0.67	0.75	0.94	0.78	0.63	0.70
Threonine	%	0.68	0.57	0.37	0.47	0.64	0.53	0.35	0.44
Tryptophan	%	0.17	0.14	0.11	0.12	0.16	0.13	0.10	0.11
Valine	%	0.62	0.52	0.41	0.46	0.59	0.49	0.38	0.43
Fat									
Linoleic acid	%	1.00	1.00	1.00	1.00	1.00	1.00	1.00	1.00

Macrominerals									
Calcium	%	0.90	0.80	0.80	2.00	0.90	0.80	0.80	1.80
Chlorine	%	0.15	0.12	0.12	0.15	0.12	0.11	0.11	0.11
Magnesium	mg	600.0	500.0	400.0	400.0	570	470	370	370
Nonphytate phosphorus	%	0.40	0.35	0.30	0.32	0.40	0.35	0.30	0.35
Potassium	%	0.25	0.25	0.25	0.25	0.25	0.25	0.25	0.25
Sodium	%	0.15	0.15	0.15	0.15	0.15	0.15	0.15	0.15
Trace minerals									
Copper	mg	5.0	4.0	4.0	4.0	5.0	4.0	4.0	4.0
Iodine	mg	0.35	0.35	0.35	0.35	0.33	0.33	0.33	0.33
Iron	mg	80.0	60.0	60.0	60.0	75.0	56.0	56.0	56.0
Manganese	mg	60.0	30.0	30.0	30.0	56.0	28.0	28.0	28.0
Selenium	mg	0.15	0.10	0.10	0.10	0.14	0.10	0.10	0.10
Zinc	mg	40.0	35.0	35.0	35.0	38.0	33.0	33.0	33.0
Fat soluble vitamins									
A	IU	1500	1500	1500	1500	1420	1420	1420	1420
D_3	ICU	200	200	200	300	190	190	190	280
E	IU	10	5	5	5	9.5	4.7	4.7	4.7
K	mg	0.5	0.5	0.5	0.5	0.47	0.47	0.47	0.47
Water soluble vitamins									
B_{12}	mg	0.009	0.003	0.003	0.004	0.009	0.003	0.003	0.003
Biotin	mg	0.15	0.10	0.10	0.10	0.14	0.09	0.09	0.09
Choline	mg	1300	900	500	500	1225	850	470	470
Folacin	mg	0.55	0.25	0.25	0.25	0.52	0.23	0.23	0.23
Niacin	mg	27	11	11	11	26.0	10.3	10.3	10.3
Pantothenic acid	mg	10	10	10	10	9.4	9.4	9.4	9.4
Pyridoxine	mg	3.0	3.0	3.0	3.0	2.8	2.8	2.8	2.8
Riboflavin	mg	3.6	1.8	1.8	2.2	3.4	1.7	1.7	1.7
Thiamin	mg	1.0	1.0	0.8	0.8	1.0	1.0	0.8	0.8

Table 3 : Nutrient requirements of leghorn - Type laying hens as Percentages or units per Kilogram of diet (90% dry matter), NRC - 1994, USA

		Dietary concentration required by white-egg layers at different feed intakes		
Nutrient	**Unit**	**80 a,b**	**100 a,b**	**120 a,b**
Crube protein	%	18.8	15	12.5
Arginine	%	0.88	0.70	0.58
Histidine	%	0.21	0.17	0.14
Isoleucine	%	0.81	0.65	0.54
Leucine	%	1.03	0.82	0.68
Lysine	%	0.86	0.69	0.58
Methionine	%	0.38	0.30	0.25
Methionine + Cystine	%	0.73	0.58	0.48

Phenylalanine	%	0.59	0.47	0.39
Phenylalanine + tyrosine	%	1.04	0.83	0.69
Threonine	%	0.59	0.47	0.39
Tryptophan	%	0.20	0.416	0.13
Valine	%	0.88	0.70	0.58
Fat				
Linoleic acid	%	1.25	1.0	0.83
Macrominerals				
Calcium	%	4.06	3.25	2.71
Chloride	%	0.16	0.13	0.11
Magnesium	mg	625	500	420
Nonphytate phosphorus	%	0.31	0.25	0.21
Potassium	%	0.19	0.15	0.13
Sodium	%	0.19	0.15	0.13
Trace minerals				
Copper	mg			
Iodine	mg	0.044	0.035	0.029
Iron	mg	56	45	38
Manganese	mg	25	20	17
Selenium	mg	0.08	0.06	0.05
Zinc	mg	44	35	29
Fat soluble vitamins				
A	IU	3750	3000	2500
D_3	IU	375	300	250
E	IU	6	5	4
K	mg	0.6	0.5	0.4
Water soluble vitamins				
B_{12}	mg	0.004	0.004	0.004
Biotin	mg	0.13	0.10	0.08
Choline	mg	1310	1050	875
Folacin	mg	0.31	0.25	0.21
Niacin	mg	12.5	10	8.3
Pantothenic acid	mg	2.5	2.0	1.7
Pyridoxine	mg	3.1	2.5	2.1
Riboflavin	mg	3.1	2.5	2.1
Thiamin	mg	0.88	0.70	0.60

a Grams feed intake per hen daily
b Based on dietary MEn concentrations of approximately 2900 kcal/kg and an assumed rate of egg production of 90% (90 eggs per 100 hens daily).

Source : NRC (1994) National Research Council, Nutrient Requirements of Poultry Ninth Revised Edition, National Academy Press, Washington, D.C., Subcommittee on Poultry Nutrition, Committee on Animal Nutrition.

b. Indian Standards Institution (BIS) Specification for Mineral Mixture

Now-a-days, several Industries are involved in the manufacture of mineral mixture, but they should formulate the mineral mixture as per conformity to the Indian Standards Institution specifications for supplementing cattle feeds.

Table 4 : Requirements for mineral mixture containing salt for supplementing cattle feeds. Type I (*Source :* ISI, 1968, IS : 1664)

	Characteristic	Requirements
1.	Moisture, per cent by Wt.. Max.	7
2.	Calcium, per cent by wt. Min.	22
3.	Phosphorus, per cent by wt. Min.	9
4.	Salt (chlorine as sodium chloride) per cent by wt., Min.	22
5.	Iron, per cent by weight	0.4 to 0.6
6.	Iodine, (as KI), per cent by weight	0.02 to 0.10
7.	Copper, per cent by weight	0.06 to 0.10
8.	Manganese, per cent by weight	0.09 to 0.12
9.	Cobalt, per cent by weight	0.01 to 0.02
10.	Fluorine, per cent by weight, Max.	0.03
11.	Spores of *Bacillus anthracis, clostridium* sp.	Nil

Table 5 : Requirements for mineral mixture without salt for supplementing Cattle feeds: Type II (*Source :* ISI, 1968, IS : 1664), (BIS)

	Characteristic	Requirement
1.	Moisture, per cent by wt., Max.	7
2.	Calcium, per cent by wt., Min.	28
3.	Phosphorus, per cent by wt. Min.	12
4.	Iron, per cent by wt.	0.50 to 0.75
5.	Iodine, (as KI), per cent by wt.	0.026 to 0.130
6.	Copper, per cent by wt.	0.077 to 0.130
7.	Manganese, per cent by wt.	0.12 to 0.15
8.	Cobalt, per cent by wt.	0.013 to 0.026
9.	Flourine, per cent by wt. Max.	0.04
10.	Spores of *Bacillus anthracis, clostridium* sp.	Nil

As per ISI (BIS), (1968 : IS : 1664) specifications, each container should provide the following information.

a. Name and type of the material
b. Name of the manufacturer
c. *Percentage of dicalcium phosphate in mineral mixture*
d. Batch or code number
e. Net weight
f. Date of manufacture

A leaflet should also be attached with each container, consisting the following information.

a. Name and type of the material
b. Ingredients
c. Guaranteed composition
d. Directions for use.
e. In the case of type II mineral mixture, the quantity of salt required to be added before use, should be indicated.

Importance of Protein Quality Tests

Feeds formulation for non ruminants require pre information on amino acid contents and their availability as well as total protein content, Amino acid analysis of protein concentrate is a costly analysis and only large commercial feed manufacturing organisations could afford such type of expenditure. *Actual assay of available lysine is necessary. This is beacuse damage to proteins during processing or subsequent storage can render a proportion of lysine nutritionally unavailable, and it is therefore particularly dangerous to rely on figures for total lysine given in compositional tables. Regular determination of available lysine in protein concentrates should be carried out, this will aid to assess the protein quality of human foods as well as animal feeds.*

Deleterious Substances

There are many examples of endogenous toxins viz. gossypol in cottonseed, glucosinolates in rapeseed and cyanogenetic glycosides (liberating hydrogen cyanide) in linseed and Cassava, mowrin (Mahua cake) aflatoxin produced by the growth of fungi *Aspergillus flavus*. These endogenous toxins produces interferences in the biochemical transformations usually occur in the body. We should remember by heart that tests for toxic substances are of greater importance when the materials are to be included in the ration of Pig, poultry, calf or lamb feeds. *Mature ruminants are more tolerant to these toxins, however routine tests for these toxins are not strictly necessary.*

Liquid feed Ingredients (Molasses)

We should estimate total sugar in molasses. Since molasses contains higher concentration of potassium, therefore it should be checked in routine analysis. Moisture may be estimated by "Dairy search" method according to Krishna *et al.* (1972), referred in Volume I of compendium.

Minerals and Vitamins

Since in the developing countries, non conventional resources available from Agro-Industries are being included in the compounded feed, therefore these ingredients should be analysed for important major minerals viz. calcium, phosphorus, sulphur, sodium, potassium etc. and minor minerals viz. copper, zinc, cobalt, iron and manganese. Among the vitamins, Carotene estimation is necessary.

Information on Compounded Rations Bags Packing

Feed manufactures should provide the following information with every bag.

1. *The name and purpose of the feed.*
2. *The net or gross weight.*
3. *The calculated nutrient content.*
4. *Details of any special additives, specifying chemical name, common name, level of inclusion in grams per ton or grams or milligrams per kilo.*
5. *Age of stock for which the food is designed.*
6. *Batch number.*
7. *The name of manufacturer.*

Table 6 : Indian standards Institution (BIS) specifications of animal feed ingredients

Name of ingredient	Crude protein (Min.)	Ether extract (Min.)	Crude fiber (Max.)	Total ash	Acid Insoluble ash	ISI specification number
I. Cotton seed oil cake						IS : 1712 - 1970
1. Decorticated, solvent extracted cake						
Grade 1	42	1.5	16	-	2.0	
Grade 2	40	2.0	18	-	2.5	
2. Decorticated oil cake						
Grade 1	40	7.0	12	-	2.0	
Grade 2	35	6.0	15	-	2.5	
3. Undecorticated oil cake						
Grade 1	24	7.0	22	-	2.0	
Grade 2	20	5.0	26	-	2.5	
II. Groundnut oil cake						
Decorticated cake (solvent extracted)						
Grade 1	51	-	7.0	-	2.5	
Grade 2	47	-	10.0	-	2.5	
Expeller or hydraulic pressed oil cakes (Decorticated)						IS : 1713-1970
Grade HF	50	8.0	7.0	7.0	1.5	
Grade LF	48	5.0	9.0	8.0	2.0	
Ghani pressed oil cakes	45	10	6	6	2.5	
III. Decorticated safflower cake						
(KARDI) oil cake Expeller or hydraulic pressed	48	5	15	9	2.0	
Ghani pressed oil cake	45	8	15	9	2.0	
IV. Fish meal						
Grade 1	60	10	-	-	3.0	
Grade 2	50	10	-	-	5.0	
V. Gram Churi	18	3.5	12	4.5	0.8	IS : 3161-1965
VI. Gram husks	3	-	50	6.0	1.0	IS : 3162-1965
VII. Guar meal	40	3-0	12	7.0	0.5	IS : 4193-1967

VIII. Linsed oil cake						
Grade HF	29.0	8.0	10.0	8.0	1.5	
Grade LF	31.0	5.0	10.0	8.0	1.2	
Maize bran						IS : 2153-1962
Coarse bran	7.5	2.0	12.5	1.5	0.5	
Fine bran	14.0	2.5	9.5	1.5	0.5	
Maize gluten						IS : 2152-1972
Grade 1	45	4	3.5	4.0	0.5	
Grade 2	23	3	8.0	6.0	0.5	
Mustard and rapeseed oil cake						
Rotary pressed oil cake						
LF grade	35	5	9.0	8.0	1.5	
HF grade	37	8	10.0	9.0	2.0	
Ghani pressed	33	12	7.0	8.0	2.5	
I. Rice bran (ordinary)	11	12	12.0	13.0	4.0	IS : 3648-1975
II. Rice polish	11	15	4.0	10.0	1.5	IS : 3163-1965
V. Sesamum (Til) oil cake						
Rotary pressed						
Grade HF	40	8	7.0	13.0	1.5	
Grade LF	42	5	7.0	13.0	2.0	
Ghani pressed	36	14	7.0	13.0	2.0	
Solvent extracted						
Rice bran						IS : 3593-1979
Grade 1	15	1.5	14.0	6.0	-	
Grade 2	14	1.5	16.0	10.0	-	
I. Solvent extracted coconut oil cake						
Grade 1	23	1.0	14.0	-	1.5	
Grade 2	21	1.5	15.0	-	2.0	
II. Decorticated Sunflower oilcake	45	12	6	6	1.0	IS : 10165-1982
III. Tur husk	5	-	44.0	6	1.0	IS : 5063-1969
X. Wheat bran	14.5	3.0	11.0	6.5	0.25	IS : 2239-1971

List of ISI (BIS) specifications related to Animal feeds

1. Animal feeds and feedingstuff, methods of tests for : Part I : General methods, IS : 7874 (Part I), 1975
   Part II. Minerals and trace elements, IS : 7874 (Part II), 1975.
   Part III. Microbiological methods, IS : 7874 (Part III), 1975.

2. Blood meal as livestock feed, IS : 7060-1973
3. Bone meal as livestock feed supplement (first revision), IS : 1942-1968.
4. Calcined bone meal as livestock feed supplement, IS : 7061-1973
5. Coconut oil cake as livestock feed (first revision), IS : 2154-1972.
6. Common salt and Cattle licks for animal consumption (first revision), (Superseding IS : 1291-1958), IS : 1291-1958.
7. Compounded feeds for Cattle (third revision), IS : 2051-1979.
8. Compounded feeds for young stock, IS : 5560-1970.
9. Cottonseed, oilcake as livestock feed (first revision), IS : 1712-1982.
10. Decorticated groundnut oil cake as livestock feed (first revision), IS: 1713-1970.
11. Decorticated saflower (Kardi) oilcake as livestock feed, IS : 2503-1963.
12. Dicalcium phosphate, animal feed grade, IS : 5470-1969.
13. Dried silk worm pupae as livestock feed, IS : 6107-1971.
14. Fish meal as livestock feed (first revision), IS : 4307-1973.
15. Fodder yeast, IS : 3198-1965.
16. Gram chuni, IS : 3161-1965.
17. Gram husks, IS : 3162-1965.
18. Guar meal as livestock feed, IS : 4193-1967.
19. Linseed oilcake as livestock feed, IS : 1935-1982.
20. Maize bran, IS : 2153-1962.
22. Maize gluten feed (first revision), IS : 2152-1972.
23. Meat meal and meat-cum bone meal as livestock feed, IS : 5065-1969.
24. Mineral mixture for supplementing cattle feeds (first revision), IS : 1664-1968.
25. Mustard and rapeseed oilcake as livestock feed (first revision), IS : 1932-1972.
26. Pig feeds, IS : 7472-1974.
27. Rice bran as livestock feed (first revision), IS : 3648-1975.

    Rice bran (Par boiled) as livestock feed ingredient, IS : 9867-1981.
28. Rice polish, IS : 3163-1965.
29. Rubber seed cake as livestock feed, IS : 9599-1980.
30. Sesamum (Til) oil cake as livestock feed, IS : 1934-1982.

31. Solvent extracted coconut oilcake (meal) as livestock feed (first revision), IS : 3591-1968.
32. Solvent extracted cottonseed oilcake (meal)_ as livestock feed (first revision), IS : 3592-1968.
33. Solvent extracted groundnut oilcake (meal)_ as livestock feed (first revision), IS : 3441-1982.
34. Solvent extracted linseed oilcake (meal)_ as livestock feed (first revision), IS : 3440-1966.
35. Solvent extracted nigerseed oilcake (meal)_ as livestock feed (first revision), IS : 5862-1970.
36. Solvent extracted rice bran (meal)_ as livestock feed (first revision), IS : 3593-1979.
37. Solvent extracted safflower oilcake (meal)_ as livestock feed (first revision), IS : 6242-1971.
38. Solvent extracted salseed (meal) for feeding livestock, IS : 7059-1973.
39. Sunflower oilcake (Decorticated) as livestock feed ingredient, IS : 10165-1982.
40. Tapioca as livestock feed (first revision), (Superseding IS : 1510-1959) IS: 1509-1972.
41. Tapioca spent pulp as livestock feed (first revision), IS : 5064-1980.
42. Tur chuni, IS : 3160-1965.
43. Tur husk, IS : 5063-1969.
44. Wheat bran (first revision), IS : 2239-1971.

A New Invention in the World

Indigenous Kit based on Novel CLE Complex Process for Assessing Nutritive Value and Detection of Adulterant in Animal Feed (Original Innovation)

(Method of Krishna, G. Certified by ISA Authority, Patent office Vienna, registered with WIPO H.Q., Geneva) Patent application field at Indian Patent Office, Delhi

Background

Animal Feed manufacturers always face a crucial problem to obtain Animal feed ingredients free from adulterants viz. extraneous Sand and Silica, saw dust from wood processing industries, Expeller mud from oil seed processing industries, Rice husk from paddy processing Industries and high quantity of urea.

The above limitation is the main hurdle before animal Feed manufacturers to produce high quality animal feed as per BIS standards, Manak Bhavan, Delhi (India).

To solve this problem of animal Feed manufacturers, this kit has been designed and any extraneous adulterants could be detected using ordinary Laboratory facility.

There is no need of maintaining surgical modified Cattle/Buffalo as Government of India has banned rumen fistulation as this Act comes under the category of prevention of cruelty Act as per Animal Welfare Board of India approved by Indian Parliament.

Components of Kit

1. Novel cud liquor enzyme complex (CLE complex)
   (Innovator - Prof. Dr. Gopal Krishna, CCS-HAU, Hisar (Haryana-India) invention Registered with WIPO, Head quarter GENEVA. Excellent ISA report issued by Patent Office Vienna (Austria), Indian Patent application field at Indian Patent Office, Delhi (India).
2. Pepsin (1 : 10000) E. Merck
3. 6 N HCl, E. Merck.

Equipment Required

1. *In Vitro* glass tubes fitted with Bunsen valve (100 ml capacity)
2. Expandable laboratory supplies Beakers, Erlenmeyer flask, funnel, desiccator, Graduated cylinder, cheese cloth, Thermos flask.
3. Whatman filter Paper No. 54
4. Analytical balance
5. Centrifuge having container for 100 ml centrifuge Tube and Tube stand
6. Incubator-Provision to maintain 39°C temperature

Procedure for Testing

1. Weigh 250 mg finely grinded feed material in an *in Vitro* Tube
2. Add 25 ml of Novel CLE complex supplying 0.625 unit cellulase per mg of testing material (1 ml Novel CLE complex provide 6.24 units cellulase)
3. Prepare three blank tubes with 25 ml Novel CLE complex without any substrate
4. The said tube is then kept in incubator at 39°C for 48 hours
5. After 48 hours of incubation, add 0.2 g of pepsin and 2 ml of 6 N Hcl, incubate for another 48 hrs.
6. Centrifuge the tube contents at 200 g speed for 15 minutes
7. Filter the contents of Tube using whatman filter paper No. 54

8. Wash the residue with warm water (six times)
9. Keep the filter paper with residue in the oven for 12 hours
10. Remove the filter paper with residue and keep in desiccator
11. Weigh the filter paper and residue three times at 02 hours interval till the constant weight is obtained
12. Weigh 02 g of substrate in moisture cup and keep in the oven for 24 hours at 85°C for calculating results of DM disappearance on DM basis.

Calculation

1. *In Vitro* matter disappearance percent (IVDMD%)

$$\frac{\text{Sample d.m. wt - residual d.s. wt - residual d.m. of blank}}{\text{Sample dry matter weight}}$$

2. Prediction of Crude protein disappearance percent (Y) using newly developed prediction equation (Using triplicate samples observations of 51 samples of animal Feed of India and Germany).

Cattle

Y = 51.434 + 0395x

r^2 = 0.608, Sxy (%) = 2.970

Where Y = Crude protein disappearance percent

X = dry matter disappearance percent

(Prediction percent = 101, Actual Value (Y) = 67 and predicted value 68.03)

Buffalo

Y = 50.350 + 0437x

r^2 = 0.643, Sxy (%) = 3.323

Where Y = Crude protein disappearance percent

X = dry matter disappearance percent

(Prediction percent = 99.79, Actual Value (Y) = 62 and predicted value 61.87)

Practical Application of Invention

How to Judge that Animal Feed is Adulterated with Extraneous Material

Please see the standard values of dry matter and crude protein disappearance obtained by using Novel CLE Complex of newly designed kit on 51 samples (Triplicate) of Animal Feed commonly used in routine feeding in India and Germany (Table 17.6) the efficiency of kit was also tested using Pure Sigma cellulose type 101 (Catalogue No. S-6790), Casein (raw and protected) (E. Merck) and Fungal cellulase based on *Trichoderma viride* (Sigma Cat No. E 9422).

Perfection of KIT was also assessed by comparing the *in vitro* value with the *In Vivo* published data in International Journals, Siddons *et al.* (1985 J. Dairy Sci, 68: 829-39) and NIR Spectroscopy values (Garg *et al.*, 2006; Indian Journal Animal Nutrition **23** : 63-68).

Table 7 : Standard values of *in vitro* dry matter and crude protein disappearance percent (based on triplicate observations of 51 samples of India and Germany), National Index

Name of Feed	NovelCLE Complex prepared from			
	Cattle		Buffalo	
	Disappearance percent			
	DM	CP	DM	CP
Mustard cake	67	77	66	83
Cottonseed cake	44	75	41	76
Soybean meal	89	88	89	88
Groundnut cake	71	87	66	86
Fish meal	89	86	89	85
Maize	78	84	72	76
Barley	83	76	61	73
Maize Gluten	87	84	72	85
Rice polish	55	61	51	60
Cotton seed	42	67	36	62
Gram churi	65	80	63	75

The results related to Rumen protein degradability are presented in Table 17.7. The results obtained were compared with published data (AFRC 1993, Sampath 1990 and Straahlen and Tamminga, 1990). The values obtained were found at par with the published values.

Before marketing bypass feed, it is essential to confirm the amount of undegradable protein which will convince the Dairy owner to use and pay the money accordingly.

We may calculate bypass protein values as a percentage of soybean Meal (India) based on *in vitro* cud liquor enzyme complex method (Byass x Crude protein) = (Soybean meal equivalent).

The data are presented in Table 17.8 which are based on *"Soybean meal equivalent"* recommended under Nebraska Growth System by Klopfenstein *et al.* (1982) of USA.

Signals of Adulteration

1. If dry matter/crude protein disappearance percent values and degradability percent are below 30 to 35 percent of standard values mentioned in Table 17.6 and 17.7 indicate adulteration with extraneous materials is confirmed.
2. If crude protein disappearance percent value is more than 30 to 32.5 percent of standard values mentioned in Table 17.6 and 17.7 then adulteration with urea is confirmed.

Cost of Analysis

Rs. 50/- for testing one feed sample in Triplicate.

Accuracy of Results Tested in Triplicate

Standard error between triplicates of tested Feed sample was almost negligible which prove the perfection of process to prepare novel CLE complex as per WIPO (Geneva) International publication, simultaneously ISA report has been confirmed by Patent Office, Vienna.

Animal Feed Tested by Newly Designed Kit at CCS - HAU Hisar, Haryana (India) by Author of this Compendium

51 Sample (30 from India and 21 from Germany) of Common Feeds fed to Cattle/Buffalo, were taken for study.

Batch I (India)

Groundnut cake, Mustard cake, Soybean meal, Fish meal, Cotton seed, Cottonseed cake, Maize, Barley, Rice polish and Gram Chuni.

Batch II (India)

Mustard Cake - 10 (different locations samples)

Cottonseed cake - 10 (different locations samples)

Batch III (Germany)

Mustard cake - (10 different locations samples)

Soybean Meals (08 different locations samples)

Maize Gluten meal (03 different location samples)

Batch IV

Sigma cellulose Type 101 (Catalogue No. S-6790)

Batch V

Raw casein and Protected Casein

Table 8 : Ruminal Protein degradability, Crude Protein (CP) Rumen degradable protein (RDP) and undegradable protein (UDP) Content of Indian & Germany Animal Feeds. (Based on Novel CLE Complex), National Index.

S.No.	Feedstuffs	Crude Protein g/kg/DM	Cattle	Buffalo	RDP g/kg DM		UDP g/kg/DM		AFRC (1993) (1)	Sampath (1990) (2)	Straalen and Tamminga (3)
					Cattle	Buffalo	Cattle	Buffalo			
1.	Gram Churi	238.4	dg8(0.52)	dg8(0.55)	123.97	131.12	114.43	107.28	-	-	-
2.	Soybean meal (India)	416.2	dg5(0.66)	dg5(0.66)	274.69	274.69	141.51	141.51	dg8[3](0.60)	0.66	-
	(Germany)	568.8	-do-	-do-	375.41	375.41	193.39	193.39	-do-	-do-	0.61
3.	Cottonseed cake	268.7	dg8(0.57)	dg8(0.56)	153.16	150.47	115.54	118.23	dg8(0.59)	0.51	0.57
4.	Rice polish	134.1	dg8(0.65)	dg8(0.65)	87.16	87.16	46.94	46.94	dg6(0.66)	0.45	0.66
5.	Mustard cake (India)	362.72 ± 4.336	dg8(0.74)	dg8(0.72)	268.41	261.16	94.31	101.56	dg8(0.69)	0.75	-
	(Germany)	438.95 ± 8.588	dg8(0.72)	dg8(0.72)	316.04	316.04	122.91	122.91	dg8[3](0.73)	0.69	0.66
6.	Maize	115.1	dg8(0.25)	dg8(0.32)	28.77	36.83	86.33	78.27	dg8(0.31)	-	0.43
7.	Barley	102.3	dg8(0.86)	dg8(0.86)	87.98	87.98	14.32	14.32	dg8(0.82)	0.82	0.66
8.	Groundnut cake	423.4	dg5(0.69)	dg5(0.69)	292.14	292.14	131.26	131.26	dg6(0.69)	0.68	0.74
9.	Cottonseed	207.0	dg8(0.54)	dg8(0.61)	111.78	126.27	95.22	80.73	-	-	0.73
10.	Fish meal	428.4	dg8(0.31)	dg8(0.32)	132.80	137.09	295.60	291.31	dg8(0.42)	0.41	0.44
11.	Maize gluten Feed	245.833	dg(0.70)	dg5(0.69)	172.08	169.62	73.75	76.21	dg6(0.69)	0.75	0.68

1. AFRC (1993) *Energy and protein requirements of Ruminants. An advisory manual prepared by the AFRC Technical Committee on Responses to nutrients. CAB INTERNATIONAL*, Wallingford, U.K.
2. Sampath, K.T. (1990) *Rumen degradable protein and undegradable crude protein Content of feeds and fodders.* The Indian Journal of Dairy Science, 43 : 1-10.
3. Straalen, W.M. Van and Tamminga, S. (1990). *Protein degradation of ruminant diet. In : feedstuffs Evaluation*, Wiseman, J. Scale D.J.A (Eds) Butterworths, London pp. : 55-72.

Table 9 : Bypass protein* values as a percentage of Soybean Meal (India) based on In-vitro CLE Complex (Bypass x Crude protein) = "Soybean Meal equivalent"
Based on Nebraska Growth System, National Index.

S. No.	Name of Feed	UDP (Bypass protein) g/1000g DM		Bypass as a percentage "Soybean Meal equivalent"	
		C	B	C	B
1.	Gram Churi	114.43	107.28	81.24	76.17
2.	Soybean meal (India)	141.51	141.51	100.00	100.00
	(Germany)	193.39	**193.39**	**137.31**	**137.31**
3.	Cottonseed cake	115.54	118.23	82.03	83.94
4.	Rice Polish	46.94	46.94	33.33	33.33
5.	Mustard cake (India)	94.31	101.56	66.96	72.11
	(Germany)	122.91	122.91	87.26	87.26
6.	Maize	86.33	78.27	61.29	55.57
7.	Barley	14.32	14.32	10.16	10.16
8.	Groundnut cake	131.26	131.26	**93.19**	**93.19**
9.	Cotton seed	95.22	80.73	67.60	57.32
10.	Fish meal	295.60	291.31	**209.87**	**206.83**
11.	Maize gluten feed	73.75	76.21	52.36	54.11

Grading

	Name of feed	**Scoring Position**
1.	Fish meal	I
2.	Soybean meal (Germany)	II
3.	Groundnut cake	III

- *Bypass protein is that protein which escapes digestion in the rumen and is digested in the small intestine. "Soybean Meal Equivalent" (Klopfen Stein et al., 1982 of USA)*

References

Cockerell, D.H. and Morgan, D.J. (1975). *Quality control in the animal feedstuffs manufacturing industry, G 97, Tropical products Insititute 56/62 Gray's Inn Road,* London., WCI X 8 LU, Ministry of Overseas development.

Indian Standards Institution, (BIS) (1981). *Sectional lists of Indian standards Institution, I. Agricultural and food products,* ISI, Manak Bhavan, 9, Bahadur Shah Zafar Marg, New Delhi (India).

Klopfenstein, T.J., Britton, R.A. and Stock, R.A. (1982). Nebraska growth system. Protein requirements for cattle, Symposium. Owens, F.N., ed. Oklahoma State Univ., Stillwater.

Krishna, G., Razdan, M.N. and Ray, S.N. (1972). *"Dairy Search" method for moisture determination in molasses,* Proc. second world congress on Animal feeding, Madrid (Spain) cited in volume I of this compendium.

Krishna, G. (2002a). International index of rumen protein degradability assessed by cud liquor (Cattle/buffalo) based *in vitro* method in feedstuffs of India and Germany. *Proc. Soc. Nutr. Physiologie.* 11: 151 (Germany).

Krishna, G. (2002b). Bypass protein Soybean Meal equivolent index of Indian and Germany feedstuffs assessed by Cud liquor (Cattle/Buffalo) based *in vitro* method Proc. Soc. Nutr. Physiologie. 11: 152.

Bibliography : Tracer Techniques

Abou-Akkada, A.R., D.A. Messmex. L.R. Fina, and E.E. Bartley, (1968). *J. Dairy Sci,*. 51: 78.

Annison, E.F. (1954). *Biochem. J.,* 57: 400.

Ash, R.W. (1961a). *J. Physiol.,* 157: 93.

Ash, R.W. (1961b). *J. Physiol.,* 157: 185.

Balch. C.C. (1961). *Movement of digesta through the digestive tract. In D. Lewis's Digestive Physiology and Nutrition of the Ruminant. London: Butterworth.*

Bergrman, E.N., R.S. Reid, M.G. Murry, J.M. Brockway, and F.G Whitelaw, (1965). *Biochem. J.,* 97:53.

Beever, D.E., D.G. Harrison, D.J. Thomson, S.B. Cammell, and D.F. Osbourn, (1974). *Brit. J. Nutr.,* 32:99.

Bernard, G.C., C.V. Boucque, (1968). *J. Agric. Food Chem.,* 16: 105.

Binnerts, W.T., A. T. Klooster, VanT and A.M. Frens, (1958). *Vety. Record.,* 82: 470.

Birks, J.B. (1964). *The Theory and Practice of Scintillation Counting. Oxford: Pergamon Press.*

Black, A.L. (1968). *In isotope studies on the nitrogen chain, pp. 287. (Proc. Symp. Vienna,* 1967).

Blackbum, T.H. and P.N. Hobson, (1960). *Brit. J. Nutr.,* 14: 445.

Blaxter, K.L., N.M. Graham and F.W. Wainman, (1956). *Brit. J. Nutr.*, 10: 69.

Bray, G.A. (1960). Analytical Biochemistry, 1: 279.

Bris, E.J., I.A. Dyer, and I.D. Teare, (1967). Agronomy 59:255.

Bryant, E.A. J.E. Sattizahn, and B. Warren, (1959). Analytical Chem., 31: 334.

Castle, (1956a). *Brit. J. Nutr.*, 10: 15.

Cocimano, M.R.and R.A. Leng, (1966). Proc. Aust. Soc, Amin. Prod., 6: 378.

Conrad, H.R., R.C. Miles, and J. Butdorf, (1967). *J. Nutrition.*, 91: 337.

Conard, H.R. (1972). *Urea kinetics and amino acid entry rates in dairy cows. In Tracer studies on non protein nitrogen for ruminants. Proc. of a panel, IAEA, Vienna*, pp. 69.

Corbett, J.L. Miller, T.D., E.W. Clarke, and E. Florence, (1956). *Proc. Nutr. Soc.*, 15: V.

Corbett, J.L., J.F.D., Greenhalgh, E. Florence, (1959). *Brit. J. Nutr.*, 13: 337.

Corbett, J.L., J.F.D. Greenhalgh, Gwynn, P.E. and D. Walker, (1958). *Brit, J. Nutr.* 12: 266.

Curie, Marie, Pierre Curie, (1923). New York: The Macmillan Co., cited Quimby *et al.*, 1970.

Donefer. E., E.W. Crampton and L.E. Lloyd, (1960). *J. Anim. Sci.*, 19: 545.

Downes, A.M. and I.W. McDonald. *Brit. J. Nutr.*, 18: 153.

Ellis, W.C. andW.H. Pfander, (1965). *Nature*, 205:974.

Ellis, W.C. and J.E.Huston, (1968). *J. Nutr.*, 95: 67.

Ely, D.G., C.O. Little, P.G. Woolfolk, and G.E. Mitchell, Jr. (1967). *J. Nutr.* 91: 314.

el-shazly, K. and R.E. Hungate, (1966). Applied Microbiol., 14: 27.

el-Shaly, K.and A.R. Abou Akkada, (1972). *Techniques for studying protein synthesis by rumen micro-organisms. In Tracer studies on non-protein nitrogen for ruminants.Proc. of a panel IAEA, Vienna*, pp. 47.

Erfle, J.D., F.D. Sauer, and S. Mahadeven, (1977). *J. Dariy Sci.*, 60:1064.

Esdale, W.J., G.A. Broderick, and L.D Salter, (1968). *J. Dair Sci.*, 51: 1823.

Folch, J., M. Lees, and G.H. Solane Stanley, (1957). *J. Biol. Chem.*, 226: 497.

Francois, E., R. Compe're, and G. Rondia, (1968). Bulletin des researche Agronomiques de Gembloux. 3(4) 655. Cited by Kotb, A.R. and Luckey, T.D., 1972, Nutr. Abstr. and Reviews, 42: 28.

Garner, R.J., H.G. Jones, and L. Ekman, (1960). *J. Agric. Sci. Camb.*, 55: 107.

Gibbs, F.O., R.W Rice, and C.J. Kercher, (1969). *J. Anim. Sci.*, 28: 858.

Goodall, E. and R.N.B. Kay, (1962). *Digestion and absorption in the large intestine of the sheep.* Proc. XXII Int. Physiol Congr., Leiden.

Gray. F.V. G.B. Jones, and A.F. Pilgrim, (1960). *Aust. J. Agric. Res.*, 11: 383.

Gray, F.V., R.A. Weller, A.F. Pilgrim, and G.B. Jones, (1966). *Austral. J. Agric. Res.*, 17: 69.

______, (1967). *Aust J. Agric.Res.*, 18: 107.

Gray, F.V., R.A. Weller, and A.F. Pilgrim, (1966). *Austr. J. Agric. Res.*, 17:69.

Halvorsen, A.W., G.D. Williams, and G.D. Paulson, (1968). *J. Nutr.*, 95:363.

Harmeyer, J. and J. Varady, (1972). *Measurements of nitrogen recycling in sheep and goats under various conditions. In Tracer studies on non-protein nitrogen for ruminants. Proc. of a panel IAEA, Vienna*, pp, 91.

Hecker, J.F. (1971). *J. Agri. Sci. Camb.*, 77: 151.

Henderickx, H.K., D.I. Demeyer, and C.J. Van Nevel, (1972). *Problem in estimating Microbial Protein synthesis in the rumen. In Tracer studies on non-protein nitrogen for ruminants. Proc. of a panel IAEA, Vienna*, pp. 57.

Hevesy, G.V. and E. Hofer, (1934). *Nature*, 134: 879.

Hogan, J.P. (1964). *Austr J. Agric. Res.*, 15: 384.

Horiguchi, M. and M. Kandatsu, (1960). *Bull. Agr. Chem. Sec.* Japan, 24: 565.

Hungate, R.E. (1968). *The rumen and its microbes* New York and London: Academic Press.

Huston, J.E. and W.C. Ellis, (1968). *J. Agr. Food Chem.*, 16: 225.

Hyden, S. (1955a). Kungl. Lantbrukshogskolans, Annaler, 22: 139.

________, (1955b), Kungl. Lantbrukshogskolans Annaler. 22: 411.

________, (1961), Kungl. Lantbrukshogskolans Annaler., 27: 51.

Ibrahim, E.A., J.R. Ingalls, and N.E. Stanger, (1970). *J. Anim. Sci.*, 50: 101.

International Atomic Energy Agency, (1969). *Laboratory Training manual on the use of Isotope and Radiation in Animal Research Technical Reports series No. 60, IInd Edn. Vienna*: IAEA.

James, A.T. and A.J.P Martin, (1951). *Biochem. J. Proc.*, 48: VII.

Jayasuriya, G.C.N. and R.E Hungate, (1959). Arch. Biochem. Biophys., 82: 274.

King, W.A, J. Lee, H.J. Webb, and D.B. Roderick, (1960). *J. Dairy Sci.*, 43:388.

Klooster, A.T., Van T and P.A.M Rogers, (1970). *Neth. J Vet. Sci.*, 3:114.

Knox., K.L., A.L. Black, and M. Kleiber, (1967). *J. Dairy Sci.*, 50: 1716.

Krishna, G and A. Ekern (1974a). *Z. Tierphysiol. Tierernährg. U. Futtermittelkde*, 33: 275.

________, (1974b). *Z . Tierphysiol., Tierernährg. U. Futtermittelkde*, 33: 281.

________, (1974c). *Z . Tierphysiol., Tierernährg. U. Futter-mittelkde*, 33: 323.

________, (1974d), Acta Agricultural Scandinavica 24: 211.

________, (1976). *India Vet . J.,* 53: 265.

Kromann, R.P., J.H. Meyer, and W.J. Stielau, (1967). *J Dairy Sci.,* 50: 73.

Landis, J. (1963). *Z. Tierphysiol. Tierernährg. U Futtermittelkde,* 18: 357.

Leng, R.A. and G.J. Leonard, (1965). *Brit. J. Nutr.,* 19: 469.

Leng, R.A. and D.J. Brett. (1966). *Brit. J. Nutr.,* 20: 541.

Leng, R.A., J.L. Corbett, and D.J. Bret (1968). *Br. J. Nutr.,* 22: 57.

Leng, R.A. (1969). Formation and production of volatile fatty acids in the rumen. In Physiology of digestion and metabolism in the ruminant, pp. 406. Phillipson, A.T. (ed.) New Castle upon Tyne: Oriel Press.

Leng, R.A. and R.M. Murray, (1972). Estimation of the fermentation rate in the rumen of sheep using VFA production, carbon dioxide production and methane production. In Tracer studies on non protein nitrogen for ruminants, Proc. of a panel, IAEA. Vienna. pp.25.

Lueker, C.E. and G.P. Lofgreen, (1961). *J. Nutr.* 74: 233.

Lutwak, L. (1959). *Analytical Chem.,* 31: 341.

Markham, R. (1942). *Biochem. J.,* 36: 790.

Mason, V.C. (1969). *J. Agric. Sci. Camb.,* 73: 99.

Mathison, G.W. and L.P. Milligan, (1970). *Brit. J. Nutr.,* 25: 351.

McAllan, A.B. and R.H. Smith, (1969). *Br. J. Nutr.,* 23: 671.

________, (1973). *Br. J. Nutr.,* 29: 467.

Mc Anally, R.A., (1944). *J. Exp. Biol.,* 20: 130.

Mc Donald, I.W. (1954). *Biochem. J.,* 56: 120.

Mc Donald, I.W. and R.J. Hall, (1957). *Biochem. J.,* 67: 400.

Mc Dougall, E.I. (1949). *Biochem. J.,* 43: 99.

Morries, M.P. and J. Garcia-Rivera, (1955). *J. Dairy Sci.,* 38: 1169.

Muller, G., L. Von Erishsen, (1952). *Z. Tierzucht. Zuchtbiol.,* 60: 20.

Nagel, S. and B. Piatkowski, (1972). Archiv. für Tierernährung, 10: 749.

Nolan, J.V.W.B. Norton, and R.A. Leng. (1972). Dynamic aspects of nitrogen metabolism in sheep. In Tracer studies on non-protein nitrogen for ruminants. Proc. of a panel, IAEA. Vienna, pp. 13.

Olbrich, S.E., F.A. Martz, J.R. Vogt, and E.S. Hilder Brand, (1971). *J. Anim. Sci.,* 33: 899.

O Mea, E.K. and G.A. Leveille, (1968). Comp. Biochem. Physiol., 26: 111.

Panic, B., M., Jovanovic, M., Cuperlovic, D. Djardjevic, (1967). Thioamino acids to indicate the synthetic activity of the rumen in in vitro experiments. In Proc. of symposium on "Isotope studies on the nitrogen chain", IAEA. Vienna.

Phillipson, A.T., M.J. Dobson, T.H. Black-burn, M. Brown, (1961). *Brit. J. Nutr.*, 16: 151.

Pilgrim, A.F., F.V. Gray, R.A. Weller, and C.B. Belling, (1970). *Brit. J. Nutr.*, 24: 589.

Quicke, G.V., O.G. Bentley, H.W. Scott, and A.L. Moxon, (1959). *J. Anim. Sci.*, 18: 275.

Quimby. E.H. S. Feitelberg. and W. Gross, (1970). Radioactive nuclide in Medicine and Biology, Philadelphia : Lea and Feliger.

Rittenberg, D. and G.L. Foster, (1940). *J. Biol. Chem.*, 133: 737.

Roberts, S.A. And E.L. Miller, (1969). *Proc. Nutr. Soc.*, 28: 32.

Sayre, E. (1963). Methods and applications of activation analysis. Ann. Rev. Nuclear Science, 13: 145-62.

Singh, U.B., D.N. Verma, A. Varma and S.K. Ranjhan, (1974). *J. Agric. Sci. Camb.*, 83: 13.

_________, (1974). *J. Dairy Res.*, 41: 299.

Sheppard, A.J, R.M. Forbes, and B.C. Johnson, (1959). *Proc. .Soc. Exp. Biol. Med.*, 101: 715.

Shultz, T.A. and E. Shultz, (1970). *J. Dairy Sci.* 53: 781.

Sinha, K.N., F.A. Martz. H.D. Johnson, and L Hahn, (1970). *J. Anim. Sci.* 30: 467.

Smith, R.H. (1969). *J. Dairy Res.*, 36: 313.

___________, (1979). *J. Anim. Sci.*, 49: 1604.

Smith, R.H., D.N. Salter, and K. Daneshvar, (1977). *J. Nuclear Agric. Biol.*, 6: 8.

Sperber, I., S. Hyden and J. Ekman, (1953). Kungliga Lantbrukshog skolans Annaler., 20: 337.

Steele, R., J.S. Wall. R.C. De Bodo, and N. Altszuler, (1956). *Am. J. Physiol.*, 187: 15.

Temler-Kucharski, A. and B. Gausseres, (1965). *Ann. Biol. Anim. Bioch. Biophys.*, 5: 207.

Till, A.R. and A.M. Downes, (1965). *Brit. J. Nutr.*, 19: 435.

Tulloh, N.M. J.W. Hughes, and R.P. Newthe, (1965). *New Zealand J. Agric. Res.*, 8: 636.

Ulyatt, M.J. (1964a). *Newzealand J. Agric Res.*, 7: 713.

________, (1964b). *Newzealand J. Agric. Res.*, 7: 774.

Vaughan, M. (1961). *J. Lipid Research.*, 2: 293.

Visek, W.J., R.A. Monroe, E.W. Swanson, and C.L. Comer, (1953). *J. Nutr.*, 50: 23.

Walker, D.M. and K.E. Hawley, (1965). Proc. IX th Intern. Grassland Congress, 759.

Walker, D.J. and C.J. Nader, (1968). *Appl. Microbiol.*, 16: 1124.

Warner, A.C.I. and B.D. Stacy, (1968b). *Brit. J. Nutr.*, 22: 389.

Wotts, P.S. (1957). *Aust. J. Agric. Sci.*, 8: 266.

Weller, R.A., A.F. Pilgrim, and F.V. Gary, (1962). *Brit. J. Nutr.* 16: 83.

________, (1969). *Brit. J. Nutr.*, 21: 97.

Weller R.A., F.V. Gray, A.F. Pilgrim and G.B. Jones, (1967). *Aust J. Agric. Res.* 18: 107.

Weston, R.H. and J. P. Hogan, (1967). *Aust J. Agri. Res.*, 18: 789.

________, (1968). *Aust J. Agric. Res.*, 19: 419.

Whitelaw, F.G. J. Hyldgaard-Jenson, R.S. Reid, and M.G. Kay, (1970). *Brit, J. Nutr.*, 24:179.

William, W.M. and A.P. George, (1971). *J. Wildlife Management*, 35: 723.

Wiseman, H.G. and H.M. Irvin, (1957). *J. Agric. Food. Chem.*, 5: 213.

Zilversmit, D.B. (1960). *Am. J. Med.*, 29: 832.

References for Further Study

Aronoff, S. (1965). *Techniques of Radiobiochemistry*. Iowa State: College Press.

Benyon, J.H. (1967). *Mass spectrometry and its application to organic chemistry*, Elsevier, London.

Chase, G.D. and J.L Rabinowitz, (1962). *Principles of Radioistope Methodology*, Minneapolis: Burgess Publishing Co.

Faires. R.A. and B.H. Parks, (1973). *Radioisotope Laboratory Techniques*, 3rd Edn., London: Buterworths.

Hill, H.C. (1971). *Introduction of mass spectrometry*. Heyden.

International Atomic Energy Agency, (1971). *Mineral studies with isotopes in domestic animals. Proc. of a panel on the use of Nuclear Techniques in studies of mineral metabolism and disease in domestic animals.* FAO/IAEA, Vienna.

Rakovic, M. (1963). *Ionising Radiations, Precautions for Industrial users*. HMSO. London.

________, (1970). Activation analysis. lliffe.

Wolf, G. (1964). *Isotopes in Biology*, Ist Edn. New York and London: Academic Press.